THE LATEST NANDA DIAGNOSES THROUGH THE 11th CONFERENCE

1. Acute Confusion
2. Altered Family Process: Alcoholism
3. Chronic Confusion
4. Decreased Adaptive Capacity: Intracranial
5. Disorganized Infant Behavior
6. Effective Management of Therapeutic Regimen: Individual
7. Energy Field Disturbance
8. Impaired Environmental Interpretation Syndrome
9. Impaired Memory
10. Ineffective Community Coping
11. Ineffective Management of Therapeutic Regimen: Community
12. Ineffective Management of Therapeutic Regimen: Families
13. Potential for Enhanced Community Coping
14. Potential for Enhanced Organized Infant Behavior
15. Potential for Enhanced Spiritual Well-Being
16. Risk for Disorganized Infant Behavior
17. Risk for Loneliness
18. Risk for Parent/Infant/Child Attachment
19. Risk for Perioperative Positioning Injury

Helen C. Cox, RN, C, EDD, FAAN
Interim Executive Associate Dean, Professor of Nursing
Texas Tech University Health Sciences Center School of Nursing
Lubbock, Texas

Mittie D. Hinz, RN, C, MSN
Clinical Nurse Specialist,
Arnot Ogden Medical Center
Elmira, New York

Mary Ann Lubno, RN, PhD, CNAA
Associate Dean for the Undergraduate Program, Associate Professor of Nursing
Texas Tech University Health Sciences Center School of Nursing
Lubbock, Texas

Susan A. Newfield, RN, MSN, CS
Assistant Professor
West Virginia University School of Nursing
Morgantown, West Virginia

Nancy A. Ridenour, RN, C, PhD, FNP
Associate Dean for the Graduate Program, Professor of Nursing
Texas Tech University Health Sciences Center School of Nursing
Lubbock, Texas

Mary McCarthy Slater, RN, C, MSN
Assistant Professor of Clinical Nursing
Texas Tech University Health Sciences Center School of Nursing
Lubbock, Texas

Kathryn L. Sridaromont, RN, C, MSN
Assistant Professor of Clinical Nursing
Texas Tech University Health Sciences Center School of Nursing
Lubbock, Texas

Clinical Applications of Nursing Diagnosis

Adult, Child, Women's, Mental Health, Gerontic and Home Health Considerations

Second Edition

F. A. Davis Company · Philadelphia

F. A. Davis Company
1915 Arch Street
Philadelphia, PA 19103

Printed in the United States of America

Last digit indicates print number: 10 9 8 7 6 5 4

Publisher, Nursing: Robert Martone
Production Editor: Gail Shapiro
Cover Design By: Steven Ross Morrone

As new scientific information becomes available through basic and clinical research, recommended treatments and drug therapies undergo changes. The authors and publisher have done everything possible to make this book accurate, up to date, and in accord with accepted standards at the time of publication. The authors, editors, and publisher are not responsible for errors or omissions or for consequences from application of the book, and make no warranty, expressed or implied, in regard to the contents of the book. Any practice described in this book should be applied by the reader in accordance with professional standards of care used in regard to the unique circumstances that may apply in each situation. The reader is advised always to check product information (package inserts) for changes and new information regarding dose and contraindications before administering any drug. Caution is especially urged when using new or infrequently ordered drugs.

Library of Congress Cataloging-in-Publication Data

Clinical applications of nursing diagnosis : adult, child, women's,
  mental health, gerontic, and home health considerations / Helen C. Cox
  . . . [et al.]. — 2nd ed.
     p.   cm.
  Includes bibliographical references and index.
  ISBN (invalid) 0-8036-1999-5 (alk. paper) :
  1. Nursing diagnosis.   2. Nursing assessment.   3. Nursing.
  I. Cox, Helen C.
  [DNLM: 1: Nursing Assessment.   2. Nursing Diagnosis.   3. Nursing
Process.   WY 100 C6403 1993]
  RT48.6.C6   1993
  610.73 — dc20
  DNLM/DLC
  for Library of Congress   93-17764
                                                                       CIP

To the administration, faculty, students
and staff of Texas Tech University
Health Sciences Center School of
Nursing for support and encouragement
above and beyond the usual.

Consultants

Barbara Brown, RN, MN, CCRN
Professor of Nursing
Community College of Allegheny County-North Campus
Pittsburgh, Pennsylvania

Margo Neal, RN, MN
Malibu, California

Norma L. Pinnell, BSN, MSN, RN
Instructor
Southern Illinois University — Edwardsville
Edwardsville, Illinois

Sharilyn Robinson, RN, MN
Nursing Faculty
Glendale Community College
Glendale, Arizona

Janet Weber, RN, EdD
Assistant Professor of Nursing
Southeast Missouri State University
Cape Girardeau, Missouri

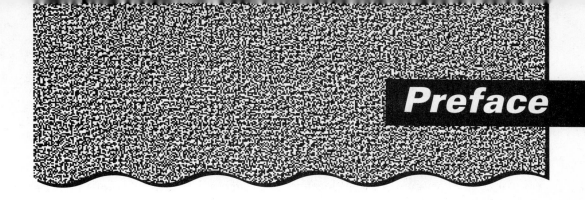

The North American Nursing Diagnosis Association (NANDA) has been identifying, classifying, and testing diagnostic nomenclature since the early '70s. In our opinion, use of nursing diagnosis helps to define the essence of nursing and to give direction to care that is uniquely nursing care.

In this second edition we have made numerous changes to stay abreast of changes in national standards and criteria. In doing so we have moved from talking about specific care plan forms to talking about the process of planning care. This allows the reader to adapt information in this book to a variety of care documentation formats and to focus on the full process of planning care to meet the individual needs of the patient.

If nurses (in all instances we are referring to registered nurses) enter the medical diagnosis of acute appendicitis as the patient's problem, they have met defeat before a start can be made. A nurse cannot intervene for this medical diagnosis; intervention requires a medical practitioner who can perform an appendectomy. However, if the nurse enters the nursing diagnosis "Pain", then a number of nursing interventions come to mind.

Several books use nursing diagnosis to contribute to planning care. However, these books generally focus outcome and nursing interventions on the related factors; that is, nursing interventions deal with resolving, to the extent possible, the causative and contributing factors that result in the nursing diagnosis. We have chosen to focus nursing intervention on the nursing diagnosis. To focus on the nursing diagnosis promotes the use of concepts in nursing rather than worrying about a multitude of specifics; for example, there are common nursing measures that can be used to relieve pain regardless of the etiologic pain factor involved. Likewise, the outcomes focus on the nursing diagnosis. The main outcome nurses want to achieve when working with the nursing diagnosis, "Pain," is control of the patient's response to pain to the extent possible. Again, the outcome allows the use of a conceptual approach rather than a multitude-of-specifics approach. To clarify further, we ask you to look again at the medical diagnosis of appendicitis. The physician's first concern is not related to whether the appendicitis is caused by a fecalith, intestinal helminths, or *Escherichia coli* run amok. The physician focuses first on intervening for the appendicitis, which usually results in an appendectomy. The physician will deal with etiologic factors following the appendectomy, but the appendectomy is the first level of intervention. Likewise, the nurse can deal with the related factors through nursing actions, but the first level of intervention is directed to resolving the patient's problem that is reflected by the nursing diagnosis. With the decreasing length of stay for the majority of patients entering a hospital, we may indeed do well to complete the first level of nursing actions.

Additionally, there is continuing debate among NANDA members as to whether the current list of diagnoses that are accepted for testing are nursing diagnoses or a list of diagnostic categories or concepts. We therefore have chosen to focus on concepts. Using a conceptual approach allows focus on independent nursing functions and helps avoid focusing on medical intervention. This book has been designed to serve as a guide to using NANDA accepted nursing diagnoses as the primary base for the planning of care. The expected outcomes, target dates, nursing actions, and evaluation algorithms (flowcharts) are not meant to serve as standardized plans of care but rather as guides and references in promoting the visibility of nursing's contribution to health care.

Marjory Gordon's "Functional Health Patterns" are used as an organizing framework for the book. The functional health patterns allow grouping of the nursing diagnoses into specific groups, which in our opinion, promotes a conceptual approach to assessment and formulation of a nursing diagnosis.

Chapter 1 serves as the overview-introductory chapter and gives basic content related to the process of planning care and information regarding the relationship between nursing process and nursing models (theories). Titles for Chapters 2 through 12 are taken from the functional patterns. Included in each of these chapters is a pattern description, pattern assessment, a list of diagnoses within the pattern, conceptual information, and developmental information related to the pattern.

The pattern description gives a succinct summary of the pattern's content and assists in explaining how the diagnoses within the pattern are related. The pattern assessment serves to pinpoint information from the initial assessment base and was specifically written to direct the reader to the most likely diagnosis within the pattern. Each assessment factor is designed to allow an answer of "Yes" or "No". If the patient's answer or signs are indicative of a diagnosis within the pattern, the reader is directed to the most likely diagnosis or diagnoses. The list of diagnoses within the pattern is given to simplify location of the diagnoses. The conceptual and developmental information is included to provide a quick, ready reference to the physiological, psychological, sociological and age related factors that could cause modification of the nursing actions in order to make them more specific for your patient. The conceptual and developmental information can be used to determine the rationale for each nursing action.

Each nursing diagnosis within the pattern is then introduced with accompanying information of definition, defining characteristics, and related factors. We have added a section titled Related Clinical Concerns. This section serves to highlight the most common medical diagnoses or cluster of diagnoses that could involve the individual nursing diagnosis. Immediately after the related clinical concerns section is a section titled "Have you selected the correct diagnosis?"

The "Have you selected the correct diagnosis?" section was included as a validation check because we realize that several of the diagnoses appear very closely related and that it can be difficult to distinguish between these diagnoses. A part of this problem is related to the fact that the diagnoses have been accepted for testing, not as statements of absolute, discrete diagnoses. Thus, having this section assists the reader in learning how to pinpoint the differences between diagnoses and in feeling more comfortable in selecting a diagnosis that most clearly reflects a patient's problem area that can be helped by nursing actions.

After the diagnosis validation section are Expected Outcomes. Expected Outcomes serve as the end point against which progress can be measured. Also called objectives, patient goals, and outcome standards, the expected outcomes are connected by the words "and/or," signifying that the reader may choose to use only one of the outcomes or to use both of the outcomes. Readers might also choose to design their own patient-specific expected outcomes using the given expected outcomes as guidelines.

Target dates are suggested following the expected outcomes. The target dates DO NOT indicate the time or day the outcome must be fully achieved; instead, the target date signifies the time or day when evaluation should be completed in order to measure the patient's progress TOWARD achievement of the expected outcome. Target dates are given in reference to short-term care. For home health, particularly, the target date would be in terms of weeks and months rather than days.

Nursing actions/interventions and rationales are the next information given. In each instance the adult health nursing actions serve as the generic nursing actions. Subsequent sets of nursing actions (child health, women's health, mental health, gerontic health, and home health) show only the nursing actions that are different from the generic nursing actions. The different nursing actions make each set specific for the target population, but MUST BE used in conjunction with the adult health nursing actions to be complete. Gerontic health nursing actions are new to the second edition in recognition of our aging population. Gerontology will be a major practice arena for nurses in the very near future. Rationales have been included to assist the student in learning the reason for particular nursing actions. While some of the rationales are scientific in nature, that is, supported by documented research, others could be more appropriately termed common sense or usual practice rationales. These rationales are reasons nurses have cited for particular nursing actions and result from nursing experience BUT, research has not been conducted to document these rationales. After the home health actions, evaluation algorithms are shown that help judge the patient's progress toward achieving the expected outcome.

Evaluation of the patient's care is based on the degree of progress the patient has made toward achieving the expected outcome. For each stated outcome, there is an evaluation flowchart (algorithm). The flowcharts provide minimum information, but demonstrate the decision-making process that must be used.

In all instances, the authors have used the definitions, major and minor defining characteristics, and related factors that have been accepted by NANDA for testing. A grant was provided to NANDA by F.A. Davis for the use of these materials. All of these materials may be ordered from NANDA (1211 Locust Street, Philadelphia, PA 19107).

In some instances, additional information is included following a set of nursing actions. The additional information includes material that either needs to be highlighted or does not logically fall within the defined outline areas.

Throughout the nursing actions we have used "patient" and "client" interchangeably. The terms refer to the system of care and include the individual as well as the family and other social support systems. The nursing actions are written very specifically. This specificity aids in communication between and among nurses and promotes consistency of care for the patient.

We have written this book for any nurse or nursing student who is beginning to work with nursing diagnosis. We hope to promote the use of nursing diagnosis to the end that nursing itself is advanced. If you, our readers, begin to feel more comfortable with using nursing diagnosis nomenclature and begin to use nursing diagnosis more in your practice, then our hope will have become reality.

Helen Cox, RNC, EdD, FAAN

Acknowledgments

The publication of a book necessitates the involvement of many persons beyond the authors. We wish to acknowledge the support and assistance of the following persons who indeed made this book possible.

Our families, who supported our taking time away from family activities.

Margo Neal and Rose Mary Carroll-Johnson, who helped us clarify and refine so that the first edition of this book became even more than we had envisioned it could be.

Sue Glover, Nursing Editor, of Williams & Wilkins, who was most facilitative for the first edition of the book.

Bob Martone, Publisher, Nursing, of F.A. Davis, whose enthusiasm for a new edition and belief in the book were most gratifying and helpful.

AND

A special acknowledgement to Dr. Marjory Gordon, a most gracious lady who freely shared ideas, materials, support, and encouragement.

To each of these persons we wish to say a heartfelt "Thank You". Please accept our deepest gratitude and appreciation.

Contents

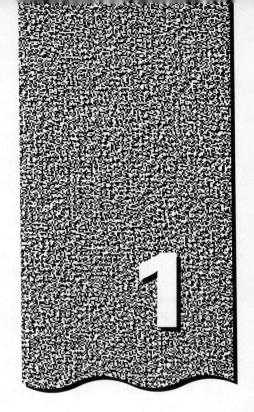

Introduction

Why This Book?

At the time the first edition of this book was written, all of the authors were faculty members at the same school of nursing. We had become frustrated with the books that were available for teaching nursing diagnosis to students, and we found that the students were expressing some of the same frustrations.

The students felt the need to bring several books to the clinical area because the books related to nursing diagnosis had limited information regarding pathophysiology, psychosocial, or developmental factors that definitely impacted individualized care planning. The students were also expressing confusion regarding the different definitions, defining characteristics, and related factors each of the authors was using. The students were having difficulty in writing individualized nursing actions for their patient because the various authors appeared to focus on specifics related to the etiology or signs and symptoms of the nursing diagnosis rather than the concept represented by the nursing diagnosis that had been emphasized to our students. We were also concerned about the number of books our students were having to buy since the majority of books relating to the use of nursing diagnosis in the clinical area focused on just one clinical area such as adult health or pediatrics but not both. Thus, as the students progressed through the school, they had to buy different books for different clinical areas even though each of the books had the common theme of the use of nursing diagnosis. Another concern we, as faculty, had was the lack of information in the various books regarding the final phase of the nursing process, evaluation. This most vital phase was briefly mentioned, but very little guidance was given in how to do this phase. For these reasons we have written this book, and for these reasons the book is particularly geared to student use. The final concern that led to the writing of the book was our desire to focus on nursing actions and nursing care, not medical care and medical diagnosis. We strongly believe in and support the vital role that nurses play in the provision of health care for our nation and so have focused, in this book, strictly on nursing. After all, statistics show that the largest number of health care providers are nurses and that the general public has a high respect for nurses. Therefore, let us work on developing our profession and its contributions.

Specifically, this book was written to assist students in learning how to apply nursing diagnosis in the clinical area. By using the framework of the nursing process and the materials generated by the North American Nursing Diagnosis Association (NANDA), we believe this book makes it easier for you, the student, to learn and use nursing diagnosis in planning care for your patients.

The Nursing Process

PURPOSE

Gordon[1] indicates that Lydia Hall was one of the first nurses to use the term "nursing process" in the early 1950s. Since that time the term "nursing process" has been used to describe the accepted method of delivering nursing care. Iyer, Taptich, and Bernocchi-Losey[2] state, "The major purpose of the nursing process is to provide a framework within which the individualized needs of the client, family, and community can be met."

It may be easier to think of a "framework" as a blueprint or an outline that guides the planning of care for a patient.* As Doenges and Moorhouse write,[3] "The nursing process is central to nursing actions in any setting because it is an efficient method of organizing thought processes for clinical decision making and problem solving." Use of the nursing process framework is beneficial for both the patient and the nurse because it helps ensure that care is planned, individualized, and reviewed over the period of time that the nurse and patient have a professional relationship. It is important to emphasize that the nursing process requires the involvement of the patient throughout all the phases. If the patient is not involved in all phases, then the plan of care is not individualized.

DEFINITION

Alfaro[4] defines "nursing process" as "an organized, systematic method of giving individualized nursing care that focuses on identifying and treating unique responses of individuals or groups to actual or potential alterations in health." This definition fits very nicely with the American Nurses Association (ANA) Social Policy Statement[5] that states specifically that "nursing is the diagnosis and treatment of human responses to actual and potential health problems." Alfaro's definition is further supported by the ANA Standards of Clinical Nursing Practice[6] (Table 1 – 1), practice standards written by several boards of nursing,[7] and the definition of nursing that is written into the majority of nurse practice acts in the United States. (The Board of Nurse Examiners for the State of Texas Nursing Practice Standards are used as an example. See Table 1 – 2.)

Basically, the nursing process provides each nurse a framework to utilize in working with the patient. The process begins at the time the patient needs assistance with health care through the time the patient no longer needs assistance to meet health care maintenance. The nursing process represents the cognitive (thinking, reasoning), psychomotor (physical), and affective (emotion, feelings, and values) skills and abilities used by the nurse to plan care for a patient.

---

*Note: Throughout this book we use the terms "patient" and "client" interchangeably. In most instances these terms refer to the individual who is receiving nursing care; however, a patient can also be a community, such as in the community – home health nursing actions, or the patient can be a family, such as in the nursing diagnosis Ineffective Family Coping: Compromised.

Table 1 – 1 STANDARDS OF CARE

Standard I. Assessment
　The nurse collects client health data.
Standard II. Diagnosis
　The nurse analyzes the assessment data in determining diagnoses.
Standard III. Outcome Identification
　The nurse identifies expected outcomes individualized to the client.
Standard IV. Planning
　The nurse develops a plan of care that prescribes interventions to attain expected outcomes.
Standard V. Implementation
　The nurse implements the interventions identified in the plan of care.
Standard VI. Evaluation
　The nurse evaluates the client's progress toward attainment of outcomes.

Source: Reprinted with permission from Standards of Clinical Nursing Practice,[6] © 1991, American Nurses Association, Kansas City, MO, p 9.

Table 1–2 **STANDARDS OF NURSING PRACTICE**

The Registered Professional Nurse shall:

1. Know and conform to the laws and regulations governing the practice of professional nursing in the State of Texas.
2. Utilize the nursing process to provide individualized, goal-directed nursing care by:
    a. Performing nursing assessments regarding the health status of the patient/client.
    b. Making nursing diagnoses which serve as the basis for the strategy of care.
    c. Developing a plan of care based on assessment and nursing diagnoses.
    d. Implementing nursing care.
    e. Evaluating the patient's/client's responses to nursing interventions.
3. Institute appropriate nursing intervention which might be required to stabilize a patient's/client's condition and/or prevent complications.
4. Know the rationale for, the effects of, and the proper administration of the medications and/or treatments he/she administers.
5. Accurately report and document the patient's/client's symptoms, responses, and progress.
6. Respect the patient's/client's right to privacy by protecting confidential information unless obligated or allowed by law to disclose the information.
7. Promote and participate in patient/client education and counseling based on health needs.
8. Collaborate with members of health disciplines in the interest of the patient's/client's health care.
9. Consult and utilize community agencies and resources for continuity of patient/client care.
10. Consult with the appropriate licensed practitioner to clarify any order or treatment regimen that the nurse has reason to believe is inaccurate and/or contraindicated.
11. Make assignments to other nursing personnel that take into consideration patient safety and that are commensurate with the personnel's educational preparation, experience, and knowledge.
12. Supervise nursing care provided by nursing personnel for which he/she is administratively responsible.
13. Accept only those nursing assignments that are commensurate with his/her educational preparation, experience, and knowledge of patient safety.
14. Be responsible for his/her continuing competence in nursing practice and individual professional growth.

Source: Adapted from Board of Nurse Examiners for the State of Texas,[7] p 37, with permission.

ROLE IN PLANNING CARE

Perhaps the important question is, why do we need to plan care? There are several answers to this question that range from the individual needs of a patient to the legal aspects of nursing practice.

First, the patient has a right to expect that the nursing care received will be complete and of high quality. If care planning is not done, then gaps are going to exist in the patient's care. At this time, we are seeing patients being admitted to the hospital more acutely ill than in the past. We are now caring for patients on a general medical-surgical unit who would have been in a critical care unit 10 years ago. We are now sending patients home in 3 to 5 days that we would have kept in the hospital another 5 to 10 days 10 years ago. A variety of factors have led to this situation, including the advent of Diagnosis Related Groups (DRGs), prospective payment plans, movement from acute care to longer-term care settings such as home health, nursing homes, and rehabilitation units, and, most importantly, the desire to contain the rapidly rising costs of health care. With this problem, which has been labeled the "quicker, sicker" phenomenon, in combination with a national shortage of registered nurses, contact time with a patient is being cut to a minimum. If care planning is not done, given this set of circumstances, then there is no doubt that gaps will exist in the nursing care given to a patient and that such care will be incomplete, inconsistent, and certainly not of high quality.

Second, care planning and its documentation provide a means of professional communication. This communication promotes consistency of care for the patient and provides a comfort level for the nurse. Any patient admitted to a health care agency is going to have some level of anxiety. Imagine how this anxiety increases when each nurse who enters the room does each procedure differently, answers questions differently, or uses different time lines for care (e.g., a surgical dressing that has been changed in the morning every day since surgery is not changed until the afternoon). Care planning provides a comfort level for the nurse because it gives the nurse a ready reference to help ensure that care is complete. Care planning also provides a guideline for documentation and promotes practicing within legally defined standards.

Third, care planning provides legal protection for the nurse. We are practicing in one of the most litigious societies that has ever existed. In the past, nurses were not frequently named in legal actions; however, this has changed as a brief review of suits being filed these days would show. In a legal suit, the nursing care is measured against the idea of what a reasonably prudent nurse would do in the same circumstances. The accepted standards of nursing practice, as published by the ANA[6] (Table 1–1) and the individual boards of nursing[7] (Table 1–2), are the accepted definitions of reasonable, prudent nursing care.

Finally, accrediting and approval agencies such as the Joint Commission on Accreditation of Healthcare Organizations (JCAHO), the National League for Nursing (NLN), Medicare, and Medicaid have criteria that specifically require documentation of planning of care. The accreditation status of a health care agency can depend on consistent documentation that planning of care has been done. Particularly with third-party payers such as Medicare, Medicaid, and insurance companies, lack of documentation regarding the planning and implementation of care means no reimbursement for care. Ultimately, nonreimbursement for care can lead to a lack of new equipment and/or salary increases; it can even lead to hospital closures.

CARE PLAN VERSUS PLANNING OF CARE

Recent revisions of nursing standards by the JCAHO created questions regarding the necessity of nursing care plans. Some have predicted the rapid demise of the care plan, according to Brider,[8] but review of the revised nursing standards shows that the standards require not less but more detailed care planning documentation in the patient's medical record.

Review of the new criteria indicates that the standards require documentation related to the nursing process. For example, JCAHO[9] Nursing Care Standard 1.3.5 requires:

> Nursing care data related to patient assessments, the nursing care planned,
> nursing interventions, and patient outcomes are permanently integrated into the
> clinical information system (for example, the medical record).

Rather than eliminating care plans, the new JCAHO requirements call for more specific, as well as more permanent, documentation of the plan of care. This documentation must be in the medical record. The standard indicates a separate care plan form is no longer necessary; however, the standard also still allows a separate care plan form. Various institutions are now testing flexible ways of documenting care planning. The care plan is not dead . . . it is rather revised to more clearly reflect the important role of nursing in the patient's care. No longer a separate, often discarded, and irrelevant page, the plan of care must be part of the permanent record. The flow sheets developed for this book offer guidelines for computerizing information regarding nursing care.

Faculty can use the revised JCAHO standards to assist students in developing expertise beyond writing extensive nursing care plans. This additional expertise requires the new graduate to integrate all phases of the nursing process into the permanent record. Rather than eliminating the need for care planning and nursing diagnosis, the new standards have reinforced the importance of nursing care and nursing diagnosis.

Nursing Process Steps

There are five steps, or phases, in the nursing process: assessment, diagnosis, planning, implementation, and evaluation. These steps are not discrete steps but overlap and build on each other. To accurately carry out the entire nursing process, you must be sure to accurately complete each step and then use the information in that step to build upon in order to complete the next step.

ASSESSMENT

The first step, or phase, of the nursing process is assessment. During this phase you are collecting data (factual information) from several sources. The collection and organization of this data allow you to:

1. Determine the patient's current health status
2. Determine the patient's strengths and problem areas (both actual and potential)
3. Prepare for the second step of the process—diagnosis

Data Sources and Types

The sources for data collection are numerous, but it is essential to remember that the patient is the primary data source. No one else can explain as accurately as the patient the start of the problem, the reason for seeking assistance, or the exact nature of the problem and what it is doing to the patient. Other sources include the patient's family or significant others, the patient's admission sheet from the admitting office, the physician's history, physical, and orders, laboratory and x-ray results, information from other caregivers, and current nursing literature.

Assessment data can be further classified as types of data. According to Iyer et al.,[2] the data types are subjective, objective, historical, and current.

Subjective data are the facts presented by the patient that show his or her perception, understanding, and interpretation of what is happening. An example of subjective data is the patient's statement, "The pain begins in my lower back and runs down my left leg."

Objective data are those facts that are observable and measurable by the nurse. These data are gathered by the nurse through physical assessment, interviewing, and observing, and they involve the use of the senses of seeing, hearing, smelling, and touching. An example of objective data is the measurement and recording of vital signs. Objective data are also gathered through such diagnostic examinations and procedures as laboratory tests and x-rays.

Historical data are those health events that happened prior to this admission or health problem episode. An example of historical data is the patient statement, "The last time I was in a hospital was 1984 when I had an emergency appendectomy."

Current data are those facts specifically related to this admission or health problem episode. An example of this type of data is vital signs on admission — T 99.2°F, P 78, R 18, BP 134/86. Please note that just as there is overlapping of the nursing process steps, there is also overlapping of the data types. Both historical and current data may be either subjective or objective. Historical and current data assist in establishing time references and can give an indication of the patient's usual functioning.

Essential Skills

Assessment requires use of the skills of interviewing, physical assessment, and observation. As with the nursing process itself, these skills cannot be separated into three discrete skills. While you are interviewing the patient, you are also observing and determining physical areas requiring a detailed physical assessment. While completing a physical assessment, you are asking questions (interviewing) and observing the patient's physical appearance as well as the patient's response to the physical examination.

Interviewing generally starts with gathering data for the nursing history. In this interview, you ask general demographic questions such as name, address, date of last hospitalization, age, allergies, current medications, and why the patient was admitted. Depending on the agency's admission form, you may then progress to other specific questions or a physical assessment. An example of an admission assessment specifically related to the Functional Health Patterns is given in Appendix A.

The physical assessment calls for four skills: inspection, palpation, percussion, and auscultation. *Inspection* means careful and systematic observation throughout the physical examination such as observation for and recording of any skin lesions. *Palpation* means assessment by feeling and touching. Assessing the differences in temperature between a patient's upper and lower arm would be an example of palpation. Another common example of palpation is breast self-examination. *Percussion* involves touching, tapping, and listening. Percussion allows determination of size, density, organ locations, and boundaries. Percussion is usually performed by placing the index or middle finger of one hand firmly on the skin and striking with the middle finger of the other hand. The resultant sound is dull if the body is solid under the fingers (such as the presence of the liver) and hollow sounding if there is a body cavity under the finger (such as the abdominal cavity). *Auscultation* involves listening with a stethoscope and is used to help assess respiratory, circulatory, and gastrointestinal status.

The physical assessment may be performed using a head-to-toe approach or a body system approach, or it may be performed according to the Functional Health Patterns. In the head-to-toe approach, you begin with the patient's general appearance and vital signs. Progression then proceeds, as the title indicates, from the head to the extremities.

The body system approach to physical assessment focuses on the major body systems. As the nurse is conducting the nursing history interview, he or she will get a firm idea of which body systems will need detailed examination. An example of this type of examination is a cardiovascular examination where the apical and radial pulses, blood pressure (BP), point of maximum intensity (PMI), heart sounds, and peripheral pulses are examined.

The Functional Health Pattern approach is based on Gordon's Functional Health Pattern typology and allows the collection of all types of data according to each pattern. This is the approach used by this book and leads to three levels of assessment. First is the overall admission assessment, where each pattern is assessed through the collection of objective and subjective data. This assessment will indicate patterns that need further attention, which requires implementation of the second level of pattern assessment. The second level of pattern assessment indicates the nursing diagnoses within the pattern that might be pertinent to this patient, which leads to the third level of assessment, the defining characteristics for each individual nursing diagnosis. Having a three-tiered assessment might seem complicated, but each assessment is so closely related that completion of the assessment is easy. A primary advantage in using this type of assessment is the validation it gives to the nurse that the resulting nursing diagnosis is the most correct diagnosis. Another benefit of using this type of assessment is that grouping of data is already accomplished and does not have to be a separate step.

Data Grouping

Data grouping simply means organizing the information into sets or categories that will assist you to identify the patient's strengths and problem areas. A variety of organizing frameworks are available such as Maslow's hierarchy of needs, NANDA's Human Response Patterns, and Gordon's Functional Health Patterns. Each of the nursing theorists (e.g., Roy, Levine, and Orem) speak to assessment within the framework of their theories.

Organizing the information allows you to identify the appropriate Functional Health Pattern and will also allow you to spot any missing data. If you cannot identify the pertinent Functional Health Pattern, then you need to collect further data. The goal of data grouping is to arrive at a nursing diagnosis.

Diagnosis

Diagnosis means reaching a definite conclusion regarding the patient's strengths and problems. The problems are the primary focus for planning care, and the strengths are used to assist you in implementing this care. In this book, we concentrate the diagnosis phase of the nursing process on nursing diagnosis and use the diagnoses accepted by NANDA for testing

NURSING DIAGNOSIS

The North American Nursing Diagnosis Association (NANDA), formerly the National Conference Group for Classification of Nursing Diagnosis, has been meeting since 1973 to identify, develop, and classify nursing diagnoses. Setting forth a nursing diagnosis nomenclature articulates nursing language, thus promoting the identification of nursing's contribution to health, and facilitates communication between nurses. In addition, the use of nursing diagnosis provides a clear distinction between nursing diagnosis and medical diagnosis and establishes a direction for the remaining aspects of care planning.

NANDA accepted its first working definition of "nursing diagnosis" in 1990:[10]

A nursing diagnosis is a clinical judgment about individual, family or community responses to actual or potential health problems/life processes. Nursing diagnoses provide the basis for selection of nursing interventions to achieve outcomes for which the nurse is accountable.

Much debate occurred during the ninth conference regarding this definition, and it is anticipated that this debate will continue. The debate centers on a multitude of issues related to the definition that are beyond the purpose of this book. Readers are urged to read the official journal of NANDA, *Nursing Diagnosis*, to keep themselves updated on this debate.

The definition of "nursing diagnosis" distinguishes the primary ways nursing diagnosis differs from medical diagnosis. Another way nursing diagnosis is different from medical diagnosis is in the area of focus. Kozier, Erb, and Olivieri[11] write that nursing diagnoses focus on patient response while medical diagnoses focus on disease process. As indicated by the definition of "nursing diagnosis," nurses also identify potential problems while physicians place primary emphasis on identifying the current problem.

Nursing diagnosis and medical diagnosis are similar in that the same basic procedures are used to derive the diagnosis (i.e., physical assessment, interviewing, and observing). Likewise, according to Kozier et al.,[11] both types of diagnoses are designed for essentially the same reason—planning care for a patient.

A nursing diagnosis is based on the presence of the major and minor defining characteristics. According to NANDA,[12] "defining characteristics" are clinical criteria that represent the presence of the diagnostic category (nursing diagnosis). For actual nursing diagnoses (the problem is present), 80 to 100 percent of the major defining characteristics must be present and 50 to 79 percent of the minor defining characteristics should be present. For high-risk diagnoses (risk factors indicate the problem might develop), the risk factors must be present.

DIAGNOSTIC STATEMENTS

According to the literature, complete nursing diagnostic statements include, at a minimum, the human response and an indication of the factors contributing to the response. The following is a rationale for the two-part statement:[13]

> Each nursing diagnosis, when correctly written, can accomplish two things. One, by identifying the unhealthy response, it tells you what should change. . . . And two, by identifying the probable cause of the unhealthy response, it tells you what to do to effect change.

While there is no consensus on the phrase that should be used to link the response and etiologic factors, perusal of current literature indicates that the most commonly used phrases are:

Related to
Secondary to
Due to

The phrase "related to" is gaining the most acceptance because it does not imply a direct cause-and-effect relationship. Kieffer[14] believes using the phrases "due to" and "secondary to" could reflect such a cause-and-effect relationship that could be hard to prove. Thus a complete nursing diagnostic statement would read: Pain related to surgical incision.

Gordon[1] identifies three structural components of a nursing diagnostic statement: The problem (P), the etiology (E), and the signs and symptoms (S). The problem describes the patient's response or current state (the nursing diagnosis). The etiology describes the cause or causes of the response (related to), and the symptoms delineate the defining characteristics or observable signs and symptoms demonstrated or described by the patient. The S component can be readily connected to the P and E statements through the use of the phrase "as evidenced by." Using this format, a complete nursing diagnostic statement would read: Pain related to surgical incision as evidenced by verbal comments and body posture.

As discussed in the preface, we recommend starting with stating the nursing diagnosis only. Therefore, the nursing diagnosis would be listed in the patient's chart in the same manner as it is given in the nomenclature: Pain. Remember that the objective and subjective data related to the patient's pain have already been recorded in the health record in the assessment section, so there is no need to repeat it again.

The nursing diagnostic statement examples given previously describe the existence of an actual problem. Professional nurses are strong supporters of preventive health care — cases in which a problem does not yet exist and in which measures can be taken to ensure that the problem does not arise. In such instances the nursing diagnostic statement is prefaced by the words "High Risk for." Nursing diagnoses that carry the preface "High Risk for" also carry with them Risk Factors rather than defining characteristics.

While other books include a variety of nursing diagnoses, this book will use only the actual and high-risk (formerly labeled "potential") diagnoses accepted by NANDA for testing. Probable related factors (formerly "etiologic factors") will be grouped, as will the defining characteristics (formerly "signs and symptoms"), under each specific nursing diagnosis. As indicated in the preface, nursing actions in this book reflect a conceptual approach rather than a specific (to related factors or defining characteristics) approach.

To illustrate this approach, let us use the diagnosis Pain. There are common nursing orders related to the incidence of pain regardless of whether the pain is caused by surgery, labor, or trauma. You can take this conceptual approach and make an individualized adaptation according to the etiologic factors affecting your patient and the reaction your patient is exhibiting to pain.

Identifying and specifying the nursing diagnoses leads to the next phase of the process — planning. Now that you know what the problems and strengths are, you can decide how to resolve the problem areas while building on the areas of strength.

Planning

Planning involves three subsets: setting priorities, writing expected outcomes, and establishing target dates. Planning sets the stage for writing nursing actions by establishing where you are going with the plan of care. Planning further assists in the final phase of evaluation by defining the standard against which progress will be measured.

SETTING PRIORITIES

With the sicker, quicker problem discussed earlier, you are going to find yourself in the situation of having identified many more problems than can possibly be resolved in a 3- to 5-day (today's average length of stay) hospitalization. In long-term care facilities, such as home health, rehabilitation, and nursing homes, long-range problem solving is possible, but setting priorities of care is still necessary.

Several methods of assigning priorities are available. Some nurses will assign priorities based on the life threat posed by a problem. For example, Ineffective Airway Clearance would pose more of a threat to life than the diagnosis High Risk for Impaired Skin Integrity. Some nurses will base their prioritization on Maslow's hierarchy of needs. In this instance, physiologic needs would require attention before social needs. One simple way to establish priorities is to simply ask the patient which problem he or she would like to pay attention to first. Another way to establish priorities is to analyze the relationships between problems. For example, a patient has been admitted with a medical diagnosis of headaches and possible brain tumor. The patient exhibits the defining characteristics of both Pain and Anxiety. In this instance you might want to implement nursing actions to reduce anxiety, knowing that if the anxiety is not reduced, pain control actions will not be successful. Once priorities have been established, you are ready to establish expected outcomes.

EXPECTED OUTCOMES

"Outcomes," "goals," and "objectives" are terms that are frequently used interchangeably because all indicate the end point you will use to measure the effectiveness of the plan of care. Because so many published sets of standards and the JCAHO talk in terms of "outcome standards" or "criteria," we have chosen to use the term "expected outcomes" in this book.

Several authors[11,15,16] give guidelines that assist in writing clinically useful expected outcomes:

1. Clearly stated in terms of patient behavior or observable assessment factors:

   EXAMPLE:
   POOR   Will increase fluid balance by time of discharge.
   GOOD   Will increase oral fluid intake to 1500 ml per 24 hours by 9/11.

2. Realistic, achievable, safe, and acceptable from the patient's viewpoint:

   EXAMPLE:
   Mrs. Braxton is a 28-year-old female who has delayed healing of a surgical wound. She is to receive discharge instructions regarding a high-protein diet. She is a widow with three children under the age of 10. Her only source of income is Social Security.
   POOR   Will eat at least two 8-oz servings of steak daily
            [unrealistic, nonachievable, unacceptable, etc.].
   GOOD   Will eat at least two servings from the following list each day:
            Lean ground meat
            Eggs
            Cheese
            Pinto beans
            Peanut butter
            Fish
            Chicken

3. Written in specific, concrete terms depicting patient action:

   EXAMPLE:
   POOR   Maintains fluid intake by (date).
   GOOD   Will drink at least 8 oz of fluid every hour from 7 a.m. to 10 p.m.
            by (date).

4. Directly observable by use of at least one of the five senses:

EXAMPLE:
POOR   Understands how to self-administer insulin by (date).
GOOD   Accurately return-demonstrates self-administration of insulin by (date).

5. Patient centered rather than nurse centered:

EXAMPLE:
POOR   Teaches how to measure blood pressure by (date).
GOOD   Accurately measures own blood pressure by (date).

ESTABLISHING TARGET DATES

Writing a target date at the end of the expected outcome statement facilitates the plan of care in several ways:[11,15]

1. Assists in "pacing" the care plan. Pacing helps keep focus on the patient's progress.
2. Serves to motivate both patients and nurses toward accomplishing the expected outcome.
3. Helps patient and nurse to see accomplishments.
4. Alerts nurse when to evaluate care plan.

Target dates can be realistically established by paying attention to the usual progress and prognosis connected with the patient's medical and nursing diagnoses. Additional review of the data collected during the initial assessment will help indicate individual factors to be considered in establishing the date. For example, one of the previous expected outcomes was stated as: Accurately return-demonstrates self-administration of insulin by (date).

The progress or prognosis according to the patient's medical and nursing diagnosis will not be highly significant. The primary factor will be whether diabetes mellitus is a new diagnosis for the patient or is a recurring problem for a patient who has had diabetes mellitus for several years.

For the newly diagnosed patient, you would probably want the deadline day to be 5 to 7 days from the date of learning the diagnosis. For the recurring problem, you might establish the target date to be 2 to 3 days from the date of diagnosis. The difference is, of course, the patient's knowledge base.

Now look at an example related to the progress issue. Mr. Kit is a 19-year-old college student who was admitted early this morning with a medical diagnosis of acute appendicitis. He has just returned from surgery following an appendectomy. One of the nursing diagnoses for Mr. Kit would, in all probability, be: Pain. The expected outcome could be: Will have decrease in number of requests for analgesics by (date). In reviewing the general progress of a young patient with this medical and nursing diagnosis, we know that generally analgesic requirements start decreasing within 48 to 72 hours. Therefore, you would want to establish the target date as 2 to 3 days following the day of surgery. This would result in the objective reading (assume the date of surgery was 11/1): Will have decrease in number of requests for analgesics by 11/3.

To further emphasize the target date, it is suggested that the date be underlined, highlighted by using a different-colored pen, or circled to make it stand out.

Pinpointing the date in such a manner emphasizes that evaluation of progress toward achievement of the expected outcome should be made on that date. In assigning the dates, be sure not to schedule all of the diagnoses and expected outcomes for evaluation on the same date. Such scheduling would require a total revision of the plan of care, which could contribute to not keeping the plan of care current. Being able to revise single portions of the plan of care facilitates use and updating of the plan. Remember the target date does not mean the expected outcome must be totally achieved by that time; instead, the target date signifies the evaluation date.

Once expected outcomes have been written, you are then ready to focus on the next phase — implementation. As previously indicated, the title supported by this book for this section is "Nursing Actions."

Implementation

Implementation is the action phase of the nursing process; hence, why we chose the term "nursing actions." Two important steps are involved in implementation. First is determining the specific nursing actions that will assist the patient to progress toward the expected outcome, and second is the documentation of the care administered.

Nursing action is defined as nursing behavior that serves to help the patient achieve the expected outcome. Nursing actions include both independent and collaborative activities. *Independent actions* are those activities the nurse performs using his or her own discretionary judgment. These activities require no validation or guidelines from any other health care practitioner. Examples of independent actions are choosing which noninvasive technique to use for pain control or deciding when to teach the patient self-care measures. *Collaborative actions* are those activities that involve mutual decision making between two or more health care practitioners, for example, a physician and nurse's deciding which narcotic to use when meperidine is ineffective in controlling the patient pain or a physical therapist and nurse's deciding on the most beneficial exercise program for a patient. Implementing a physician's order or referral to a dietitian are other common examples of collaborative actions. Written nursing actions guide both actual patient care and proper documentation.

Written nursing actions should be detailed and exact. Written nursing actions should be even more definite than what is generally found in physician orders. For example, a physician writes the order, "Increase ambulation as tolerated," for a patient who has been immobile for 2 weeks. The nursing actions should reflect specified increments of ambulation as well as ongoing assessment:

11/2 1. a. Prior to activity assess BP, P, and R. After activity assess: (1) BP, P, R; (2) presence/absence of vertigo; (3) circulation; (4) presence/absence of pain.
   b. Assist to dangle on bedside for 15 minutes at least four times a day on 11/2.
   c. If BP, P, or R changes significantly or vertigo present or impaired circulation present or pain present, return to supine position immediately. Elevate head of bed 30 degrees for 1 hour; then to 45 degrees for 1 hour; then to 90 degrees for 1 hour. If tolerated with no untoward signs or symptoms, initiate order 1*b* again.
   d. Assist up to chair at bedside for 30 minutes at least four times a day on 11/3.
   e. Assist to ambulate to bathroom and back at least four times a day on 11/4.
   f. Supervise ambulation of one-half length of hall at least four times a day on 11/5 and 11/6.
   g. Supervise ambulation of length of hall at least four times a day on 11/7.

S. J. Smith, RN

Nursing actions further differ from physician orders in that the patient's response is directly related to the implementation of the action. It is rare to see a physician's order that includes alternatives if the first order has minimal, negative, or no effect on the patient.

A complete written nursing action incorporates at least the following five components according to Sorensen and Luckmann:[15]

1. Date the action was initially written
2. A specific action verb that tells what the nurse is going to do (e.g., "assist," "supervise")
3. A prescribed activity (e.g., ambulation)
4. Specific time units (e.g., for 15 minutes at least four times a day)
5. Signature of the nurse who writes the initial action order (i.e., accepting legal and ethical accountability)

A nursing action should not be implemented unless all five components are present. A nurse would not administer a medication if the physician's order read, "Give Demerol"; neither should a nurse be expected to implement a nursing action that reads, "Increase ambulation gradually."

Additional criteria that should be remembered to ensure complete, quality nursing action include:

1. Consistency between the prescribed actions, the nursing diagnosis, and expected outcome (including numbering).

   FOR EXAMPLE:
   Nursing Diagnosis 1: Impaired physical mobility, level 2.
   Expected Outcome 1: Will ambulate length of hall by 11/8.
   Nursing Action 1:

11/2 a. Prior to activity assess BP, P, and R. After activity assess: (1) BP, P, R; (2) presence/absence of vertigo; (3) circulation; (4) presence/absence of pain.
   b. Assist to dangle on bedside for 15 minutes at least four times a day on 11/2.
   c. If BP, P, or R changes significantly or vertigo present or impaired circulation present or pain present, return to supine position immediately. Elevate head of bed 30 degrees for 1 hour; then to 45 degrees for 1 hour; then to 90 degrees for 1 hour. If tolerated with no untoward signs or symptoms, initiate action 1b again.
   d. Assist up to chair at bedside for 30 minutes at least four times a day on 11/3.
   e. Assist to ambulate to bathroom and back at least four times a day on 11/4.
   f. Supervise ambulation of one-half length of hall at least four times a day on 11/5 and 11/6.
   g. Supervise ambulation of length of hall at least four times a day on 11/7.

S. J. Smith, RN

---

2. Consideration of both patient and facility resources. It would be senseless to make referrals to physical and occupational therapy services if these were not available. Likewise, from the patient's resource viewpoint, it would be foolish to teach him or her and his or her family how to manage his or her care in a hospital bed if this bed were not available to the patient at home.
3. Careful scheduling to include the patient's significant others and to incorporate his or her usual activities of daily living (i.e., rest, meals, sleep, and recreation).
4. Incorporation of patient teaching and discharge planning from the first day of care.

5. Individualization and updating in keeping with the patient's condition and progress.

Including the key components and validating the quality of the written nursing actions help to promote thorough documentation. In essence, the written nursing actions can give an outline for documentation.

Properly written nursing actions demonstrate to the nurse both nursing actions and documentation to be done. Referring to the example on page 13, we can see that the nurse responsible for this patient's care should chart the patient's BP, P, and R rates prior to the activity, the patient's BP, P, and R rates after the activity, the presence or absence of vertigo, the presence or absence of pain, and the results of a circulatory check. Additionally, the nurse knows to chart that the patient dangled, sat up, or ambulated for a certain length of time or distance. Further, the nurse has guidelines of what to do and chart if an untoward reaction occurs in initial attempts at ambulation.

EXAMPLE:

1000	BP 132/82, P 74, R 16. Up on side of bed for 5 minutes. Complained of vertigo and nausea. Returned to supine position with head of bed elevated to 30-degree angle. BP 100/68, P 80, R 24.
1100	BP 122/74, P 76, R 18. No complaints of vertigo or nausea. Head of bed elevated to 45-degree angle.

Writing nursing actions in such a manner automatically leads to reflection of the quality of care planning in the chart. Documentation of care planning in the patient's chart is essential to meet national standards of care and criteria for agency accreditation.

Documentation

Just as development of the nursing process as a framework for practice has evolved, so documentation of that process has become an essential link between the provision of nursing care and the quality of the care provided. Several nursing documentation systems have emerged that make it easier to document the nursing process. Three of these systems will be discussed here. You will note that the narrative system is not discussed as it tends to be fragmented, disjointed, and presents problems in retrieval of pertinent information about the patient response to and outcomes of nursing care.

The *Problem Oriented Record (POR)*, with its format for documenting progress notes, provides a system for documenting the nursing process. Additionally, the **POR** is an interdisciplinary documentation system that can be used to coordinate care for all health care providers working with the patient.

The POR consists of four major components:

1. The database
2. The problem list
3. The plan of care
4. The progress notes

The database is that information which has been collected through patient interview, observation, physical assessment, and the results of diagnostic tests. The database provides the basis for developing the problem list.

The problem list is an inventory of numbered, prioritized patient problems. Patient problems may be written as nursing or medical diagnoses. Problems may be actual or high-risk diagnoses. Because each problem is numbered, information about each problem is easily retrieved.

The plan of care incorporates the expected outcomes, target dates, and prescribed nursing actions as well as other interventions designed to resolve the problem. The plan of care reflects multidisciplinary care and should be agreed to by the health care team.

The progress note provides information about the patient's response to or outcomes of the care provided. The full format for documenting progress is based on the acronym *SOAPIER*, which stands for *subjective data, objective data, analysis/ assessment, plan, intervention, evaluation, and revision*. As the plan of care is implemented for each numbered, prioritized problem, it is documented using the SOAPIER format. For example, recall the case of Mr. Kit, the 19-year-old college student who is recovering from an appendectomy. The problem list inventory would probably show Problem 1: Pain. His plan of care would state as an expected outcome: Will have decrease in number of requests for analgesics by 11/3. Some of the written nursing actions read:

1. Monitor for pain at least every 2 hours and have patient rank pain on a scale of 0 to 10.
2. Administer pain medications as ordered. Monitor response.
3. Spend at least 30 minutes once a shift teaching patient deep muscle relaxation. Talk patient through relaxation every 4 hours, while awake, at (list times here) once initial teaching is done.

The progress note of 11/3 would appear as follows:

Problem 1

S "I have had only one pain medication during the last 24 hours and that relieved my pain." "I would rank my pain as a 1 on a scale of 0 to 10."

O Relaxation exercises taught and return-demonstration completed on 11/2. No request for pain medication within past 12 hours.

A Pain relieved.

P None.

I None.

E Expected outcome met. Problem resolved. Discontinue problem.

R None.

The POR with its SOAPIER progress note emphasizes the problem-solving process inherent in the nursing process and provides documentation of the care provided. For further information about the POR system, you are directed to the Weed[17] reference.

FOCUS charting is a documentation system that uses the nursing process to document care and is an offshoot of POR. Unlike the interdisciplinary POR, FOCUS charting is entirely oriented to nursing documentation. Like the POR system,

FOCUS charting has a database, a problem list (FOCUS), a plan of care, and progress notes. However, the FOCUS (problem list) is broader than a POR. In addition to nursing and medical diagnoses, the FOCUS of care may also be treatments, procedures, incidents, patient concerns, change in condition, or other significant events. The medical record incorporates the plan of care in a three-column format (in addition to date/signature) labeled "FOCUS," "Expected Patient Outcomes," and "Nursing Interventions." To illustrate, again with Mr. Kit:

Date/Signature	FOCUS	Expected Pt. Outcome	Nursing Intervention
11/1 J. Jones, RN	Pain	Will have decrease in number of requests for analgesics by 11/3	Monitor for pain at least every 2 hours. Have pt. rate pain on 0 to 10 scale. Administer pain med. as ordered. Monitor response. Teach pt. use of noninvasive pain relief techniques as appropriate.

The progress notes incorporate a flow sheet for documenting daily interventions and treatments and a narrative progress note using, again, a three-column format. The three-column format for the progress note includes a column for date/time/signature; a FOCUS column; and a patient care note column. When the progress note is written in the patient care note column, it is organized using the acronym *DAR—data, action, and response*. To illustrate, again using Mr. Kit:

Date/Time Signature	FOCUS	Patient Care Note	
11/1 1500 J. Jones, RN	Pain	D:	C/o pain "My side hurts. It is a 9 on a 0 to 10 scale." BP 130/84, P 88, R 22.
1/1 1530 J. Jones, RN		A:	Demerol 100 mg given in rt. gluteus. Turned to left side. Back rub given.
11/1 1615 J. Jones, RN		R:	States pain is better. Rates it 2 on a 0 to 10 scale. BP 120/80, P 82, R 18.

FOCUS charting provides a succinct system for documenting the nursing process. It reflects all the elements required by JCAHO. It is flexible, provides cues to documentation with its DAR format, and makes for easy retrieval of pertinent data. For more information on FOCUS, use the information written by Lampe.[18]

The PIE documentation system emphasizes the nursing process and nursing diagnosis. *PIE* is the acronym for *problem, intervention, and evaluation.* A time-saving aspect of this system is that PIE does not require a separate plan of care. The initial database and ongoing assessments are recorded on special forms or flow sheets. Assessment data are not included in the progress note unless a change in the patient's condition occurs. If a change occurs, A for *assessment* would be recorded in the progress note. Routine interventions are recorded on a flow sheet, and the progress note is used for specific numbered problems.

When a problem is identified, it is entered into the progress note as a nursing diagnosis. Each problem is numbered consecutively during a 24-hour period, for example, P#1, P#2, and so on. Therefore, the nurse may refer to the number rather than having to restate the problem. *Interventions* (I) directed to the problem are documented relative to the problem number (e.g., IP#1 and IP#2). *Evaluations* (E) reflect patient response to or outcomes of nursing intervention and are labeled according to the problem number (EP#1, EP#2, and so on). To illustrate, again using Mr. Kit:

Date	Time	Nurses' Notes
11/1	1500	P#1: Pain. IP#1: BP 130/84, P 88, R 22. J. Jones, RN.
11/1	1530	IP#1: Demerol 100 mg given IM in rt. gluteus. Turned to left side. Back rub given. J. Jones, RN.
11/1	1615	EP#1: States pain relieved. Rates pain as 2 on a 0 to 10 scale. BP 120/80, P 82, R 18. J. Jones, RN.

Each problem is evaluated at least every 8 hours, and all problems are reviewed and summarized every 24 hours. Continuing problems with appropriate interventions and evaluation are renumbered and redocumented daily, thus promoting continuity of care. When a problem is resolved, it no longer is documented.

The PIE documentation system reflects the nursing process and simplifies documentation by integrating the plan of care into the progress notes. This saves time and promotes easy retrieval of pertinent data. Siegrist, Deltor, and Stocks[19] are the originators of the PIE system.

To complete the nursing process cycle and, depending on its outcome, perhaps start another cycle, the final phase of the process must be done. The last phase of the nursing process is evaluation.

Evaluation

Evaluation simply means assessing what progress has been made toward meeting the expected outcomes; it is the most ignored phase of the nursing process. The evaluation phase is the feedback and control part of the nursing process. Evaluation requires continuation of assessment that was begun in the initial assessment phase. In this instance, assessment is the data collection form we use to measure patient progress.

DATA COLLECTION

The data collection should initially be aimed at collecting the specific data needed to measure the progress made toward achieving the stated expected outcome. As an example, let us return to the outcome written for Mr. Kit, the 19-year-old college student who had an appendectomy. The expected outcome is "Will have decrease in number of requests for analgesics by 11/3." It is now 11/3, and the nurse caring for Mr. Kit notes the date and initiates evaluation of the stated outcome. He or she first checks the chart and counts the number of complaints of pain, number of analgesics given, and Mr. Kit's response to the pain medication. The nurse looks for any change in medication or a change in Mr. Kit's condition. He or she then interviews Mr. Kit regarding his perception of pain acuity and level of relief. At the same time the nurse will be completing other assessments such as wound condition, ease of ambulation, or presence of any other untoward signs or symptoms. The nurse then studies the data to see what action is necessary.

ACTION FOLLOWING DATA COLLECTION

Action following data collection simply means making a nursing judgment of what modifications in the plan of care are needed. There are essentially only three judgments that can be made:

1. Resolved
2. Revise
3. Continue

Resolved means that the evaluative data indicate the health care problem reflected in the nursing diagnosis and its accompanying expected outcome no longer exist; that is, the expected outcome has been met. The nurse documents the data collected and records the judgment: Resolved. To illustrate, let us return to Mr. Kit.

The nurse first reviews the chart. He or she finds that Mr. Kit requested pain medication every 3 to 4 hours for the first 18 hours after surgery. The nurses taught Mr. Kit relaxation exercises and turned him, positioned him, and gave him a back rub immediately after the administration of each analgesic. Mr. Kit has requested only one analgesic in the past 24 hours and none in the past 12 hours. He can return-demonstrate relaxation exercises and states that he has only a mild "twinge" when he gets out of bed. He is looking forward to returning to school next week.

The nurse returns to the patient's chart and records the following: "11/3 Data: 1 analgesic in past 24 hours; none in past 12 hours. Ambulates without pain; states having no pain. Resolved." He or she then will draw one line through the nursing diagnosis, related expected outcome(s), and nursing actions to show they have been discontinued.

Revise can indicate two actions. In one instance, the initial nursing diagnosis was not correct so the diagnosis itself is revised. For example, the nurse may have made an initial diagnosis of Self-Esteem Disturbance. Upon collecting evaluation data, the patient and his or her family share further information that indicates the more appropriate diagnosis is Powerlessness: moderate. The plan of care is then modified to reflect the change in the nursing diagnosis. For evaluation purposes, the nurse again records the data and the word "Revised." He or she then adds the new nursing diagnosis and marks one line through the initial nursing diagnosis.

In the second instance, while the nurse is collecting evaluation data for one nursing diagnosis and expected outcome, he or she finds assessment factors that show another problem has arisen. He or she simply records the appropriate judgment for the initial diagnosis and expected outcome (e.g., Resolved) and revises the plan to include the new nursing diagnosis with its appropriate expected outcome and nursing actions.

Continue indicates that the expected outcome has not been met. The nurse again collects the appropriate data and, based on the data, makes the nursing judgment that the expected outcome has not been met. He or she records the data and adds the phrase, "Continue, reevaluate on (date)." He or she then modifies the plan of care by going back to the stated expected outcome, marking one line through the date, and adding a new date. Likewise, the nursing actions would be modified as necessary.

With evaluation, the nursing process cycle is completed (see Fig. 1–1). Another cycle can begin with both the nurse and the patient being sure that quality care is being given and received.

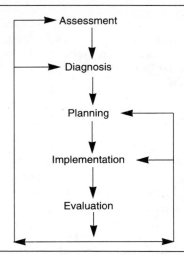

Figure 1—1 Nursing process flowchart.

Nursing Process and Conceptual Frameworks

NURSING MODELS

Many nurses do not see a direct relationship between nursing models (nursing theories) and nursing process, but a direct relationship does exist. Nursing models present a systematic method for assessing and directing nursing practice through promoting organization and integration of what is known about human beings, health, illness, and nursing. Nursing models are based on purposeful orientations;[20] therefore, the nursing process is the action phase of a nursing model. In essence, models guide the use of the nursing process,[21] and, as previously stated, the care planning presented in this book is a result of the nursing process.

For further clarification, let us look at a few examples. If you are a supporter of Levine's conservation model, you would assess your patient in keeping with this model and then design your care plan to reflect the prioritizing of the nursing diagnoses and nursing actions in a manner that would best promote conservation principles. Likewise, if you are a proponent of Roy's adaptation model, you would assess the four adaptation modes, then prioritize your diagnoses in an order that would best promote adaptive responses. In summation, current nursing models affect care planning in terms of assessing and prioritizing nursing diagnoses rather than requiring different diagnostic statements and different nursing actions.

PATTERNS

Several typologies have emerged as a result of the work done with nursing diagnosis. The typologies are representative of another step in theory development and are designed to facilitate the use of nursing diagnosis. The typologies provide an organizational framework that enables the nurse to focus on the pattern description and assessment rather than on trying to remember all the details of individual diagnoses. The nurse can easily locate the individual diagnosis by being familiar with the patterns.

Functional Health Patterns

Gordon[1] writes that the Functional Health Patterns were identified, circa 1974, to assist in the teaching of assessment and diagnosis at the Boston College School of Nursing. The Functional Health Patterns organize the individual diagnoses into categories, thus providing for the organized collection of assessment data.

The advantages[1] offered by assessment, according to the Functional Health Patterns, include having a standardized method that does not have to be relearned if the setting, patient's age, or condition changes; having an assessment tool specifically designed to lead to identification of pertinent nursing diagnoses; and having an assessment method that is holistic in nature.

Functional Health Patterns focus on the client's usual ways of living[1] and direct attention to all the factors that impact the individual in these ways of living. Gordon[1] defines a pattern as "a sequence of behavior across time." The Functional Health Patterns allow the nurse to assess these behaviors by promoting the patient's describing his or her own perception as well as incorporating the nurse's observations. Both the patient's description and the nurse's observations must be included to ensure a complete assessment.

Use of the Functional Health Patterns for assessment allows identification of three major types of data:

1. **Functional patterns:** The functional patterns are client strengths that can be used to deal with either dysfunctional or potentially dysfunctional patterns; for example, assessment of the Coping–Stress Tolerance Pattern shows no problem areas. The nurse can then use this functional pattern to assist the patient in learning to cope with the identified problem areas.
2. **Dysfunctional patterns:** The dysfunctional health patterns identify problem areas and the nursing diagnoses related to the problem areas; for example, in assessing the Elimination Pattern, a nurse may have identified problems with urination, and specifically with Urinary Retention. Knowing that the patient has effective individual coping, the nurse then plans teaching that will utilize this strength rather than interventions that are totally nursing-focused such as intermittent catheterization. The nurse could teach the patient to use Crede's maneuver, pouring warm water over the genital area, running tap water, and so on, to use the client's already demonstrated strength.
3. **Potential dysfunctional patterns:** The potential dysfunctional patterns are high-risk conditions, for example, in a client who has urinary retention, risk factors for the development of Excess Fluid Volume would also be highly likely. Utilizing this knowledge, the nurse would identify areas of observation to monitor and to teach the patient to monitor.

Use of the Functional Health Patterns in assessment focuses on a nursing model of assessment, diagnosis, planning, intervention, and evaluation rather than on a medical model. Thus, the nurse can readily differentiate between areas for independent nursing intervention and areas requiring collaboration or referral.

Table 1–3 lists the Functional Health Patterns along with a brief description of each pattern as designed by Gordon.[22] The titles of the patterns are, in essence, self-explanatory. Because the titles are self-explanatory, the Functional Health Patterns are easy to use. The chapters in this book are organized using the Functional Health Patterns, and each chapter includes more detail regarding each Functional Health Pattern as introductory information for the specific chapter.

Table 1–3 FUNCTIONAL HEALTH PATTERNS

Pattern	Description
Health perception–health management	The patient's awareness of personal health and well-being; health practices; understanding of how health practices contribute to health status.
Nutritional-metabolic	The patient's description of food and fluid intake; relationship of intake to metabolic needs; includes indicators of ineffectual nutrition on metabolic functioning, for example, healing.
Elimination	Description of all routes and routines of output. Includes any aids to excretion.
Activity-exercise	Patient's overall activities of daily living, including recreational activity.
Sleep-rest	Patient's 24-hour routine of rest, relaxation, and sleep.
Cognitive-perceptual	Cognitive functional performance and sensory performance.
Self-perception–self-concept	Patient's self-assessment; attitudes, ability, worth; verbal and nonverbal communication.
Role-relationship	Patient's assessment of all roles, related responsibilities, and interrelatedness between these factors and other people.
Sexuality-reproductive	Satisfaction-dissatisfaction with sexuality. Any dysfunction in sexuality or reproduction.
Coping–stress tolerance	Effectiveness or noneffectiveness in dealing with difficult situations; how handles; reaction to; support available.
Value-belief	Ideas held in esteem by patient. Guiding principles for overall lifestyle.

Source: From Gordon,[22] p 2, with permission.

Human Response Patterns

Patterns of Unitary Persons was first presented at the Fourth National Conference of NANDA. A group of nursing theorists met in between, as well as during, conferences to design a framework for classification of nursing diagnoses.[23,24] The NANDA Taxonomy Committee and Special Interest Group on Taxonomy[25] reviewed, clarified, and relabeled the patterns as Human Response Patterns. These revisions were presented at the Fifth and Sixth National Conferences. The patterns proposed by the theorist group describe clustering factors that represent person-environment interaction.[26] The Unitary Persons categories were not mutually exclusive; that is, one nursing diagnosis might relate to one, two, or even three of the patterns. From the Fifth through the Ninth National Conferences, refinement of the Human Response Patterns has continued. At the Seventh National Conference the Human Response Patterns were presented as the framework for "NANDA Nursing Diagnosis Taxonomy I,"[27] and the taxonomy was endorsed by NANDA members attending this conference. To assist you in applying this typology, each diagnosis has information regarding its category and coding place in the Human Response Pattern.

This endorsement indicated acceptance of Taxonomy I as a working document that would require further testing, revision, refinement, and expansion. Additional input regarding Taxonomy I Revised was solicited at the Eighth National Conference. Much of the discussion at the eighth conference focused on the various levels of the taxonomy with specific questions about the clinical usefulness of Level I.

The first level of abstraction in Taxonomy I is the Human Response Patterns.

Table 1–4 HUMAN RESPONSE PATTERNS

Pattern	Description
Exchanging	To give, relinquish, or lose something while receiving something in return; the substitution of one element for another; the reciprocal act of giving and receiving.
Communicating	To converse; to impart, confer, or transmit thoughts, feelings, or information, internally or externally, verbally or nonverbally.
Relating	To connect, to establish a link between, to stand in some association to another thing, person, or place; to be borne or thrust in between things.
Valuing	To be concerned about, to care; the worth or worthiness; the relative status of a thing, or the estimate in which it is held, according to its real or supposed worth, usefulness, or importance; one's opinion of, like for a person or thing; to equate in importance.
Choosing	To select between alternatives; the action of selecting or exercising preference in regard to a matter in which one is a free agent; to determine in favor of a course; to decide in accordance with inclinations.
Moving	To change the place or position of a body or any member of the body; to put and/or keep in motion; to provoke an excretion or discharge; the urge to action or to do something; leave in; to take action.
Perceiving	To apprehend with the mind; to become aware of by the senses; to apprehend what is not open or present to observation; to take in fully or adequately.
Knowing	To recognize or acknowledge a thing or person; to be familiar with by experience or through information or report; to be cognizant of something through observation, inquiry, or information; to be conversant with a body of facts, principles, or methods of action; to understand.
Feeling	To experience a consciousness, sensation, apprehension, or sense; to be consciously or emotionally affected by a fact, event, or state.

Source: From Fitzpatrick, JJ: Taxonomy II: Definitions and development. In Carroll-Johnson, RM (ed): Classification of Nursing Diagnosis: Proceedings of the Ninth Conference. Lippincott, Philadelphia, 1991.

The second level is Alterations in Functions. Levels II through V become increasingly concrete, with levels IV and V reflecting the diagnostic labels. Table 1–4 lists the Human Response Patterns with accompanying brief definitions. In this book we have focused on Level II and include Levels IV and V in the conceptual information and "Have You Selected the Correct Diagnosis?" section.

Diagnostic Divisions

Doenges, Moorhouse, and Geissler[28] designed the diagnostic divisions for use in their book *Nursing Care Plans: Guidelines for Planning Patient Care*. The diagnostic divisions group nursing diagnoses into related categories. These related categories are the result of a blending of Maslow's hierarchy of needs and a self-care philosophy. Table 1–5 lists the diagnostic divisions with an explanation of each division.[29]

Valuing Planning of Care and Care Plans

The nursing process and the resultant plan for nursing care have not been given the attention or credit that they deserve. Part of the problem is that planned nursing care has not had value attached to it. All of us will make time or a place for those things that are of value to us, and as the planning of nursing care becomes a more important aspect of nursing, we will "find" time to do it. It is only recently that completing and evaluating the quality-of-care planning has begun to show up on

Table 1-5   **DIAGNOSTIC DIVISIONS AND NURSING DIAGNOSES**

Diagnostic Divisions	Description
Activity/rest	Ability to engage in necessary/desired activities of life (work and leisure), and to obtain sleep/rest.
Circulation	Ability to transport oxygen and nutrients necessary to meet cellular needs.
Ego integrity	Ability to develop and use skills and behaviors to integrate and manage life experiences.
Elimination	Ability to excrete waste products.
Food/fluid	Ability to maintain intake of and utilize nutrients and liquids to meet physiologic needs.
Hygiene	Ability to perform activities of daily living.
Neurosensory	Ability to perceive, integrate, and respond to internal and external cues.
Pain/comfort	Ability to control internal/external environment to maintain comfort.
Respiration	Ability to provide and utilize oxygen to meet physiologic needs.
Safety	Ability to provide safe, growth-promoting environment.
Sexuality (component of Ego integrity and Social interaction)	Ability to meet requirements/characteristics of male/female role.
Social interaction	Ability to establish and maintain relationships.
Teaching/learning	Ability to incorporate and use information to achieve health lifestyle/optimal wellness.

Source: From Doenges, Moorhouse, and Geissler,[28] p 13, with permission.

employee evaluation forms. Likewise, it is still rare to see "complete nursing care plan" or "update care plan" on the patient assignment form.

With the changes that are occurring in health care due to federal and state legislated mandates, completion and use of nursing care planning is going to increase in importance. Several insurance companies now audit charts, care plans, and the like in detail. No documentation of care means no reimbursement for care. Likewise, one of the first places a lawyer looks when hunting evidence for health-related court cases is the patient's chart. The basic principle in lawsuits has been "not charted, not done." Planning care, as proposed in this book, would furnish additional documentation that reasonably prudent care was given as well as providing a guideline for better charting.

Use of nursing diagnoses helps ensure that teaching and discharge planning are considered from the start of care. As we increase our knowledge and begin to think in terms related to nursing nomenclature, a natural nursing action for many of the diagnoses is going to relate to teaching and planning for home care.

Many of the standards supported by the JCAHO, the ANA, and state boards of nursing are automatically implemented when the nursing process is completed, implemented, and documented. A review of these standards by the reader will reveal that several standards in the nursing process and planning of care can be met just by writing a nursing care plan.

It is not uncommon to hear, "I don't do care plans because I don't have time to do them." It is true that there is an investment of time in completing and documenting the nursing process, but over a long-term period, such planning of care actually saves time. To illustrate, we know one nurse who works full time in nursing education but works part time at a local hospital to keep her clinical skills current. One afternoon she went to work at the hospital, received her patient assignments and a brief report, then began to implement patient care. One nursing order read, "Change dressing as needed." Assessment of the dressing showed a change was needed. In the patient's room were all kinds of dressings, fluids, and ointments. There were no instructions for changing the dressing on the care plan or the patient's chart. The nurse then requested information from the patient, who stated, "I don't like to look at it, so I don't know." The nurse then began to search for a staff member who had cared for this patient and could teach her the routine for the special dressing change. After 30 minutes, she finally found a nurse who had cared for the patient. Learning the proper dressing change took only a few minutes. The nurse then went back to the care plan, and in 3 minutes recorded the way to change the dressing under nursing action.

Comparing the time it took to locate the information and the time it took to record the information gives a graphic example of how time can be saved by completing and documenting the nursing process. Consider the time saved if the written nursing actions are used as an outline for charting or the time that could be saved in between-shift reports if documentation of the nursing process were complete. Last, consider the time that could be saved by not having to go to court when questions arise over reasonable prudent care. Making time to use and document the nursing process because we can see its value to us actually saves us time in the long run.

Summary

The nursing process provides a strong framework that gives direction to the practice of nursing. By completing each phase, you can reassure yourself that you are providing quality, individualized care that meets local, state, and national standards. By using the NANDA nomenclature and by providing feedback to NANDA, you can help develop this nomenclature and help ensure that nursing is recognized for the contributions it makes to our nation's health.

References

1. Gordon, M: Nursing Diagnoses: Process and Application, ed 2. McGraw-Hill, New York, 1987.
2. Iyer, PW, Taptich, BJ and Bernocchi-Losey, D: Nursing Process and Nursing Diagnosis. WB Saunders, Philadelphia, 1986.
3. Doenges, ME and Moorhouse, MF: Nurse's Pocket Guide: Nursing Diagnosis with Interventions. FA Davis, Philadelphia, 1991.
4. Alfaro, R: Applying Nursing Diagnosis and Nursing Process: A Step-by-Step Guide. JB Lippincott, Philadelphia, 1990.
5. American Nurses Association: Nursing: A Social Policy Statement. Author, Kansas City, MO, 1980.
6. American Nurses Association: Standards of Clinical Nursing Practice. Author, Kansas City, MO, 1991.
7. Board of Nurse Examiners for the State of Texas: Standards of Nursing Practice. Texas Nurse Practice Act. Author, Austin, TX, 1991.
8. Brider, P: Who killed the nursing care plan? Am J Nurs 91:35, 1991.
9. Joint Commission on Accreditation of Healthcare Organizations: Accreditation Manual for Hospitals. Author, Chicago, 1991.
10. Carroll-Johnson, R: Reflections on the ninth biennial conference. Nurs Diagn, 1:50, 1990.
11. Kozier, BB, Erb, GH and Olivieri, R: Fundamentals of Nursing, ed 4. Addison-Wesley Nursing, Redwood City, CA, 1991.
12. North American Nursing Diagnosis Association: Taxonomy I: Revised 1990. Author, St. Louis, 1990.
13. Tartaglia, MJ: Nursing diagnosis: Keystone of your care plan. Nursing, 15:34, 1985.
14. Kieffer, JS: Nursing diagnosis can make a critical difference. Nurs Life, 4:18, 1984.
15. Sorensen, KC and Luckmann, J: Basic Nursing: A Psychophysiologic Approach, ed 2. WB Saunders, Philadelphia, 1986.
16. Cox, HC: Developing Nursing Care Plan Objectives: A Programmed Unit of Study. Texas Tech

University Health Sciences Center School of Nursing, Continuing Education Program, Lubbock, TX, 1982.

17. Weed, LM: Medical records that guide and teach. N Engl J Med 27:593, 1986.
18. Lampe, S: FOCUS Charting, ed 4. Creative Nursing Management, Minneapolis, 1988.
19. Siegrist, L, Deltor, R and Stocks, B: The PIE system: Planning and documentation of nursing care. Quality Review Bulletin. June, 1986.
20. Flynn, JM and Heffron, PB: Nursing: From Concept to Practice, ed 2. Appleton-Lange, Norwalk, CT, 1988.
21. Yura, H and Walsh, MB: The Nursing Process: Assessing, Planning, Implementing, Evaluating, ed 5. Appleton-Century-Croft, East Norwalk, CT, 1988.
22. Gordon, M: Manual of Nursing Diagnosis: 1991–1992. CV Mosby, St. Louis, 1991.
23. Roy, C, Sr.: Historical perspective of the theoretical framework for the classification of nursing diagnosis. In MJ Kim & DA Moritz (eds): Classification of Nursing Diagnosis: Proceedings of the Third and Fourth National Conferences. McGraw-Hill, St. Louis, 1982, p 235.
24. Roy, C, Sr.: Framework for classification system development: Progress and issues. In MJ Kim, GK McFarland, and AM McLane (eds): Classification of Nursing Diagnosis: Proceedings of the Fifth National Conference. McGraw-Hill, St. Louis, 1984, p 29.
25. Kritek, PB: Report of the group who worked on taxonomies. In MJ Kim, GK McFarland, and AM McLane (eds): Classification of Nursing Diagnosis: Proceedings of the Fifth National Conference. McGraw-Hill, St. Louis, p 46, 1984.
26. Newman, MA: Looking at the whole. Am J Nurs 84:1496, 1984.
27. North American Nursing Diagnosis Association: Taxonomy I with Complete Diagnoses. Author, St. Louis, 1987.
28. Doenges, ME, Moorhouse, MF, and Geissler, AC: Nursing Care Plans: Guidelines for Planning Patient Care, ed 2. FA Davis, Philadelphia, 1989.
29. Doenges, ME and Moorhouse, MG: Application of Nursing Process: An Interactive Text. FA Davis, Philadelphia, 1992.

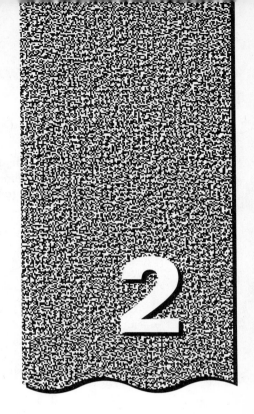

2

Health Perception – Health Management Pattern

PATTERN INTRODUCTION

Pattern Description

Nurses assist individuals and families who have limited knowledge or understanding of:

1. Their current health status
2. How to achieve a good health status
3. How to maintain a good health status

This lack of perception (awareness) leads to the individual or family's having problems with management (control) of their health status. The nursing diagnoses in this pattern are the results of this lack of perception and management.

Pattern Assessment

1. Review the patient's vital signs. Is the temperature within normal limits?
   a. Yes
   b. No (High Risk for Infection; Altered Protection)
2. Review the results of the *complete blood cell (CBC)* count. Are the cell counts within normal limits?
   a. Yes
   b. No (High Risk for Infection; Altered Protection)
3. Review sensory status (sight, hearing, touch, smell, and taste). Is the patient's sensory status within normal limits?
   a. Yes
   b. No (Potential for Injury)
4. Was patient or family satisfied with the usual health status?
   a. Yes
   b. No (Health-Seeking Behavior; Altered Health Maintenance)
5. Did the patient or family describe the usual health status as good?
   a. Yes
   b. No (Health-Seeking Behavior; Altered Health Maintenance)
6. Had the patient or family sought any health care assistance in the past year?
   a. Yes (Health-Seeking Behavior)
   b. No (Altered Health Maintenance)
7. Did the patient or family follow the routine the (doctor, nurse, dentist, and so on) prescribed?
   a. Yes
   b. No (Ineffective Management of Therapeutic Regimen)
8. Did the patient or family have any accidents or injuries in the past year?
   a. Yes (Potential for Injury)
   b. No

Nursing Diagnoses in This Pattern

1. Health Maintenance, Altered (page 38)
2. Health-Seeking Behaviors (Specify) (page 49)
3. Infection, High Risk for (page 56)
4. Injury, High Risk for (page 65)
   a. High Risk for Injury: Suffocation
   b. High Risk for Injury: Poisoning

    c. High Risk for Injury: Trauma
5. Management of Therapeutic Regimen (Individual): Ineffective (page 80)
6. Noncompliance (page 80)
7. Protection, Altered (page 92)

Conceptual Information

A person who practices health management techniques, for example, regular exercise, attention to diet, balance of rest and activity, has an accurate view of his or her or the family's level of personal health status and will also identify other ways to maintain health. These persons will be accurate in reporting the current health status level. They also will readily identify alterations (changes) in health status and will take active steps to correct these changes to increase their movement toward optimal health. Additionally, they will also initiate measures to prevent further alterations in health status. The goal in health management is to assist all patients to achieve this level of health maintenance.

Various factors influence a person's ability to achieve optimal health perception (understanding) and health management (control). One major factor is individual and/or family interaction with the environment.[1] This interaction increases the likelihood that environmental hazards will play a role in health management by increasing exposure to problem areas. Health protection activities can reduce environmental hazards and increase optimal health management. Examples of such activities include individual and community efforts to clean up air and water pollution and to manage sewage and hazardous waste disposal.

Another major factor is an intact sensory system. Sensory organs provide information to the individual regarding the environment. An intact nervous system is also required since it provides for optimum functioning of sensory, motor, and cognitive activities. An accurate cognitive-perceptual pattern and self-perception–self-concept pattern are also necessary to achieve the optimal level of health perception and management. The ability to think and understand greatly impacts basic knowledge of health and illness. Likewise the individual's feeling of self-worth and interpretation of the meaning of health and illness to the self will influence the individual's health practices. Knowledge related to health promotion and disease prevention is essential for the individual to fully maintain health management.

Cultural, societal, and familial values and beliefs also influence the capacity to achieve positive health perception and health management. Values and beliefs influence what is identified as optimal health.

The *Health Belief Model*[2] (see Fig. 2–1) provides a framework in which to study actions taken by individuals to avoid illness. A basic assumption of the model is that the subjective state of the individual is more important in determining actions than is the objective reality of the situation. The health belief model states that for an individual to take action to avoid a disease, she or he needs to believe the following:

1. That she or he is personally susceptible to disease
2. That the occurrence of the disease will have at least a moderate impact on some part of her or his life
3. That taking action will be beneficial
4. That such action will not involve overcoming psychological barriers such as cost, pain, or embarrassment

These beliefs can be described as variables under the headings of "Perceived Susceptibility" and "Severity" and as the variables that define perceived benefits

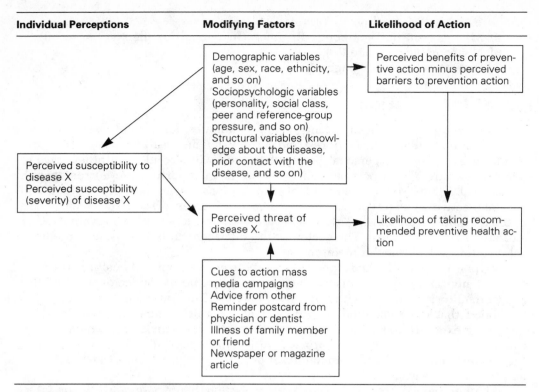

Individual Perceptions

Perceived susceptibility to disease X
Perceived susceptibility (severity) of disease X

Modifying Factors

Demographic variables (age, sex, race, ethnicity, and so on)
Sociopsychologic variables (personality, social class, peer and reference-group pressure, and so on)
Structural variables (knowledge about the disease, prior contact with the disease, and so on)

Perceived threat of disease X.

Cues to action mass media campaigns
Advice from other
Reminder postcard from physician or dentist
Illness of family member or friend
Newspaper or magazine article

Likelihood of Action

Perceived benefits of preventive action minus perceived barriers to prevention action

Likelihood of taking recommended preventive health action

Figure 2–1 The Health Belief Model. (From Becker, MH, et al: Selected psychosocal models and correlates of individual health-related behaviors. Medical Care 15:27, 1977 [Supplement], with permission.)

and barriers to taking action. Because these variables do not account for the activation of the behavior, the originators of the Health Belief Model have added another class of variable called "cues to action." The individual's level of readiness provides the energy to act, and the perception of benefits provides a preferred manner of action that offers the path of least resistance. A cue to action is required to set off this appropriate action. The model suggests that by manipulating any combination of variables affecting action, the inclination to seek preventive care can be altered.

The Health Belief Model does not contain concepts related to knowledge of disease as a potential factor in determining an individual's decision to engage in preventive behavior. Several authors point out that knowledge of health consequences has only a limited relationship to the occurrence of the desired health behavior.[3,4,5] Yet, quite often, imparting knowledge about diseases to the patient, in an effort to encourage future preventive behavior, is the main method employed by nurses.

The Health Belief Model is disease-specific. The model does not adequately explain positive health actions designed to maximize wellness, fulfillment, and self-actualization. Although the Health Belief Model is useful in predicting preventive behavior, it does not fully explain behavior motivated by health promotion.[6] More research is needed to identify the determinants of health-promoting behavior to increase our ability to assist the patient in achieving health promotion.

The Health Belief Model does provide the nurse with the conceptual notion that by working with the patient's perception of the situation, increasing an individual's cues to action, and decreasing an individual's barriers to action, the nurse can enhance the possibility that the patient will engage in disease prevention and early detection activities.

Pender[6] points out that while health promotion and disease prevention are complementary concepts, they are not congruent (identical). Health promotion is directed toward growth and improvement in well-being, while disease prevention conceptually operates to maintain the status quo.[7]

The Health Promotion Model as developed by Pender[6] (see Fig. 2–2) provides the framework for nursing research and practice. This model emphasizes the importance of cognitive-perceptual factors in behavior regulation. Cognitive-perceptual factors such as importance of health, definition of health, perceived self-competency, and perceived control of health are primary motivational mechanisms for health-promoting behavior.

Healthy People 2000[8] describes the national health promotion and disease prevention objectives. Three major goals are addressed by this document:

1. Prevent the premature onset of disease and disability
2. Help all Americans achieve healthier, more productive lives
3. Cut health care costs

The document presents baseline epidemiological data and projected goals for health promotion, health protection, and preventive services. Special emphasis is placed on vulnerable populations, for example, lower socioeconomic, disabled, elderly, and ethnic groups. This document is recommended as a guide for identifying factors that

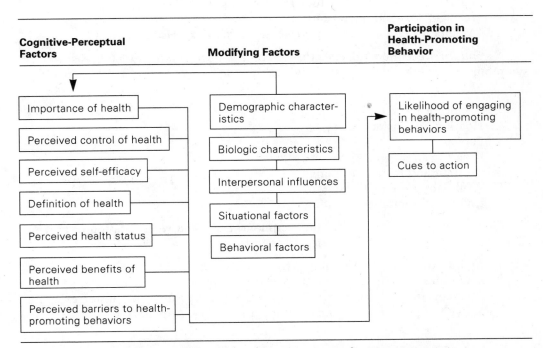

Figure 2–2 Health Promotion Model. (From Pender,[6] p 58, with permission.)

influence the health perception–health management pattern. Strategies for intervention and evaluation are also included in this document.

Whether working with individuals, families, or aggregates (groups such as the elderly), the nurse should plan interventions appropriate for the learning needs of those being targeted. Mass-media campaigns are useful when conveying general information, but information specific to a particular situation or person is best done individually.

The concepts of primary, secondary, and tertiary prevention[9] are also useful to the nurse when using the health management pattern. It is important for the nurse to recognize that a focus on the patient's strengths, and not just on the patient's problems, is an integral part of health promotion.[10,11]

Primary prevention consists of activities that prevent a disease from occurring. A patient engaged in primary prevention activities would:

1. Maintain up-to-date immunizations.
2. Have adequate water supply and sanitation facilities.
3. Use seat belts and infant car seats and properly store household poisons to minimize accident fatalities.
4. Eliminate tobacco products.
5. Maintain adequate nutrition, elimination, and exercise; also maintain social and personal relationships.
6. Employ regular oral care and dental examinations.
7. Demonstrate safe sun exposure.
8. Maintain weight within normal range for age, sex, and height.
9. Maintain an environment free of chemical, biological, and physical hazards.
10. Maintain regular sleep and rest patterns.
11. Practice healthy nutritional intake (e.g., low salt, sugar, and fat intake with balanced intake of basic four food groups and total calories as appropriate for age, sex, and condition).
12. Maintain regular relaxation, recreation, and exercise activities.

Secondary prevention indicates those activities designed to detect disease before symptoms are recognized. These activities include:

1. Glaucoma screening
2. Hypertensive screening
3. Hearing and vision testing
4. Pap smears
5. Breast examinations
6. Prostate and testicle examinations
7. Well-baby examinations
8. Colon and rectal examinations

Tertiary prevention refers to the treatment, care, and rehabilitation of current illness. This area indicates the patient's need to:

1. Adhere to medical and nursing treatments.
2. Make lifestyle changes necessitated by condition.
3. Seek consultation from experts in area requiring intervention, for example, individual practitioners and support groups. See Appendix B.

Developmental Considerations

Care providers can encourage the acceptance of responsibility for health-promoting activities and adherence to agreed-on treatment plans by giving appropriate attention to the impact that developmental levels have on the individual or on the primary caregiver.

INFANT AND TODDLER

Since the neonate is totally dependent on others for care, it is the primary caregiver who is entrusted with carrying out the therapeutic interventions. As the infant grows and develops, self-care abilities increase. The following information outlines developmental milestones from birth to approximately 24 months as described by Piaget's sensorimotor stage of cognitive development.[12] During this period of development the individual must be protected from hazards in the environment, and the primary caregiver must assume major responsibility for compliance with the treatment program.

Providing a safe environment includes the following accident prevention strategies: (1) turning pot handles away from edge of stove; (2) storing medicines, matches, alcohol, plastic bags, and house and garden chemicals in child-proofed areas; (3) using cold-water, not hot-water, humidifier; (4) avoiding heating formula in microwave; (5) using protection screens on heaters, fireplaces, and electrical outlets; (6) using nonflammable clothing; (7) protecting stairways and windows; (8) supervising children at play, while bathing, in car, or in shopping cart; (9) controlling pets or stray animals; (10) avoiding items hung around neck; (11) providing a smoke-free environment; (12) avoiding small objects that can be inserted in mouth or nose; (13) avoiding pillows and plastic in crib; (14) removing poisonous plants from house and garden; and (15) removing lead-based paint.

Children should be screened at birth for congenital anomalies, phenylketonuria (PKU), thyroid function, cystic fibrosis, vision, and hearing. A newborn assessment should be performed, and anticipatory guidance should be provided for patients regarding growth and development, safety, health promotion, and disease prevention.

Well-baby examinations and developmental assessments are recommended at 2, 4, 6, 15, and 18 months.[13] Height and weight should be recorded on growth charts, with hemoglobin and hematocrit checked at least once during infancy. Parent counseling includes discussion of nutrition with attention paid to iron-rich foods; safety and accident prevention; oral, perineal, and perirectal hygiene; sensory stimulation of the infant; baby-bottle tooth decay; and the effects of passive smoking. Immunizations are given during the well-baby checks according to the following schedule:[14]

1. Diphtheria, pertussis, and tetanus (DPT) at 2, 4, and 6 months
2. Oral polio vaccine at 2 and 4 months, with an additional dose at 6 months in geographic areas where polio is endemic
3. Measles, mumps, and rubella (MMR) vaccine and tuberculin test at 15 months. (The MMR may be given at 12 months in areas of recurrent measles.)
4. Haemophilus b conjugate vaccine (HbCV) may be included at 18 months.

New vaccines (HbOC or PRP-OMP) have been developed for the haemophilus b vaccination, beginning as early as 2 months with repeats at 4, 6, 12, or 15 months.[15] For children who have not been immunized during the first year of life, you will need to consult the latest established standards for appropriate timetables.[14] The Center for Disease Control (CDC) now also recommends incorporating the hepatitis B vaccine (HBv) into childhood vaccination schedules. The HBv can be administered at the same time as the DTP and/or HbCV.[16]

Host factors such as age and behavior will affect the susceptibility to infectious disease. In general, most infectious diseases produce the greatest morbidity and mortality in the very old and the very young.[17] It is also important to note that the normal newborn will have a white blood cell count that is higher than that of the normal adult. The normal white blood cell count decreases gradually throughout childhood until reaching the adult norms.[18] It is essential that the nurse be very familiar with the blood cell count norms for this age group.

During fetal life, the fetus has been protected by maternal antibodies to diseases such as diphtheria, tetanus, measles, and polio, assuming the mother has developed antibodies to these diseases. This temporary immunity lasts 3 to 6 months. Colostrum contains antibodies that provide protection against enteric pathogens. Some infections can cross the placental barrier, leading to the development of congenital (present at birth) infections. Syphilis, HIV, and rubella are examples of such infections. Pathogenic organisms such as herpes simplex may be acquired during passage through the birth canal. Because the infant does not begin to produce its own immunoglobulins until 2 to 3 months after birth, it is susceptible to infections for which it has not gained passive immunity.

TORCH infections (toxoplasmosis, hepatitis B, rubella, cytomegalovirus, and herpes) can be of serious concern during the perinatal period.[19] When caring for a pregnant female or a newborn, it is important to teach techniques to prevent acquisition and transmission of these disorders and to recognize signs and symptoms so that early interventions can be instituted. For newborns exposed prenatally, the HBv series should be initiated at birth before discharge from the hospital.[16]

Child care practices must include hygienic disposal of soiled diapers and cleaning of the perineum. Proper handwashing technique is required of the care provider. Proper formula preparation and storage are also critical if the newborn is to be bottle-fed. Anatomically the newborn and infant's eustachian tube facilitates the passage of infection-causing organisms into the middle ear. It is important for care providers not to prop bottles but rather to hold the newborn or infant while feeding. Passive exposure to tobacco smoke irritates the bronchial tree and increases the possibility of respiratory infection.

The infant may respond to an infection with a very high fever. Care providers should be taught how to take axillary and rectal temperatures, to provide hydration to an ill infant, to give tepid baths when fever is elevated, and to seek professional evaluation when an infant has a febrile illness.

TODDLER AND PRESCHOOLER

During the preoperational period, children learn how to teach themselves through trial and error, exploration, and repetition. From age 2 to 4 years, the child is egocentric, using himself or herself as a standard for others; he or she can categorize on the basis of a single characteristic. Because of the child's curiosity and exploration of the environment, it is important for the caregiver to provide a safe environment.

During this period the concepts of "no," "hot," "sharp," and "hurt" should be introduced and repeatedly reinforced by the care provider. Safety rules should be taught and reinforced repeatedly.

From age 4 to 7 years the child can begin to see simple relationships and can begin to think in logical classes. The child can learn his or her own address and can follow directions of three steps. Rules need to be reinforced. The child can be responsible for personal hygiene with instruction and coaching.

Strategies used to provide a safe environment for the infant should also be employed during childhood. Discipline, accident prevention, and the development of self-care proficiency related to eating, dressing, bathing, and dental hygiene are important areas of concern. Developmental assessments with emphasis on hearing, vision, and speech are recommended. The DPT and OPV are given once between ages of 4 and 6, at or before school entry. Consult guidelines if the child has not been immunized during the first year of life.[14] The Immunizations Practices Advisory Committee (IPAC) of the United States Public Health Service[20] recommends that a second dose of the MMR vaccine be given at 4 to 5 years, when the child enters kindergarten.

Anticipatory guidance regarding growth and development includes the development of initiative and guilt, nutrition and exercise, safety and accident prevention, toothbrushing and dental care, effects of passive smoking, and skin protection from ultraviolet light.[12] Additionally, the parents should be taught that, as the child begins to explore the environment and put objects and foods into his or her mouth, it will be important to ensure that contact with infectious pathogens or foreign bodies is controlled. Foreign-object-induced infection should be considered in childhood infections of the external ear, nose, and vagina.

If the preschooler has been exposed to other children, he or she most likely will have experienced several middle ear, gastrointestinal, and upper respiratory tract infections. If the child has not been around other children, he or she will likely experience such infections when entering preschool or kindergarten. Prevention of injury will also assist in the prevention of infection. The adenoidal and tonsillar lymphoid tissue may normally enlarge during the early school years partly in response to the exposure to pathogens in school.

The child will require assistance with toileting hygiene until 4 to 5 years of age. Handwashing techniques can be introduced along with toilet training and followed with consistent role modeling by the adults and older children with assistance to the child. Bubble baths and other scented soaps and toilet tissue may irritate the urethra in the female and lead to urinary tract or vaginal infections. Parents, grandparents, and the child should be taught to avoid such items. In addition, proper dental hygiene can be taught to the child to help in preventing tooth and gum infections.

SCHOOL-AGE CHILD

This period is characterized by developing logical approaches to concrete problems; the concepts of reversibility and conservation are developed, and the child can organize objects and events into classes and arrange them in order of increasing values. The child can be responsible for personal hygiene and simple household tasks. The child will need assistance when ill, but he or she can be taught self-care activities as required, such as insulin injections or taking medications on a regular basis. The child can distinguish and describe physical symptoms and report them to the appropriate caregiver, and he or she can follow instructions.

Strategies employed by care providers to provide a safe environment, prevent disease, and promote health can be taught to the child. The child can perform many of these functions with supervision. Emphasis is placed on health education of the child in safety and accident prevention, nutrition, substance abuse, and anticipated changes with puberty. Anticipatory guidance for both the parents and their child should include the development of industry and inferiority.

ADOLESCENT

True logical thought is developed and abstract concepts can be manipulated by the person in this developmental level. A scientific approach to problem solving can be planned and implemented. The adolescent can develop, with guidance, responsibility for total self-care. With experience the adolescent requires less guidance and can assume full responsibility for self-care and decision making.

Emphasis should be placed on health education of the adolescent in healthy living habits, safe driving, sexuality, skin care, substance abuse, career choices, relationships, dating and marriage, breast self-examination for females, and testicular self-examination for males. Screening for pregnancy, sexually transmitted diseases, depression, high blood pressure, and substance abuse can be done. Anticipatory guidance for parents and adolescents should include the development of identity, role confusion, and formal operational thought.[12]

The hormonal changes of puberty may lead to acne vulgaris. If severe, proper hygiene and dermatologic evaluation will prevent serious complications. The changes in the vaginal tissue secondary to hormonal changes provide an environment conducive to yeast infections. If the adolescent is engaging in sexual activity, he or she is at risk for exposure to sexually transmitted diseases. Irritants such as soap and bubble bath may increase the possibility of urinary tract infection in females. Improper genital hygiene also predisposes the female to urinary tract infection.

The American Academy of Pediatrics[14] recommends the second dose of MMR at entry into middle school (at approximately 11 to 12 years of age). Persons born after 1956 who lack evidence of immunity to measles should receive the MMR vaccine. The MMR vaccine should not be given during pregnancy. Individuals susceptible to mumps should be vaccinated.[21] A diphtheria and tetanus vaccination (TD) should be given at age 14 to 15. Adolescents may be living in group settings, for example, a dormitory, which increases the risk of contracting a communicable disease. Good personal hygiene is important in decreasing this risk.

Risk-taking behavior of adolescents may increase the risk of infection and accidents. Examples of these risk-taking behaviors include intravenous (IV) drug use; use of tobacco; traumatic injury that breaks the skin, allowing a portal of entry for pathogenic organisms; fad diets or other activities that decrease the overall health status; improper technique or equipment in water sports; motor vehicle accidents; running a vehicle or other combustion engine with improper ventilation; substance abuse; choking on food; smoke inhalation; improper storage and handling of guns, ammunition, and knives; excessive risk-taking behavior; smoking in bed; improper use or storage of flammable items, hazardous tools, and equipment; drug ingestion; playing or working around toxic vegetation; improper preparation and storage of food; and improper precautions and use of insecticides, fertilizers, cleaning products, medications, alcohol, and other toxic substances.

ADULT

Adult thought is more refined than adolescent thought because experience and education allow the adult to differentiate among many points of view and potential outcomes in an objective and realistic manner. The adult can consider more options and can apply inductive as well as deductive approaches to problem solving. The adult assumes total responsibility for the care of a child. In middle adult years, the adult may also care for an elderly parent.

The adult is concerned about many of the same health promotion and disease prevention issues that adolescents worry about. Emphasis should be placed on lifestyle counseling related to family planning, parenting, stress management, career advancement, relationship enhancement, hazards at work, and development of intimacy and generativity.

Regular breast self-examination and Pap smear (female) and testicular self-examination (male) should be taught and encouraged. Screening for glaucoma, high blood pressure, blood cholesterol, rubella antibodies, sexually transmitted diseases, and colon, endometrial, oral, or breast cancer should be done if the patient is in a risk category.

As the body develops more and more antibodies to pathogens, the adult may find that he or she does not have as many colds as he or she used to. Some viral infections (mumps, for example) may present serious consequences to adults (males in the case of mumps). The adult female is as susceptible to genitourinary infections as the adolescent. Sexually active adults are at risk for sexually transmitted diseases.

Tetanus-diphtheria (TD) boosters should be given every 10 years. The hepatitis B vaccine should be given to people at risk of exposure. Remember, persons born after 1956 who lack evidence of immunity to measles should receive the MMR vaccine, but the MMR vaccine should not be given during pregnancy. Individuals susceptible to mumps should be vaccinated. Pneumococcal and influenza vaccines are given based upon susceptibility and at-risk status.[22] Advanced age, conditions associated with decline in antibody levels, Native American ethnicity, and institutional settings such as military training camps, jails, and boardinghouses are all identified as risk factors[21,23,24] for the development of pneumonia and influenza.

OLDER ADULT

In the absence of illness affecting cognitive functioning, the older adult maintains formal operational abilities. The older adult can assume total responsibility for decision making and self-care. The older adult also often assumes responsibility for the care of others such as a spouse, child, or grandchild. As with other developmental levels, illness or physical disability can alter the cognitive functioning and lead to self-care deficits.

Emphasis is on health education related to grandparenting, retirement, and home safety. Anticipatory guidance is related to the development of ego integrity. Breast self-examination, Pap smear, mammography (female), and testicular self-examination (male) should be taught and encouraged. Glaucoma, blood pressure, and colon cancer screening should also be done. Podiatry care should be given as needed. Tetanus-diphtheria (TD) boosters, hepatitis B vaccine, and pneumococcal and influenza vaccines are given according to the same conditions discussed in the adult section.[21,22,23,24]

The elderly person may have decreased ability to remove himself or herself from hazardous situations due to decreased mobility. They also may have a decreased ability to recognize smoke- or gas-related odors secondary to a decreased olfactory sense. Sensory, motor, and perceptual deficits as well as orthostatic hypotension may increase the risk for injury and increase self-care deficits.

There is an increase in frequency and severity of infections with aging. Normally the immunologic defenses decline with aging.[16] Skin changes may provide easier access to infecting organisms since increased dryness and thinning of the dermis makes the skin more injury prone.

Motility and secretion, for example, of hydrochloric acid, decrease in the gastrointestinal (GI) tract. Esophageal and gastric peristalsis are decreased. Renal filtration, absorption, and excretion diminish. Incomplete emptying of the bladder provides a medium for the growth of organisms. The respiratory muscles are weaker, and there is decreased elasticity of lung tissue. Diminished cough and gag reflexes may increase the possibility of aspiration. The skin becomes thinner and less elastic. Poor circulation related to vascular insufficiency, peripheral neuropathy, and the increased fragility of the skin increase the possibility of tissue trauma and resulting invasion by microorganisms.

There is decreased production of T lymphocytes, leading to impaired ability to destroy infectious organisms. The production of antibodies by B lymphocytes is also decreased. These changes make the elderly more susceptible to infection and unable to recover as quickly as when they were younger; some may not develop immunity after an infection.

Chronic illness and hospitalization or nursing home placement additionally increase the risk of infection.[17] An important point to remember is that the elderly adult may not demonstrate an increased body temperature in response to an infection. An additional point to emphasize is that infection in the older adult may be manifested by mental status changes such as confusion or restlessness.

APPLICABLE NURSING DIAGNOSES

Health Maintenance, Altered

DEFINITION

Inability to identify, manage, and/or seek out help to maintain health.[25]

NANDA TAXONOMY: MOVING 6.4.2

DEFINING CHARACTERISTICS

1. Major defining characteristics:
   a. Demonstrated lack of knowledge regarding basic health practices
   b. Demonstrated lack of adaptive behaviors to internal or external environmental changes
   c. Reported or observed inability to take responsibility for meeting basic health practices in any or all functional pattern areas
   d. History of lack of health-seeking behavior
   e. Expressed interest in improving health behaviors
   f. Reported or observed lack of equipment, financial, and/or other resources

g. Reported or observed impairment of personal support systems
2. Minor defining characteristics:
   None given

RELATED FACTORS

1. Lack of, or significant alteration in, communication skills (written, verbal, and/or gestural)
2. Lack of ability to make deliberate and thoughtful judgments
3. Perceptual or cognitive impairment (complete or partial lack of gross and/or fine motor skills)
4. Ineffective individual coping
5. Dysfunctional grieving
6. Unachieved developmental tasks
7. Ineffective family coping
8. Disabling spiritual distress
9. Lack of material resources

RELATED CLINICAL CONCERNS

1. Dementias such as Alzheimer's disease and multi-infarct
2. Mental retardation
3. Any condition causing an alteration in level of consciousness, for example, closed head injury, carbon monoxide poisoning, or cerebrovascular accident
4. Any condition impacting the person's mobility level, for example, hemiplegia, paraplegia, fractures, muscular dystrophy
5. Chronic diseases, for example, rheumatoid arthritis, cancer, chronic pain, or multiple sclerosis

HAVE YOU SELECTED THE CORRECT DIAGNOSIS?

Spiritual Distress   A problem in the Value-Belief Pattern could result in variance in health maintenance. If the therapeutic regimen causes conflict with cultural or religious beliefs or with the individual's value system, then it is likely some alteration in health maintenance will occur. Interviewing the patient regarding individual values, goals, or beliefs that guide personal decision making will assist in clarifying whether the primary diagnosis is Altered Health Maintenance or a problem in the Value-Belief Pattern. (See page 923.)

Ineffective Coping   Either Ineffective Individual Coping or Ineffective Family Coping could be suspected if there are major differences between the patient and family reports of health status, health perception, and health care behavior. Verbalizations by the patient or family regarding in ability to cope also indicate ineffective coping. (See pages 874 and 892.)

Altered Family Process   Through observing family interactions and communication, the nurse may assess that Altered Family Process exists. Rigidity of family functions and roles, poorly communicated messages, and failure to ac-

Continued

HAVE YOU SELECTED THE CORRECT DIAGNOSIS?—*Continued*

complish expected family developmental tasks are a few observations to alert the nurse to this possible diagnosis. (See page 710.)

Activity Intolerance or Self-Care Deficit   The nursing diagnosis of Activity Intolerance or Self-Care Deficit should be considered if the nurse observes or validates reports of inability to complete the required tasks because of insufficient energy or because of the patient's inability to feed, bathe, toilet, dress, and groom himself or herself. (See pages 327 and 472.)

Powerlessness   The nursing diagnosis of Powerlessness is considered if the patient reports or demonstrates having little control over situations, expresses doubt about ability to perform, or is reluctant to express feelings to health care providers. (See page 657.)

Knowledge Deficit   A Knowledge Deficit may exist if the patient or family verbalizes less-than-adequate understanding of health management or recalls inaccurate health information. (See page 536.)

Impaired Home Maintenance Management   This diagnosis is demonstrated by the inability of the patient or family to provide a safe living environment. (See page 438.)

EXPECTED OUTCOMES

1. Will describe at least (number) contributing factors that lead to health maintenance alteration and at least one measure to alter each factor by (date) and/or
2. Will design a positive health maintenance plan by (date)

TARGET DATE

Assisting patients to adapt their health maintenance will require a significant investment of time and will also require close collaboration with home health caregivers. For these reasons it is recommended the target date be no less than 7 days from the date of admission.

NURSING ACTIONS/INTERVENTIONS WITH RATIONALES

Adult Health

Actions/Interventions	Rationales

• Assist patient to identify factors contributing to health maintenance alteration through one-to-one interviewing and value clarification strategies. Factors may include:
  ○ Stopping smoking[26,27,28]
  ○ Ceasing drug and alcohol use
  ○ Establishing exercise patterns[29]
	Healthy living habits reduce risk. Assistance is often required to develop long-term change. Identification of the factors significant to the patient will provide the foundation for teaching positive health maintenance.

○ Following good nutritional habits
○ Using stress management techniques
○ Using family and community support systems
○ Using over-the-counter medications
○ Use of herb, vitamins, food supplements, or cleansing programs[30]

- Develop with the patient a list of assets and deficits as he or she perceives them. From this list, assist the patient in deciding what lifestyle adjustments will be necessary.

Increases patient's sense of control and keeps the idea of multiple changes from being overwhelming.

- Identify, with patient, possible solutions, modifications, and so on to cope with each adjustment.
- Develop a plan with the patient that shows both short-term and long-term goals. For each goal specify the time the goal is to be reached.

The more the patient is involved with decisions, the higher is the probability that the patient will incorporate the changes. Avoids overwhelming the patient by indicating that not all goals have to be accomplished at the same time.

- Have patient identify at least two support persons. Arrange for these persons to come to the unit and participate in designing the health maintenance plan.

Provides additional support for patient in maintaining plan.

- Assist patient and significant others to develop a list of *potential* strategies that would assist in the development of the lifestyle changes necessary for health maintenance. (This list should result from a brainstorming process and should include those solutions that appear to be very unrealistic as well as those that appear most realistic.) After the list is developed, review each item with the patient, combining and eliminating strategies when appropriate.

People most often approach change with "more-of-the-same" solutions. If the individual does not think that the strategy will have to be implemented, he or she will be more inclined to develop creative strategies for change.[31]

- Develop with the patient a list of the benefits and disadvantages of behavior change. Discuss with the patient the strength of motivation that each listed item has.

Placing items in priority according to patient's motivation increases probability of success.

- Develop a behavior change contract with the patient, allowing the patient to identify appropriate rewards and consequences. Remember to establish modest goals and short-term rewards. Note reward schedule here.

Positive reinforcement enhances self-esteem and supports continuation of desired behaviors. This also promotes patient control, which in turn increases motivation to implement the plan.[32]

- Teach patient appropriate information to improve health maintenance (e.g., hygiene, diet, medication administration, relaxation techniques, and coping strategies).

Provides the patient with the basic knowledge needed to enact the health maintenance changes.

- Review activities of daily living (ADL) with patient and support person. Incorporate

Incorporation of usual activities personalizes the plan.

Continued

Actions/Interventions	Rationales
these activities into the design for a health maintenance plan. (*Note:* May have to either increase or decrease the ADL).	
• Assist patient and support person to design a monthly calendar that reflects the daily activities needed to succeed in health maintenance.	Provides a visual reminder.
• Have patient and support person return-demonstrate health maintenance procedures at least once a day for at least 3 days before discharge. Times and types of skills should be noted here.	Permits practice in a nonthreatening environment where immediate feedback can be given.
• Set a time to reassess with the patient and support person progress toward the established goals. (This should be on a frequent schedule initially and can then be gradually decreased as the patient demonstrates mastery.) Note evaluation times here.	Provides an opportunity to evaluate and to give the patient positive feedback and support for achievements.
• Provide the patient with appropriate positive feedback on goal achievement. Remember to keep this behaviorally oriented and specific.	
• Communicate the established plan to the collaborative members of the health care team.	Provides continuity and consistency in care.
• Refer patient to appropriate community health agencies for follow-up care. Be sure referral is made at least 3 to 5 days before discharge. (See Appendix B.)	Ensures the service can complete their assessment and initiate operations before the patient is discharged from the hospital. Use of the network of existing community services provides for effective utilization of resources. Facilitates patient's keeping of appointments and reinforces importance of health maintenance.
• Schedule appropriate follow-up appointments for patient before discharge. Notify transportation service and support persons of these appointments. Write appointment on brightly colored cards for attention. Include date, time, appropriate name (physician, physical therapist, nurse practitioner, and so on), address, telephone number, and name and telephone number of person who will provide transportation.	

Child Health

NOTE: Developmental consideration should always guide the health maintenance planned for the child patient. Also, identification of primary defects is stressed to reduce the likelihood of secondary and tertiary delays.

Actions/Interventions	Rationales
• Teach patient and family essential information to establish and maintain health according to age, development, and status.	An individualized plan of care will more definitively reflect specific health maintenance needs and will increase the value of the plan to the patient and family. Reinforcement in a more tangible mode facilitates compliance with the plan of health maintenance, especially in long-term situations.
• Assist patient and family in designing a calendar to monitor progress in meeting goals. Offer developmentally appropriate methods, for example, toddlers enjoy stickers of favorite cartoon or book characters.	
• Identify risk factors that will impact health care maintenance, for example, prematurity, congenital defects, altered neurosensory functioning, errors of metabolism, or altered parenting.	Identification of risk factors allows for more appropriate anticipatory planning of health care, assists in minimizing crises and escalation of simple needs, and serves to reduce anxiety.
• Begin to prepare for health maintenance on initial meeting with child and family.	A holistic plan of care realistically includes futuristic goals, not merely immediate health needs.
• Provide appropriate phone numbers for health team members and clinics to child and/or parents to assist in follow-up.	Anticipatory planning for potential need for communication allows the patient and family realistic methods for assuming health care responsibility while enjoying the back-up of resources.

Women's Health

Actions/Interventions	Rationales
• Assist the patient to describe her perception and understanding of essential information related to her individual life-style and the adjustment necessary to establish and maintain health in each cycle of reproductive life.	Allows assessment of the patient's basic level of knowledge so that a plan can begin at the patient's current level of understanding.
• Develop with the patient a list of stress-related problems at work and at home as she perceives them. From this list, assist the patient in deciding what life-style adjustments will be necessary to establish and maintain health.	Provides essential information to assist patient in planning a healthy life-style.
• Identify with the patient possible solutions and modification to facilitate coping with adjustments. Develop a plan that includes short-term goals and long-term goals. For each goal specify the time the goal is to be reached.	Provides sequential steps to alternate health maintenance within a defined time period. Keeps the patient from being overwhelmed by all the changes that might be necessary.

Continued

Actions/Interventions	Rationales
• Provide factual information to the patient about menstrual cycle patterns throughout the life span. Include prepubertal, menarcheal, menstrual, premenopausal, menopausal, and postmenopausal phases.	Provides basic information and knowledge that is needed throughout life span.
• Teach patient how to record accurate menstrual cycle, obstetric, and sexual history. Assist patient in recognizing life-style changes that occur as a part of normal development.	Provides the patient with the information necessary to cope with changes throughout the reproductive cycle.
• Discuss pregnancy and the changes that occur during pregnancy and childbearing. Stress the importance of a physical examination *before* becoming pregnant— to include a Pap smear, rubella titer, AIDS profile, and genetic workup (if indicated by family history).	Provides patient with the information needed to plan for a healthy pregnancy.
• Describe and assist the patient in planning routines that will maintain well-being for the mother and fetus including reducing fatigue, eating an adequate diet, obtaining early prenatal care, and attending classes to obtain information about the birthing experience.	Provides the basic information to allow the patient and her family to plan for extension of their family.
• Provide information and support during the postpartum period to assist the new mother in establishing and maintaining good infant nutrition, whether breast-feeding or formula feeding.	
• Refer to appropriate groups for support and encouragement after birth of baby, for example, La Leche League or parenting groups. (See Appendix B.)	
• Teach terminology and factual information related to spontaneous abortion or the interruption of pregnancy. Encourage expression of feelings by the patient and her family. Provide referrals to appropriate support groups within the community.	Allows patient to grieve and reduces fear regarding subsequent pregnancies.
• Provide contraceptive information to the patient, including describing different methods of contraception and their advantages and disadvantages.	Allows patient to plan appropriate contraceptive measures according to personal values and beliefs.
• Emphasize the importance of lifestyle changes necessary to cope with postmenopausal changes in the body, such as estrogen replacement therapy, calcium	Provides patient with basic information that will assist in planning a healthy life-style during and following menopause.

supplements, balanced diet, exercise, and
routine sleep patterns.

- Teach the patient the importance of routine physical assessment throughout the reproductive life cycle, including breast self-examination, Pap smear, and routine exams by the health care provider of her choice, for example, nurse midwife, nurse practitioner, or physician.

Provides knowledge that allows the patient to plan a healthy lifestyle.

Mental Health

Actions/Interventions	Rationales
• Include the client in group therapy to provide positive role models, provide peer support, and permit assessment of goals and exposure to differing problem solutions.	Group provides opportunities to relate and react to others while exploring behavior with one another.

Gerontic Health

NOTE: Major emphasis here is on educating the client. Due to stereotypes about aging, there is a misconception that older adults cannot learn new information. This is untrue. The majority of elderly people are still capable of cognitive growth and intellectual development, and there are ways to enhance the learning experience for older adults exposed to new information.[33]

Actions/Interventions	Rationales
• Ensure privacy, comfort, and rapport prior to teaching sessions. • Avoid presenting large amounts of information at one time. • Monitor energy level as teaching session progresses. • Present small units of information, with repetition, and encourage patient to use cues that enhance ability to recall information.	Reduces anxiety and provides a nondistracting environment that enhances learning ability. This allows patient an increased opportunity to process and store new information. The most ideal way to present new material to the older adult is through self-paced instruction. The cues should be highly personalized for the individual patient. An older woman learning to do a dressing change might relate the steps involved to a recipe for baking: "First I do this, then this, and so on."

Home Health

Actions/Interventions	Rationales
• Assist the client and family to identify home and workplace factors that can be modified to promote health maintenance, for example, ramps instead of steps, tacking down throw rugs, or nonsmoking environment.[34]	This action will enhance safety and assist in preventing accidents. Promoting a nonsmoking environment helps reduce the damaging effects of passive smoke.
• Involve the client and family in planning, implementing, and promoting a health maintenance pattern through: ○ Helping establish family conferences ○ Teaching mutual goal setting ○ Teaching communication ○ Assisting family members in specified tasks as appropriate (e.g., cooking, cleaning, transportation, companionship, or support person for exercise program)	Involvement improves motivation and improves the outcome.
• Teach the client and family health promotion and disease prevention activities: ○ Relaxation techniques ○ Nutritional habits to maintain optimal weight and physical strength ○ Techniques for developing and strengthening support networks (e.g., communication techniques and mutual goal setting) ○ Physical exercise to increase flexibility, cardiovascular conditioning, and physical strength and endurance[35] ○ Evaluation of occupational conditions[34] ○ Control of harmful habits (e.g., control of substance abuse) ○ Therapeutic value of pets[36]	These activities promote a healthy lifestyle.

FLOW CHART EVALUATION
Flow Chart Expected Outcome 1

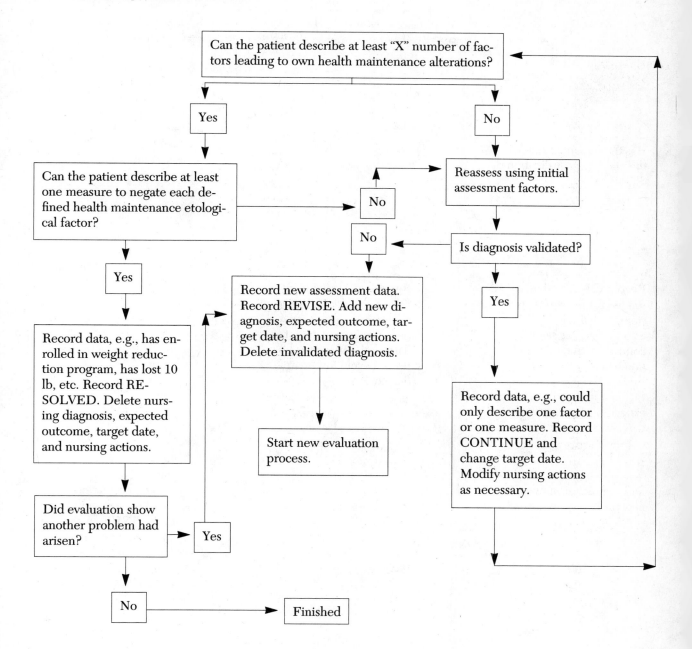

Can the patient describe at least "X" number of factors leading to own health maintenance alterations?

Yes

No

Can the patient describe at least one measure to negate each defined health maintenance etological factor?

No

Reassess using initial assessment factors.

No

Is diagnosis validated?

Yes

Yes

Record data, e.g., has enrolled in weight reduction program, has lost 10 lb, etc. Record RESOLVED. Delete nursing diagnosis, expected outcome, target date, and nursing actions.

Record new assessment data. Record REVISE. Add new diagnosis, expected outcome, target date, and nursing actions. Delete invalidated diagnosis.

Record data, e.g., could only describe one factor or one measure. Record CONTINUE and change target date. Modify nursing actions as necessary.

Start new evaluation process.

Did evaluation show another problem had arisen?

Yes

No

Finished

Flow Chart Expected Outcome 2

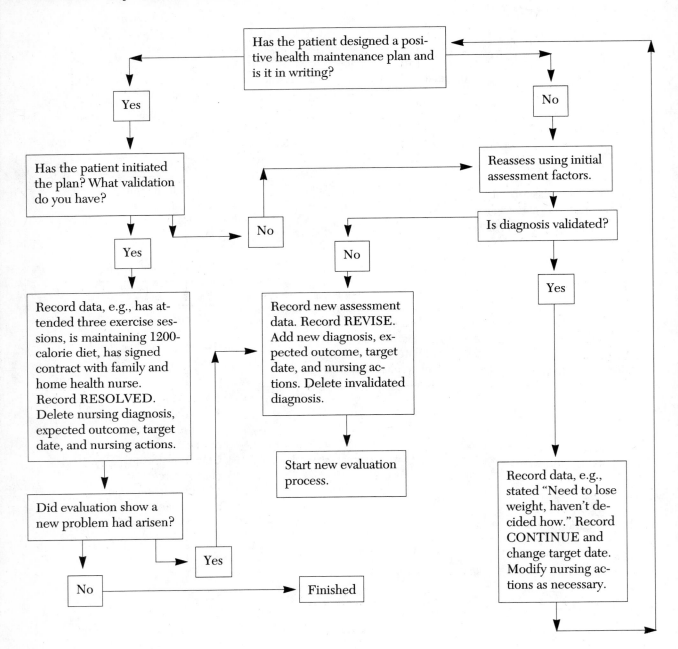

Has the patient designed a positive health maintenance plan and is it in writing?

Yes

No

Has the patient initiated the plan? What validation do you have?

Reassess using initial assessment factors.

Yes

No

Is diagnosis validated?

No

Yes

Record data, e.g., has attended three exercise sessions, is maintaining 1200-calorie diet, has signed contract with family and home health nurse. Record RESOLVED. Delete nursing diagnosis, expected outcome, target date, and nursing actions.

Record new assessment data. Record REVISE. Add new diagnosis, expected outcome, target date, and nursing actions. Delete invalidated diagnosis.

Start new evaluation process.

Record data, e.g., stated "Need to lose weight, haven't decided how." Record CONTINUE and change target date. Modify nursing actions as necessary.

Did evaluation show a new problem had arisen?

No

Yes

Finished

Health-Seeking Behaviors (Specify)

DEFINITION

A state in which an individual in stable health is actively seeking ways to alter personal health habits and/or the environment in order to move toward a higher level of health.*

NANDA TAXONOMY: CHOOSING 5.4

DEFINING CHARACTERISTICS

1. Major defining characteristics:
   a. Expressed or observed desire to seek a higher level of wellness.
2. Minor defining characteristics:
   a. Expressed or observed desire for increased control of health practice.
   b. Expression of concern about current environmental conditions on health status.
   c. Stated or observed unfamiliarity with wellness community resources.
   d. Demonstrated or observed lack of knowledge in health promotion behaviors.

RELATED FACTORS

None given.

RELATED CLINICAL CONCERNS

Since this diagnosis, as indicated by the definition, relates to individuals in stable health, there are no related medical diagnoses.

HAVE YOU SELECTED THE CORRECT DIAGNOSIS?

Impaired Home Maintenance Management   This diagnosis may be involved if the individual or family is unable to independently maintain a safe, growth-promoting immediate environment. (See page 438.)

Powerlessness   If the client expresses the perception of lack of control or influence over the situation and potential outcomes or does not participate in care or decision making when opportunities are provided, the diagnosis of Powerlessness should be investigated. (See page 657.)

EXPECTED OUTCOMES

1. Will describe or write realistic plans to modify habit (name) by (date) and/or
2. Will (increase/decrease) (habit) by (amount) by (date)

Stable health status is defined as age-appropriate illness prevention measures have been achieved, client reports good or excellent health, and signs and symptoms of disease, if present, are controlled. Altered Health Maintenance should be considered if the individual is not able to identify, manage, or seek out help to maintain health.

EXAMPLES:
Will decrease smoking by 75 percent by (date)
Will increase exercise by walking 2 miles three times per week by (date)

TARGET DATE

Changing a habit involves a significant investment of time and energy, regardless of whether the change involves starting a new habit or stopping an old habit. Therefore, the target dates should be expressed in terms of weeks and months.

NURSING ACTIONS/INTERVENTIONS WITH RATIONALES

Adult Health

Actions/Interventions	Rationales
• Initiate discharge plans soon after admission to facilitate posthospital follow-up.	Allows adequate time to complete discharge planning and teaching required for home care.
• Note potential risk factors that should be dealt with regarding actual health status (for example, financial status, coping strategies, or resources).	Provides basic knowledge that will contribute to individualized discharge planning.
• Teach patient about activities for promotion of health and prevention of illness (for example, well-balanced diet, including restricted sodium and cholesterol intake; need for adequate rest and exercise; effects of air pollutants, including smoking; and stress management techniques).	Provides the patient and family with the essential knowledge needed to modify behavior.
• Review patient's problem-solving abilities and assist patient to identify various alternatives, especially in terms of altering his or her environment.	Promotes shared decision making and enhances patient's feeling of self-control.
• Provide appropriate teaching to assist patient and family in becoming confident in self-seeking health care behavior, for example, teach assertiveness techniques to patient and family.	Increases sense of self-control and reduces feelings of powerlessness.
• Assist patient and family to list benefits of high-level wellness and health-seeking behavior.	Makes visible the reasons these activities will help the family.
• Help patient and family develop a basic written plan for achieving individual high-level wellness. Provide time for questions before dismissal to solidify plans for follow-up care. A minimum of 30 minutes per day for 2 days prior to discharge should be allowed for this question-and-answer period. Note times here.	Demonstrates importance of follow-up care.

• Give and review pamphlets about wellness community resources.	Reinforces teaching and provides ready reference for patient and family after discharge from agency.
• Support patient in his or her health-seeking behavior. Advocate when necessary.	Provides supportive environment and underlines the importance of health-seeking activities.
• Refer to appropriate health care providers and various community groups as appropriate for assistance needed by the patient and his or her family. (See Appendix B.)	Provides professional support systems that can assist in health-seeking behavior.

Child Health

Actions/Interventions	Rationales
• Monitor child and family for perceived value of health. Incorporate into any plan personal and family needs identified through this monitoring.	Values are formulated in the first 6 years of life and will serve as primary factors in how health is perceived and enjoyed by the individual and family. If values are in question, there is greater likelihood that how health is able to be maintained will be subject to this values conflict. Until health-seeking behavior is identified as a value, follow-up care will not be deemed beneficial.
• Assist child and family to identify appropriate health maintenance needs and resources, for example, immunizations, nutrition, daily hygiene, basic safety, obtaining medical services when needed (including health education), instructions on how to take temperature of an infant, basic skills and care for health problems, health insurance, Medicaid, and/for Crippled Children's Services.	Knowing of available resources and incorporating them into the plan for health care will facilitate long-term attention to health.

Women's Health

Actions/Interventions	Rationales
• Teach the patient the importance of seeking information and support during the reproductive life cycle. Include information about prepubertal, menarcheal, menstrual, childbearing, menopausal, and postmenopausal periods of the life cycle.	Provides the basic information needed to support health-seeking behaviors.

Actions/Interventions	Rationales
• Assign client a primary care nurse.	Provides increased individuation and continuity of care, facilitating the development of a therapeutic relationship. The nursing process requires that a trusting and functional relationship exist between nurse and client.[32]
• Primary care nurse will spend 30 minutes twice a day with client (note times here). The focus of these interactions will conform to the following schedule:	Promotes client's perception of control.
○ *Interaction 1:* Have the client identify specific areas of concern. List the identified concerns on the care plan. Also identify the primary source of this concern (i.e., client, family member, member of the health care team, or other members of the client's social system).	
○ *Interaction 2:* List specific goals for each concern the client has identified. These goals should be achievable within a 2- to 3-day period. (One way of setting realistic, achievable goals is to divide the goal described by the client by 50 percent.)	Promotes client's self-esteem when goals can be accomplished.
○ *Interaction 3:* Have the client identify steps that have been previously taken to address the concern.	Promotes client's self-esteem and provides motivation for continued efforts.
○ *Interaction 4:* Determine the client's perceptions of abilities to meet established goals and areas where assistance may be needed. (If client indicates a perception of inability to pursue goals without a great deal of assistance, the alternative nursing diagnoses of Powerlessness and Knowledge Deficit may need to be considered.)	
• All future interactions will be spent assisting the client in developing strategies to achieve the established goals, developing action plans and evaluating the outcome of these plans, and then revising future actions.	
• Provide positive verbal reinforcement for client's achievement of goals. This reinforcement should be specific to the client's goals. Note those things that are rewarding to the client here and the kind of behavior to be rewarded.	

Gerontic Health

Actions/Interventions	Rationales
• Nursing actions for this diagnosis and the older adult are essentially the same as those in adult health.	
• Encourage patient to participate in health-screening and health promotion programs such as Senior Wellness Programs. These programs are often offered by hospitals and senior citizens' centers.	Provides a cost-effective, easily accessible, long-term support mechanism for the patient.

Home Health

Actions/Interventions	Rationales
• Help the client identify his or her personal definition of health, perceived personal control, perceived self-efficacy, and perceived health status.	Facilitates awareness of definition of health, locus of control, perceived efficiency and health status. Identifies potential facilitators and barriers to action.
• Assist the client in identifying required life-style changes. Assist the client to develop potential strategies that would assist in the life-style changes required.	Life-style changes require change in behavior. Self-evaluation and support facilitate these changes.
• Refer to Altered Health Maintenance for additional actions that would also be applicable with this diagnosis.	

FLOW CHART EVALUATION
Flow Chart Expected Outcome 1

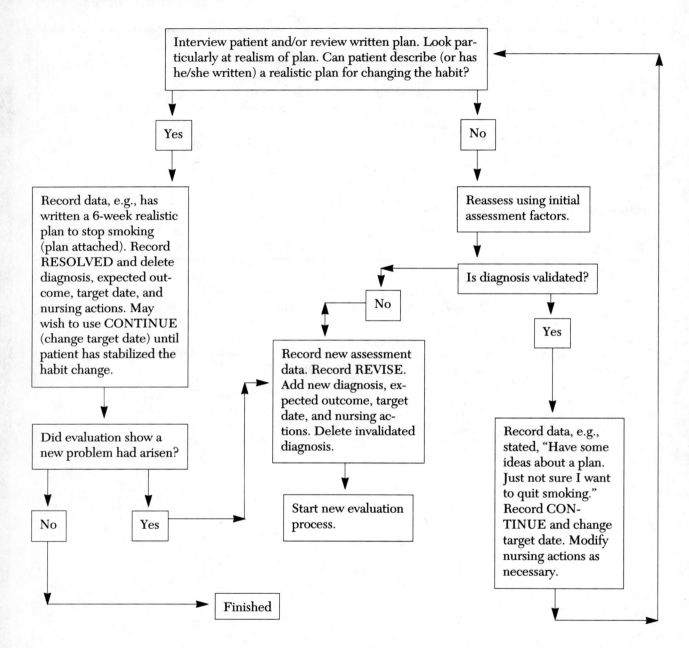

Flow Chart Expected Outcome 2

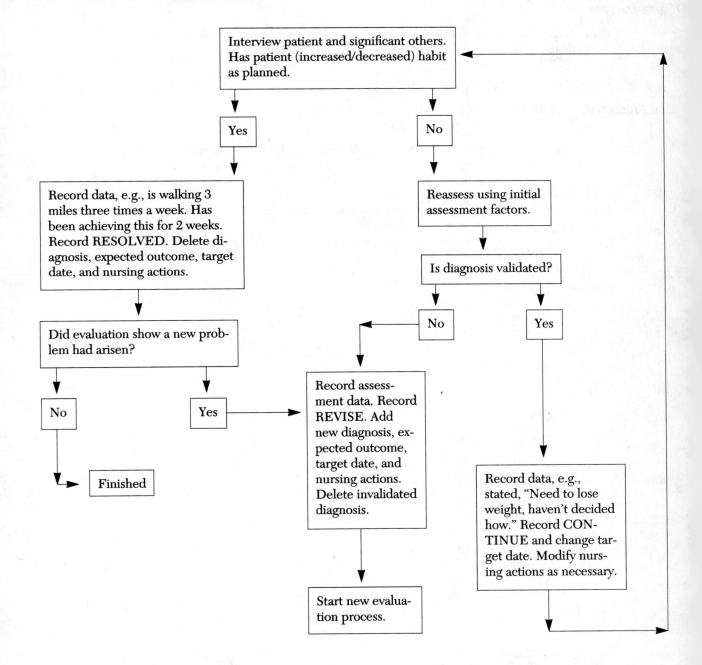

Infection, High Risk for

DEFINITION

The state in which an individual is at increased risk for being invaded by pathogenic organisms.

NANDA TAXONOMY: EXCHANGING 1.2.1.1

DEFINING CHARACTERISTICS

1. Major risk factors:
   a. Inadequate primary defenses (broken skin, traumatized tissue, decrease in ciliary action, stasis of body fluids, change in pH secretions, or altered peristalsis).
   b. Inadequate secondary defenses (e.g., decreased hemoglobin, leukopenia, or suppressed inflammatory response) and immunosuppression.
   c. Inadequate acquired immunity.
   d. Tissue destruction and increased environmental exposure.
   e. Chronic disease.
   f. Invasive procedures.
   g. Malnutrition.
   h. Pharmaceutical agents.
   i. Trauma.
   j. Rupture of amniotic membranes.
   k. Insufficient knowledge to avoid exposure to pathogens.
2. Minor risk factors:
   None given.

RELATED FACTORS

The risk factors serve also as the related factors.

RELATED CLINICAL CONCERNS

1. AIDS
2. Burns
3. COPD
4. Diabetes mellitus
5. Any surgery and any condition where steroids are used as a part of the treatment regimen
6. Substance abuse/dependence
7. Premature rupture of membranes

HAVE YOU SELECTED THE CORRECT DIAGNOSIS?

Self-Care Deficit   Self-Care Deficit, especially in the areas of toileting, feeding, and bathing-hygiene, may need to be considered if improper handwashing, personal hygiene, toileting practice, or food preparation and storage have increased the risk of infection. (See page 472.)

> **Impaired Skin Integrity, Impaired Tissue Integrity, Altered Nutrition**
> Less Than Body Requirements or Altered Oral Mucous Membrane may be
> predisposing the client to infection. (See page 239.)
>
> **Impaired Physical Mobility**   This diagnosis should be considered if skin
> breakdown is secondary to lack of movement. Skin breakdown always predis-
> poses the patient to High Risk for Infection. (See page 460.)
>
> **Altered Body Temperature: High Risk for, or Hyperthermia**   These diag-
> noses should be considered when the body temperature increases above nor-
> mal, which is common in infectious processes. (See pages 125 and 177.)
>
> **Ineffective Management of Therapeutic Regimen (Noncompliance)**
> This diagnosis may be occurring in cases of inappropriate antibiotic usage or
> inadequate treatment of wounds or chronic diseases. (See page 80.)

EXPECTED OUTCOMES

1. Will return-demonstrate measures to decrease the high risk for infection by
   (date) and/or
2. Will remain free from any symptoms of an infection by (date).

TARGET DATE

An appropriate target date would be within 3 days from the date of diagnosis.

NURSING ACTIONS/INTERVENTIONS WITH RATIONALES

Adult Health

Actions/Interventions	Rationales
• Monitor vital signs every 4 hours around the clock. State times here.	Provides a baseline that allows quick recognition of deviations in subsequent measurements.
• Use universal precautions and teach patient and family the purpose and techniques of universal precautions.[37,38,39,40,41]	Protects patient and family from infection.
• Maintain adequate nutrition and fluid and electrolyte balance. Provide a well-balanced diet with increased amounts of vitamin C, sufficient iron, and 2400 to 2600 ml of fluid daily.	Helps prevent disability that would predispose the patient to infection.
• Collaborate with physician regarding screening specimens for culture and sensitivity, for example, blood, urine, spinal fluid.	Allows accurate determination of the causative organism and identification of the antibiotic that will be most effective against the organism.
• Monitor the administration of antibiotics for maintenance of blood levels and for side effects, for example, diarrhea.	Antibiotics have to be maintained at a consistent blood level, usually 7 to 10 days, to kill causative organisms. Antibiotics may

Continued

Actions/Interventions	Rationales
	destroy normal bowel flora, predisposing the patient to the development of diarrhea and increasing the chance of infection in the lower GI tract.
• Maintain a neutral thermal environment.	Avoids overheating or overcooling of room, which would contribute to complications for the patient.
• Assist patient with a thorough shower at least once daily (dependent on age) or total bed bath daily.	Reduces microorganisms on the skin.
• Wash your hands thoroughly between each treatment. Teach patient the value of frequent handwashing.	Prevents cross-contamination and nosocomial infections.
• Provide good genital hygiene, and teach patient how to care for the genital area.	Prevents spread of opportunistic infections.
• Use reverse or protective isolation as necessary.	Protects the patient from exposure to pathogens.
• Use sterile technique when changing dressings or performing invasive procedures.	Protects the patient from exposure to pathogens.
• Turn every 2 hours on (odd/even) hour.	Prevents inadequate tissue perfusion and stasis of blood.
• Have patient cough and deep-breathe every 2 hours on (odd/even) hour.	Mobilizes static pulmonary secretions.
• Perform passive exercises, or have patient perform active range-of-motion (ROM) exercises every 2 hours on the (odd/even) hour. Remember that patient may have decreased tolerance of activity.	Prevents inadequate tissue perfusion and stasis of blood.
• Teach the patient and family about the infectious process, routes, pathogens, environmental and host factors, and aspects of prevention.	Provides basic knowledge for self-help and self-protection.
• Consult with appropriate assistive resources as indicated. (See Appendix B.)	Appropriate use of existing community services is efficient use of resources.

Child Health

Actions/Interventions	Rationales
• Monitor axillary temperature every 2 hours on the (odd/even) hour.	Is the most appropriate route for frequent measurements for the very young child. Oral temperature measurements would not be accurate.
• Encourage child and parents to verbalize fears, concerns, or feelings related to infection by scheduling at least 30 minutes per shift to counsel with family. Note times here.	Provides support, decreases anxiety and fears, and provides teaching opportunity.

Women's Health

Actions/Interventions	Rationales
• In the presence of ruptured amniotic membranes, monitor for signs of infection at least every 4 hours at (state times here), for example, elevated temperature or vaginal discharge odor.	Provides clinical data needed to quickly recognize the presence of infection.
• Use aseptic technique when performing vaginal examinations, and limit the number of vaginal examinations during labor.	Reduces the opportunities to introduce infection.
• Teach mother to take only showers (no tub baths) and how to monitor and record temperature. Have her take temperature at least every 4 hours on a set schedule.	Teaching patient basic information to recognize and prevent infection.
• Keep linens and underpads clean and changed as necessary during labor.	Reduces the likelihood of nosocomial infections.
• Monitor incisions (C-section or episiotomy) at least every 4 hours at (state times here) for redness, drainage, oozing, hematoma, or loss of approximation.	Provides clinical data needed to quickly recognize the presence of infection.
• During postpartum period, monitor fundal height at least every 4 hours at (state times here) around the clock for 48 hours.	Provides database necessary to screen for infection.
• During postpartum period, monitor at least every 4 hours at (state times here) for any signs of foul-smelling lochia, uterine tenderness, or increased temperature.	Provides clinical data needed to quickly recognize the presence of infection.
• In instances of abortion, obtain a complete obstetric history.	
• Monitor abdomen at least every 4 hours at (state times here) for any swelling, tenderness, or foul-smelling vaginal discharge following an abortion.	
• If meconium present in amniotic fluid, immediately clear airway of infant by suctioning (preferably done by physician immediately upon delivery of infant's head).	Helps prevent aspiration pneumonia in infant.
• Suction gastric content immediately. Observe for sternal retractions, grunting, trembling, jitters, or pallor. If any of these signs are present, notify the physician at once.	Indicates development of respiratory complications secondary to meconium.
• Wash hands before and after each time baby is handled.	Prevents development of nosocomial infections.
• Avoid wearing sharp jewelry that could scratch the baby.	
• Keep umbilical cord clean and dry by	Gives parents basic information regarding

Continued

Actions/Interventions	Rationales

cleansing at each diaper change or at least every 2 hours on (odd/even) hour.
• Monitor circumcision site for swelling, odor, or bleeding at each diaper change or at least every 2 hours on (odd/even) hour.
• Demonstrate and have parent return-demonstrate:
  ○ How to take baby's temperature measurement
  ○ How to properly care for the umbilical cord and circumcision
	prevention of infection and monitoring for the development of infection.

Mental Health

Actions/Interventions	Rationales
• Monitor the temperature of clients receiving antipsychotic medications twice a day, and report any elevations to physician. Note times for temperature measurement here.	These clients are at risk for developing agranulocytosis. The greatest risk is 3 to 8 weeks after therapy has begun.
• Monitor the client for the presence of a sore throat in the absence of a cold or other flu-like symptoms at least daily. Report any occurrence.	This could be a symptom of agranulocytosis.
• Teach the client to report temperature elevations and sore throats in the absence of other symptoms to the physician.	Provides a baseline for comparison after the client has begun antipsychotic therapy.
• During the first 8 weeks of treatment with an antipsychotic, report any signs of infection in the client to the physician for assessment of white cell count. • Review the client's CBC before antipsychotics are started, and report any abnormalities on this and any subsequent CBCs to the physician.	
• Teach the client and family handwashing techniques, nutrition, appropriate antibiotic use, hazards of substance abuse, and universal precautions.	These measures can help prevent or decrease the risk of infection.

Gerontic Health

Actions/Interventions	Rationales
• Avoid shearing forces when repositioning patient.	Dermal fragility leads to frequent skin tears when patients are repositioned or transferred from bed to chair, and so on.
• Monitor any incidents of nausea, vomiting, or diarrhea.	The GI tract of the older adult is more sensitive to the effects of contaminated food; therefore, these patients are more susceptible to GI infections.
• Encourage frequent handwashing by the patient.	Hands may serve as fomites due to more frequent contact with contaminated items, for example, wheelchair wheels.

Home Health

Actions/Interventions	Rationales
• Teach client and family measures to prevent transmission of infectious disease to others. Assist patient and family with life-style changes that may be required: ○ Handwashing ○ Isolation as appropriate ○ Proper disposal of infectious waste (e.g., bagging) ○ Proper use of disinfectants ○ Appropriate medical intervention (e.g., antibiotics or antipyretics) ○ Immunization ○ Signs and symptoms of infection ○ Treatment for lice and removal of nits ○ Asepsis for wound care.	Many infectious diseases can be prevented by appropriate measures. Client and family members require this information and the opportunity to practice these skills.

NOTE: Items can be sterilized at home by immersing in boiling water for 10 minutes. The water needs to be boiling for the entire 10 minutes.

• Participate in tuberculosis screening and prevention program.	This action serves as the database to identify the need for interventions to prevent infections.
• Monitor for factors contributing to the high risk for infection.	
• Involve the client and family in planning, implementing, and promoting reduction in the high risk for infection: ○ Family conference ○ Mutual goal setting ○ Communication	Family involvement is important to ensure success. Communication and mutual goals improve the outcome.

Continued

Actions/Interventions	Rationales
• Teach the client and family measures to prevent or decrease potential for infection: ○ Handwashing techniques ○ Universal precautions for blood and body fluids ○ Personal hygiene and health habits ○ Nutrition; immunization schedule ○ Proper food storage and preparation ○ Elimination of environmental hazards such as rodents or insects ○ Proper sewage control and trash collection ○ Appropriate antibiotic use ○ Hazards of substance abuse ○ Preparation and precautions when traveling to areas in which infectious diseases are endemic ○ Signs and symptoms of infectious diseases for which the client and family are at risk ○ Preparation for disaster (water storage, canned or dried food, emergency waste disposal)	These measures reduce the risk of infection.

FLOW CHART EVALUATION
Flow Chart Expected Outcome 1

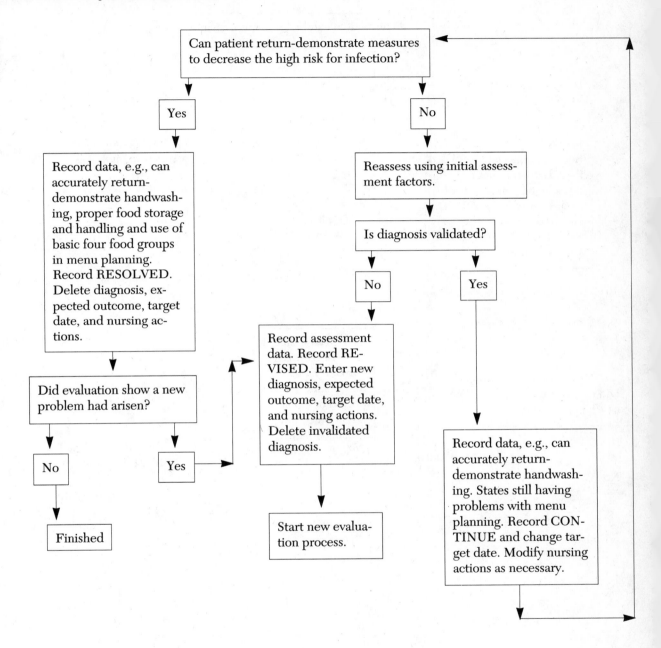

Can patient return-demonstrate measures to decrease the high risk for infection?

Yes

No

Record data, e.g., can accurately return-demonstrate handwashing, proper food storage and handling and use of basic four food groups in menu planning. Record RESOLVED. Delete diagnosis, expected outcome, target date, and nursing actions.

Reassess using initial assessment factors.

Is diagnosis validated?

No

Yes

Did evaluation show a new problem had arisen?

No

Yes

Record assessment data. Record REVISED. Enter new diagnosis, expected outcome, target date, and nursing actions. Delete invalidated diagnosis.

Finished

Start new evaluation process.

Record data, e.g., can accurately return-demonstrate handwashing. States still having problems with menu planning. Record CONTINUE and change target date. Modify nursing actions as necessary.

Flow Chart Expected Outcome 2

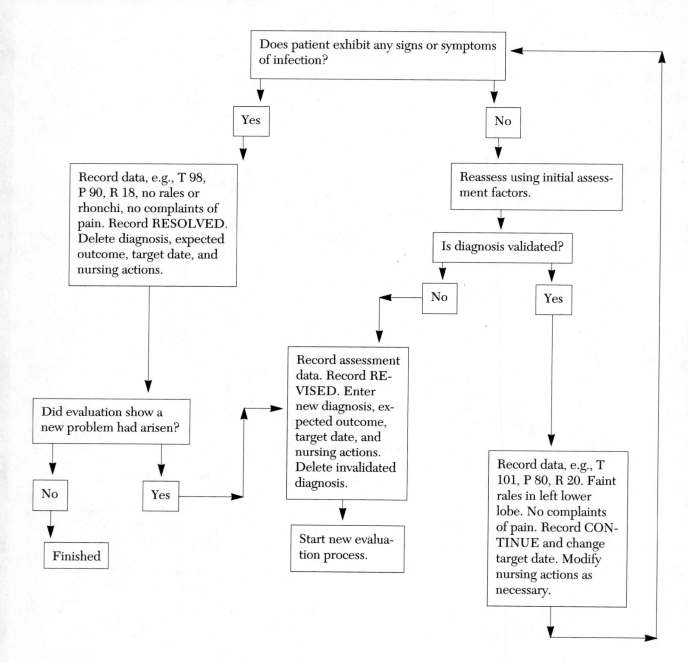

Injury, High Risk for

DEFINITION

A state in which the individual is at risk of injury as a result of environmental conditions interacting with the individual's adaptive and defensive resources.[25]

NANDA TAXONOMY: EXCHANGING 1.6.1

DEFINING CHARACTERISTICS

NOTE: According to the NANDA Taxonomy, High Risk for Injury is a level 3 diagnosis. Level 4 diagnoses under High Risk for Injury are Suffocation, Poisoning, and Trauma. To assist you in making the most specific diagnosis, the definitions, defining characteristics, and related factors for these level 4 diagnoses are also included.

A. High Risk for Injury

1. Major risk factors:
   a. Internal:
   (1) *Biochemical, regulatory function*: Sensory dysfunction, integrative dysfunction, effector dysfunction, tissue hypoxia
   (2) Malnutrition
   (3) Immuno-autoimmune
   (4) *Abnormal blood profile*: Leukocytosis or leukopenia, altered clotting factors, thrombocytopenia, sickle cell, thalassemia, decreased hemoglobin
   (5) *Physical*: Broken skin, altered mobility
   (6) *Developmental age*: Physiological, psychosocial
   (7) *Psychological*: Affective, orientation
   b. External:
   (1) *Biological*: Immunization level of community, microorganism
   (2) *Chemical*: Pollutants, poisons, drugs, pharmaceutical agents, alcohol, caffeine, nicotine, preservatives, cosmetics, and dyes
   (3) *Nutrients*: Vitamins, food types
   (4) *Physical*: Design, structure, and arrangement of community building, and/or equipment
   (5) Mode of transport or transportation
   (6) *People or provider*: Nosocomial agents; and staffing patterns; and cognitive, affective, and psychomotor factors
2. Minor risk factors:
   None given.

B. High Risk for Injury: Suffocation

1. *Definition*: Accentuated risk of accidental suffocation (inadequate air available for inhalation)[25]
2. Major risk factors:
   a. Internal (individual):
   (1) Reduced olfactory sensation

      (2) Reduced motor abilities
      (3) Lack of safety education
      (4) Lack of safety precautions
      (5) Cognitive or emotional difficulties
      (6) Disease or injury process
   b. External (environmental):
      (1) Pillow placed in an infant's crib
      (2) Propped bottle placed in an infant's crib
      (3) Vehicle warming in a closed garage
      (4) Children playing with plastic bags or inserting small objects into their mouths or noses
      (5) Discarded or unused refrigerators or freezers without removed doors
      (6) Children left unattended in bathtubs or pools
      (7) Household gas leaks
      (8) Smoking in bed
      (9) Use of fuel-burning heater not vented to outside
      (10) Low-strung clothesline
      (11) Pacifier hung around infant's head
      (12) Consuming large mouthfuls of food
 3. Minor risk factors:
   None given.

C. High Risk for Injury: Poisoning

   1. *Definition*: Accentuated risk of accidental exposure to or ingestion of drugs or dangerous products in doses sufficient to cause poisoning.[25]
   2. Major risk factors:
   a. Internal (individual):
      (1) Reduced vision
      (2) Verbalization of occupational setting without adequate safeguards
      (3) Lack of safety or drug education
      (4) Lack of proper precaution
      (5) Cognitive or emotional difficulties
      (6) Insufficient finances
   b. External (environmental):
      (1) Large supplies of drugs in house
      (2) Medicines stored in unlocked cabinet accessible to children or confused persons
      (3) Dangerous products placed or stored within the reach of children or confused persons
      (4) Availability of illicit drugs potentially contaminated by poisonous additives
      (5) Flaking, peeling paint or plaster in presence of young children
      (6) Chemical contamination of food and water
      (7) Unprotected contact with heavy metals or chemicals
      (8) Paint, lacquer, and so on in poorly ventilated areas or without effective protection
      (9) Presence of poisonous vegetation
      (10) Presence of atmospheric pollutants

3. Minor risk factors:
None given.

D. High Risk for Injury: Trauma

1. *Definition*: Accentuated risk of accidental tissue injury, for example, wound, burn, or fracture.[25]
2. Major risk factors:
   a. Internal (individual):
      (1) Weakness
      (2) Poor vision
      (3) Balancing difficulties
      (4) Reduced temperature or tactile sensation
      (5) Reduced large- or small-muscle coordination
      (6) Reduced hand-eye coordination
      (7) Lack of safety education
      (8) Lack of safety precautions
      (9) Insufficient finances to purchase safety equipment or effect repairs
      (10) Cognitive or emotional difficulties
      (11) History of previous trauma
   b. External (environmental):
      (1) Slippery floors (for example, wet or highly waxed)
      (2) Snow or ice collected on stairs or walkways
      (3) Unanchored rugs
      (4) Bathtub without handgrip or antislip equipment
      (5) Use of unsteady ladders or chairs
      (6) Entering unlighted rooms
      (7) Unsteady or absent stair rails
      (8) Unanchored electric wires
      (9) Litter or liquid spills on floors or stairways
      (10) High beds
      (11) Children playing without a gate at the top of the stairs
      (12) Obstructed passageways
      (13) Unsafe window protection in homes with young children
      (14) Inappropriate call-for-aid mechanisms for bedresting patient
      (15) Pot handles facing toward front of stove
      (16) Bathing in very hot water (for example, unsupervised bathing of young children)
      (17) Potential igniting gas leaks
      (18) Delayed lighting of gas burner or oven
      (19) Experimenting with chemical or gasoline
      (20) Unscreened fires or heaters
      (21) Wearing plastic apron or flowing clothes around open flame
      (22) Children playing with matches, candles, or cigarettes
      (23) Inadequately stored combustibles or corrosives (for example, matches, oily rags, or lye)
      (24) Highly flammable children's toys or clothing
      (25) Overloaded fuse boxes
      (26) Contact with rapidly moving machinery, industrial belts, or pulleys
      (27) Sliding on coarse bed linen or struggling within bed restraints

        (28) Faulty electric plugs, frayed wires, or defective appliances
        (29) Contact with acids or alkalis
        (30) Playing with fireworks or gunpowder
        (31) Contact with intense cold
        (32) Overexposure to sun, sunlamps, or radiotherapy
        (33) Use of cracked dinnerware or glasses
        (34) Knives stored uncovered
        (35) Guns or ammunition stored unlocked
        (36) Large icicles hanging from roof
        (37) Exposure to dangerous machinery
        (38) Children playing with sharp-edged toys
        (39) High-crime neighborhood and vulnerable clients
        (40) Driving a mechanically unsafe vehicle
        (41) Driving after partaking of alcoholic beverages or drugs
        (42) Driving at excessive speed
        (43) Driving without necessary visual aid
        (44) Children riding in the front seat of car
        (45) Smoking in bed or near oxygen
        (46) Overloaded electric outlet
        (47) Grease waste collected on stoves
        (48) Use of thin or worn potholders
        (49) Misuse of necessary headgear for motorized cyclists or young children carried on adult bicycles
        (50) Unsafe road or road-crossing conditions
        (51) Play or work near vehicle pathways (for example, driveways, laneways, or railroad tracks)
        (52) Nonuse or misuse of seat restraints
  3. Minor risk factors:
    None given.

RELATED FACTORS

The risk factors serve as the related factors for high-risk diagnoses.

RELATED CLINICAL CONCERNS

1. AIDS
2. Dementias such as Alzheimer's disease or multi-infarct
3. Diseases of the eye such as cataracts or glaucoma
4. Medications, for example, hallucinogens, barbiturates, opioids, or benzodiazepines
5. Epilepsy
6. Substance abuse or dependence

STOP

HAVE YOU SELECTED THE CORRECT DIAGNOSIS?

Activity Intolerance   This diagnosis should be considered if the nurse observes or validates reports of the patient's inability to complete required tasks because of insufficient energy. Insufficient energy could lead to accidents through falling or dropping of items, and so on. (See page 327.)

Impaired Physical Mobility This diagnosis is appropriate if the patient has difficulty with coordination, range of motion, muscle strength and control, or activity restrictions related to treatment. This could be manifested by the frequent occurrence of accidents or injury. (See page 460.)

Knowledge Deficit This diagnosis may exist if the client or family verbalizes less-than-adequate understanding of injury prevention. (See page 536.)

Impaired Home Maintenance Management This diagnosis is demonstrated by the inability of the patient or the family to provide a safe living environment. (See page 000.)

Altered Thought Process This diagnosis should be considered if the patient exhibits impaired attention span; impaired ability to recall information; impaired perception, judgment, and decision making; or impaired conceptual reasoning abilities. This diagnosis could certainly be reflected in increased accidents or injuries. (See page 577.)

High Risk for Violence This diagnosis exists if the accidents or injuries can be related to the risk factors for self-inflicted or other-directed physical trauma (for example, self-destructive behavior, substance abuse, rage or hostile verbalizations). (See page 801.)

EXPECTED OUTCOMES

1. Will identify hazards (list) contributing to high risk for injury and at least one corrective measure (list) for each hazard by (date) and/or
2. Will have no incidents of injury by (date)

TARGET DATE

While preventing injury may be a lifelong activity, establishing a mindset to avoid injury can be begun rapidly. An appropriate target date would be within 3 days of admission.

NURSING ACTIONS/INTERVENTIONS WITH RATIONALES

Adult Health

Actions/Interventions	Rationales
• Check on patient at least once an hour. If high risk for injury exists, do not leave patient unattended. Schedule sitters around the clock. If the patient has been identified as being at high risk for injury, for example, falls, place green dot on armband, chart, and head of bed.	Primary preventive measures to ensure patient safety. Green dot serves to alert other health care personnel of patient's status.
• Check respiratory rates, depth, and chest sounds at least every 4 hours at (state times here).	Ongoing monitoring of risk factors.

Continued

Actions/Interventions	Rationales
• Do not leave medications, solutions, or any type of liquids in the room. Use only paper cups and containers that can be disposed of immediately in patient's room. Use "Mr. Yuk" on bottle labels of poisonous substances. Teach patient and family to use this type of labeling at home.	Basic safety measures to prevent poisoning.
• Keep continuous check on airway patency. Keep suctioning equipment, ventilation equipment, and lavage setup on standby.	Ongoing monitoring of risk factors.
• Keep bed wheels locked and bed in low position. Keep head of bed elevated at least 30 degrees at all times.	Basic safety measures to prevent injury.
• Pad siderails and keep siderails up when patient is in bed.	
• Make sure handrails are in place in the bathroom and that safety strips are in tub and shower. Do not leave patient unattended in bathtub or shower.	
• Keep the patient's room free of clutter.	
• Orient the patient to time, person, place, and environment at least once a shift.	Keeps patient aware of environment.
• Provide night light.	Safety measure to prevent falling at night. Correction of vision and so on will assist in accident prevention.
• Assist in correcting, to the extent possible, any sensory-perceptual problems through appropriate referrals.	
• Assist the patient with all transfer and ambulation. If the patient requires multiple pillows for rest or positioning, tape the bottom layer of pillows to prevent dislodging.	Assists in preventing suffocation or tripping on pillows.
• Teach patient and family safety measures for use at home:	
○ Use nonskid rugs or tack down throw rugs.	
○ Use handrails.	
○ Install ramps.	
○ Use color contrast for steps, door knobs, electric outlets, and light switches.	
○ Avoid surface glare (for example, floors or table tops), maintain clean, nonskid floors, and keep rooms and halls free of clutter.	
○ Change physical position slowly.	
○ Use covers for electric outlets.	
○ Position pans with handles toward back of stove.	
○ Have family post poison control phone number for ready reference.	

- ○ Provide extra lighting in room and night light.
- Teach patient and significant other:
  - ○ Alterations in lifestyle that may be necessary (for example, stopping smoking, stopping alcohol ingestion, decreasing or ceasing drug ingestion, or ceasing driving)
  - ○ Use of assistive devices (for example, walkers, canes, crutches, or wheelchairs)
  - ○ Heimlich maneuver
  - ○ CPR
  - ○ Recognition of signs and symptoms of choking and carbon monoxide poisoning
  - ○ Necessity of chewing food thoroughly and cutting food into small bites
- Refer to appropriate agency for safety check of home. Make referral at least 3 days prior to discharge. (See Appendix B.)

Basic safety measures.

Allows time for checking and correction of problem areas.

Child Health

Actions/Interventions	Rationales
• Maintain appropriate supervision of infant at all times. Allow respite time for parents. *Do not* leave infant unattended. Have bulb syringe available in case of need to suction oropharynx. If regular equipment for suctioning is required, validate by checking label that all safety checks have been completed on equipment. Be aware of potential for young children to answer to any name. Validate identification for procedures in all young children.	Will prevent medication or treatment errors.
• Keep siderails of crib up, and monitor safety of all attachments for crib or infant's bassinet.	Infants and small children are prone to putting small pieces in mouth, nose, or ears. Basic safety measures.
• Check temperature of water before bathing and formula or food before feeding. *Do not* microwave formula.	Helps prevent scalding or chilling of infant.
• Maintain contact at all times during bathing. Infants unable to sit must be held constantly. Older children should be monitored as well, with special attention given to mental or physical needs for a handicapped child.	Helps prevent aspiration in case of vomiting.
• Place infant on abdomen with face turned	

Continued

Actions/Interventions	Rationales
to one side or the other until capable of rolling from side to side.	
• Investigate any signs and symptoms that warrant potential child protective service referral.	Provides assistance for child and family in instances of child abuse.
• Teach family basic safety measures:	Ensures environmental safety for infant or child.
○ Store plastic bags in cabinet out of child's reach.	
○ Do not cover infant or child's mattress or pillows with plastic.	
○ Make certain crib design follows federal regulations and that mattress has appropriate fit with crib frame.	
○ Discourage sleeping in bed with infant.	
○ Avoid use of homemade pacifiers (use only those of one-piece construction with loop handle).	
○ *Do not* tie pacifier around infant's neck.	
○ Untie bibs, bonnets, or other garments with snug fit around neck of infant before sleep.	
○ Inspect toys for removable parts, and check for safety approval.	
○ *Do not* feed infant foods that do not readily dissolve, such as grapes, nuts, or popcorn.	
○ Keep doors of large appliances, especially refrigerators, closed at all times.	
○ Maintain fence and constant supervision with swimming pool.	
○ Exercise caution while cleaning, with attention to pails of water and cleaning solutions.	
○ As infant or child is able, encourage swimming lessons with supervision and foster water safety.	
○ Use caution in exposure to sun for periods greater than 10 minutes.	
○ Use appropriate seat belts and car seats according to weight and development.	
○ Keep matches and pointed objects, such as knives, in a safe place, out of child's reach.	
○ Use lead-free paint in child's furniture and environment.	
○ Keep toxic substances locked in cabinet and out of child's reach.	

- Hang plants and avoid placement on floor and tables.
- Discard used poisonous substances.
- *Do not* store toxic substances in food or beverage containers.
- Administer medication as a drug, not as candy.
- Use child-proof medication containers.
- Keep Syrup of Ipecac accessible and use it appropriately.
- Use special monitoring equipment as applicable.
- Use appropriate meal-time safety precautions to prevent aspiration with giggling.

Women's Health

Actions/Interventions	Rationales
• Teach patient and family the high risk for injury to the fetus and patient when the pregnant woman smokes, is exposed to smoke, or engages in substance abuse, for example, alcohol or drugs (legal or illegal).	Provides initial safety information regarding the well-being of the fetus.
• Report to proper authorities any suspicion of family violence. (See Chapters 9 and 10 and Appendix B for more detailed nursing actions.)	A legal requirement in most states.
• Provide atmosphere that allows the patient considering abortion to relate her concerns and experiences and to obtain detailed information about the method of abortion that is being considered.	Allows patient to receive nonjudgmental information about the pros and cons of all choices available.
• Encourage questions and verbalization of patient's life expectations.	
• Provide information on options available to patient.	
• Assist patient in identifying life-style adjustments that her decision could entail.	
• Involve significant others, if so desired by patient, in discussion and problem-solving activities regarding life-style adjustments.	
• In instances where the patient has performed a self-induced abortion, obtain detailed information regarding the method used. Provide atmosphere that allows patient to relate her experience.	In self-induced abortion, there is high probability of injury and subsequent infection. This information will provide the health team with basic data to begin assessing the degree of injury.

Continued

Actions/Interventions	Rationales
• Ascertain if abortifacients (castor oil, turpentine, lye, ammonia, and so on) or mechanical means (coat hanger, knitting needles, broken bottle, knife) were used.	

• Regardless of the type of abortion, obtain a history from patient that includes:
  ○ Date of last menstrual period
  ○ Method of contraception, if any
  ○ Previous obstetric history
  ○ Known allergies to anesthetics, analgesics, antibiotics, or other drugs
  ○ Current drug usage
  ○ Past medical history
	Provides basic database to initiate planning of care.

• Note patient's mental state, for example, anxious, frightened, or ambivalent.	

• Perform physical assessment with special notice of:
  ○ Amount and character of vaginal discharge
  ○ Temperature elevation
  ○ Pain
  ○ *Bleeding*: Consistency, amount, and color	

• Teach patient importance of proper storage of birth control pills, spermicides, and medications.	
• Assist patient in identifying drugs that are teratogenic to the fetus.	Provides information that allows the patient to plan for safety during pregnancy.
• Assist patient in becoming aware of environmental hazards when pregnant, such as x-rays, people with infections, cats (litter boxes), and hazards on the job (surgical gases and industrial hazards).	

Mental Health

Actions/Interventions	Rationales
• Orient client to person, place, and time on each interaction.	Disorientation can increase the client's risk for injury if the environment is perceived as dangerous.
• Provide appropriate assistance to client as he or she moves about the environment.	Prevents falls and possible injury.
• Monitor level of consciousness every 15 minutes when the client is acutely disoriented following special treatments or when consciousness is affected by drugs or	Patient safety is of primary importance. Provides information about client's current status so interventions can be adapted appropriately. Prevents aspiration by

alcohol. If level of consciousness is impaired, place client on side to prevent aspiration of vomitus, and withhold solid food until level of consciousness improves. Place client in bed with siderails and keep siderails raised.

- Do not allow client to smoke without supervision when disoriented or when consciousness is clouded.
- Provide supervision for clients using new tools that could precipitate injury in special activities such as occupational therapy.
- Teach client and support system:
  - Risks associated with excessive use of drugs and alcohol
  - Appropriate methods for compensating for sensory-perceptual deficits (for example, use of pictures or colors to distinguish environmental cues when ability to read is lost)
- Remove all environmental hazards, for example, personal grooming items that could produce a hazard, cleaning agents, foods that produce a hazard when taken with certain medicines, plastic bags, clothes hangers, belts and ties, and shoestrings. Remove unnecessary pillows and blankets from the bed.
- Maintain close supervision of client. (If client is suicidal, refer to nursing actions for High Risk for Violence, Chapter 9, for specific interventions.)
- Check client's mouth carefully after oral medicines are given for any amounts that might be held in the mouth to be used at a later date.
- If client is at risk for holding pills in the mouth to be used later, collaborate with physician to have doses changed to liquids or injections.
- Keep lavage setup and airway and oxygen equipment on standby.
- Talk with client and support system about situations that increase the risk for poisoning, and develop a list of these situations.
- Label all medicines and poisonous substances appropriately.

facilitating drainage of fluids away from airway and prevents falls and possible injury.

Prevents client from acting impulsively to injure self with items easily found in environment. This allows staff time to offer alternative coping strategies when clients are experiencing difficulty with coping.

Prevents client from acting impulsively.

Basic safety precautions.

Gerontic Health

Actions/Interventions	Rationales
• Refer the independent elder to home health for home safety assessment at least 3 days prior to discharge from hospital.	Provides timely home care planning and allows implementation of safety measures before patient is discharged.
• Instruct patient on safe administration of medication. Monitor for knowledge of drug dosage, reason for medication, expected effect, and possible side effects. Reinforce teaching on a daily basis.	Basic medication safety measures.
• If patient suffers from dementia, teach the caregiver the following safety adaptations:[42]	Older adults with the diagnosis of dementia often display signs of poor judgment. The teaching factors that are listed here decrease the risk for injury in the home setting.
○ Place in a locked closet articles such as power tools, medications, or appliances that the individual may misuse, causing injury to self or others.	
○ Ensure that water temperature is low enough to prevent scalding.	
○ Remove knobs from stove if cooking is a fire hazard.	
○ Install gates at the top of stairs to prevent falls.	
○ Tape door latches or remove tumblers from locks to prevent patient from being accidentally locked in a room.	
○ Place two locks on entry or exit doors if the individual is prone to wandering.	
○ Ensure that furnishings do not have sharp edges or large areas of glass that could cause injury during a fall.	

Home Health

Actions/Interventions	Rationales
• Involve client and family in planning, implementing, and promoting reduction in the high risk for injury:	Involvement of the client and family enhances motivation and increases the possibility of positive outcomes and the long-term lifestyle changes required.
○ Arrange family conferences.	
○ Assist family to define mutual goals.	
○ Promote communication.	
○ Assist family members with specific tasks as appropriate to reduce the high risk for injury. (*Note*: Restraining the client may increase — not decrease — the risk for injury.[43]) It is important to arrange the environment so that the client can avoid injury, for example, installing a bedside commode or raised toilet seat; removing	

unnecessary furniture; picking up objects that may be blocking pathway;[44] removing unsafe or improperly stored chemicals, weapons, cooking utensils, and appliances; safely using and storing toxic substances; acquiring certification in first aid and CPR; properly storing food; acquiring knowledge of poisonous plants; learning to swim; removing fire hazards from environment; designing and practicing an emergency plan for action if fire occurs; and properly operating machines that use petroleum products.

- Teach client and family about injury prevention activities and equipment as appropriate:
  - Proper lifting techniques
  - Back exercises to prevent back injury
  - Removal of hazardous environmental conditions such as improper storage of hazardous substances, improper use of electrical appliances, smoking in bed, open heaters and flames, and congested walkways
  - Proper ventilation when using toxic substances
  - First aid for poisoning
  - Proper labeling, storage, and disposal of toxic materials such as household cleaning products, lawn and garden chemicals, and medications
  - Proper food preparation and storage
  - Proper skin, lung, and eye protection when using toxic substances
  - Toxic substances out of reach of infants and young children
  - Recognition of toxic plants and removal from environment as indicated
  - Plan of action if accidental poisoning occurs
- Assist client and family in life-style adjustments that may be required.

- Refer to appropriate assistance resources as indicated. (See Appendix B.)
- Participate in early return-to-work programs.[45]
- Participate in local, state, and national immunization initiatives.[46]

Prevention activities reduce the risk of injury. Many people either do not know these prevention strategies, or they may need to have them reinforced.

For long-term change, life-style adjustments are often required. Many people require assistance with these changes.
Use of existing community services is efficient use of resources.
Such programs lead to better client outcomes.

Community participation in immunization initiatives improves the rate of appropriate immunization and reduces the risk of outbreak of these diseases.

FLOW CHART EVALUATION
Flow Chart Expected Outcome 1

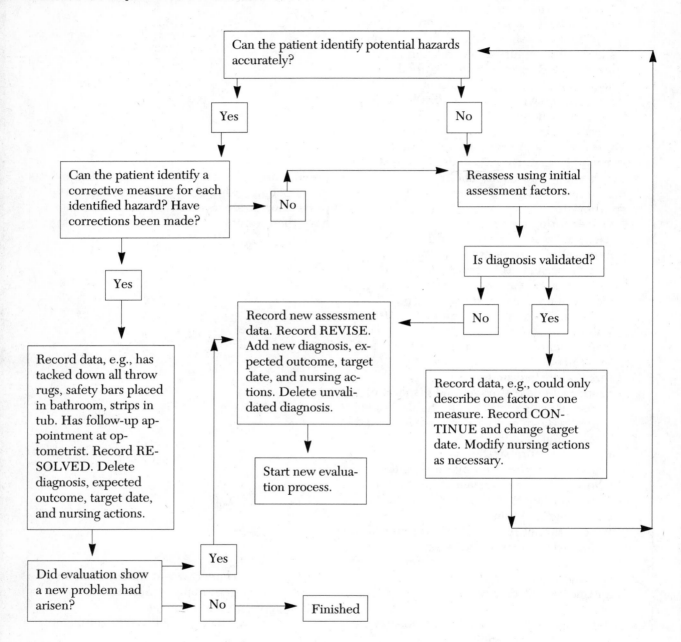

Can the patient identify potential hazards accurately?

Yes

No

Can the patient identify a corrective measure for each identified hazard? Have corrections been made?

No

Reassess using initial assessment factors.

Yes

Is diagnosis validated?

No

Yes

Record new assessment data. Record **REVISE**. Add new diagnosis, expected outcome, target date, and nursing actions. Delete unvalidated diagnosis.

Record data, e.g., has tacked down all throw rugs, safety bars placed in bathroom, strips in tub. Has follow-up appointment at optometrist. Record **RESOLVED**. Delete diagnosis, expected outcome, target date, and nursing actions.

Start new evaluation process.

Record data, e.g., could only describe one factor or one measure. Record **CONTINUE** and change target date. Modify nursing actions as necessary.

Did evaluation show a new problem had arisen?

Yes

No

Finished

Flow Chart Expected Outcome 2

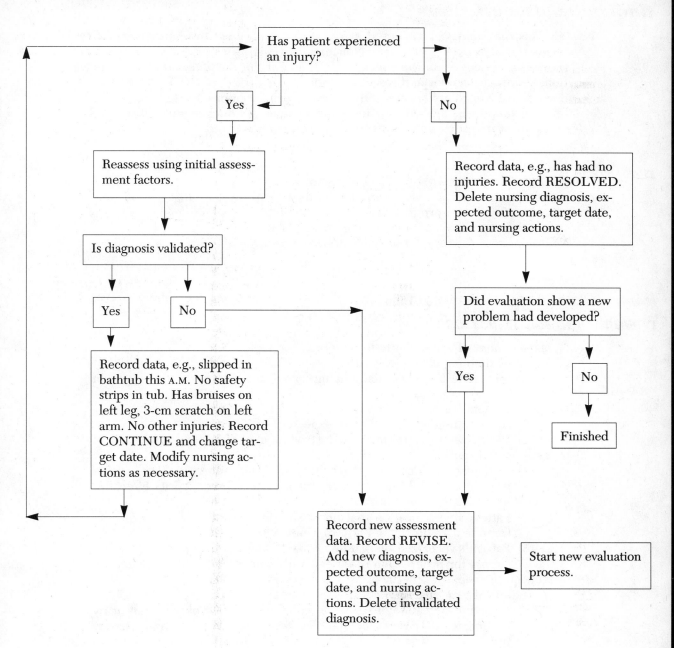

Management of Therapeutic Regimen (Individuals): Ineffective

NOTE: This diagnosis was proposed at the Tenth NANDA Conference with the result that a proposal to delete Noncompliance is expected to be presented shortly. As discussed in the conceptual section of this chapter and in the additional information later in this section, there are many people who object to the diagnosis of Noncompliance. For this reason, we will not provide nursing actions for Noncompliance but will provide the definition, defining characteristics, and related factors for this diagnosis until it is officially deleted.

DEFINITION

Ineffective Management of Therapeutic Regimen: A pattern of regulating and integrating into daily living a program for treatment of illness and the sequelae of illness that is unsatisfactory for meeting specific health goals.[47]

Noncompliance (Specify): A person's informed decision not to adhere to a therapeutic recommendation.[25]

NANDA TAXONOMY: CHOOSING 5.2.1

DEFINING CHARACTERISTICS

1. Management of Therapeutic Regimen:
   a. Major defining characteristics:
   Inappropriate choices of daily living for meeting the goals of a treatment or prevention program.
   b. Minor defining characteristics:
      (1) Acceleration (expected or unexpected) of illness symptoms.
      (2) Verbalized desire to manage the treatment of illness and prevention of sequelae.
      (3) Verbalized difficulty with regulation and/or integration of one or more prescribed regimens for treatment of illness and its effects or prevention of complications.
      (4) Patient's verbalization that he or she did not take action to include treatment regimens in daily routines.
      (5) Patient's verbalization that he or she did not take action to reduce risk factors for progression of illness and sequelae.
2. Noncompliance:
   a. Major defining characteristics:
      (1) Behavior indicative of failure to adhere (by direct observation or by statements of patient or significant others). *Note*: critical characteristic.
      (2) Objective tests (physiologic measures or detection of markers).
      (3) Evidence of development of complications.
      (4) Evidence of exacerbation of symptoms.
      (5) Failure to keep appointments.
      (6) Failure to progress.
   b. Minor defining characteristics:
   None given.

RELATED FACTORS

1. Ineffective Management of Therapeutic Regimen:
   a. Complexity of health care system
   b. Complexity of therapeutic regimen
   c. Decisional conflicts
   d. Economic difficulties
   e. Excessive demands made on individual or family
   f. Family patterns of health care
   g. Inadequate number and types of cues to action
   h. Knowledge deficits
   i. Mistrust of regimen and/or health care personnel
   j. Perceived seriousness
   k. Perceived susceptibility
   l. Perceived barriers
   m. Perceived benefits
   n. Powerlessness
   o. Social support deficits
2. Noncompliance:
   a. *Patient value system*: Health beliefs, cultural influences, spiritual values
   b. Client-provider relationships

RELATED CLINICAL CONCERNS

1. Any diagnosis new to the patient, that is, patient does not have education or experience in dealing with this disorder
2. Any diagnosis of a chronic nature, for example, pain, migraine headaches, or rheumatoid arthritis
3. Any diagnosis that has required a change in physicians, for example, referred from long-time family physician to cardiologist

HAVE YOU SELECTED THE CORRECT DIAGNOSIS?

Knowledge Deficit This is the most appropriate diagnosis if the patient or family verbalizes less-than-adequate understanding of health management or recalls inaccurate health information. (See page 536.)

Ineffective Individual Coping or Ineffective Family Coping These diagnoses are suspected if there are major differences between the patient and family reports of health status, health perception, and health care behavior. Verbalizations by the patient or family regarding inability to cope also indicate this differential nursing diagnosis. (See pages 874 and 892.)

Altered Family Processes Through observing family interactions and communication, the nurse may assess that Altered Family Processes is a consideration. Poorly communicated messages, rigidity of family functions and roles, and failure to accomplish expected family developmental tasks are a few observations to alert the nurse to this possible diagnosis. (See page 710.)

Continued

HAVE YOU SELECTED THE CORRECT DIAGNOSIS?—*Continued*

Activity Intolerance or Self-Care Deficit   These diagnoses should be considered if the nurse observes or validates reports of inability to complete the tasks required because of insufficient energy or because of inability to feed, bathe, toilet, dress, and groom self. (See pages 327 and 472.)

Altered Thought Process   If the patient exhibits impaired attention span, impaired ability to recall information, impaired perception, judgment, and decision making, or impaired conceptual and reasoning abilities, the nursing diagnosis of Altered Thought Process should be considered. (See page 577.)

Impaired Home Maintenance Management   This diagnosis is demonstrated by the inability of the patient or family to provide a safe living environment. (See page 438.)

ADDITIONAL INFORMATION

NOTE: Some nursing authors object to the term "Noncompliance."[48,49,50,51] Compliance can become the basis for a power-oriented relationship in which one is judged and labeled "compliant" or "noncompliant" based on the hierarchical position of the professional in relation to the patient. The diagnosis of Noncompliance is to be used for those patients who wish to comply with the therapeutic recommendations but are prevented from doing so by the presence of certain factors. The nurse can in such situations strive to lessen or eliminate the factors that preclude the willing patient from complying with recommendations.

The principles of informed consent and autonomy[54] are critical to the appropriate use of this diagnosis. A person may freely choose not to follow a treatment plan. The nursing diagnosis Noncompliance should not carry a connotation of the ability of the patient to obey but rather that the patient has attempted the prescribed plan and has found it difficult to implement. The area of noncompliance must be specified. A patient may follow many aspects of a treatment program very well and find only a small part of the plan difficult to manage. Such a patient is noncompliant only in the area of difficulty.

Several nursing authors have recognized the interdependent nature of illness and healing.[52,55,56,57] This interdependence is especially pronounced in chronic illness. As a patient and his or her family adapts to a chronic condition, noncompliance with prescribed treatment regimens may actually be constructive and therapeutic, not detrimental.[53] The nurse who learns to listen to the patient and plan treatments in collaboration with the patient will benefit from the wisdom of people experiencing illness.[58]

EXPECTED OUTCOMES

1. Will identify barriers to implementing regimen and devise at least one way to overcome each barrier (list) by (date) and/or
2. Will return-demonstrate appropriate technique or procedures (list) for self-care by (date)

TARGET DATE

The specific target dates for these objectives will be directly related to the barriers identified, the patient's entering level of knowledge, and the comfort the patient feels in expressing satisfaction or dissatisfaction. The target date could range from 1 to 5 days following the date of admission.

NURSING ACTIONS/INTERVENTIONS WITH RATIONALES

Adult Health

Actions/Interventions	Rationales
• Help the patient and family identify potential areas of conflict, for example, values, religious beliefs, cultural mores, or cost.	Assesses motivation and decreases risk of ineffective management of therapeutic regimen.
• Start instructions for self-care within 24 hours of admission.	Provides time to incorporate changes into lifestyle and to practice as necessary before day of discharge from hospital.
• Assist the patient and family in identifying factors that actually or potentially may impede the desired therapeutic regimen plan: ○ Sense of control ○ Language barriers (provide translators, assign nursing personnel to care for patient who speak the patient's language) ○ Cultural concerns (cultural mores, religious beliefs, and so on; design a plan that will allow incorporation of the therapeutic regimen within the cultural norms of the patient) ○ Financial constraints ○ Knowledge deficits ○ Time constraints ○ Entry to health care system	Assesses motivation and decreases risk of diagnosis development.
• Make a list of these potential areas of conflict, and help patient and family problem solve each area one area at a time.	
• Allow opportunities for the patient and family to vent feelings about therapeutic regimen. Schedule at least 30 minutes at least once per day for this activity. Note times here.	
• Teach the patient and significant others knowledge and skills needed to implement the therapeutic regimen (for example, measuring blood pressure, counting calories, administering medications, or weighing self).	

Continued

Health Perception–Health Management Pattern

Actions/Interventions	Rationales
• Have the patient and significant others return-demonstrate or restate principles at least daily for at least 3 consecutive days prior to discharge.	Allows sufficient practice time that provides immediate feedback on skills, and so on.
• Design a chart to assist the patient to visually see the effectiveness of therapeutic regimen (for example, weight-loss chart, days without smoking, blood pressure measurements). Begin the chart in hospital within 1 day of admission.	Visualization of actual progress promotes implementation of prescribed regimen.
• Assist in the development of a schedule that will allow the patient to keep appointments and not miss work. Forward plan to employer and physician.	Demonstrates importance of schedule to patient, employer, and physician. Coordinated effort encourages adherence to regimen.
• Assist the patient in developing time-management skills to incorporate time for relaxation and exercise. Have patient develop a typical 1-week schedule; then work with patient to adapt schedule as needed.	Individualizes schedule and highlights need for relaxation and exercise.
• Contract, in writing, with the patient and significant others for specifics regarding regimen. Follow up 1 week after discharge; recheck 6 weeks following discharge.	Demonstrates, in writing, the importance of the plan. Also, listing definitive follow-up times enhances the probability of regimen implementation.
• Design techniques that encourage the patient's implementation of the regimen, such as setting single, easy-to-accomplish, short-term goals first and progressing to long-term goals as the short-term goals are met. For example, if the idea of stopping smoking is too overwhelming, help patient design a personal adaptive program such as (1) changing to a lower tar and nicotine cigarette, (2) timing smoking (only one cigarette per 30 or 60 minutes), (3) stabilizing, and (4) making further reductions.	Prevents multiple changes from overwhelming patient, thus avoiding one major contributor to ineffective management of therapeutic regimen.
• Teach the patient and significant others assertive techniques that can be used to deal with dissatisfaction with caregivers.	Long waiting periods in offices, unanswered questions, being rushed, and so on increase the likelihood of abandoning the regimen. Assertiveness helps the patient and family overcome the feelings of powerlessness and increases the sense of control.
• Allow time for the patient and family to verbalize fears related to therapeutic regimen (for example, body image, cost, side effects, pain, or dependency) by devoting at least 30 minutes per day to this activity. List times here.	Increases patient's sense of control. Facilitates continuity and consistency of plan.

- Assist in correction of sensory, motor, and similar deficits to the extent possible through referrals to appropriate consultants (for example, occupational therapist, physical therapist, ophthalmologist, or audiologist).
- Have patient design a home care plan. Assist the patient to modify the plan as necessary. Forward the plan to home health service, social service, physician, and so on.
- Relate any information regarding dissatisfaction to appropriate caregiver (for example, to physician — problems with the time spent in waiting room, cultural needs, privacy needs, costs, or need for generic prescriptions).
- Make follow-up appointments prior to the patient's leaving the hospital. Do it from the patient's room, and put appropriate information regarding appointment on brightly colored card (i.e., name, address, time, date, and telephone number).

Demonstrates exactly how to make appointments for patient.

- Refer the patient to appropriate follow-up personnel, for example, nurse practitioner, visiting nurse service, social service, or transportation service. Make referral at least 3 days prior to discharge.

Allows time for home care assessment and initiation of service.

- Request follow-up personnel to remind the patient of appointments via card or telephone.

Shares the responsibility for implementing the regimen and demonstrates the importance attached to follow-up care by those providers.

- For the last 2 to 3 days of hospitalization, let the patient perform all of his or her own care. Supervise performance, critique, and reteach as necessary.

Child Health

Actions/Interventions	Rationales
• Assist in developing health values of regimen adherence before the infant's birth through emphasis on these aspects in childbirth education classes.	Initiates idea of individual health management for child's health before birth. Allows sufficient time for parents to incorporate theses ideas.
• Allow for the infant or child's schedule in appointment scheduling (for example, respect for naps and meal times). Involve the family in planning care for the infant or child.	Facilitates comfort for child, parents, and health care provider. Demonstrates individuality and increases likelihood of regimen implementation.
• Reward progress in the appropriate manner for age and development.	

Women's Health

Actions/Interventions	Rationales
• Develop a sensitivity for cultural differences of women's roles and their impact on implementation of a therapeutic regimen.	Demonstration of understanding of the patient's culture and inclusion of these differences in planning increase the probability of effective management of the therapeutic regimen.
• Encourage family to share views of childbirth with health care personnel through classes and interviews.[59]	
• Discuss with family their traditions and taboos for mother and baby during transitional period after childbirth, for example, in some Far Eastern cultures, the mother does not touch the infant for several days after birth. The grandmother or aunts become the primary caregivers for the infant.[59]	

Mental Health

NOTE: It is important to remember that the mental health client is influenced by a larger social system and that this social system plays a crucial role in the client's ongoing participation with the health care team. The conceptualization that may be most useful in intervention with and assessment of the client who does not follow the recommendations of the health care team in this area may be "system persistence." Hoffman[60] uses this concept to communicate the idea that the system is signaling that it desires to continue in its present manner of organization. This could present a situation in which the individual client indicates to the health care team that he or she desires change, and yet change is not demonstrated due to the constraints placed on the individual by the larger social system (i.e., the family). This places the responsibility on the nurse to initiate a comprehensive assessment of the client system when the diagnosis of Ineffective Management of the Therapeutic Regimen or Noncompliance is considered.

Actions/Interventions	Rationales

• Involve the client system in discussions on the treatment plan. This should include:
  ○ Family
  ○ Individuals the client identifies as important in making decisions related to health (i.e., cultural healers, social institutions such as probation officers, public welfare workers, officials in the school system, and so on)
	Promotes client's perceived control and increases potential for client's involvement in the treatment plan.

• Discuss with the identified system those factors that inhibit system reorganization:
    ○ Knowledge and skills related to necessary change
    ○ Resources available
    ○ Ability to use these resources
    ○ Belief system about treatment plan
    ○ Cultural values related to the treatment plan.
	Recognition of those factors that inhibit change can facilitate the development of a plan that eliminates these problems.

• Assist the system in making the appropriate adjustments in system organization. • Enhance current patterns that facilitate system reorganization.	Affirms and promotes client's strengths.
• Make small changes in those patterns that inhibit system change; for example, ask the client to talk with the family in the group room instead of in an open public area on the unit, or ask the client who washes his or her hands frequently to use a special soap and towel and then gradually introduce more changes in the patterns.	Promotes client's control and provides realistic, achievable goals for the client, thus preserving self-esteem when change can be accomplished.
• Advise the client to make changes slowly. It is important not to expect too much too soon.	Increases self-esteem and increases desire to continue those behaviors that elicit this response.
• Provide the appropriate positive verbal feedback to all parts of the system involved in assisting with the changes. It is important not to focus on the demonstration of old patterns of behavior at this time. The smallest change should be recognized.	
• Communicate the plan to all members of the health care team.	Promotes continuity of care and builds trust.

Gerontic Health

Actions/Interventions	Rationales
• Refer to mental health specialist to rule out depression. • Refer to community resources. (See Appendix B.)	Depression in the elderly is frequently underdiagnosed and undertreated. The older patient may have concerns related to availability of support systems, financial concerns regarding medication costs, and availability of transportation. Use of already available community resources provides a long-term, cost-effective support system.

Home Health

Actions/Interventions	Rationales

• Assist the client to delineate factors contributing to ineffective therapeutic regimen management by helping the client to assess:
  ○ Level of knowledge and skill related to treatment plan
  ○ Resources available to meet treatment plan objectives
  ○ Appropriate use of resources to meet treatment plan objectives
  ○ Complexity of treatment plan
  ○ Current response to treatment plan
  ○ Use of nonprescribed interventions
  ○ Barriers to compliance
	Barriers and facilitators to ineffective management can be altered to improve outcomes.

• Involve the client and family in planning, implementing, and promoting the treatment plan through:[53,58,61]
  ○ Assisting with family conferences
  ○ Coordinating mutual goal setting
  ○ Promoting increased communication
  ○ Assigning family members specific tasks as appropriate to assist in maintaining the therapeutic regimen plan (for example, support person for patient, transportation, companionship in meeting mutual goals, and so on).
	Involvement increases motivation and improves the probability of success.

• Support the client in eliminating barriers to implementing the regimen by:
  ○ Providing for privacy
  ○ Referring to community services (for example, church, home health volunteer, transportation service, or financial assistance)
  ○ Alerting other health care providers and social service personnel of the problem that long waiting periods create
  ○ Providing for interpreters and for community-based language classes for English speakers to learn other languages as well as for non-English speakers to learn English
• Assign one health care provider or social service worker, as much as possible, to avoid lack of continuity in care provision.
• Assist health care providers and social
	Many barriers are institutional and can be eliminated or reduced.

service workers to understand the
constructive nature of noncompliance in
chronic illness[62]

- Make timely phone calls to clients to
discuss care (for example, 1 day after being
seen in clinic for minor acute infection, or
weekly or monthly on a routine schedule
for a chronically ill person[63]).
- Collaborate with other health care
professionals and social service workers to
reduce the number and variety of
medications for chronically ill clients.[62]
- Reteach the client and family appropriate
therapeutic activities as need arises.

Reinforcement of information and continued
assistance may be required to improve
implementation of the therapeutic regimen.

FLOW CHART EVALUATION
Flow Chart Expected Outcome 1

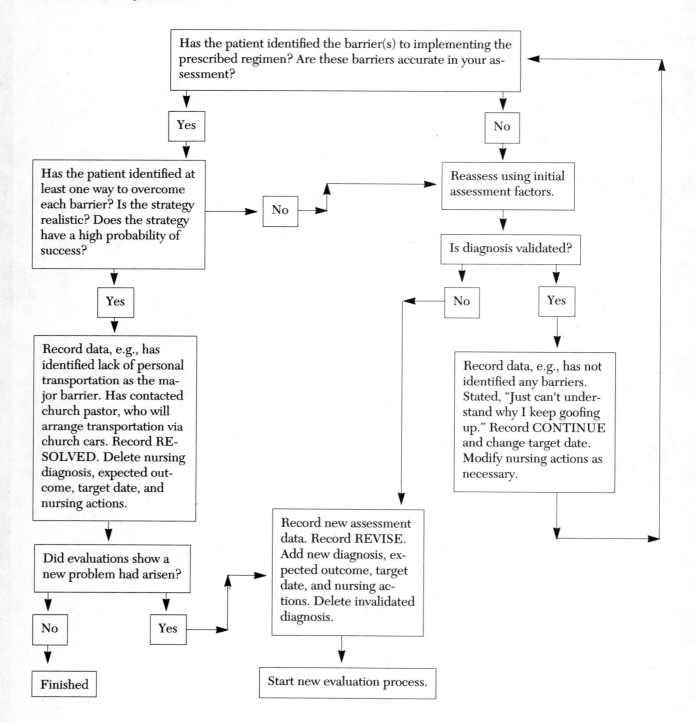

Flow Chart Expected Outcome 2

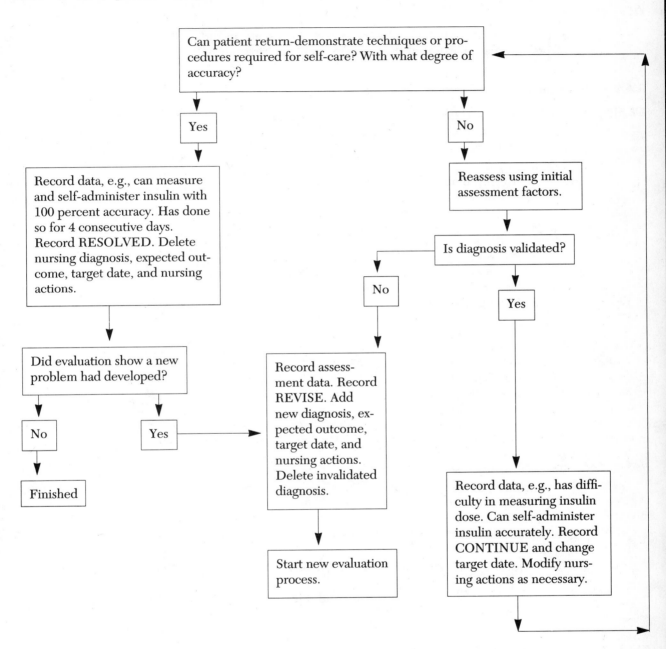

Can patient return-demonstrate techniques or procedures required for self-care? With what degree of accuracy?

Yes

No

Record data, e.g., can measure and self-administer insulin with 100 percent accuracy. Has done so for 4 consecutive days. Record RESOLVED. Delete nursing diagnosis, expected outcome, target date, and nursing actions.

Reassess using initial assessment factors.

Is diagnosis validated?

No

Yes

Did evaluation show a new problem had developed?

Record assessment data. Record REVISE. Add new diagnosis, expected outcome, target date, and nursing actions. Delete invalidated diagnosis.

No

Yes

Finished

Record data, e.g., has difficulty in measuring insulin dose. Can self-administer insulin accurately. Record CONTINUE and change target date. Modify nursing actions as necessary.

Start new evaluation process.

Health Perception–Health Management Pattern

Protection, Altered

DEFINITION

The state in which an individual experiences a decrease in the ability to guard the self from internal or external threats such as illness or injury.[25]

NANDA TAXONOMY: EXCHANGING 1.6.2

DEFINING CHARACTERISTICS

1. Major defining characteristics:
   a. Deficient immunity
   b. Impaired healing
   c. Altered clotting
   d. Maladaptive stress response
   e. Neurosensory alterations
2. Minor defining characteristics:
   a. Chilling
   b. Perspiring
   c. Dyspnea
   d. Cough
   e. Itching
   f. Restlessness
   g. Insomnia
   h. Fatigue
   i. Anorexia
   j. Weakness
   k. Immobility
   l. Disorientation
   m. Pressure sores

RELATED FACTORS

1. Extremes of age
2. Inadequate nutrition
3. Alcohol abuse
4. Abnormal blood profiles (leukopenia, thrombocytopenia, anemia, or coagulation)
5. Drug therapies (antineoplastic, corticosteroid, immune, anticoagulant, or thrombolytic)
6. Treatments (surgery, radiation, and disease such as cancer or immune disorders)

RELATED CLINICAL CONCERNS

1. AIDS
2. Diabetes mellitus
3. Anorexia nervosa
4. Cancer
5. Clotting disorders, for example, disseminated intravascular coagulation, thrombophlebitis, or anticoagulant medications

6. Substance abuse or dependence
7. Any disorder requiring use of steroids

 HAVE YOU SELECTED THE CORRECT DIAGNOSIS?

High Risk for Infection   This diagnosis would most likely be a companion diagnosis. "High risk" means the individual is not presenting the actual defining characteristics of the diagnosis but there are indications that the diagnosis could develop. Altered Protection is an actual diagnosis. (See page 65.)

EXPECTED OUTCOMES

1. Will return-demonstrate measures to increase self-protection by (date) and/or
2. Will exhibit, via lab tests, no worsening of condition by (date)

TARGET DATE

Altered Protection is a long-lasting diagnosis. Therefore, a date to totally meet the expected outcome could be weeks or months. However, since the target date signals the time to check progress, a date 3 days from the date of the original diagnosis would be appropriate.

NURSING ACTIONS/INTERVENTIONS WITH RATIONALES

Adult Health

Actions/Interventions	Rationales
• Place patient in protective isolation but *do not* promote an isolated feeling for the patient. Encourage frequent telephone calls and visits from significant others.	Lessens sense of isolation and maintains therapeutic relationship.
• Check patient at least every 30 minutes while awake. Spend 30 minutes with client every 2 hours on (odd/even) hour while awake to answer questions and provide emotional support while in reverse isolation. Note times for these interactions here.	
• Collaborate with occupational therapist regarding diversionary activity.	
• Protect patient from injury and infection. (See appropriate nursing actions and rationales under the diagnoses High Risk for Injury and High Risk for Infection.)	Protects patient from infection or spread of infection.
• Use universal precautions in caring for the patient.	

Continued

Actions/Interventions	Rationales

• Monitor:
  ○ Vital signs, mucous membranes, skin integrity, and response to medications at least once per shift
  ○ Unexplained blood in the urine
  ○ Prolonged bleeding after blood being drawn or from injection sites
  ○ *Side effects of blood and blood products*: Monitor for possibility of blood reaction. Take vital signs every 15 minutes × 4, then every 30 minutes until transfusion completed. In event of transfusion reaction, stop the transfusion immediately, maintain IV line with saline, and notify physician while monitoring patient for further anaphylactic signs and symptoms.
  ○ *Effects and side effects of steroids*: Improved general status, decreased inflammatory signs and symptoms versus untoward effects, including bleeding, Na or K imbalance. Calculate and record intake and output at least once per shift.
  ○ *Effects and side effects of antineoplastics such as nausea, cardiac arrhythmias, extrapyramidal signs and symptoms*: These side effects will vary according to the specific agents used. Take vital signs every 5 to 10 minutes during actual administration and use a cardiac monitor.
  ○ Signs and symptoms of infection such as lymphoid interstitial pneumonia or recurrent oral candidiasis.
	Allows comparison to baseline at admission and evaluation of effectiveness of therapy.

• Apply pressure after each injection and after removal of IV needle.	Assists in stopping of bleeding.
• Provide oral hygiene or assist patient with oral hygiene at least three times per day.	Prevents opportunistic infection.
• Provide body hygiene or assist patient with body hygiene at least once daily at time of patient's choosing.	
• Measure and record intake and output at end of each shift.	Monitors effectiveness of bowel and bladder function.
• Encourage patient to eat nutritious meals. Collaborate with diet therapist regarding patient's likes, dislikes, and planning for dietary needs after hospital discharge.	Ensures balanced intake of necessary vitamins, minerals, and so on to assist in tissue repair. Assists in lessening impact of infections.
• Collaborate with physician regarding repeat	Gives guidelines for future therapeutic

laboratory examinations (CBC, blood coagulation studies, urinalyses, drug levels, and so on).

- Collaborate with psychiatric nurse practitioner as necessary.
- Teach patient and significant others:
  ○ Medication administration
  ○ Signs and symptoms to be reported
  ○ Special laboratory or other procedures to be done at home
  ○ Anticipatory safety needs
  ○ Routine daily care
  ○ Appropriate clean and sterile technique
  ○ Isolation or reverse-isolation technique
  ○ Common antigens or allergens and seasonal variations
  ○ How to avoid or reduce exposure to antigens or allergens (alteration of environment)
  ○ Type and use of protective equipment
  ○ Universal precautions
  ○ Rationale for compliance with prescribed regimen
  ○ Resources available for assistance with health care, legal questions, or ethical questions
- Collaborate with other health professionals regarding ongoing care. (See Appendix B.)
- Identify community resources for patient and family. Make referrals at least 3 days before discharge from hospital. (See Appendix B.)

regimen as well as assessing effectiveness of current regimen.

Provides source for assistance with interventions for maladaptive stress response. Provides basic knowledge needed by patient and family to make modifications necessitated by alteration in protective mechanisms.

Care required is interdisciplinary in nature.

Allows time for agencies to initiate service. Use of existing community services is effective use of resources.

Child Health

NOTE: Infants at high risk for this diagnosis are: premature infants, infants with family history of hemophilia or sickle cell anemia, infants whose mothers have a history of drug abuse or HIV, and children who have histories of medication reaction.

In infants especially, incubation for HIV depends on acquisition time. The infant may be exposed any time during pregnancy, but sero-con/retroversion to a negative HIV status may occur, with a later positive HIV again. The more symptomatic the mother, the greater the effect in the infant due to constant reinfection in the infant. For infants whose mothers are HIV positive, 26 percent will be HIV positive in the first 5 months of life, an additional 24 percent will be HIV positive by 12 months of life, and the remaining 50 percent will be HIV positive by 2 years of age. Key symptoms are intercurrent infection and weight loss. Other conditions noted include failure to thrive, hepatomegaly, cardiomegaly, lymphoid interstitial pneumonia, chronic diarrhea, cardiomyopathy, encephalopathy, and opportunistic infections. Even tuberculosis may be seen in these infants, with a tendency to progress from primary to miliary phase. In these infants there may be disseminated BCG infection. It is important to be aware of lab studies requiring large amounts of blood to study the course of sero HIV status. This blood drawing is problematic in the already depressed immune–reticulo-endothelial systems of these infants. It is imperative that these infants *not be given* live polio vaccine due to their HIV positive status.

Actions/Interventions	Rationales

• Maintain monitoring for:
  ○ Observable lesions of ecchymotic nature or evidence of tendency toward bruising
  ○ Decreased absorption of nutrients (especially the premature infant because of the possibility of necrotizing enterocolitis)
	Essential monitoring to avoid overwhelming of child's system by infection and so on.

• Provide at least one 30- to 60-minute opportunity per day for family to vent feelings about the specific illness of their child.	Reduces anxiety, fear, and anger and provides an opportunity for teaching.
• Teach child and family essential care.	Basics of home care for child with diagnosis of altered protection.
• Provide diversionary therapy according to child's status, developmental level, and interests.	Prevents boredom and restlessness and fosters continued development of child in spite of illness.
• Be aware of current frustration with use of DDS (Dideoycytidene) and AZT (Zidovidine) in children. At this time protocols dictate doses.	Avoid unrealistic hope. Ideally toxicity is balanced against the need to reach therapeutic CNS dosage levels.

• Remind family that current treatment for AIDS is only palliative. Be sensitive to the unique nature of this health concern for all involved. Promote attention to the need for:
  ○ Spiritual and emotional support
  ○ Nutritional support
  ○ Treatment of HIV-related infections
  ○ Administration of IV immune globulin
  ○ Treatment of tumors and end organ failure
  ○ Chronic pain
	Avoids unrealistic hope while providing knowledge and support necessary to deal with a fatal illness.

Women's Health

Actions/Interventions	Rationales

• Maintain monitoring for defining characteristics of Altered Protection:
  ○ HELLP Syndrome (a severe form of Pregnancy Induced Hypertension): Monitor lab results for low platelets (less than 100,000/cc), elevated liver enzymes, elevated SGOT/SGPT, intravascular hemolysis, Schistocytes or Burr cells on peripheral smear, low HCT (without evidence of significant blood loss), and hypertension[64]
  ○ Other high-risk history in the mother such as history of preterm labor chronic hypertension or sickle cell anemia and other blood disorders
  ○ Signs and symptoms of infection
	Provides basic knowledge base for planning of care.

Mental Health

NOTE: Clients receiving antipsychotic neuroleptic drugs are at risk for development of agranulocytosis. This can be a life-threatening side effect and usually occurs in the first 8 weeks of treatment. Any rapid onset of sore throat and fever should be immediately reported and actively treated. Tricyclic antidepressants can cause blood dyscrasias with long-term therapy. Initial symptoms of these dyscrasias include fever, sore throat, and aching.

Actions/Interventions	Rationales
• Immediately report client's complaint of sore throat or development of temperature elevation to physician. Institute nursing actions for hyperthermia (Chapter 3).	Alterations could be symptoms of agranulocytosis or blood dyscrasias and could place client at risk for infection. Prompt recognition and intervention prevents progression and improves client outcome.
• Teach clients who have had this type of response to antipsychotic neuroleptics or tricyclic antidepressants that they should not take this drug again.	
• If client is experiencing severe alterations in thought processes, provide one-to-one observation until mental status improves or until client can again participate in unit activities.	Client safety is of primary importance. Provides opportunity for ongoing assessment of the quality of the content of the client's thought and provides ongoing reality orientation.

Gerontic Health

Actions/Interventions	Rationales
• Monitor sensory status. Ensure that adaptive equipment (glasses, hearing aids, and so on) is functioning appropriately and being used appropriately.	Pyrexia and elevated WBCs may not be present with infection. The first indicator of infection may be restlessness, confusion, an alteration in mental status, incontinence, irritability, or falls.
• Monitor mobility level. Ensure that adaptive equipment (brace, walker, and so on) is available. • Monitor for subtle changes in condition. • Avoid use of soaps that may cause dry skin.	Daily bathing may not be appropriate due to skin dryness associated with aging.
• Initiate measures to maintain skin integrity such as egg crate mattresses or specialized beds.	Assists in preventing the development of skin breakdown.

Home Health

Actions/Interventions	Rationales

• Develop with client, family and caregiver plans for dealing with emergency situations, for example:
  ○ Decision making regarding calling ambulance
  ○ Decision tree for calling nurse or physician
	Advanced planning improves the response and outcomes in crisis situations.

• Assist client and family to identify learning needs such as:
  ○ Universal precautions
  ○ How to disinfect surfaces contaminated with blood or body fluids (use 1:10 solution of bleach)
  ○ Protective isolation
  ○ Proper handwashing
  ○ Use of separate razors, toothbrushes, eating utensils, and so on
  ○ Proper cooking of food
  ○ Avoidance of pet excrement
  ○ Avoidance of others with infection
  ○ Skin care, oral hygiene, and wound care
  ○ Use of protective equipment
  ○ Signs and symptoms of infection, fluid and electrolyte imbalance, malnutrition, and pathological changes in behavior and underlying disease process
	This action describes knowledge required to protect the client and the family.

○ CPR and first aid
○ Hazardous waste disposal, for example, soiled dressings, needles, or chemotherapy vials
○ Advanced directive, for example, living wills and durable power of attorney for health care
○ Financial and/or estate planning
○ Symptom management and pain control
○ Administration of required medications
○ Nutrition
○ Care of catheters, IVs, respiratory therapy equipment, and so on
○ Laundry and dishwashing
○ Environmental cleanliness

• Assist client and family to identify resources to meet learning needs identified.

Involvement of the client and the family improves their ability to identify resources and to function more independently. Involvement of the client and the family improves motivation and outcomes.

• Involve client and family in planning and implementing environmental, social, and family adaptations to protect the client.

• Plan with family and client for safe as well as meaningful activities according to client's level of functioning and interests.

Provides for activity while protecting the client and family.

• Assist client and family in life-style adjustments that may be required.

Life-style changes often require support.

FLOW CHART EVALUATION
Flow Chart Expected Outcome 1

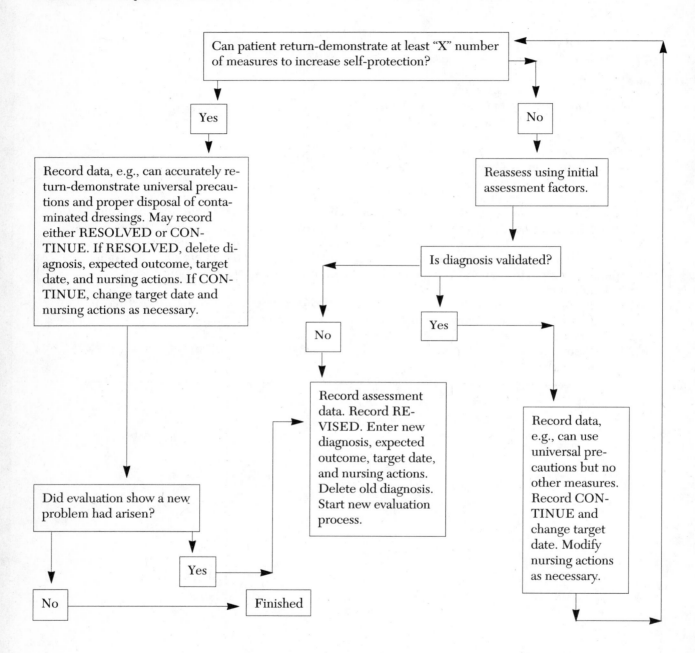

Flow Chart Expected Outcome 2

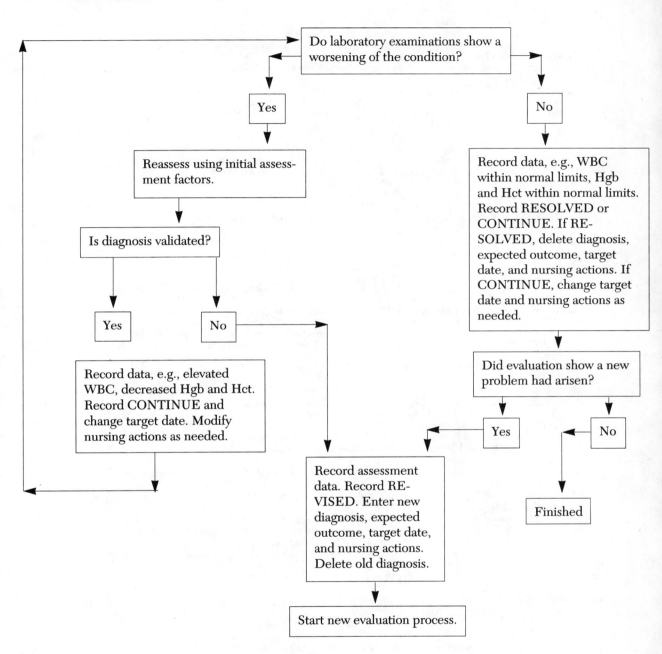

References

1. Rogers, ME: An Introduction to the Theoretical Basis for Nursing. FA Davis, Philadelphia, 1970.
2. Rosenstock, I: Historical origins of the health belief model. In Becker, M (ed): The Health Belief Model and Personal Behavior. Charles B. Slack, Thorofare, NJ, 1974.
3. Arya, O and Bennett, P: Venereal disease control: Case study of university students in Uganda. Int J Health Educ 17:53, 1974.
4. Sackett, DL and Haynes, RB: Compliance with Therapeutic Regimens. John Hopkins Press, Baltimore, 1976.
5. Ridenour, N: Health beliefs, preventive behavioral intentions and knowledge of gonorrhea: Predictors of recidivism? In Monograph 1983 Proceedings of 2nd Annual Sigma Theta Tau Conference, The World of Work: Research in Nursing Practice. Sigma Theta Tau, Indianapolis, 1983.
6. Pender, NJ: Health Promotion in Nursing Practice, ed 2. Appleton-Century-Crofts, East Norwalk, CT, 1987.
7. Brubaker, B: Health promotion: A linguistic analysis. Adv Nurs Sci 5:1, 1983.
8. U.S. Department of Health and Human Services: Healthy People 2000: National Health Promotion and Disease Prevention Objectives. U.S. Government Printing Office, Washington, DC, 1990.
9. Shortridge, L and Valanis, B: The epidemiological model applied in community health nursing. In Stanhope, M and Lancaster, J (eds): Community Health Nursing: Process and Practice for Promoting Health, ed 3. CV Mosby, St. Louis, 1992.
10. Gleit, C and Tatro, S: Nursing diagnosis for healthy individuals. Nurs Health Care 32:151, 1981.
11. Popkess-Vawter, S: Wellness nursing diagnoses: To be or not to be? Nurs Diagn, 2:19, 1991.
12. Schuster, CS and Ashburn, SS: The Process of Human Development: A Holistic Life-Span Approach, ed 3. JB Lippincott, New York, 1992.
13. U.S. Preventive Services Task Force: Guide to Clinical Preventive Services. Williams & Wilkins, Baltimore, 1989.
14. American Academy of Pediatrics: Report of the Committee on Infectious Diseases. Author, Elk Grove Village, IL, 1991.
15. Reece, S: New protection against Haemophilus Influenzae type b infections in infants and young children. The Nurse Practitioner: The Amer J Prim Health Care 16:27, 1991.
16. Centers for Disease Control: Hepatitis B virus: A comprehensive strategy for eliminating transmission in the United States through universal childhood vaccination. Morb Mort Weekly Report 40:RR-13, 1991.
17. Baron, M and Tafuro, P: The extremes of age: The newborn and the elderly. Nurs Clin North Am 20:181, 1985.
18. Schuster, CS: Normal physiological parameters through the life cycle. Nurse Pract 2:25, 1977.
19. Devore, N, Jackson, V, and Peining, S: TORCH infections. Am J Nurs 83:1600, 1983.
20. Immunizations Practices Advisory Committee: Measles prevention: Recommendations of the Immunizations Practices Advisory Committee. Morb Mort Weekly Report 38:1, 1989.
21. American College of Physicians: Guide for Human Immunizations, ed 2. Author, Philadelphia, 1990.
22. Centers for Disease Control: Update on adult immunization. Morb Mort Weekly Report 40:RR-12, 1991.
23. Immunizations Practices Advisory Committee: Pneumococcal polysaccaride vaccine. Morb Mort Weekly Reports 38:64, 1989.
24. Shapiro, E, et al: The protective efficacy of polyvalent pneumococcal polysaccharide vaccine. N Engl J Med 325:1453, 1991.
25. North American Nursing Diagnosis Association: Taxonomy I, Revised 1990. Author, St. Louis, 1990.
26. Anderson, R and Anderson, K: Success and failure attributions in smoking cessations among men and women. Am Assoc Occup Health Nurs J 38:180, 1990.
27. Wewers, M and Gonyon, D: Cigarette craving during the immediate postcessation period. Appl Nurs Res 2:46, 1989.
28. Frost, C: Implications of smoking bans in the workplace. Am Assoc Occup Health Nurs J 39:270, 1991.
29. Volden, C, Langemo, D, Adamson, M, and Oeschsel, L: The relationship of age, gender and exercise practices to measures of health, life-style, and self-esteem. Appl Nurs Res 3:20, 1990.
30. Brown, J and March, S: Use of botanicals for health purposes by members of a prepaid health plan. Res Nurs Health 14:330, 1991.
31. Watzlawick, P, Weakland, J, and Fisch, R: Change: Principles of Problem Formation and Problem Resolution. WW Norton, New York, 1974.
32. Erickson, HC, Tomlin, EM, and Swain, MP: Modeling and Role-Modeling: A Theory and Paradigm for Nursing. Prentice-Hall, Englewood Cliffs, NJ, 1983.
33. Rendom, DC, Davis, DK, Giorella, EC, and Tranzillo, MJ. The right to know, the right to be taught. J Gerontol Nurs 12:33, 1986.
34. Briasco, M: Indoor air pollution: Are employees sick from their work? Am Assoc Occup Health Nurs J 38:375, 1990.
35. Bonheur, B and Young, S: Exercise as a health-promoting lifestyle choice. Appl Nurs Res 4:2, 1991.

36. Rosenkoetter, M: Health promotion: The influence of pets on life patterns in the home. Holist Nurs Pract 5:42, 1991.
37. Centers for Disease Control: Recommendations for the prevention of HIV transmission in health-care setting. Morb Mort Weekly Report 36:1, 1987.
38. Centers for Disease Control: Update: Universal precautions for prevention of transmission of human immunodeficiency virus, hepatitis B virus, and other bloodborne pathogens in health-care settings. Morb Mort Weekly Report 37:377, 1988.
39. Centers for Disease Control: Recommendations for preventing transmission of human immunodeficiency virus and hepatitis B virus to patients during exposure-prone invasive procedures. Morb Mort Weekly Report 40:1, 1991.
40. Benenson, A: Control of communicable disease in man, ed 15. American Public Health Association, Washington, DC, 1990.
41. Dooley, S, et al: Guidelines for preventing the transmission of tuberculosis in health-care settings, with special focus on HIV-related issues. Morb Mort Weekly Report 39:RR-17, 1990.
42. Mace, N and Rabin, P: The 36-hour Day: A Family Guide. John Hopkins Press, Baltimore, 1991.
43. Evans, L and Strumpf, N: Myths about elder restraint. Image 22:124, 1990.
44. Kilpack, V, et al: Using research-based interventions to decrease patient falls. Appl Nurs Res 4:68, 1991.
45. Williams, J: Employee experiences with early return to work programs. Am Assoc Occup Health Nurs 39:64, 1991.
46. National Immunization Campaign: Community Leader's Guide for the National Immunization Campaign. Author, Washington, DC, 1991.
47. North American Nursing Diagnosis Association: Proposed New Nursing Diagnoses: NANDA 10th Conference. Author, St. Louis, 1992.
48. Ridenour, N: View of illness and approaches to therapy: Paradigm and paradox. Unpublished material, 1986.
49. Hagey, R and McDonough, P: The problem of professional labeling. Nurs Outlook 32:151, 1984.
50. Edel, M: Noncompliance: An appropriate nursing diagnosis? Nurs Outlook 33:183, 1985.
51. Breunig, K, et al: Noncompliance as a nursing diagnosis: Current use in clinical practice. In Hurley, M (ed): Classification of Nursing Diagnosis: Proceedings of the Sixth Conference. CV Mosby, St. Louis, 1986.
52. Cooper, M: Chronic illness and nursing's ethical challenge. Holist Nurs Pract 5:10, 1990.
53. Thorne, S: Constructive noncompliance in chronic illness. Holist Nurs Pract 5:62, 1990.
54. Beauchamp, T and Childress, J: Principles of Biomedical Ethics, ed 3. Oxford University Press, New York, 1989.
55. Benner, PE and Wrubel, J: The Primacy of Caring: Stress and Coping in Health and Illness. Addison-Wesley, Menlo Park, CA, 1989.
56. Gadow, S: Covenant without cure: Letting go and holding on in chronic illness. In Watson, J and Ray, M (eds): The Ethics of Care and the Ethics of Cure: Synthesis in Chronicity. National League for Nursing, New York, 1988.
57. Watson, J: Nursing, Human Science and Human Care: A Theory of Nursing. National League for Nursing, New York, 1991.
58. Kontz, M: Compliance redefined and implications for home care. Holist Nurs Pract 3:54, 1989.
59. Clark, AL: Culture and Childbearing. FA Davis, Philadelphia, 1981.
60. Hoffman, L: A co-evolutionary framework for systemic family therapy? In Hansen, JC and Keeney, BP (eds): Diagnosis and Assessment in Family Therapy. Aspen Systems, Rockville, MD, 1983.
61. Smith, F and Knice-Ambinder, M: Promoting medication compliance in clients with chronic mental illness. Holist Nurs Pract 4:70, 1989.
62. Gravely, E and Oseasohn, C: Multiple drug regimens: Medication compliance among veterans 65 years and older. Res Nurs Health 14:51, 1991.
63. Jones, S, Jones, P, and Katz, J: A nursing intervention to increase compliance in otitis media patients. Appl Nurs Res 4:68, 1989.
64. Mandeville, LK and Troiano, N: High-Risk Intrapartum Nursing. JB Lippincott, Philadelphia, 1992.

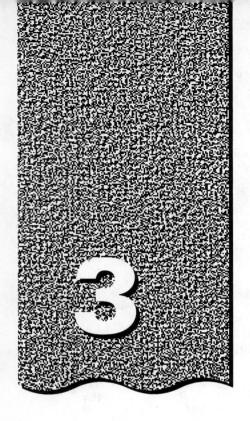

Nutritional-Metabolic Pattern

PATTERN INTRODUCTION
Pattern Description

This pattern focuses on food and fluid intake, the body's use of this intake (metabolism), and problems that might influence intake. Problems in this pattern may arise from a physiologic, psychologic, or sociologic base. Physiologic problems may be primary in nature, for example, vitamin deficiency, or they may arise secondary to another pathophysiologic state, such as a peptic ulcer. Psychologic factors, such as eating to cope with stress or anorexia nervosa, result in an alteration in the nutritional-metabolic pattern. Sociologic factors such as low income, inadequate storage, social isolation, and cultural food preferences may result in an altered nutritional-metabolic state.

A popular saying is "You are what you eat." This is a truism; what we eat is converted to our cellular structure and its functioning. The nutritional-metabolic pattern allows us to look at the whole of this relationship.

Pattern Assessment

1. Weigh patient. Does patient weigh more than the recommended range for his or her height, age, and sex?
   a. Yes (Altered Nutrition: More than Body Requirements, High Risk for or Actual; Fluid Volume Excess; Altered Body Temperature, High Risk for)
   b. No
2. Does the patient weigh less than the recommended range for his or her height, age, and sex?
   a. Yes (Altered Nutrition: Less than Body Requirements; Fluid Volume Deficit, High Risk for or Actual; Altered Body Temperature, High Risk for)
   b. No
3. Have the patient describe a typical day's intake of both food and fluid, including snacks and the pattern of eating. Is the patient's food intake above the average for age, sex, height, weight, and activity level?
   a. Yes (Altered Nutrition: More than Body Requirements, High Risk for or Actual)
   b. No
4. Is the patient's food intake below the average for age, sex, height, weight, and activity level?
   a. Yes (Altered Nutrition: Less than Body Requirements)
   b. No
5. Is the patient's fluid intake sufficient for age, sex, height, weight, activity level, and fluid output?
   a. Yes
   b. No (Fluid Volume Deficit, High Risk for or Actual; Altered Body Temperature, High Risk for)
6. Does the patient show evidence of edema?
   a. Yes (Fluid Volume Excess)
   b. No
7. Is the patient's gag reflex present?
   a. Yes
   b. No (Impaired Swallowing; High Risk for Aspiration)

8. Does the patient cough or choke during eating?
   a. Yes (Impaired Swallowing; High Risk for Aspiration)
   b. No
9. Assess patient's mouth, eyes, and skin. Are these assessments within normal limits (e.g., no lesions, soreness, or inflamed areas)?
   a. Yes
   b. No (Impaired Tissue Integrity; Altered Oral Mucous Membrane)
10. Is patient able to move freely in bed? Ambulate easily?
    a. Yes
    b. No (Impaired Tissue Integrity; Impaired Skin Integrity, High Risk for or Actual)
11. Review patient's temperature measurement. Is the temperature within normal limits?
    a. Yes
    b. No (Ineffective Thermoregulation; Hyperthermia; Hypothermia)
12. Is patient's temperature above normal?
    a. Yes (Ineffective Thermoregulation; Hyperthermia)
    b. No
13. Is patient's temperature below normal?
    a. Yes (Ineffective Thermoregulation; Hypothermia)
    b. No
14. Is patient exhibiting signs or symptoms of infection? Vasoconstriction? Vasodilation? Dehydration?
    a. Yes (Altered Body Temperature: High Risk for)
    b. No
15. Ask patient, "Do you have any problems swallowing food? Fluids?"
    a. Yes (Impaired Swallowing; High Risk for Aspiration)
    b. No

The next questions pertain only to a mother who is breast-feeding.

16. Weigh infant. Is infant's weight within normal limits for his or her age?
    a. Yes (Effective Breast-feeding)
    b. No (Ineffective Breast-feeding)
17. Ask patient, "Do you have any problems or concerns about breast-feeding?"
    a. Yes (Ineffective Breast-feeding)
    b. No (Effective Breast-feeding)

Nursing Diagnoses in This Pattern

1. Aspiration, High Risk for (page 117)
2. Body Temperature, Altered: High Risk for (page 125)
3. Breast-Feeding, Effective (page 134)
4. Breast-Feeding, Ineffective (page 140)
5. Breast-Feeding, Interrupted (page 148)
6. Fluid Volume Deficit (page 155)
   a. High Risk for
   b. Actual
7. Fluid Volume Excess (page 166)
8. Hyperthermia (page 177)

9. Hypothermia (page 186)
10. Infant Feeding Pattern, Ineffective (page 194)
11. Nutrition, Altered: Less than Body Requirements (page 200)
12. Nutrition, Altered: More than Body Requirements (page 215)
    a. High Risk for
    b. Actual
13. Swallowing, Impaired (page 226)
14. Thermoregulation, Ineffective (page 234)
15. Tissue Integrity, Impaired (page 239)
    a. Skin Integrity, Impaired
       (1) High Risk for
       (2) Actual
    b. Oral Mucous Membrane, Altered

Conceptual Information

The nutritional-metabolic pattern requires looking at four separate but closely aligned aspects: nutrition, fluid balance, tissue integrity, and thermoregulation. All four functionally interrelate to maintain the integrity of the overall nutritional-metabolic functioning of the body.

Food and fluid intake provides carbohydrates, proteins, fats, vitamins, and minerals that are metabolized by the body to meet energy needs, maintain intracellular and extracellular fluid balances, prevent deficiency syndromes, and act as catalysts for the body's biochemical reactions.[1]

NUTRITION

Nutrition refers to the intake, assimilation, and use of food for energy, maintenance, and growth of the body.[2] Assisting the patient in maintaining a good nutritional-metabolic status facilitates health promotion and illness prevention and provides dietary support in illness.[1]

Swallowing is associated with the intake of food or fluids. Swallowing is a complex activity that integrates sensory, muscular, and neurological functions. Swallowing generally occurs in four phases: (1) oral preparatory phase, where the food is chewed, mixed with saliva, and prepared for digestion; (2) oral phase, which involves movement of the food backward past the hard palate and downward to the pharynx; (3) pharyngeal phase, when the larynx closes and the food enters the esophagus; and (4) esophageal phase, which includes the peristaltic movement of the food through the esophagus to the stomach. The first two phases are under voluntary control, and the last two phases are involuntarily controlled.

Many factors affect a person's nutritional status. Included in these factors are food availability; food cost; the meaning food has for the individual; cultural, social, and religious mores; and physiologic states that might alter the individual's ability to eat.[3]

In essence, we are initially concerned with the adequacy or inadequacy of the patient's nutritional state. If the diet is adequate, there is no major reason for concern; but we must be sure that all of us are defining "adequacy" in a similar manner.

Most people probably define an adequate diet as lack of hunger; however, professionals look at an adequate diet as being one in which nutrient intake balances with body needs. The diet is adequate if it meets either MDR (minimum daily requirements) or RDA (recommended dietary allowances) standards. The MDR standards are lesser in amount than the RDA standards but do provide enough nutrients to prevent deficiency problems. The RDA standards are the ones more widely used and are the ones that provide us the well-known basic four food groups.[3] The basic four food groups are the best standards to use in assessing dietary adequacy and call for:

Meat group	Meat, eggs, fish, and poultry. Two or more 2- to 3-oz servings per day.
Milk and dairy product group	Milk, ice cream, yogurt, and cheese. Adults: Equivalent of two 8-oz glasses of milk per day. Children: Equivalent of two to three 8-oz glasses of milk per day.
Bread and cereals group	Enriched or whole-grain products. At least four servings daily.
Fruits and vegetables group	At least four servings daily, including at least one vitamin C source daily and a dark green or deep yellow vegetable at least three times a week.

NOTE: Many adults may be lactate intolerant. Lactate enzymes are now available over the counter as a digestive aid for lactase intolerance.

An inadequate nutritional state may be reflective of intake (calories) or use of the intake (metabolism) or a change in activity level. Underweight and overweight are the most commonly seen conditions that reflect alteration in nutrition.[4]

Underweight can be caused by inadequate intake of calories. In some instances, the intake is within the RDA, but there is malabsorption of the intake. The malabsorption or inadequate intake can be due to physiologic reasons (pathophysiology), psychologic reasons (anorexia or bulimia), or cultural factors (lack of resources or religious proscriptions).[4]

Special notice needs to be taken regarding the maternal nutritional needs during the postpartum period. The nutritional needs of the mother are especially important during this fourth trimester. New mothers need optimal nutrition to promote healing of the tissues traumatized during labor and delivery, to restore balance in fluid and electrolytes created by all the rapid changes in the body, and, if the mother is breast-feeding, to produce adequate amounts of milk containing fluid and nutrients for the infant.[5]

The breast-feeding woman can generally meet the nutritional needs of herself and her infant through adequate dietary intake of food and fluids; however, since the energy demand is greater during lactation, RDA standards recommend an additional 500 cal per day above the norm to prevent catabolism of lean tissue.[5] Studies have shown that the caloric intake of breast-feeding women should range from 2460 Kcal to 3060 Kcal per day and that successful breast-feeding may be related to the nutritional status during pregnancy.[6]

Overweight is rarely due to a physiologic disturbance, although a genetic predisposition may exist. Overweight is most commonly due to an imbalance between food and activity habits (that is, increased intake and decreased activity).[4] However, recent research is indicating that there is a metabolic set point and, in actuality, overweight people may be eating less than normal-weight people.

Either underweight or overweight may be a sign of malnutrition (inadequate nutrition) with the result that the patient exhibits signs and symptoms of more than body requirements or less than body requirements. In either instance, the nurse must assess carefully for the overall concept of malnutrition.

FLUID VOLUME

Fluid volume incorporates the aspects of actual fluid amount, electrolytes, and metabolic acid-base balance. Regardless of how much or how little a patient's intake or how much or how little a patient's output is, the fluid, electrolyte, and metabolic acid-base balances are maintained within a relatively narrow margin. This margin is essential for normal functioning in all body systems, and so it must receive close attention in providing care.

Approximately 60 percent of an adult's weight is body fluid (liquid plus electrolytes plus minerals plus cells), and approximately 75 percent of an infant's weight is body fluid. These various parts of body fluid are taken in daily through food and drink and are formed through the metabolic activities of the body.[1,3] The body fluid distribution includes intracellular (within the cells), interstitial (around the cells), and intravascular (in blood cells) fluids. The combination of interstitial and intravascular is known as *extracellular* (outside the cells) *fluid*. Distribution of body fluid is influenced by both the fluid volume and the concentration of electrolytes. Body fluid movement between the compartments is constant and occurs through the mechanisms of osmosis, diffusion, active transport, and osmotic and hydrostatic pressure.[1,3]

Body fluid balance is regulated by intake (food and fluid), output (kidney, gastrointestinal tract, skin, and lungs), and hormonal control (antidiuretic hormone, glucocorticoids, and aldosterone). The largest amount of fluid is located in the intracellular compartment, with the volume of each compartment being regulated predominantly by the solute (mainly the electrolytes).

Electrolytes are either positively or negatively charged particles (ions). The major positively charged electrolytes (cations) are sodium (the main extracellular electrolyte), potassium (the most common intracellular electrolyte), calcium, and magnesium. The major negatively charged electrolytes (anions) are chloride, bicarbonate, and phosphate. The electrolyte compositions of the two extracellular compartments (interstitial and intravascular) are nearly identical. The intracellular fluid contains the same number of electrolytes as the extracellular fluid does, but the intracellular electrolytes carry opposite electrical charges from the electrolytes in the extracellular fluid. This difference between extracellular and intracellular electrolytes is necessary for the electrical activity of nerve and muscle cells.[1,3] Therefore, the electrolytes help regulate cell functioning as well as the fluid volume in each compartment.

Usually the body governs intake through thirst and output through increasing or decreasing body fluid excretion via the kidneys, gastrointestinal tract, and respiration. Because of the way the body governs intake and output, in addition to the effects of pathophysiologic conditions such as shock, hemorrhage, diabetes, and vomiting on intake and output, the patient may enter a state of metabolic acidosis or alkalosis.

Acid-base balance reflects the acidity or alkalinity of body fluids and is expressed as the pH. In essence, the pH is a function of the carbonic acid : bicarbonate ratio.[3] Acid-base balance is regulated by chemical, biologic, and physiologic mechanisms. The chemical regulation involves buffers in the extracellular fluid, while the biologic regulation involves ion exchange across cell membranes. The physiologic regulation is governed in the lungs by carbon dioxide excretion and in the kidneys through metabolism of bicarbonate, acid, and ammonia.[1]

Metabolic acidosis is caused by situations in which the cellular production of acid is excessive (for example, diabetic ketoacidosis), high doses of drugs have to be metabolized (for example, aspirin), or excretion of the produced acid is impaired (for example, renal failure).[3] Weight reduction practices can contribute to the development of acidosis (fad diets or diuretics), as can chemical substance abuse.[1]

Fluid volume is affected by regulatory mechanisms, body fluid loss, or increased fluid intake. Because fluid volume is so readily affected by such a variety of factors, continuous assessment for alterations in fluid volume must be made.

TISSUE INTEGRITY

Nutrition and fluid are vitally important to tissue maintenance and repair. Underlying tissues are protected from external damage by the skin and mucous membranes. Thus, the integrity of the skin is extremely important in the promotion of health because the skin and mucous membranes are the body's first line of defense. The skin also plays a role in temperature regulation and in excretion.

The skin and mucous membranes act as protection through their abundant supply of nerve receptors that alert the body to the external environment (for example, temperature, pressure, or pain). The skin and mucous membrane also act as barriers to pathogens, thus protecting the internal tissues from these organisms.[3]

The skin's superficial blood vessels and sweat glands (eccrine, apocrine) assist in thermoregulation. As the body temperature rises, the superficial blood vessels dilate and the sweat glands increase secretion. These two actions result in increased perspiration which, through evaporation, cools the body. During instances of excessive perspiration, water, sodium chloride, and nonprotein nitrogen are excreted through the skin; this affects fluid volume and osmotic balance. As the body temperature drops, the opposite reactions occur; there is vessel constriction and decreased sweat gland secretion so that body heat is retained internally.

To fulfill its protective function of the underlying tissues, the skin and mucous membranes must be intact. Any change in skin or mucous membrane integrity can allow pathogen invasion and will also allow fluid and electrolyte loss. Skin and mucous membrane integrity rely on adequate nutrition and removal of metabolic wastes internally and externally, cleanliness, and proper positioning. A recent study[7] found that the length of a surgical procedure and extracorporeal circulation were associated with increased risk of skin breakdown for elective procedures. In emergency surgical settings or in cases of patients in poor health (very elderly and medically indigent), age and serum albumin levels might also be predictive of increased risk for skin breakdown.[7] Any factor that compromises nutrition, fluid, or electrolyte balance can result in impairment of skin or mucous membrane integrity or, at least, a high risk for impairment of skin integrity or mucous membrane integrity.

THERMOREGULATION

Thermoregulation refers to the body's ability to adjust its internal core temperature within a narrow range. The core temperature must remain fairly constant for metabolic activities and cellular metabolism to function for the maintenance of life. The core temperature rarely varies more than 1°C (less than 2°F). In fact, the range of temperature that is compatible with life ranges only from approximately 32.2 to 40°C (90 to 104°F).

Both the hypothalamus and the thyroid gland are involved in thermoregulation. The hypothalamus regulates temperature by responding to changes in electrolyte balances. Both the extracellular cations sodium and calcium affect the action potential and depolarization of cells. When there is an imbalance of sodium and calcium within the hypothalamus, hypothermia or hyperthermia can result. The thyroid gland regulates core body temperature by increasing or decreasing metabolic activities and cellular metabolism, thus altering heat production.

Many factors influence thermoregulation. The skin has previously been mentioned as a thermoregulatory organ. Heat is gained or lost to the environment by evaporation, conduction, convection, and radiation. *Evaporation* occurs when body heat transforms the liquid on a person's skin to vapor. *Conduction* is the loss of heat to a colder object through direct contact. When heat is lost to the surrounding cool air, it is called *convection*. *Radiation* occurs when heat is given off to the environment, helping to warm it.

A person generally loses approximately 70 percent of heat from radiation, convection, and conduction. Another 25 percent is lost through insensible mechanisms of the lungs and evaporation from the skin, and about 5 percent is lost in urine and feces. When the body is able to produce and dissipate heat within a normal range, the body is in "heat balance."[8]

The interrelationship of nutrition, fluid balance, thermoregulation, and tissue integrity explains the nursing diagnoses that have been accepted in the nutritional-metabolic pattern. Indeed, if there is an alteration in any one of these four factors, it would be wise for the nurse to assess the other three factors to ensure a complete assessment.

Developmental Considerations

INFANT

Swallowing is a reflex present before birth, since during intrauterine life the fetus swallows amniotic fluid. Following the transition to extrauterine life, the infant learns very rapidly (within 12 to 24 hours) to coordinate sucking and swallowing. There are really no developmental considerations of the act of swallowing since it is a reflex.

The normal process for swallowing involves both the epiglottis and the true vocal cords. These two structures move together to close off the trachea and to allow saliva or solid and liquid foods to pass into the esophagus. The respiratory system is thus protected from foreign bodies.

Salivation is adequate at birth to maintain sufficient moisture in the mouth. However, maturation of many salivary glands does not occur until the third month and corresponds with the baby's learning to swallow at other than a reflex level.[9] Tooth eruption begins at about 6 months of age and stimulates saliva flow and chewing. The infant has a small amount of the enzyme ptyalin, which breaks down starches.

Water constitutes the greatest proportion of body weight of the infant. Approximately 75 to 78 percent of an infant's body weight is water, with about 45 percent of this water found in the extracellular fluid. The newborn infant loses significant water through insensible methods (approximately 35 to 45 percent) because of relatively greater body surface area to body weight. The respiratory rate of an infant is approximately two times that of the adult; therefore, the infant is also losing water through insensible loss from the lungs. The newborn also loses water through direct excretion in the urine (50 to 60 percent) and through fairly rapid peristalsis due to the immaturity of the gastrointestinal (GI) tract.

The newborn is unable to concentrate urine well and is thus more sensitive to inadequate fluid intake or uncompensated water loss.[10] The body fluid reserve of the infant is less than that of the adult, and since the infant excretes a greater volume per kilogram of body weight than the adult, infants are very susceptible to fluid volume deficit. The infant needs to consume fluids equal to 10 to 15 percent of body weight. Fluid and electrolyte requirements for the newborn are 70 to 100 ml per kilogram per 24 hours, 2 mEq of sodium and potassium per kilogram per 24 hours, and 2 to 4 mEq of chloride per kilogram per 24 hours.

The kidney function of the infant does not reach adult levels until 6 months to 1 year of age.[10] The functional capacity of the kidneys is limited, especially during stress. In addition, the glomerular filtration rate is low, tubular reabsorption or secretory capacity is limited, sodium reabsorption is decreased, and the metabolic rate is higher. Therefore, there is a greater amount of metabolic wastes to be excreted. The infant's kidney is less able to excrete large loads of solute-free water than the more mature kidney.[11]

Feeding behavior is important not only for fluid but also for food. The caloric need of the infant is 117 calories per kilogram of body weight.[4]

Breast milk contains adequate nutrients and vitamins for approximately 6 months of life. Some bottle formulas are overly high in carbohydrates and fat (especially cholesterol), which may lead to a potential for increasing fat cells.

The introduction of solid foods should not occur until 4 to 6 months of age. Studies have indicated that there is a relationship between the early introduction of solid food (less than 4 months of age) and overfeeding of either milk or food leading to infant and adult obesity.[4] The infant should be made to feel secure, loved, and unhurried at feeding time. Skin contact is very important for the infant for both physiologic and psychologic reasons.

The skin of an infant is functionally immature, and thus the baby is more prone to skin disorders. Both the dermis and the epidermis are loosely connected, and both are relatively thin, which easily leads to chafing and rub burns.[9] Epidermal layers are permeable, resulting in greater fluid loss. Sebaceous glands, which produce sebum, are very active in late fetal life and early infancy, causing milia and cradle cap, which go away at about 6 months of age. Dry, intact skin is the greatest deterrent to bacterial invasion. Sweat glands (eccrine or apocrine) are not functional in response to heat and emotional stimuli until a few months after birth, and their function remains minimal through childhood. The inability of the skin to contract and shiver in response to heat loss causes ineffective thermal regulation.[4] Also, the infant has no melanocytes to protect against the rays of the sun. This is true of dark-skinned infants as well as light-skinned infants.

Core body temperature in the infant ranges from 97 to 100°F. Temperature in the infant fluctuates considerably because the regulatory mechanisms in the hypothalamus are not fully developed. (It is not considered abnormal for the newborn infant to lose 1 to 2° F immediately after birth.) The infant is unable to shiver to produce heat, nor does the infant have much subcutaneous fat to insulate the body.

However, the infant does have several protective mechanisms by which he or she is able to conserve heat to keep the body temperature fairly stable. These mechanisms include vasoconstriction so that heat is maintained in the inner body core, an increased metabolic rate which increases heat production, a closed body position (the so-called fetal position) which reduces the amount of exposed skin, and the metabolism of adipose tissue.

This particular adipose tissue is called "brown fat" because of the rich supply of blood and nerves. Brown fat composes 2 to 6 percent of body weight of the infant. This brown fat aids in adaptation of the thermoregulation mechanisms.[9] The ability of the body to regulate temperature at the adult level matures at approximately 3 to 6 months of age.

TODDLER AND PRESCHOOLER

By the end of the second year, the child's salivary glands are adult size and have reached functional maturity.[9] The toddler is capable of chewing food, so it stays longer in his or her mouth and the salivary enzymes have an opportunity to begin breaking down the food. The saliva also covers the teeth with a protective film that helps prevent decay. Drooling no longer occurs, since the toddler easily swallows saliva.

Dental caries occur infrequently in children under 3 years; but rampant tooth decay in very young children is almost always related to prolonged bottle feeding at naptime and bedtime (bottle mouth syndrome). The toddler should be weaned from the bottle or at least not allowed to fall asleep with the bottle in her or his mouth.[12] Parents should be taught that the adverse effects of bedtime feeding are greater than thumb sucking or the use of pacifiers.

Affected teeth remain susceptible to decay after nursing stops. If deciduous teeth decay and disintegrate early, spacing of the permanent teeth is affected, and immature speech patterns develop. Discomfort is felt and emotional problems may result.[12]

The first dental examination should be between the ages of 18 and 24 months. Dental hygiene should be started when the first tooth erupts by cleansing the teeth with gauze or cotton moistened with hydrogen peroxide and flavored with a few drops of mouthwash. After 18 months, the child's teeth may be brushed with a soft or medium toothbrush.[12] Fluoride supplements are believed to prevent caries.

In the toddler there is beginning to be the appropriate proportion of body water to body weight (62 percent water).[13] The extracellular fluid is about 26 percent, whereas the adult has about 19 percent extracellular fluid. Toddlers have a smaller reserve of body fluid than adults and lose more body water daily, both from sensible and insensible loss. This age group is highly predisposed to fluid imbalances.[14] These imbalances relate to the fact that the kidneys still are immature, so water conservation is poor and the toddler still has an increased metabolic rate and therefore greater insensible water loss than the adult. However, GI motility slows, so this age group is better able to tolerate fluid loss through diarrhea. The 2- to 3-year-old needs 1100 to 1200 ml (four to five 8-oz glasses) of fluid every 24 hours, whereas the preschooler needs 1300 to 1400 ml fluid every 24 hours.

The caloric need in the toddler is 1000 cal per day or 100 cal/kg at 1 year and 1300 to 1500 cal per day at 3 years. A child should not be forced to "clean the plate" at mealtime, and food should not be viewed as a reward or punishment. Instead, caloric intake should be related to the growing body and energy expenditures.

The caloric need of the preschooler is 85 cal/kg. Eating assumes increasing social significance and continues to be an emotional as well as a physiologic experience.[4] Frustrating or unsettled mealtimes can influence caloric intake, as can manipulative behavior on the part of the child or parent. The child may also be eating empty calories between meals.

In the toddler functional maturity of skin creates a more effective barrier against fluid loss; the skin is not as soft as the infant's, and there is more protection against outside bacterial invasion. The skin remains dry because sebum secretion is limited. Eccrine sweat gland function remains limited, eczema improves, and the frequency of rashes declines.

Skin, as a perceptual organ, experiences significant development during this period. Children like to "feel" different objects and textures and like to be hugged; melanin is formed during these years, and thus the toddler, preschooler, and school-age child are more protected against sun rays.[9]

In addition, small capillaries in the periphery become more capable of constriction and thus thermoregulation. Also, the child is able to sense and interpret that he or she is hot or cold and can voluntarily do something about it.

SCHOOL-AGE CHILD

The child at this age begins losing baby teeth as permanent teeth erupt. The child should not be evaluated for braces until after all 6-year molars have erupted. The permanent teeth are larger than the baby teeth and appear too large for the small face, causing some embarrassment. Good oral hygiene is important.

For the school-age child, the percentage of total body water to total body weight continues to decrease until about 12 years of age, when it approaches adult norms.[14] Changes occur in extracellular fluid from 22 percent at 6 years to 17.5 percent at age 12 due to the proportion of body surface area to mass, increasing muscle mass and connective tissue, and increasing percentage of body fat.

Water is needed for excretion of the solute load. Balance is maintained through mature kidneys, leading to mature concentration of urine and acidifying capacities. Fluid requirements can be calculated by height, weight, surface area, and metabolic activity. The school-age child needs about 1.5 to 3 qt of fluid a day. Additionally, the child needs a slightly positive water balance. The electrolyte values are similar to those for the adult except for phosphorus and calcium (due to bone growth).[14]

The caloric need of the school-age child is greater than that of an adult (approximately 80 cal/kg or 1600 to 2200 cal per day). The ages of 10 to 12 reflect the peak ages of caloric and protein needs of the school-age child (need 50 to 60 cal/kg) due to the accelerated growth, muscle development, and bone mineralization. "The school age child reflects the nutritional experiences of early childhood and the potential for adulthood."[4]

ADOLESCENT

By age 21, all 32 permanent teeth have erupted. The adolescent needs frequent dental visits because of cavities and also for orthodontic work that may be in progress. There are a growth spurt and sexual changes. A total increase in height of 25 percent and a doubling of weight are normally attained.[15] Muscle mass increases and total body water declines with increasing sexual development.[16] The adolescent needs 34 to 45 calories per kilogram per day and tends to have eating patterns based on external environmental cues rather than hunger. Eating becomes more of a social event. There is a high probability of eating disorders such as anorexia and bulimia arising during this age period.

The basal metabolic rate increases, lung size increases, and maximal breathing capacity and forced expiratory volume increase, leading to increased insensible loss of fluid through the lungs. Total body water decreases from 61 percent at age 12 to 54 percent by age 18 due to an increase in fat cells. Fat cells do not have as much water as tissue cells.[16] The water intake need of the adolescent is about 2200 to 2700 ml per 24 hours.

Sebaceous glands become extremely active during adolescence and increase in size. Eccrine sweat glands are fully developed and are especially responsive to emotional stimuli (are more active in males); and apocrine sweat glands also begin to secrete in response to emotional stimuli.[17] Stopped-up sebaceous glands lead to acne, and the adolescent's skin is usually moist.

YOUNG ADULT

The amount of ptyalin in the saliva decreases after 20 years of age; otherwise the digestive system remains fully functioning. The appearance of "wisdom teeth," or third molars, occurs at 20 to 21 years. There are normally four third molars, although some individuals may not fully develop all four. Third molars can create problems for the individual. Eruptions are unpredictable in time and presentation, and molars may come in sideways or facing any direction. This can force other teeth out of alignment, which makes chewing difficult and painful. Often these molars need to be removed to prevent irreparable damage to proper occlusion of jaws. Even normally erupting third molars may be painful. The young adult must see a dentist regularly.

Total body water in the young adult is about 50 to 60 percent. There is a difference between males and females due to the difference in the number of fat cells. Most water in the young adult is intracellular, with only about 20 percent of fluid being extracellular. Growth is essentially finished by this developmental age.

ADULT

Ptyalin has sharply decreased by age 60, as have other digestive enzymes. Total body water is now about 47 to 54.7 percent. Diet and activity indirectly influence the amount of body water by directly altering the amount of adipose tissue. In the adult the activity level is stable or is beginning to decline. The basal metabolic rate gradually decreases along with a reduced demand for calories. The adult needs to reduce calorie intake by approximately 7.5 percent.[18]

Tissues of the integumentary system maintain a healthy, intact, glowing appearance until age 50 or 55 if the individual is receiving adequate vitamins, minerals, other nutrients, and fluids and maintains good personal hygiene. Wrinkles do become more noticeable, however, and body water (from integumentary tissues) decreases, leading to thinner, drier skin that bruises more easily. Fat increases, leading to skin that is not as elastic and will not recede with weight loss; thus bags develop readily under the eyes.[9] Also, skin wounds heal more slowly because of decreased cell regeneration.

OLDER ADULT

In the older adult the mouth undergoes changes associated with aging, and these changes can affect nutrition. Tooth decay, loss of teeth, degeneration of jaw bone, progressive gum recession, and increased reabsorption of the dental arch can make eating and chewing a difficult task for the elderly person if good dental health has not been maintained. Reduced chewing ability, decrease in salivation, and perhaps poorly fitting dentures compound the problem of poor nutrition of the aged. Aging causes an atrophy of olfactory organs and a loss of taste buds. Usually salt and sweet taste buds are lost first, with bitter and sour taste buds remaining intact; therefore, food has little flavor. This leads to aged persons having a characteristic unpleasant bitter taste in their mouths called *dysgeusia*.[19]

Loss of taste is compounded by gum disease, poor teeth, or dentures. Fifty percent of the elderly have lost their teeth. Ninety percent who have natural teeth have periodontal disease.[20] The aged are especially vulnerable to oral carcinoma.[4]

Total body water of the older adult is about 45 to 50 percent. Although values are within normal, the elderly cannot tolerate extremes of temperature well because of slower response time to adapt to change. Excess heat and overexertion are not tolerated well by the older adult. The older adult naturally has drier, wrinkled skin, so assessment of skin in the elderly for alteration in fluid volume needs to be interpreted carefully. The recommended sites to use in assessing skin turgor in the older adult include the abdomen, sternum, and forehead. There is a decrease in number of body cells and adipose tissue, leading to a decrease in total body water. However, cell size increases.

Serum protein (albumin) production is decreased, but globulin is increased. Therefore, there is not much difference in blood volume. However, the nurse needs to consider the proportion of blood volume to body weight.

There is a decrease in nephrotic tubular functioning, which affects removal of waste, urine concentration, and dilution. This in turn leads to a decrease in specific gravity and urine osmolarity. There is decreased bladder capacity, leading to nocturia. Therefore, the elderly may limit fluid in the evening to offset nocturia, but limiting fluids may lead to nocturnal dehydration. Sodium and chloride levels remain constant, but potassium decreases. In the older adult the blood level and excretion of aldosterone decrease 50 percent if sodium is depleted.[21]

Gonadal hormones may influence fluid and electrolyte balance in terms of sodium and water retention. Therefore, with the loss of hormones in aging, there is a decrease in sodium and water retention.

Many changes are occurring in the GI tract (decreased enzyme secretion, general gastric irritation, decreased nutrient and drug absorption, decreased HCl secretion, decreased peristalsis and elimination, and decreased sphincter muscle tone) of the older adult that make nutrition a primary concern.[4] The older adult needs decreased calories but needs an increase in vitamins and trace elements as well as an adequate intake of protein, fat, carbohydrates, bulk, and electrolytes (sodium, potassium, calcium, and magnesium). However, financial concerns may lead the elderly to buy inappropriate foods containing empty calories.

The skin of the older adult becomes drier and thinner; skin lesions or discoloration and scaliness (keratosis) may appear. Integumentary changes in the older adult are readily noticeable because of our society's emphasis on youth and beauty.[9] The older adult has wrinkles, mostly in the face; exposure to the sun also produces and hastens formation of wrinkles. Fatty layers are lost in the trunk, face, and extremities, leading to the appearance of increased joint size throughout the body. The skin is nonelastic and may lose water to the air in low-humidity situations, which results in chapping.

Extremes of temperature are difficult for the elderly. Body temperature may increase because of a decrease in size, number, and functioning of the sweat glands; or the person may need a sweater because of decreased fat and peripheral circulation. Fragile blood vessels lead to bruising. The older adult loses melanocytes, leading to pale, light skin; hair turns gray and the elderly lose hair. Older women may have hair on the face or chin due to androgen-estrogen imbalances.

There is an absolute decrease in intracellular water and a decrease in both sebaceous and sweat glands. With age, skin becomes less effective as a tactile organ (touch, pressure, pain, and local temperature changes) because of the slowing of impulses to the brain and a decrease in the number of receptors.[22] Therefore, elderly persons may burn or have frostbite and not be cognizant of the problem.

APPLICABLE NURSING DIAGNOSES
Aspiration, High Risk for

DEFINITION

The state in which an individual is at risk for entry of gastrointestinal secretions, oropharyngeal secretions, or solids or fluids into tracheobronchial passages.[23]

NANDA TAXONOMY: EXCHANGING 1.6.1.4
DEFINING CHARACTERISTICS (RISK FACTORS)

1. Reduced level of consciousness
2. Depressed cough and gag reflexes
3. Presence of tracheostomy or endotracheal tube
4. Incompetent lower esophageal sphincter
5. Gastrointestinal tubes
6. Tube feedings
7. Medication administration
8. Situations hindering elevation of upper body
9. Increased intragastric pressure
10. Increased gastric residual
11. Decreased gastrointestinal motility
12. Delayed gastric emptying
13. Impaired swallowing
14. Facial, oral, or neck surgery or trauma
15. Wired jaws

RELATED FACTORS

The risk factors also serve as the related factors for this nursing diagnosis.

RELATED CLINICAL CONCERNS

1. Closed head injury
2. Any diagnosis with presenting symptoms of nausea and vomiting

3. Bulemia
4. Any diagnosis requiring use of a nasogastric tube
5. Spinal cord injury

HAVE YOU SELECTED THE CORRECT DIAGNOSIS?

Impaired Swallowing *Swallowing* means that when food or fluids are present in the mouth, the brain signals both the epiglottis and the true vocal cords to move together to close off the trachea so that the food and fluids can pass into the esophagus and thus into the stomach. Impaired Swallowing implies that there is a mechanical or physiologic obstruction between the oropharynx and the esophagus that prevents food or fluids from passing into the esophagus. In High Risk for Aspiration there may or may not be an obstruction between the oropharynx and the esophagus. The major pathophysiologic dysfunction that occurs in High Risk for Aspiration is the inability of the epiglottis and true vocal cords to move to close off the trachea. This inability to close off the trachea may occur because of pathophysiologic changes in the structures themselves; or because messages *to* the brain are absent, decreased, or impaired; or because messages *from* the brain are absent, decreased, or impaired. (See page 226.)

Ineffective Airway Clearance In Ineffective Airway Clearance, the patient is unable to effectively clear secretions from the respiratory tract due to some of the same related factors as are found with High Risk for Aspiration. However, in Ineffective Airway Clearance, the defining characteristics (abnormal breath sounds, cough, change in rate or depth of respirations, and so on) are associated directly with respiratory function, whereas the defining characteristics of High Risk for Aspiration are directly or indirectly related to the oropharyngeal mechanisms that protect the tracheobronchial passages from the entrance of foreign substances. (See page 338.)

EXPECTED OUTCOMES

1. Will demonstrate no risk factors of aspiration by (date) and/or
2. Will implement plan to offset High Risk for Aspiration by (date)

TARGET DATE

Aspiration is life-threatening. Initial target dates should be stated in hours. After the number of risk factors have been reduced, the target date can be moved to 2- to 4-day intervals.

NURSING ACTIONS/INTERVENTIONS WITH RATIONALES

Adult Health

Actions/Interventions	Rationales
• Have suction equipment available.	Would be required for emergency relief of aspiration.

- Sit patient up or elevate head of bed, especially during meals, if not contraindicated. If contraindicated, place patient on right side.
- Feed slowly and cut food into small bites. Instruct patient to chew thoroughly. Observe gag and cough reflexes. Monitor for food and secretion accumulation in mouth. Sit with patient during mealtime if cognitive functioning indicates a need for close observation.
- Teach patient to be cognizant of closing off trachea before attempting to swallow:
  - Have the patient clear his or her throat by coughing and expectorating. If patient is unable to expectorate, suction the secretions.
  - Have the patient inhale as food in put in the mouth.
  - Have the patient then perform a Valsalva maneuver as he or she is swallowing.
  - Have the patient cough, swallow again, and exhale deeply.
  - Start with soft, nonacidic, noncrumbly foods rather than liquids. (Liquids are more difficult to control.)
  - Discuss with patient the purpose for any alterations in care necessitated by this diagnosis, for example, upright position, small and frequent meals, or soft foods.
- Offer small, frequent feedings at least six times a day rather than three large meals per day. Offer soft foods rather than a full liquid diet.
- Delay fluids associated with meals for at least 30 minutes after each meal.
- Have patient cough and clear secretions prior to offering any food or fluid.
- Teach patient to limit conversation while either eating or drinking.
- Provide calm, relaxed atmosphere during mealtime, and assist patient with relaxation exercises as needed.
- Teach patient and family the Heimlich maneuver, and have them return-demonstrate at least daily for 3 days before discharge.
- Teach patient and family suctioning technique as needed, including appropriate ordering of supplies.
- Refer patient and family to appropriate resources. (See Appendix B.)

Decreases risk of reflux from stomach, thus decreasing risk of aspiration. Placing patient on right side facilitates food passage into the pylorus.
All of these measures are designed to reduce the risk of aspiration. Decreased sensation may allow pocketing of food in mouth.

Reduces risk of aspiration and promotes compliance by involving patient in his or her plan of care.

Liquids are more easily aspirated than soft food. Smaller and more frequent feedings reduce risk of aspiration while maintaining nutritional status.
Decreases the likelihood of coughing, gagging, and choking.

Would assist in episodes of choking and would allow patient and family to feel comfortable with level of expertise before going home.
Provides long-term teaching and support.

Child Health

Actions/Interventions	Rationales
• Determine best position for patient as determined by underlying risk factors, for example, head of bed elevated 30 degrees with infant propped on right side after feeding.	Natural upper airway patency is facilitated by upright position. Turning to right side decreases likelihood of drainage into trachea rather than esophagus in the event of choking.
• Check bilateral breath sounds every 30 minutes or with any change in respiratory status.	In the event of aspiration, increased gurgling and rales with correlated respiratory difficulty (from mild to severe) will be noted.
• Measure amount of residual, immediately before feeding, in nasogastric tube, and report any excess beyond 10 ml of volume.	Monitors the speed of digestion and indicates the patient's ability to tolerate the feeding.
• Note and record the presence of any facial trauma or surgery of face or head or any neck-associated drainage.	Monitoring for these risk factors will assist in preventing unexpected or undetected aspiration.
• Monitor for risk factors that would promote aspiration, for example, increased intracranial pressure, Reyes syndrome, nausea associated with medications, cerebral palsy, or neurologic damage.	An increased stimulation or sensitivity to the gag reflex increases the likelihood of choking and possible aspiration.
• Assist patient and family to identify factors that will help prevent aspiration, for example, avoiding self-stimulation of gag reflex, avoiding deep oral or pharyngeal suctioning, or chewing food thoroughly.	
• Provide opportunities for patient and family to ask questions or vent feelings regarding risk for aspiration by scheduling at least 30 minutes twice a day at (times) for discussing concerns.	Allows an opportunity to decrease anxiety, provides time for teaching, and allows individualized home care planning.
• Teach family and patient (if old enough) age appropriate cardiopulmonary resuscitation (CPR) method, first aid, and Heimlich maneuver.	Basic safety measures for dangers of aspiration.

Women's Health

NOTE: The following actions pertain to the newborn infant in the presence of meconium in amniotic fluid.

Actions/Interventions	Rationales
• Alert obstetrician and pediatrician to the presence of meconium in amniotic fluid.	Presence of meconium alerts health care providers to possible complications.
• Assemble equipment and be prepared for	Basic emergency preparedness.

resuscitation of the newborn at the time of delivery.
- Be prepared to suction infant's nasopharynx and oropharynx while head of infant is still on the perineum.
- Immediately evaluate and record the respiratory status of the newborn infant.
- Assist pediatrician in viewing the vocal cords of infant (have various sizes of pediatric laryngoscopes available); if meconium is present, be prepared to insert endotracheal tube for further suctioning.
- Continue to evaluate and record infant's respiratory status.

There is no designated time frame for observation; however, the nurse needs to continue to evaluate the infant for at least 12 to 24 hours for respiratory distress and the complications of pulmonary interstitial emphysema, pneumomediastinum, pneumothorax, persistent pulmonary hypertension, central nervous system (CNS) dysfunction, and renal failure. These infants should be placed in a level II or III nursery. Reduces anxiety.

- Reassure parents by keeping them informed of actions.
- Allow opportunities for parents to verbalize fears and ask questions.

Reduces anxiety and provides teaching opportunity.

Mental Health

NOTE: Clients receiving electroconvulsive therapy (ECT) are at risk for this diagnosis.

Actions/Interventions	Rationales
• Remain with client who has had ECT until gag reflex and swallowing have returned to normal. Monitor gag reflex and swallowing every 30 minutes until they return to normal.	Basic safety measures until client can demonstrate control.
• Place client who has had ECT on right side until reactive.	Lessens the probability of aspiration through the influence of gravity on stomach contents.
• Clients in four-point restraint should be placed on right side or stomach. Elevate client's head to eat, and remove restraints one at a time to facilitate eating. Request that oral medications be changed to liquid forms.	Lessens probability of aspiration due to difficulty in swallowing tablets or pills that might cause gagging.
• Observe clients receiving antipsychotic agents for possible suppression of cough reflex.	One side effect of these medications is suppression of the cough reflex. Loss of this reflex promotes the likelihood of aspiration.

Gerontic Health

Actions/Interventions	Rationales
• Older adults may develop a decreased gag reflex. To reduce the risk of aspiration: ○ Monitor gag reflex before any procedures involving anesthesia, such as bronchoscopy, esophagogastroduodenoscopy, or general surgery.	Establishes baseline data to use for comparison after the procedure is completed.
• Monitor gag reflex postprocedure prior to giving fluids or solids.	Ensuring return of gag reflex will decrease risk of aspiration once oral intake is resumed.

Home Health

The nursing actions for home health care of this diagnosis are the same as the actions enumerated in the adult health portion.

FLOW CHART EVALUATION
Flow Chart Expected Outcome 1

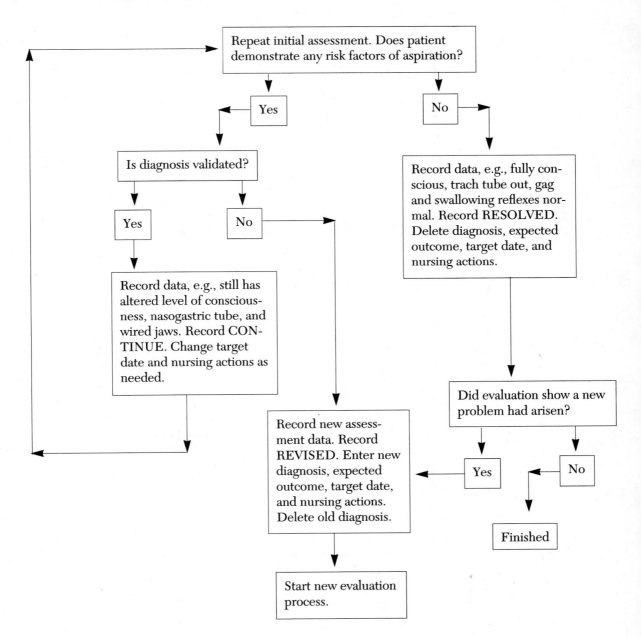

Repeat initial assessment. Does patient demonstrate any risk factors of aspiration?

Yes

No

Is diagnosis validated?

Yes

No

Record data, e.g., fully conscious, trach tube out, gag and swallowing reflexes normal. Record RESOLVED. Delete diagnosis, expected outcome, target date, and nursing actions.

Record data, e.g., still has altered level of consciousness, nasogastric tube, and wired jaws. Record CONTINUE. Change target date and nursing actions as needed.

Record new assessment data. Record REVISED. Enter new diagnosis, expected outcome, target date, and nursing actions. Delete old diagnosis.

Did evaluation show a new problem had arisen?

Yes

No

Finished

Start new evaluation process.

Flow Chart Expected Outcome 2

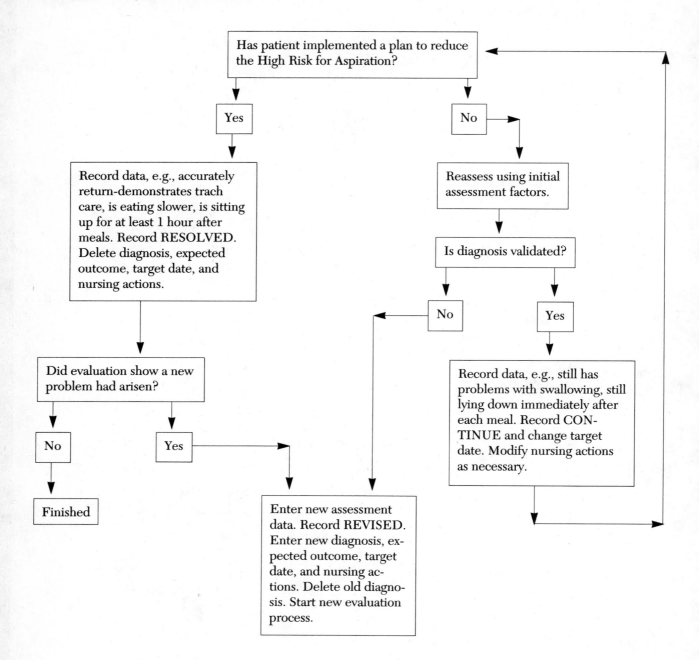

Body Temperature, Altered: High Risk for

DEFINITION

The state in which the individual is at risk for failure to maintain body temperature within normal range.

NANDA TAXONOMY: EXCHANGING 1.2.2.1

DEFINING CHARACTERISTICS (RISK FACTORS)

1. Extremes of age
2. Extremes of weight
3. Exposure to cold or cool or warm or hot environments
4. Dehydration
5. Inactivity or vigorous activity
6. Medications causing vasoconstriction or vasodilation
7. Altered metabolic rate
8. Sedation
9. Inappropriate clothing for environmental temperature
10. Illness or trauma affecting temperature regulation

RELATED FACTORS

The risk factors also serve as the related factors for this nursing diagnosis.

RELATED CLINICAL CONCERNS

1. Any infectious process
2. Hyperthyroidism/hypothyroidism
3. Any surgical procedure
4. Head injuries

HAVE YOU SELECTED THE CORRECT DIAGNOSIS?

High Risk for Altered Body Temperature needs to be differentiated from Hypothermia, Hyperthermia, and Ineffective Thermoregulation.

Hypothermia   Hypothermia is the condition under which a person maintains a temperature lower than normal for him or her. This means that the body is probably dissipating heat normally but is unable to produce heat normally. In High Risk for Altered Body Temperature, both heat production and heat dissipation are potentially nonfunctional. In Hypothermia, a lower-than-normal body temperature can be measured. In High Risk for Altered Body Temperature, temperature measurement may not show an abnormality until the condition has changed to Hyperthermia or Hypothermia. (See page 186.)

Hyperthermia   Hyperthermia is the condition under which a person maintains a temperature higher than normal. This means that the body is probably producing heat normally but is unable to dissipate the heat normally. Both

Continued

HAVE YOU SELECTED THE CORRECT DIAGNOSIS?—*Continued*

heat production and heat dissipation are potentially nonfunctional in High Risk for Altered Body Temperature. As with Hypothermia, a temperature measurement will show an abnormal measurement. (See page 177.)

Ineffective Thermoregulation   Ineffective Thermoregulation means that a person's temperature fluctuates between being too high and too low. There is nothing wrong, generally, with heat production or heat dissipation; however, the thermoregulatory systems in the hypothalamus or the thyroid are dysfunctional. Again, a temperature measurement will show an abnormality. (See page 234.)

EXPECTED OUTCOMES

1. Will have no alteration in body temperature by (date) and/or
2. Will describe at least (number) measures to keep body temperature within a range of 98 to 99° F by (date)

TARGET DATE

Initial target dates would be stated in hours. After stabilization, target dates could be extended to 2 to 3 days.

NURSING ACTIONS/INTERVENTIONS WITH RATIONALES

Adult Health

Actions/Interventions	Rationales
• Monitor for factors contributing to High Risk for Alteration in Body Temperature at least every 2 hours on (odd/even) hour. [Refer to Defining Characteristics (Risk Factors).]	Detects overproduction or underproduction of heat.
• Monitor temperature at least every 2 hours on (odd/even) hour.	
• Note pattern of temperature for last 48 hours.	Assists in ascertaining any trends. Typical viral-bacterial differentiation may be possible to detect on temperature curves.
• Monitor skin integrity and mucous membrane integrity every 2 hours on (odd/even) hour.	Allows early detection of impaired tissue integrity, which can lead to infection.
• Maintain fluid and electrolyte balance. Monitor intake and output every hour.	Adequate hydration assists in maintaining normal body core temperature.
• If temperature is above or below 98.6° F (or parameters defined by physician), take appropriate measures to bring temperature	

back to normal range. Refer to nursing actions for Hypothermia, page 186, or Hyperthermia, page 177.

- Follow up with cultures for identification of causative organisms if infection is present.

Identification of organism allows determination of most appropriate antibiotic therapy.

- Maintain consistent room temperature.

Prevents overheating or overcooling due to environment.

- Teach patient to wear appropriate clothing and modify routines to prevent alterations in body temperature:
  - Close-knit undergarments in winter to prevent heat loss
  - Hat and gloves in cold weather because heat is lost from head and hands
  - Wool in preference to synthetic fibers because wool provides better insulation
  - Socks or stockings at night
  - Light, loose, but protecting clothing in hot weather
  - Hat in hot weather to protect head
  - Use of sheet blankets rather than regular sheets
  - Staying indoors on windy days
  - Encourage patient to work outdoors in early morning and to work for limited periods of time
  - Give frequent, small meals every 3 to 4 hours and warm liquids every 2 hours on the (odd/even) hour

Regulates constant metabolism and provides warmth.

- Avoid sedatives and tranquilizers that depress cerebral function and circulation.

Risk factors for this diagnosis.

- Assist patient to learn to assess biorhythms —generally early morning is the period of lowest body metabolic activity; add extra clothes until food and physical movement stimulate increased cellular metabolism and circulation.

Helps determine peak and trough of temperature variations.

- Alternate physical and sedentary activity every 2 hours on (odd/even) hour.

Assists in maintaining consistency in metabolic functioning.

- Teach patients to use heating pads and electric blankets in a safe manner.

Basic safety measure.

- Refer to nursing diagnoses Hypothermia or Hyperthermia for interventions related to these situations once the alteration has occurred.

Child Health

Actions/Interventions	Rationales
• Monitor temperature at least every hour.	The young infant and child may lack mature thermoregulatory capacity. Temperatures either too high (102°F or above) or too low (below 97°F) may bring about spiraling metabolic demise for acid or base status. Seizures and shock may follow.
• If temperature is less than 97°F rectally (or parameters defined by physician), take appropriate measures for maintaining temperature: ○ *Infants*: Radiant warmer or isolette. ○ *Older child*: Thermoblanket. ○ Administer medications as ordered.	Young infants and children may not be able to initiate compensatory regulation of temperature, especially in premature and altered CNS-immune conditions. These basic measures must be taken to safeguard a return to homeostatic condition.
• If temperature is above 101°F, take appropriate measures to bring temperature back to normal range (or at least 98 to 100°F): ○ Administer Tylenol, antibiotics, or other medications as ordered. ○ Monitor and document related symptoms with specific regard for potential febrile seizures. ○ Monitor for the development of febrile seizures, and check for history of febrile seizures.	Young infants and childen may have febrile seizures due to immature thermoregulatory mechanisms, and they must be appropriately safeguarded against further sequelae.
○ If infant or child has reduced threshold for seizures during times of fever, be prepared to treat seizures with anticonvulsants, maintain airway, and provide for safety from injury.	Anticipatory planning promotes optimal resuscitation efforts.
○ Provide appropriate teaching to child and parents related to hyperthermia and hypothermia, for example, temperature measurement, proper clothing, use of Tylenol (not aspirin), food and fluid intake, and use of tepid baths.	Self-care will empower and foster long-term confidence as well as reduce anxiety.
○ Be cautious and do not overtax the infant or child with congestive heart failure or pulmonary problems by allowing a temperature elevation to develop.	Increased metabolic demands in the presence of an already taxed cadiopulmonary status can become severe, resulting in life-threatening conditions if left untreated.

Women's Health

Actions/Interventions	Rationales
• Assist patient in identifying life-style adjustments necessary to maintain body temperature within normal range during various life phases, for example, perimenopause, menopause.	So-called hot flashes related to changes in the body's core temperature can be somewhat controlled in women by estrogen replacement therapy; however, as hormone levels fluctuate with the aging process, some hot flashes will occur. These can be helped by adjusting the environment, for example, room temperature, amount of clothing, or temperature of fluid intake.
• Maintain house at a consistent temperature level of 70 to 72°F.	
• Keep bedroom cooler at night, and layer blankets or covers that can be discarded or added as necessary.	
• Have patient drink cool fluids, for example, iced tea or cold soda.	
• Have patient wear clothing that is layered, so that jackets can be discarded or added as necessary.	
• In collaboration with physician, assist patient in understanding role of estrogen and the amount of estrogen replacement necessary during perimenopause and menopause.	Individuals have unique, different requirements as to the amount of estrogen necessary to maintain appropriate hormone levels. It is of prime importance that each patient can recognize what her body's needs are and communicate this information to the health care provider.[5]

Mental Health

Actions/Interventions	Rationales
• Observe clients receiving neuroleptic drugs for signs and symptoms of hyperthermia. Teach clients these symptoms, and caution them to decrease their activities in the warmest part of the day and to maintain adequate hydration, especially if they are receiving lithium carbonate with these drugs.	Neuroleptic drugs may decrease the ability to sweat and therefore make it difficult for the client to reduce body temperature.[24,25]
• Observe clients receiving antipsychotics and antidepressants for loss of thermoregulation. The elderly client, especially, should be	Antipsychotics and antidepressants can cause a loss of thermoregulation. The client's learned avoidance behavior can be altered

Continued

Actions/Interventions	Rationales
monitored for this side effect. Provide the client with extra clothing and blankets to maintain comfort. Protect this client from contact with uncontrolled hot objects such as space heaters and radiators. Heating pads and electric blankets can be used with supervision.	and consciousness can be clouded due to medications.[24,25]
• Do not provide electric heating devices to the client who is on suicide precautions or who has alterations in thought processes.	Basic safety measure.
• Notify physician if client receiving antipsychotic agents has an elevation in temperature or flu-like symptoms.	Antipsychotics, especially chlorpromazine and thioridazine, can cause agranulocytosis. This risk is greatest 3 to 8 weeks after therapy has begun.[24,25] Clients who have experienced this side effect in the past should not receive the drug again since a repeat episode is highly possible.
• Review client's complete blood count (CBC) before drug is started, and report any abnormalities on subsequent CBCs to the physician.	Basic monitoring for agranulocytosis.
• Clients receiving phenothiazines should be monitored for hot, dry skin, CNS depression, and rectal temperature elevations (can be up to 108°F). Monitor client's temperature three times a day while awake at (times). Notify physician of alterations.	These medications can produce hyperthermia, which can be fatal. This hyperthermia is due to a peripheral autonomic effect.[24,25]
• Monitor clients receiving tricyclic antidepressants (TCAs) and the monoamine oxidase inhibitors (MAOIs) for alterations in temperature three times a day while awake (note times here). Notify physician of any alterations.	The side effect of a hyperpyretic crisis can be produced in clients receiving these medications.[24,25]

Gerontic Health

Nursing actions for gerontics are the same as those given in the Adult Health Section.

Home Health

Actions/Interventions	Rationales
• Teach measures to decrease or eliminate High Risk for Alteration in Body Temperature:	Appropriate environmental temperature regulation will provide support for physiologic thermoregulation.

- ○ Wearing appropriate clothing
- ○ Taking appropriate care of underlying disease
- ○ Avoiding exposure to extremes of environmental temperature
- ○ Maintaining temperature within norms for age, sex, and height
- ○ Ensuring appropriate use of medications
- ○ Ensuring proper hydration
- ○ Ensuring appropriate shelter
- • Assist client and family to identify life-style changes that may be required:
  - ○ Learn survival techniques if client works or plays outdoors.
  - ○ Measure temperature in a manner appropriate for the developmental age of the person.
  - ○ Maintain ideal weight.
  - ○ Avoid substance abuse.
- • Involve client and family in planning, implementing, and promoting reduction or elimination of the High Risk for Alteration in Body Temperature by establishing family conferences to set mutual goals and to improve communication.
- • Consult with appropriate assistive resources as indicated. (See Appendix B.)

Support is often helpful when individuals and families are considering lifestyle alterations.

Involvement of client and family provides opportunity to increase motivation and enhance self-care.

Cost-effective and appropriate use of available resources.

FLOW CHART EVALUATION
Flow Chart Expected Outcome 1

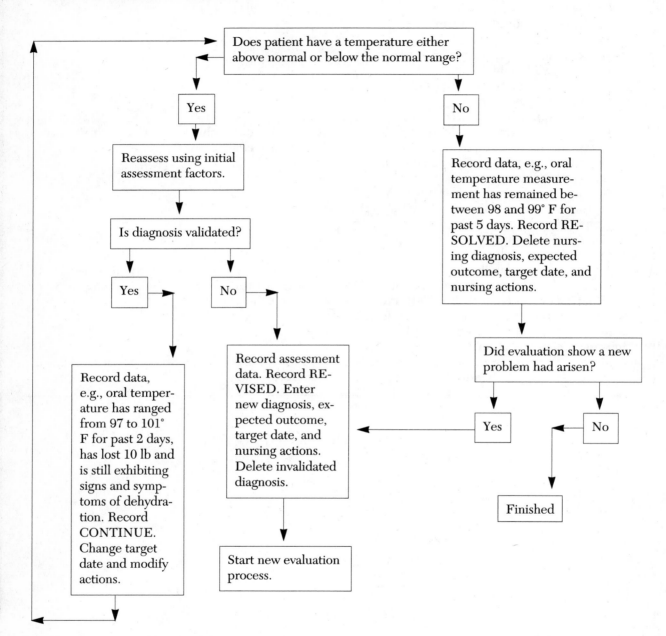

Flow Chart Expected Outcome 2

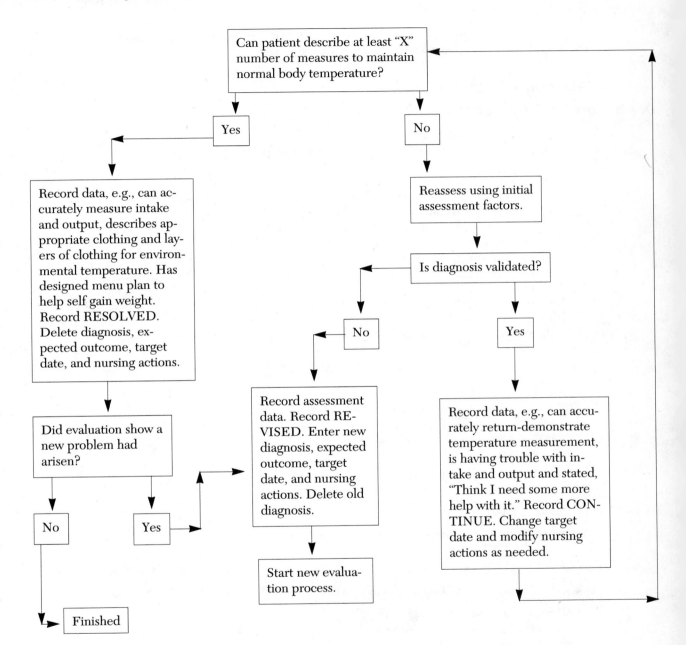

Breast-Feeding, Effective

DEFINITION

The state in which a mother-infant dyad or family exhibits adequate proficiency and satisfaction with the breast-feeding process.

NANDA TAXONOMY: MOVING 6.5.1.3

DEFINING CHARACTERISTICS

1. Major defining characteristics:
   a. Mother able to position infant at breast to promote a successful latch-on response
   b. Infant content after feeding
   c. Regular and sustained suckling and swallowing at the breast
   d. Appropriate infant weight patterns for age
   e. Effective mother-infant communication patterns (infant cues elicit maternal interpretation and response)
2. Minor defining characteristics:
   a. Signs and/or symptoms of oxytocin release (let-down or milk ejection reflex)
   b. Adequate infant elimination patterns for age
   c. Eagerness of infant to nurse
   d. Maternal verbalization of satisfaction with the breast-feeding process

RELATED FACTORS

1. Basic breast-feeding knowledge
2. Normal breast structure
3. Normal infant oral structure
4. Infant gestational age greater than 34 weeks
5. Support sources
6. Maternal confidence

RELATED CLINICAL CONCERNS

Since this is a wellness diagnosis, there will be no related clinical concerns.

HAVE YOU SELECTED THE CORRECT DIAGNOSIS?

Ineffective Breast-Feeding   Effective Breast-Feeding is a wellness diagnosis. It signifies a successful experience for both the mother and the baby. If there is a problem with breast-feeding, then the appropriate diagnosis is Ineffective Breast-Feeding (see page 140). These two diagnoses could be considered to be at opposite ends of a continuum.

Altered Parenting   Effective Breast-Feeding focuses upon the nutrition and growth of the infant rather than on breast-feeding as a mechanism of attachment with the infant. Although Effective Breast-Feeding contributes to the attachment of the infant to the mother and the mother to the infant, the supplying of the infant with nutrition by breast-feeding or by formula-feeding should be differentiated from attachment theories that are addressed in Altered Parenting: High Risk for/Actual/Role Conflict. (See page 742.)

EXPECTED OUTCOMES

1. The infant will have:
   a. Adequate weight gain and return to birth weight by 3 weeks of age
   b. Six or more wet diapers in 24 hours
   c. At least two stools every 24 hours and/or
2. Mother will recognize hunger cues of infant and demonstrate at least two breast-feeding techniques by (date).

TARGET DATE

While it usually takes 2 to 3 weeks for the mother and infant to establish a mutual pattern of feeding, an initial target date of 4 days should be set to assure an effective beginning to the breast-feeding process.

NURSING ACTIONS/INTERVENTIONS WITH RATIONALES

Adult Health

For this diagnosis, the Women's Health nursing actions serve as the generic actions. This diagnosis would probably not arise on an adult health care unit.

Child Health

It is doubtful this diagnosis would arise on a child health care unit. Please see nursing actions under Women's Health.

Women's Health

NOTE: If the diagnosis of Effective Breast-Feeding has been made, the most appropriate nursing action is continued support for the diagnosis. Successful lactation can be established in any woman who does not have structural anomalies of the milk ducts and who exhibits a desire to breast-feed. This includes adoptive mothers as well as birthmothers. The following actions serve to facilitate the development of Effective Breast-Feeding.

Actions/Interventions	Rationales
• Review the mother's knowledge base regarding breast-feeding prior to the initial breast-feeding of the infant. • Demonstrate and assist the mother and	To determine the basis for assistance and teaching. Avoid unessential repetition for the mother. Successful lactation depends upon

Continued

Actions/Interventions	Rationales
significant other with correct breast-feeding techniques, for example, positioning and latch-on.	understanding the basic "how-to's" and correct techniques for the actual feeding act.
• Teach mother and significant other basic information related to successful breast-feeding, for example, milk supply, diet, rest, breast care, breast engorgement, infant hunger cues, and parameters of a healthy infant.	
• Assess the mother's breasts for graspable nipples, surgical scars, skin integrity, and abnormalities prior to the initial breast-feeding of the infant.	Provides the assessment base for diagnosing of potential problems as well as the base for developing strategies for success.
• Assess the infant for ability to breast-feed prior to breast-feeding, for example, state of awareness and physical abnormalities.	
• Place infant to breast within the first hour after birth unless contraindicated (mother or infant instability) and on cue after this.	It is important to work with the infant's sleep-wake cycle in establishing breast-feeding after birth. If the infant can successfully suckle immediately after birth, this establishes a successful and encouraging pattern for both the mother and the infant. This assists in establishing and maintaining the milk supply. It also allows the mother to provide emotional support as well as nutritional support to the infant who cannot breast-feed due to prematurity or illness.
• To initiate and maintain lactation when unable to breast-feed infant, encourage the mother to express breast milk either manually or by using a breast pump at least every 3 hours.	
• Observe the infant at breast, noting behavior, position, latch-on, and sucking technique with the initial breast-feeding and then as necessary. Document these observations in the mother's and infant's charts.	
• Encourage the mother and significant other to identify support systems to assist her with meeting her physical and psychosocial needs at home. (See Appendix B.)	The majority of women who are successfully breast-feeding when leaving the hospital quit after 3 weeks at home. Support systems are a critical component in the maintenance of successful lactation.[30]
• Encourage mother to drink at least 2000 ml a day, or 8 oz every hour, of fluids.	
• Encourage the mother to eat a wide variety of foods from the four basic food groups, to provide sufficient amounts of calcium, protein, and calories.	Breast-feeding mothers should increase their caloric intake to 2000–2500 cal per day in order to maintain successful lactation.
• Encourage the mother to breast-feed at least every 2 to 3 hours for a minimum of 10 minutes per side to establish milk	Newborns need frequent feeding to satisfy their hunger and to establish their feeding patterns. It is important that the mother

supply; then regulate feeding according to infant's demands.

understand that the infant's suckling will determine the supply and demand of breast milk.
Helps to determine intake and nutritional status of infant.

- Monitor the infant's output for number of wet diapers. Document the number of diapers and the color of urine. (Remember, there should be at least six in a 24-hour period.)
- Weigh the infant at least every third day and record.
- Assist the mother in planning a day's activities when breast-feeding to ensure that the mother gets sufficient rest.

Helps the new mother to establish a schedule that is beneficial for both the infant and her.

- Encourage advanced planning for the working mother if she intends to continue to breast-feed after returning to work.
- Involve the father or significant other in breast-feeding by encouraging the "provider-protector" role.

The breast-feeding mother requires a lot of support and encouragement. Fathers can supply this by providing her with time for rest and assistance with infant care. For example, the father can bring the infant to the mother at night, rather than mother having to get up each time for the feeding. Fathers can intervene with family and friends to provide nursing mothers privacy and quiet.

Mental Health

This diagnosis will not be applicable in a mental health setting.

Gerontic Health

This diagnosis is not applicable in gerontic health.

Home Health

The home health nursing actions for this diagnosis are the same as those for women's health.

FLOW CHART EVALUATION
Flow Chart Expected Outcome 1

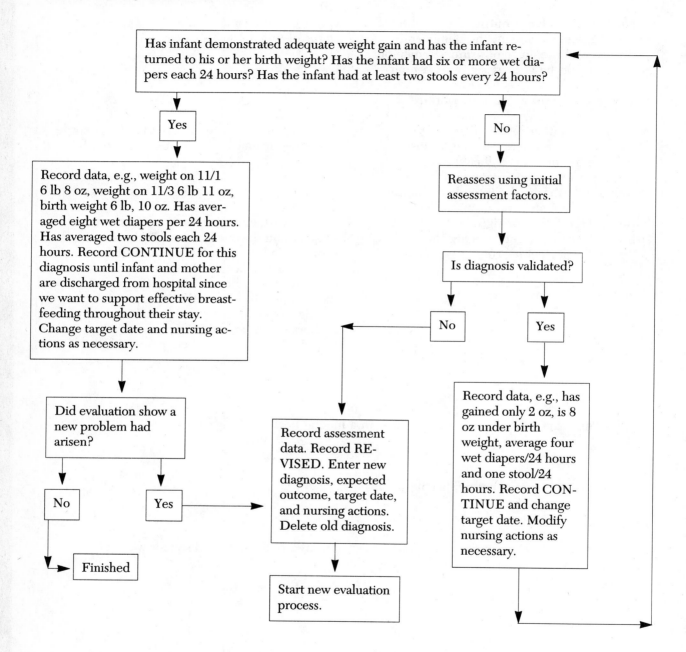

Flow Chart Expected Outcome 2

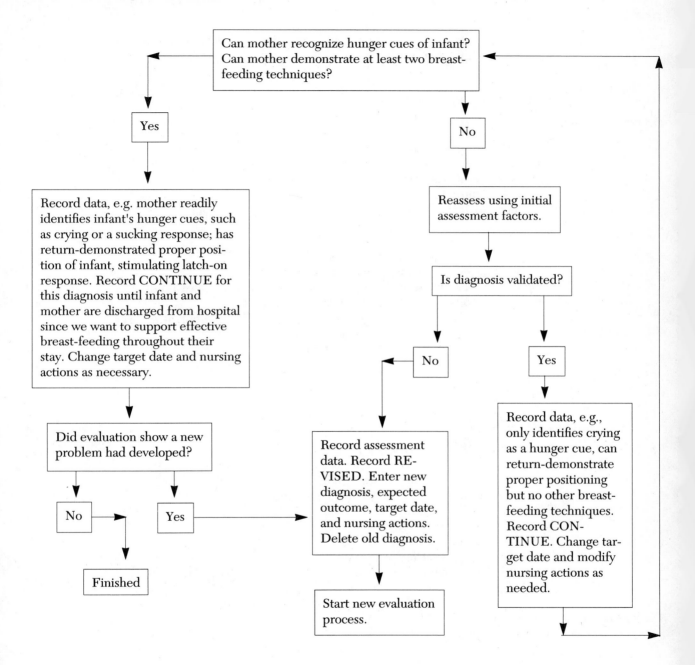

Breast-Feeding, Ineffective

DEFINITION

The state in which a mother, infant, or child experiences dissatisfaction or difficulty with the breast-feeding process.

NANDA TAXONOMY: MOVING 6.5.1.3

DEFINING CHARACTERISTICS

1. Major defining characteristics:
   a. Unsatisfactory breast-feeding process
2. Minor defining characteristics:
   a. Actual or perceived inadequate milk supply
   b. Inability of infant to attach on to maternal breast correctly
   c. No observable signs of oxytocin release
   d. Observable signs of inadequate infant intake
   e. Nonsustained sucking at the breast
   f. Insufficient emptying of each breast per feeding
   g. Persistence of sore nipples beyond the first week of breast-feeding
   h. Insufficient opportunity for sucking at the breast
   i. Infant exhibiting fussiness and crying within the first hour after breast-feeding; unresponsiveness to other comfort measures
   j. Infant arching and crying at the breast, resisting latching on

RELATED FACTORS

1. Prematurity
2. Infant anomaly
3. Maternal breast anomaly
4. Previous breast surgery
5. Previous history of breast-feeding failure
6. Infant receiving supplemental feedings with artificial nipple
7. Poor infant sucking reflex
8. Nonsupportive partner or family
9. Knowledge deficit
10. Interruption in breast-feeding
11. Maternal anxiety or ambivalence

RELATED CLINICAL CONCERNS

1. Any diseases of the breast
2. Cleft lip; cleft palate
3. Failure to thrive
4. Prematurity
5. Child abuse

HAVE YOU SELECTED THE CORRECT DIAGNOSIS?

Ineffective Breast-Feeding should be differentiated from the patient's concern over whether she wants to breast-feed or not. Although a mother who does not want to breast-feed will more than likely be ineffective in her breast-feeding attempts, Ineffective Breast-Feeding can be related to problems other than just the unwillingness to breast-feed. Other diagnoses that might need to be differentiated include:

Anxiety   Anxiety is defined as a vague, uneasy feeling, the source of which is often nonspecific or unknown to the individual. If an expression of perceived threat to self-concept, health status, socioeconomic status, role functioning, or interaction patterns is made, this would constitute the diagnosis of Anxiety. (See page 605.)

Altered Parenting   Altered Parenting is defined as the inability of the nurturing figures to create an environment that promotes optimum growth and development of another human being. Adjustment to parenting, in general, is a normal maturation process following the birth of a child. (See page 742.)

Altered Growth and Development: Self-Care Skills   This diagnosis is defined according to a demonstrated deviation from age-group norms for self-care. Inadequate caretaking would be defined according to specific behavior and attitudes of the individual mother or infant. (See page 427.)

Ineffective Individual Coping   This diagnosis is defined as the inability of the individual to deal with situations that require coping or adaptation to meet life's demands and roles. All the changes secondary to the birth of a new baby could result in this diagnosis. (See page 892.)

EXPECTED OUTCOMES

1. Will verbalize increased satisfaction with breast-feeding process by (date) and/or
2. Infant will require no supplemental feedings by (date)

TARGET DATE

Because Ineffective Breast-Feeding can be physically detrimental to the infant as well as emotionally detrimental to the mother, an initial target date of 3 days would be best.

NURSING ACTIONS/INTERVENTIONS WITH RATIONALES

Adult Health

For this nursing diagnosis, the Women's Health nursing actions serve as the generic nursing actions.

Child Health

Actions/Interventions	Rationales

• Monitor for contributory factors related to infant's ability to suck:
  ○ Structural abnormalities, for example, cleft lip or palate
  ○ Altered level of consciousness, seizures, or CNS damage
  ○ Mechanical barriers to sucking, for example, endotracheal tube or ventilator
  ○ Pain or underlying altered comfort or medication
  ○ Prematurity with diminished sucking ability
	Assessment of infant's ability to suck will assist in meeting goals for effective breast-feeding.

• Determine the effect the altered or impaired breast-feeding has on mother and infant by providing at least one 30-minute period per day for talking with mother. Monitor maternal feelings expressed, maternal-infant behaviors observed, and excessive crying or unrelenting fussiness in infant.	The maternal-infant responses will provide the essential database in determining how serious the breast-feeding issues are. This information will dictate how to approach the problem and promote realistic follow-up.
• To the degree possible, provide emotional support for infant in instances of temporary inability to breast-feed; for example, gavage feedings with appropriate cuddling. Include parents in care. Allow infant to suck on pacifier if possible. • Coordinate parents' visitation with infant to best facilitate successful breast-feeding in such areas as rest, natural hunger cycles, and comfort of all involved.	Provides temporary substitutions for breast-feeding that promote trust and sense of security for infant. Also, bonding with mother is still possible.
• Assist with plan to manage impaired breast-feeding to best provide support to all involved, for example, breast-pumping for period of time with support for this effort until normal breast-feeding can be resumed. Breast milk may be frozen or even given in gavage feeding. Support mother's choice for whatever alternatives chosen.	Maintain the mother's confidence in breast-feeding. Supporting her choice for alternative feeding demonstrates valuing of her beliefs.

Women's Health

Actions/Interventions	Rationales
• Ascertain mother's desire to breast-feed infant through careful interviewing and review of mother's knowledge regarding breast-feeding.	Provides intervention base for nursing actions. Allows planning of support, teaching, and evaluation of motives and desires to breast-feed.
• List the advantages and disadvantages of breast-feeding for the mother.	Assists the mother to make an informed decision about breast-feeding.
• Obtain a breast-feeding and bottle-feeding history from the mother; for example, did she breast-feed before, successfully or unsuccessfully?	
• Allow for uninterrupted breast-feeding periods.	Providing the mother and infant with uninterrupted breast-feeding times allows them to become acquainted with each other as well as allowing time for learning different breast-feeding techniques.
• Collaborate with physician, lactation consultant, perinatal clinical nurse specialist, and so on, to determine ways to make abnormal breast structure amenable to breast-feeding.	Assists mother who has strong desire to breast-feed to be successful.
• Observe mother with infant during breast-feeding. Explain and demonstrate methods to increase infant sucking reflex. Demonstrate to mother various positions for breast-feeding and describe how to alternate positions with each feeding to prevent nipple soreness, for example, sitting up, lying down, using football hold, holding baby "tummy-to-tummy," or using pillows for mother's comfort or for supporting baby.	Provides basic information and visible support to assist with successful breast-feeding.
• Ascertain mother's need for privacy during breast-feeding.	Promotes mother's comfort with the physical act of breast-feeding.
• Monitor for poor or dysfunctional sucking by checking: ○ Position mother is using to hold baby ○ Baby's mouth position on areola and nipple ○ Position of baby's head, for example, inappropriate hyperextension	Proper positioning facilitates satisfaction with breast-feeding for both mother and baby.
• Ascertain mother's support for breast-feeding from others, for example, husband or significant other, patient's mother, obstetrician, pediatrician, or nurses on postpartum unit.	Support from others is essential in attaining successful breast-feeding.

Continued

Actions/Interventions	Rationales

• Discuss infant's needs and frequency of feedings.
• Assist mother in planning a day's activities when breast-feeding, ensuring that the mother gets plenty of rest.
• Teach patient:
  ○ The proper diet for the breast-feeding mother, listing important food groups and necessary calories to adequately maintain milk production
  ○ The idea of advanced planning for the working mother who plans to breast-feed
  ○ That it takes time to establish breast-feeding (usually a month)
  ○ The use of various hand pumps, battery-operated pumps, and electric pumps
  ○ How to hand-express breast milk
  ○ How to properly store expressed breast milk
• Schedule specific times for consultation and support for the mother. Plan at least 30 minutes per shift (while awake) for talking with mother.
• If baby is separated from mother, such as in NICU, involve baby's nurses in planning with mother routines and times for breast-feeding infant.
• Refer mother to breast-feeding support groups. (See Appendix B.)
• For the mother who has had a cesarean section, place a pillow over the abdomen before putting infant to breast.
• Assist the mother of a premature baby to pump breast routinely to initiate milk production.
• Demonstrate proper storage and transportation of breast milk for the premature baby.
• Assist mother who has to wean a premature baby from tube feedings to breast-feeding by:
  ○ Teaching mother to place infant at the breast several times a day and during tube feeding
  ○ Encouraging mother to hold, cuddle, and interact with infant during tube feedings
  ○ Allowing mother and infant privacy to begin interaction with breast-feeding
	Provides basic information and visible support to assist with successful breast-feeding. Provides information necessary for the mother to plan the basics of her self-care.
	
	Provides basic information and visible support to assist with successful breast-feeding. Assists in keeping pressure off the incision line while breast-feeding.
	
	Basic teaching to ensure safe nutrition for infant.
	
	Provides needed support during this process.

○ Being available to assist with infant during breast-feeding interaction	
○ Reassuring mother it might take several attempts before baby begins to breast-feed.	
• Give breast-feeding mothers copies of educational materials.	Provides a readily available information source.
• If breast-feeding is not possible due to an infant physical deformity, teach the mother how to pump breasts and how to feed infant breast milk in bottles with special nipples.	Allows the mother the option of breast-feeding in the event that the deformity can be surgically corrected.
• Encourage maternal attachment behavior.	Assists mother in adjustment to parenting and effective caretaking of infant.

Mental Health

Refer to Women's Health nursing actions for interventions related to this diagnosis.

Gerontic Health

This diagnosis is not appropriate for gerontic health.

Home Health

Actions/Interventions	Rationales
• Teach measures to promote effective breast-feeding, for example, quiet environment, adequate nutrition and hydration, appropriate technique, and family support.	Knowledge and support increase the likelihood of a positive outcome.
• Assist client and family in identifying risk factors pertinent to the situation: ○ Premature infant ○ Infant anomaly ○ Maternal breast dysfunction ○ Infection ○ Previous breast surgery ○ Supplemental bottle feedings ○ Nonsupportive family ○ Lack of knowledge ○ Anxiety	Identification of and early interventions in high-risk situations provide the opportunity to prevent problems.
• Consult with or refer to appropriate resources as indicated. (See Appendix B.)	Appropriate and cost-effective use of available resources.

FLOW CHART EVALUATION
Flow Chart Expected Outcome 1

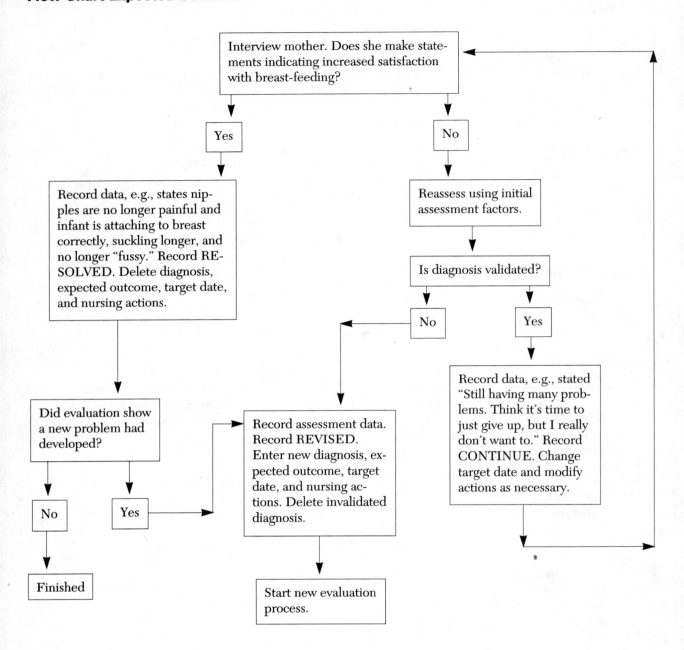

Nutritional-Metabolic Pattern

Flow Chart Expected Outcome 2

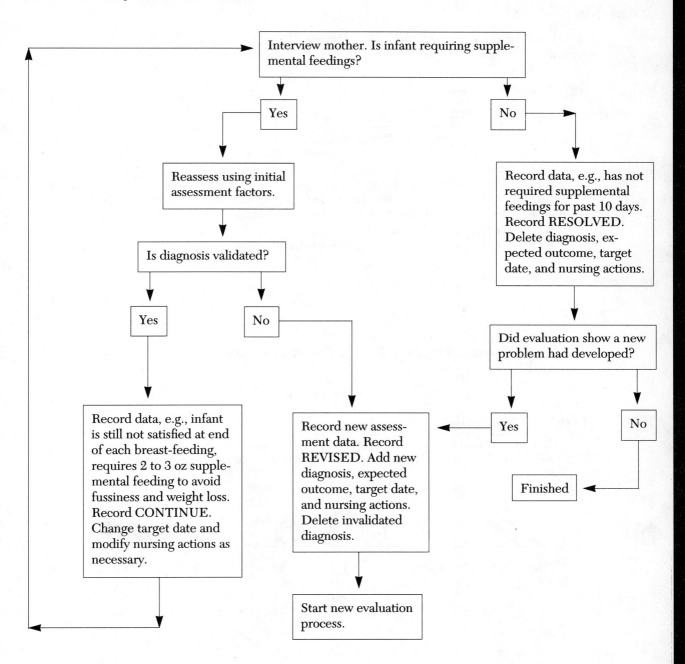

Breast-Feeding, Interrupted

DEFINITION

A break in the continuity of the breast-feeding process as a result of inability or inadvisability to put baby to breast for feeding.[26]

NANDA TAXONOMY: MOVING 6.5.1.2.1

DEFINING CHARACTERISTICS

1. Major defining characteristics:
   a. Infant does not receive nourishment at the breast for some or all of feedings.
2. Minor defining characteristics:
   a. Maternal desire to maintain lactation and provide (or eventually provide) her breast milk for her infant's nutritional needs.
   b. Separation of mother and infant.
   c. Lack of knowledge regarding expression and storage of breast milk.

RELATED FACTORS

1. Maternal or infant illness
2. Prematurity
3. Maternal employment
4. Contraindications to breast-feeding (for example, drugs or true breast milk jaundice)
5. Need to abruptly wean infant

RELATED CLINICAL CONCERNS

1. Any condition requiring emergency admission of mother to hospital
2. Any condition requiring emergency admission of infant to hospital
3. Prematurity
4. Postpartum depression

HAVE YOU SELECTED THE CORRECT DIAGNOSIS?

Ineffective Breast-Feeding With Ineffective Breast-Feeding, there is expressed dissatisfaction or problems with breast-feeding. With Interrupted Breast-Feeding, there is no expressed dissatisfaction or major problem; however, breast-feeding has temporarily ceased due to factors beyond the mother's control. (See page 140.)

Ineffective Infant Feeding Pattern In this diagnosis, there is a defined problem with the infant's ability to suck, swallow, and breathe. Breast-feeding for this infant has never been successful. With Interrupted Breast-Feeding, the infant has no problems with sucking or swallowing, and the stoppage of breast-feeding can be overcome by storing breast milk and feeding the infant via a bottle. (See page 194.)

EXPECTED OUTCOMES

1. Family will have designed a plan to overcome Interrupted Breast-Feeding by (date) and/or
2. Infant will demonstrate no weight loss secondary to adaptations for Interrupted Breast-Feeding by (date)

TARGET DATES

Since this interruption might occur as a result of an emergency, initial evaluation should occur within 24 hours after the initial diagnosis. Thereafter, target dates can be moved to every 3 days.

NURSING ACTIONS/INTERVENTIONS WITH RATIONALES

Adult Health

Actions/Interventions	Rationales
• Arrange care activities to facilitate mother's breast-feeding of infant according to feeding schedule of mother-infant dyad.	Supports continued successful breast-feeding, attachment, and bonding.
• Encourage continuation of breast-feeding: ○ Arrange special visitation privileges for infant and infant's caregiver during the time of the mother's hospitalization. ○ Provide privacy for family. ○ Collaborate with diet therapist regarding mother's nutritional needs during this time. ○ Provide breast pump for mother and assist with breast pumping as needed every 3 to 4 hours.	Helps relieve engorgement. Milk can be stored and used to feed infant.
• Collaborate with perinatal clinical nurse specialist and/or lactation consultant regarding maintenance of breast-feeding.	Provides needed consultation for nurse and patient.

Child Health

Actions/Interventions	Rationales
• Monitor for infant's ability to suck. Encourage sucking on a regular basis, especially if gavage feedings are a part of the therapeutic regimen.	Provides basic data critical to success. In times of non-breast-feeding, it is beneficial to encourage sucking to reinforce the feeding time as pleasurable and to enhance digestion unless contraindicated by a surgical or medical condition, for example, cleft repair of lip or palate, prolonged NPO with concerns for air swallowing.

Continued

Actions/Interventions	Rationales

• Provide support for the mother-infant dyad to facilitate the breast-feeding satisfaction.
• Monitor infant cues suggesting satisfaction:
  ○ Weight gain appropriate for status
  ○ Ability to sleep at intervals
	Feedback may provide essential valuing during times of stress.
	The fact that the infant's satisfaction and input is valued provides a critical component in the entire process of breast-feeding.

Women's Health

Actions/Interventions	Rationales

• Provide appropriate information on why breast-feeding needs to be interrupted. Be specific about length of time, for example, days, weeks, or months, and offer options for maintaining breast milk until able to resume breast-feeding.[27,28,29]
• Describe routine for pumping, expressing, and storing breast milk during emergency period.
• Contact lactation consultant and/or perinatal nurse to assist with plan of nursing care and with maintenance of breast milk during mother's illness, for example, emergency surgery, medical regimen (medications) that contradict breast-feeding, or injury requiring hospitalization of mother.[30,31]
• Provide mother with appropriate information about breast pumps and how to obtain one (rent or buy) to aid in expression of breast milk, for example, semiautomatic breast pump, automatic breast pump, battery-operated breast pump, or manual breast pump.
• Demonstrate and have mother return-demonstrate proper assembly and use of breast pump.
• Assist mother in learning manual expression of breast milk:[28]
  ○ Good handwashing technique before expressing milk
  ○ Correct positioning of hand and fingers so as not to damage breast tissue
  ○ Sterile wide-mouth funnel and bottle for storage of breast milk
	Assists breast-feeding families in establishing and maintaining breast-feeding capabilities when it is inadvisable or impossible to put baby to breast for feeding.

- Discuss options for maintaining breast-feeding with the mother who is returning to work. Provide assistance to help mother establish feeding schedule with work schedule, for example, breast-feed a.m. and p.m., or pumping at noon.[29,30,31]
- Provide resources, for example, printed materials or consultant, to assist mother when negotiating with employer for time and place to pump or breast-feed during working hours.[31]
- Assist mother and family to arrange schedule to bring infant to her during working hours.
- Encourage mother and significant other to verbalize their frustrations and concerns about establishing and maintaining lactation when the infant is ill or premature.[32,33,34,35]
- Refer to lactation consultant or clinical nurse specialist who can support parents and assist nurse in developing a program of breast-feeding or supplementing of infant with mother's breast milk.[36]
- Instruct parents in the proper methods of storage and transportation of breast milk.[28,35,36]

Provides basic information that assists in promoting effective breast-feeding.

Mental Health

This diagnosis will not, in all likelihood, be applicable in a mental health setting. Should a mother be admitted with a mental-health-related diagnosis, the physician would probably suggest changing the infant to bottle feedings. Should the physician agree that breast-feeding could continue, the Adult Health actions would be applicable for the mental health client.

Gerontic Health

This diagnosis is not appropriate for gerontic health.

Home Health

NOTE: If home care is needed because of either mother or infant illness or disability, the nurse will need to address the underlying problem in order to promote Effective Breast-Feeding. It is not likely that home health care would be initiated if the only diagnosis were Interrupted Breast-Feeding; however, there are lactation consultants whose entire practice is home health. This practice has been specifically designed to assist with maintenance of successful lactation.

Actions/Interventions	Rationales
• Support mother, infant, and family dynamics for successful breast-feeding. • Recognize cultural variations in feeding practices when assessing effectiveness of breast-feeding. • Provide additional education or referrals as requested or as situation changes.	Encouragement and support increases the potential for positive outcomes. Feeding patterns vary according to cultural norms. Community-based support is ongoing; early intervention as the situation changes increases the potential for continued effectiveness.

FLOW CHART EVALUATION
Flow Chart Expected Outcome 1

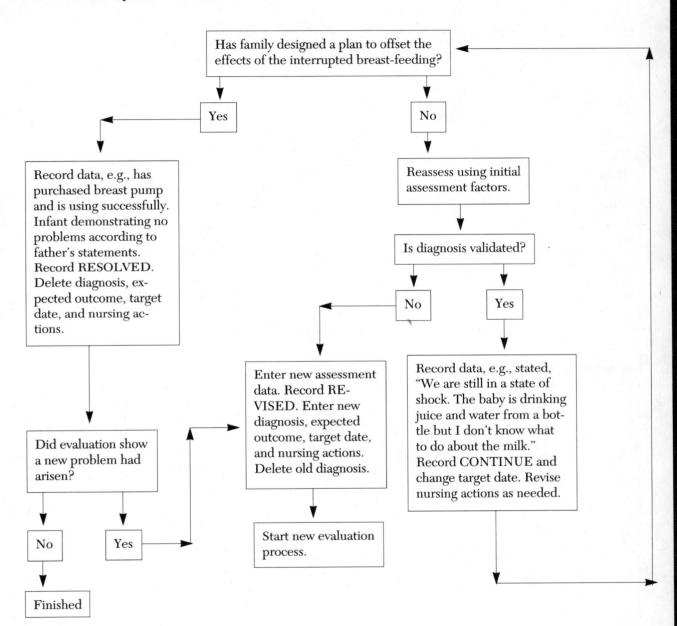

Has family designed a plan to offset the effects of the interrupted breast-feeding?

Yes

No

Record data, e.g., has purchased breast pump and is using successfully. Infant demonstrating no problems according to father's statements. Record RESOLVED. Delete diagnosis, expected outcome, target date, and nursing actions.

Reassess using initial assessment factors.

Is diagnosis validated?

No

Yes

Did evaluation show a new problem had arisen?

No

Yes

Enter new assessment data. Record REVISED. Enter new diagnosis, expected outcome, target date, and nursing actions. Delete old diagnosis.

Record data, e.g., stated, "We are still in a state of shock. The baby is drinking juice and water from a bottle but I don't know what to do about the milk." Record CONTINUE and change target date. Revise nursing actions as needed.

Start new evaluation process.

Finished

Flow Chart Expected Outcome 2

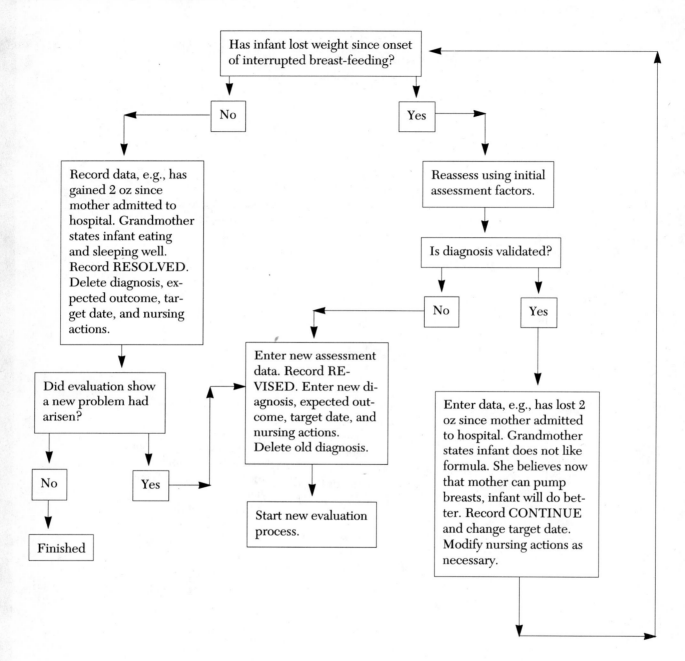

Fluid Volume Deficit, High Risk for or Actual

DEFINITION

The state in which an individual is at risk of experiencing or is experiencing vascular, cellular, or intracellular dehydration.

NANDA TAXONOMY: EXCHANGING 1.4.1.2.2.1

DEFINING CHARACTERISTICS

1. High Risk for Fluid Volume Deficit:
   a. Major defining characteristics (risk factors):
      (1) Extremes of age
      (2) Extremes of weight
      (3) Excessive losses through normal routes, for example, diarrhea
      (4) Loss of fluid through abnormal routes, for example, indwelling tubes
      (5) Deviations affecting access to or intake or absorption of fluids, for example, physical immobility
      (6) Factors influencing fluid needs, for example, hypermetabolic state
      (7) Knowledge deficiency related to fluid volume
      (8) Medications, for example, diuretics
   b. Minor defining characteristics (risk factors):
      None given.
2. Actual Fluid Volume Deficit:
   a. Major defining characteristics:
      (1) Change in urine output
      (2) Change in urine concentration
      (3) Sudden weight loss or gain
      (4) Decreased venous filling
      (5) Hemoconcentration
      (6) Change in serum sodium
   b. Minor defining characteristics (listed as other possible characteristics):
      (1) Hypotension
      (2) Thirst
      (3) Increased pulse rate
      (4) Decreased skin turgor
      (5) Decreased pulse volume or pressure
      (6) Change in mental state
      (7) Increased body temperature
      (8) Dry skin
      (9) Dry mucous membranes
      (10) Weakness

RELATED FACTORS

1. High Risk for Fluid Volume Deficit:
   The risk factors also serve as the related factors for this diagnosis.
2. Actual Fluid Volume Deficit:
   a. Active fluid volume loss.
   b. Failure of regulatory mechanisms.

RELATED CLINICAL CONCERNS

1. Addison's disease (adrenal insufficiency or crisis)
2. Hemorrhage
3. Burns
4. AIDS
5. Chron's disease
6. Vomiting and diarrhea
7. Ulcerative colitis

HAVE YOU SELECTED THE CORRECT DIAGNOSIS?

Altered Oral Mucous Membrane and Altered Nutrition: Less than Body Requirements   The client may not be able to ingest food or fluid because of primary problems in the mouth, or the client just may not be ingesting enough food from which the body can absorb fluids. (See pages 200 and 239.)

Altered Bowel Elimination: Diarrhea or Altered Urinary Elimination: Incontinence   These diagnoses may be causing an extreme loss of fluid before it can be absorbed and used by the body. (See pages 285 and 293.)

Impaired Skin Integrity   This diagnosis could be the primary problem. For example, the patient who has been burned has grossly impaired skin integrity. The skin is supposed to regulate the amount of fluid lost from it. If there is relatively little intact skin, the skin is unable to perform its regulatory function, and there is significant loss of fluid and electrolytes. (See page 239.)

Self-Care Deficit or Altered Parenting   In the infant or young child, the problem may primarily be a Self-Care Deficit or Altered Parenting. The infant or young child is not able to obtain the fluid he or she wants and must depend on others. If the parents are unable to recognize or meet these needs, then the infant or young child may have a High Risk for or Actual Fluid Volume Deficit. Even in an adult, the primary nursing diagnosis may be Self-Care Deficit. Again, if the adult is unable to obtain the fluid he or she requires because of some pathophysiologic problem, then he or she may have a High Risk for or Actual Fluid Volume Deficit. (See pages 472 and 742.)

EXPECTED OUTCOMES

1. Intake and output will balance within 200 ml by (date) and/or
2. Will describe (number) factors influencing adequate hydration and methods to prevent fluid volume deficit by (date)

TARGET DATE

Normally, intake and output will approximately balance only every 72 hours; thus, an appropriate target date would be 3 days.

NURSING ACTIONS/INTERVENTIONS WITH RATIONALES

Adult Health

Actions/Interventions	Rationales
• Measure and record total intake and output every shift: ○ Check intake and output hourly. ○ Observe and document color and consistency of all urine, stools, and vomitus. ○ Check urine specific gravity every 4 hours at (state times here).	Determines fluid loss and need for replacement.
• Take vital signs every 2 hours on (odd/even) hour, and include apical pulse. • Monitor intravenous fluids. (See Altered Nutrition: Less than Body Requirements, Additional Information, page 205.)	Permits monitoring of cardiovascular response to illness state and replacement therapy. Monitoring of fluid replacement and prevention of fluid overload.
• Monitor: ○ Skin turgor at least every 4 hours at (state times here) while awake ○ Electrolytes, blood urea nitrogen hematocrit, and hemoglobin. Collaborate with physician regarding frequency of lab tests ○ Central venous pressure every hour (if appropriate) ○ Mental status and behavior at least every 2 hours on the (odd/even) hour ○ For signs and symptoms of shock at least every 4 hours at (state times here), for example, weakness, diaphoresis, hypotension, tachycardia, or tachypnea	Essential monitoring for fluid and electrolyte imbalance.
• Weigh daily at (state time here). Teach patient to weigh at same time each day in same weight clothing.	Monitoring for fluid replacement. Allows consistent comparison of weight.
• Force fluids to a minimum of 2000 ml daily: ○ Ascertain patient's fluid likes and dislikes (list here). ○ Offer small amount of fluid (4 to 5 oz) at least every hour while awake and at every awakening during night. ○ Offer fluids at temperature that is most acceptable to patient, for example, warm or cool. ○ Interspace fluids with high-fluid-content foods, for example, popsicles, gelatin, pudding, ice cream, or watermelon. Note patient's preferences here.	

Continued

Actions/Interventions	Rationales
• Administer medications as ordered, for example, antidiarrheals or antiemetics. Monitor medication effects.	
• Assist patient to eat and drink as necessary. Provide positive verbal support for patient's consuming fluid.	Prevents dehydration and easily replaces fluid loss without resorting to intravenous (IV) feeding. Frequent fluids improve hydration; variation in fluids is helpful in encouraging patient to increase intake.
• Administer or assist with oral hygiene after each meal and before bedtime.	Cleans and lubricates the mouth. Encourages patient to eat and drink.
• Turn and properly position patient at least every 2 hours on (odd/even) hour.	
• Encourage patient to alter position frequently.	
• Provide active and passive range of motion every 4 hours at (state times here) while awake.	Prevents stasis of fluids in any one part of body. Assists in circulation of fluid.
• Schedule 1-hour rest periods for patient at least 4 times a day at (times).	Prevents overexertion and extra strain on circulatory system.

• If temperature elevation develops:
  ○ Maintain cool room temperature.
  ○ Offer cool, clear liquids.
  ○ Administer ordered antipyretics.
  ○ Give tepid sponge bath.
  ○ Remove heavy and excess clothing and bed covers.
	Assists in reducing fluid loss due to perspiration, and so on.

• If gastric tube is present:
  ○ Use only normal saline for irrigation.
  ○ Monitor amount of oral intake of water and ice chips. Avoid if at all possible. Offer commercial electrolyte replenishment solutions if permitted, for example, Gatorade, 10K.
	Avoids altering of electrolyte balance which, in turn, may alter fluid volume balance.

• Teach patient, prior to discharge, to increase fluid intake at home during:
  ○ Elevated temperature episodes
  ○ Periods when infection or elevated temperatures are present
  ○ Periods of exercise
  ○ Hot weather	

• Measures to ensure adequate hydration:
  ○ Need to drink fluids before feeling of thirst is experienced
  ○ Recognizing signs and symptoms of dehydration such as dry skin, dry lips, excessive sweating, dry tongue, and decreased skin turgor
	Support patient's self-care by pointing out measures he or she can use to control fluid imbalance. Adequate intake and early intervention will prevent undesirable outcomes.

- ○ How to measure, record, and evaluate intake and output
- Refer to other health care professionals as necessary. (See Appendix B.)

Provides support and fosters cost-effective collaboration through use of readily available resources.

Child Health

Actions/Interventions	Rationales

- Measure and record total intake every shift:
  ○ Check intake and output hourly [may require weighing diapers or insertion of a Foley catheter (infants may require use of a no. 5 or no. 8 feeding tube if size 10 Foley is too large)].
  ○ Check urine specific gravity every 2 hours on (odd/even) hour or every voiding or as otherwise ordered.
	A 24-hour fluid assessment will be meaningful for diagnosing deficits and also provide a basis for replacement needs. Specific gravity is a good indicator of degree of hydration.

- Force fluids to a minimum appropriate for size (will be closely related to electrolyte needs and cardiac, respiratory, and renal status):
  ○ *Infant*: 70 to 100 ml/kg in 24 hours
  ○ *Toddler*: 55 to 70 ml/kg in 24 hours
  ○ *School-age child*: 20 to 50 ml/kg in 24 hours
	Prompt replacement and maintenance of appropriate fluids will prevent further circulatory/systemic problems. Specific attention is also required with respect to sodium, potassium, and calorie requirements. Infants are subject to fluid volume depletion because of their relatively greater surface area, higher metabolic rate, and immature renal function.[37]

- Weigh patient daily at same time of day, on same scale, and in same clothing (infants without diaper).	Accuracy of weight cannot be overstressed. The weight often serves as a major indicator of the effectiveness of the treatment regimen. Iatrogenic problems are more likely to occur with inaccuracies.
- Assist in individualizing oral intake to best suit the patient's needs and preferences. Include parents in designing this individualization.	When options exist, honoring these will facilitate better compliance with goals and helps the patient and family to feel valued.

Women's Health

Actions/Interventions	Rationales
- Assist patient to identify life-style factors that could be contributing to symptoms of nausea and vomiting during early pregnancy:	Provides basis for treatment of symptoms and basis for teaching and support strategies.

Continued

Actions/Interventions	Rationales
○ Identify patient's support system. ○ Monitor patient's feelings (positive or negative) about pregnancy. ○ Evaluate social, economic, and cultural conditions. ○ Involve significant others in discussion and problem-solving activities regarding physiologic changes of pregnancy that are affecting work habits and interpersonal relationships (for example, nausea and vomiting). • Teach patient measures that can help alleviate pathophysiologic changes of pregnancy. • In collaboration with dietitian: ○ Obtain dietary history. ○ Assist patient in planning diet that will provide adequate nutrition for her and her fetus' needs. • Teach methods of coping with gastric upset, nausea, and vomiting: ○ Eat bland, low-fat foods (no fried foods or spicy foods). ○ Increase carbohydrate intake. ○ Eat small amounts of food every 2 hours (avoid empty stomach). ○ Eat dry crackers or toast before getting up in the morning. ○ Take vitamins and iron with night meal before going to bed. (Vitamin B, 50 mg, can be taken twice a day but never on an empty stomach.) ○ Drink high-protein liquids (for example, soups or eggnog).[5]	Provides information, education, and support for self-care during pregnancy.
• Monitor patient for: ○ Variances in appetite ○ Vomiting first 16 weeks (beyond 12 weeks) of pregnancy ○ Weight loss ○ Intractable nausea and vomiting	Provides basis for therapeutic intervention if necessary as well as support of patient which can decrease fear and feelings of helplessness.
• Collaborate with physician regarding monitoring for: ○ *Electrolyte imbalance*: Hemoconcentration, ketosis with ketonuria, hyponatremia, and hypokalemia ○ Dehydration (*Note:* "During pregnancy, gastric-acid secretion normally is reduced because of increased estrogen stimulation.	Provides support and information to increase self-awareness and self-care.

This places the women at risk for alkalosis rather than the acidosis that usually occurs in an advanced stage of dehydration."[5])

- Hydration (approximately 3000 ml per 24 hours) and providing vitamin supplements
- Restriction of oral intake and providing parental administration of fluids and vitamins. (*Note:* "Vitamin B6 has been found effective and safe for use in nausea and vomiting during pregnancy."[5])

• Allow expression of feelings and encourage verbalization of fears and questions by scheduling at least 30 minutes with patient at least once per shift.

• Provide patient and family with diet information for the breast-feeding mother to prevent dehydration:
- Increase daily fluid intake.
- Drink at least 2500 ml of fluid daily.
- Extra fluid can be taken just before each breast-feeding (for example, water, fruit juices, decaffeinated tea, or milk).
- Eat well-balanced meals to include the four basic food groups.

Provides information that allows for successful lactation and healthy recovery from childbirth.

• Teach the parents fluid intake needs of the newborn. The newborn should be taking in approximately 420 ml soon after birth and building to 1200 ml at the end of 3 months.

• Monitor newborn for fluid deficit, and teach parents to monitor via the following factors:
- "Fussy baby," especially immediately after feeding.
- Constipation (Remember, breast-fed babies have fewer stools than formula-fed babies.)
- Weight loss or slow weight gain:

Provides information and support for healthy growth and development of newborn.

• Closely monitor baby, mother, and nursing routine:
- Is baby getting empty calories (for example, a lot of water between feedings)?
- Does the baby have nipple confusion, from switching baby from breast to bottle and vice versa many times?
- Count number of diapers per day (should have 6 to 8 really wet diapers per day).
- Intolerance to mother's milk or bottle formula.

Continued

Actions/Interventions	Rationales
• Monitor baby for illness or lactose intolerances. • Monitor how often mother is nursing infant (infrequent nursing can cause slow weight gain).	

Mental Health

Actions/Interventions	Rationales
• If client is confused or is unable to interpret signs of thirst, place on intake and output measurement, and record this information every shift.	Medications and/or clouded consciousness may affect client's ability to recognize need for fluids.
• Evaluate potential for fluid deficit resulting from medication or medication interaction, for example, lithium and diuretics. If this presents a risk, place client on intake and output measurement every shift.	Estimated daily requirement for adults is 1500 to 3000 ml per day.[38]
• Evaluate mental status every shift at (times).	Basic monitoring to determine client's ability to independently take fluids.

• If client's values and beliefs influence intake:
  ○ Alter environment as necessary to facilitate fluid intake and note alterations here, for example, if client thinks fluids from cafeteria are poisonous, have client assist in making drink on unit.
  ○ Provide positive attention to client at additional times to avoid not drinking as a way of obtaining negative attention.	

Gerontic Health

Actions/Interventions	Rationales
• Encourage patient to drink at least 8 oz of fluid every hour while awake.	Older adults with cognitive deficits may forget to consume liquids. Prompting such patients to drink fluids should be an essential part of their plan of care.
• Be sure fluids are within reach of the patient confined to bed.	For those confined to bed or with restricted movement, this action is a simple, basic measure to promote fluid intake.

Home Health

Actions/Interventions	Rationales

• Assist client and family in identifying risk factors pertinent to the situation:
  ○ Diabetes
  ○ Protein malnourishment
  ○ Extremes of age
  ○ Excessive vomiting or diarrhea
  ○ Medication for fluid retention or high blood pressure
  ○ Confusion or lethargy
  ○ Fever
  ○ Excessive blood loss
  ○ Wound drainage
  ○ Inability to obtain adequate fluids because of pain, immobility, or difficulty in swallowing
	Early intervention in high-risk situations can prevent dehydration.

• Assist client and family in identifying life-style changes that may be required:
  ○ Avoiding excessive use of caffeine, alcohol, laxatives, diuretics, antihistamines, fasting, and high-protein diets
  ○ Use of salt tablets
  ○ Exercise without electrolyte replacement
	Avoidance of dehydrating activities will prevent excessive fluid loss.

FLOW CHART EVALUATION
Flow Chart Expected Outcome 1

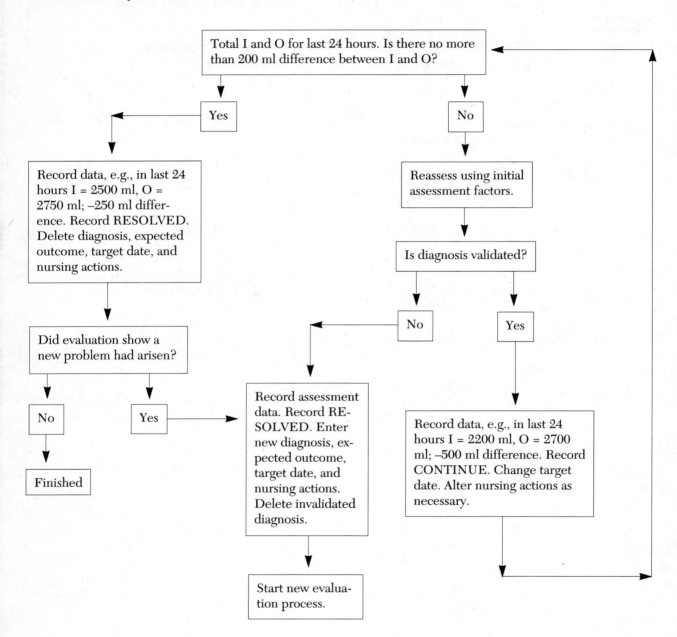

Flow Chart Expected Outcome 2

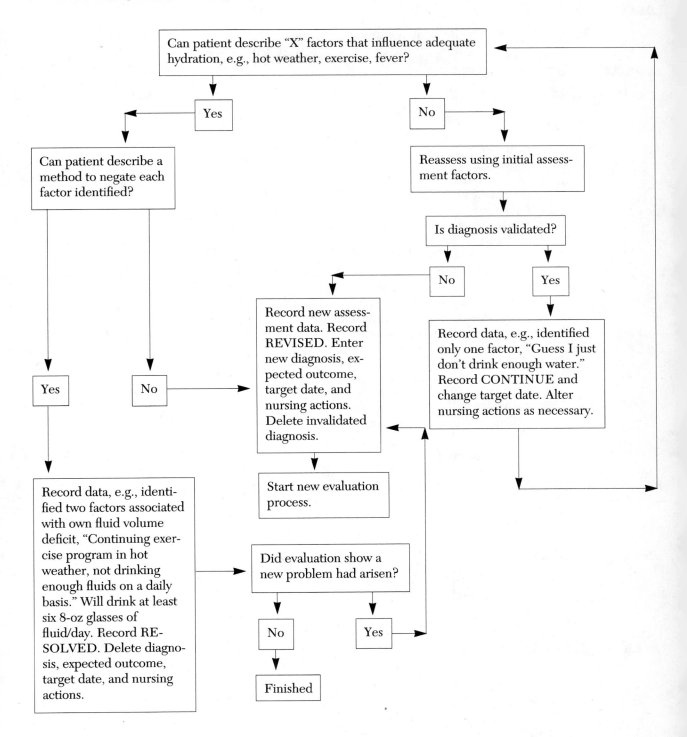

Fluid Volume Excess

DEFINITION

The state in which an individual experiences increased fluid retention and edema.

NANDA TAXONOMY: EXCHANGING 1.4.1.2.1

DEFINING CHARACTERISTICS

1. Major defining characteristics:
   a. Edema
   b. Effusion
   c. Anasarca
   d. Weight gain
   e. Shortness of breath
   f. Orthopnea
   g. Intake greater than output
   h. S3 heart sound
   i. Pulmonary congestion (chest x-ray)
   j. Abnormal breath sounds, rales (crackles)
   k. Change in respiratory pattern
   l. Change in mental status
   m. Decreased hemoglobin and hematocrit
   n. Blood pressure changes
   o. Central venous pressure changes
   p. Pulmonary artery pressure changes
   q. Jugular vein distention
   r. Positive hepatojugular reflex
   s. Oliguria
   t. Specific gravity changes
   u. Azotemia
   v. Altered electrolytes
   w. Restlessness
   x. Anxiety
2. Minor defining characteristics:
   None given

RELATED FACTORS

1. Compromised regulatory mechanisms
2. Excess fluid intake
3. Excess sodium intake

RELATED CLINICAL CONCERNS

1. Congestive heart failure
2. Renal failure
3. Cirrhosis of the liver
4. Cancer
5. Toxemia

HAVE YOU SELECTED THE CORRECT DIAGNOSIS?

Altered Cardiac Output: Decreased and Impaired Gas Exchange The body depends on both appropriate gas exchange and adequate cardiac output to oxygenate tissues and circulate nutrients and fluid for use and disposal. If either of these is compromised, then the body will suffer in some way. One of the major ways the body suffers is in the circulation of body fluid. Fluid will be left in tissue and not absorbed into the general circulation to be redistributed or eliminated. (See page 360.)

Altered Nutrition More than Body Requirements could be the primary problem. The person ingests more food and fluid than the body can metabolize and eliminate. The result is excess fluid volume in addition to the other changes in the body's physiology. (See page 215.)

Impaired Urinary Elimination: Retention One way the body compensates fluid balance is through urinary elimination. If the body cannot properly eliminate fluids, then the system "backs up" so to speak, and excess fluid remains in the tissues. (See page 304.)

Impaired Physical Mobility Besides appropriate gas exchange and adequate cardiac output, the body also needs movement of muscles to assist in transporting food and fluids to and from the tissue. Impaired Mobility might lead to an alteration in movement of food and fluids. Waste products of metabolism and excess fluid are allowed to remain in tissues, creating a fluid volume excess. (See page 460.)

ADDITIONAL INFORMATION

Fluid volume excess can occur as a result of water excess, sodium excess, or water and sodium excess. Careful assessment and monitoring is needed to recognize the difference in precipitating causes.

Edema: Mild or 1+ means that the skin can be depressed 0 to $\frac{1}{4}$ in; moderate or 2+ means that the skin can be depressed $\frac{1}{4}$ to $\frac{1}{2}$ in; severe or 3+ means that the skin can be depressed $\frac{1}{2}$ to 1 in; and deep pitting edema or 4+ means that the skin can be depressed more than 1 in and that it takes longer than 30 seconds to rebound.

EXPECTED OUTCOMES

1. Intake and output will balance within 200 ml by (date) (*Note:* May want difference to be only 50 ml for a child.) and/or
2. Will not exhibit any signs or symptoms of fluid volume excess by (date)

TARGET DATE

In a healthy person, intake and output reach an approximate balance over a span of 72 hours. An acceptable target date would then logically be the third day of admission.

NURSING ACTIONS/INTERVENTIONS WITH RATIONALES

Adult Health

Actions/Interventions	Rationales
• Take vital signs every 2 hours at (state times here) and include apical pulse. • Check lung, heart, and breath sounds every 2 hours on (odd/even) hour. • Elevate head of bed. • Measure and record total intake and output every shift. • Check intake and output hourly (urinary output not less than 30 ml per hour). • Observe and document color and character of urine, vomitus, and stools. • Check urine specific gravity at least every 2 hours on (odd/even) hour.	Permits monitoring of cardiovascular response to illness state and therapy. Essential monitoring for fluid collection in lungs and cardiac overload due to edema. Facilitates respiration. Assists in determining amount of fluid retention and need for fluid limitation.

• Monitor:
  ○ Skin turgor at least every 4 hours while awake (note times here).
  ○ Electrolytes, hemoglobin, and hematocrit. Collaborate with physician regarding frequency of lab tests.
  ○ Mental status and behavior at least every 2 hours on (odd/even) hour.
	Essential monitoring for fluid and electrolyte imbalance.

• Weigh daily at (state times here). • Weigh at same time each day and in same-weight clothing. • Administer medication (for example, diuretics) as ordered. Monitor medication effects.	Monitoring for fluid replacement. Allows consistent comparison of weight.

• Collaborate with physician regarding restricting intake:
  ○ Amount
  ○ Type, for example, clear fluids only or intravenous only
	Restricting fluids prevents cardiovascular system overload and reduces work load on renal system.

• Turn and properly position patient at least every 2 hours on (odd/even) hour.
• Check dependent parts for edema (for example, ankles, sacral area, or buttocks).
• Protect edematous skin from injury:
  ○ Avoid shearing force.
  ○ Use powder or cornstarch to avoid friction.
  ○ Use pillows, foam rubber pads, and so on to avoid pressure.
  ○ Encourage patient to alter position frequently.
	Prevents stasis of fluids in any one part of body. Assists in circulation of fluid and assists in preventing skin integrity problems.

Actions/Interventions	Rationales
○ Provide active or passive range of motion every 4 hours while awake at (state times here).	
• Administer or assist with complete oral hygiene after each meal and at bedtime.	Cleans and lubricates the mouth. Permits patient to more fully enjoy foods and fluid allowed.
• Teach patient to monitor own intake and output at home.	Supports patient's self-care by pointing out measures he or she can use to control fluid imbalance. Adequate intake and early intervention will prevent undesirable outcomes.
• In collaboration with dietitian: ○ Obtain nutritional history. ○ Begin high-protein diet (80 to 100 g of protein). ○ Reduce sodium intake (not above 6 g daily or below 2.5 g daily). ○ Refer to other health care professionals as appropriate. (See Appendix B.)	Cost-effective use of readily available resources. Promotes interdisciplinary care and, thus, better care for patient.

Child Health

Actions/Interventions	Rationales
• Measure and record total intake and output every shift: ○ Check intake and output hourly; weigh diapers. ○ Monitor specific gravity at least every 2 hours or as specified.	A strict assessment of intake and output serves to guide treatment for indication of hydration status. The specific gravity will assist in determining cardiac, renal, and respiratory function and electrolyte status.
• Reposition as tolerated every $\frac{1}{2}$ hour.	Prevents stasis of fluids in any one part of body. Assists in circulation of fluid and assists in preventing skin integrity problems.
• Weigh daily at same time under same conditions of dress (infants without clothes, children in underwear).	Accuracy of weight is critical and serves as a major indicator for treatment effectiveness and is an ongoing parameter for treatment.

Women's Health

NOTE: *Pregnancy-induced hypertension (PIH)*, often called the "disease of theories," has been documented for the last 200 years. Numerous causes have been proposed but never substantiated. However, data collected during this time does support the following:

1. Chorionic villi must be present in the uterus for a diagnosis of PIH to be made.

2. Women exposed for the first time to chorionic villi are at increased risk for developing **PIH**.
3. Women exposed to an increased amount of chorionic villi, for example, multiple gestation or hydatidiform mole, are at greater risk for developing **PIH**.
4. Women with a history of **PIH** in a previous pregnancy are at increased risk for developing **PIH**.
5. Women who change partners are more likely to develop **PIH** in a subsequent pregnancy.
6. There is a genetic predisposition for the development of **PIH** which may be a single gene or multifactorial.
7. Vascular disease places the patient at greater risk for developing superimposed **PIH**.[38]

Actions/Interventions	Rationales

• Review client's history for factors associated with PIH:
  ○ Family and personal history such as diabetes, multiple gestation
  ○ RH incompatibility, or hypertensive disorder
  ○ Chronic blood pressure 140/90 mm Hg or greater prior to pregnancy or, in the absence of a hydatidiform mole, that persists for 42 days postpartum.
	Basic database required to assess for potential of PIH.

• During current pregnancy observe for following characteristics of PIH:
  ○ Nulliparous women under 20 or over 35 years of age
  ○ Multipara with multiple gestation, renal or vascular disease
  ○ Presence of hydatidiform mole
	Increased knowledge for patient will assist the patient with earlier help-seeking behaviors.

• Monitor patient for chronic hypertension:
  ○ Increase in systolic blood pressure of 30 mm Hg or diastolic blood pressure of at least 15 mm Hg above baseline on two occasions at least 2 hours apart
  ○ Development of proteinuria	

• Monitor and teach patient to immediately report the following signs of PIH:
  ○ Increase of 30 mm in blood pressure or 140/90 blood pressure and above
  ○ *Edema:* Weight gain of 5 pounds or greater in 1 week
  ○ *Proteinuria:* 1 g/L or greater of protein in a 24-hour urine collection (2+ by dipstick)
  ○ *Visual disturbances:* Blurring of vision or headaches	

○ Epigastric pain
- Observe closely for signs of severe preeclampsia in any patient who presents with:[27]
  ○ Blood pressure greater than or equal to 160 mm Hg systolic, or greater than or equal to 110 mm Hg diastolic, on at least two occasions 6 hours apart with the patient on bed rest
  ○ Proteinuria greater than or equal to 5 g in 24 hours or 3+ to 4+ on qualitative assessment
  ○ *Oliguria:* Less than 400 ml in 24 hours
  ○ Cerebral or visual disturbances
  ○ Epigastric pain
  ○ Pulmonary edema or cyanosis
  ○ Impaired liver function of unclear etiology
  ○ Thrombocytopenia

Knowledge of the complexity and multisystem nature of the disease assists with early detection and treatment.

- Monitor, at least once per shift, for edema. Teach patient:
  ○ To monitor swelling of hands, face, legs, or feet
  ○ *Caution:* To remove rings if necessary
  ○ To wear loose shoes or a bigger shoe size if necessary
  ○ To schedule rest breaks during day and elevate feet
  ○ When lying down, to lie on left side to promote placental perfusion and prevent compression of vena cava

Increased knowledge for patient will assist the patient with earlier help-seeking behaviors.

- In collaboration with dietitian:
  ○ Obtain nutritional history.
  ○ Place patient on high-protein diet (80 to 100 g of protein).
  ○ Place patient on reduced sodium intake (not above 6 g daily or below 2.5 g daily).
- Monitor:
  ○ Intake and output: Urinary output not less than 30 ml per hour or 120 ml per 4 hours.
  ○ Effect of magnesium sulfate ($MgSO_4$) and hydralazine hydrochloride (Apresoline) therapy. Have antidote for $MgSO_4$ (calcium gluconate) available at all times during $MgSO_4$ therapy.
  ○ Deep tendon reflexes (DTR) at least every 4 hours (state times here).
  ○ Respiratory rate, pulse, and blood pressure (BP) at least every 2 hours on the (odd/even) hour.

Basic safety measures.

Continued

Actions/Interventions	Rationales
○ Fetal heart rate and well-being at least every 2 hours on the (odd/even) hour. • Institute seizure precautions. • Ensure bed rest and reduction of noise level in patient's environment.	Decreases sensory stimuli that might increase the likelihood of a seizure.

Mental Health

Actions/Interventions	Rationales

• Observe chronic psychiatric clients and clients with preexisting alcoholism[40] for signs and symptoms of polydipsia and/or water intoxication. The observations include:[40,41,42]
  ○ Frequent trips to sources of fluid and excessive consumption of fluids
  ○ Client stating, "I feel as if I have to drink water all the time" or a similar statement
  ○ Fluid-seeking behavior
  ○ Dramatic or rapid fluctuations in weight
  ○ Polyuria
  ○ Incontinence
  ○ Carrying large cups
  ○ Urine specific gravity of 1.008 or less[40]
  ○ Decreases in serum sodium
	A pattern of extreme polydipsia and polyuria can develop in clients with psychiatric disorders. This may be related to dopamine central nervous system activity and dysfunction in antidiuretic hormone activity in combination with psychosocial factors. The sense of thirst can also be increased by certain medications.[41,42]

• Discuss client's explanations for excessive drinking to determine causes of excessive fluid intake. If it is determined that drinking is a diversionary activity or an attempt to avoid interaction, implement nursing actions for Social Isolation and/or Diversional Activity Deficit as appropriate. If it is determined that fluid intake is related to testing concern of staff or testing limits, refer to nursing actions for Powerlessness or Self-Concept Disturbance.	Determining exact reason for polydipsia allows for more effective intervention.
• If it is determined that client is at risk for water intoxication, implement the following actions: ○ Monitor and document fluid intake and output and weight fluctuations on a daily basis.	Water intoxication can be life-threatening.[40]

- ○ Fluid-restrict client as ordered.
- Provide small medicine cup (30 ml) for client to obtain fluids.
- Provide fluids such as chipped ice on a schedule. Note schedule here.
- Instruct client in need for reducing nicotine consumption. If client cannot do this, it may be necessary to initiate a "rationing" plan. If so, note plan here.

Nicotine increases release of ADH, a water-conserving hormone.[40]

- Provide client with sugarless gum and/or hard candy to decrease dry mouth. Note client's preference.
- Identify with client those activities that would be most helpful in diverting attention from fluid restriction. Note specific activities here with schedule for use.
- Refer to occupational and recreational therapists.
- If client continues to have difficulty restricting fluids, provide increased supervision by limiting client to day area or other group activity rooms where he or she can be observed. Note restrictions here. If necessary, place client on one-to-one observation.
- Talk with client about feelings engendered by restrictions for 15 minutes per shift. Note times here.
- Discuss client's restriction in a community meeting if:
  - ○ Restrictions are impacting others on the unit
  - ○ Support from peers would facilitate client's maintaining restrictions
- Provide positive verbal support for client's maintaining restriction(s).
- Identify with client appropriate rewards for maintaining restrictions and reaching goals. Describe rewards and behaviors necessary to obtain rewards here.

Promotes client's self-esteem and provides motivation for continued efforts.
Promotes client's self-esteem and sense of control and provides motivation for continued efforts.

Gerontic Health

Nursing actions for the gerontic health patient with this nursing diagnosis are the same as those for adult health and home health.

Home Health

Actions/Interventions	Rationales

• Teach methods to protect edematous tissue:
  ○ Practice proper body alignment.
  ○ Use pillows, pads, and so on to relieve pressure on dependent parts.
  ○ Avoid shearing force when moving in bed or chair.
  ○ Alter position at least every 2 hours.
	Tissue is at risk for injury. Client and family can be taught to minimize risks and damage.

• Assist client and family to set criteria to help them to determine when a physician or other intervention is required.	Planned decision making to prepare for potential crisis.
• Assist client and family in identifying risk factors pertinent to the situation, for example, heart disease, kidney disease, diabetes mellitus, diabetes insipidus, liver disease, pregnancy, or immobility.	Identification of risk factors and understanding of relationship to fluid excess provides for intervention to reduce or prevent negative outcomes.

• Teach signs and symptoms of fluid excess:
  ○ Peripheral and dependent edema
  ○ Shortness of breath
  ○ Taut and shiny skin
	Early recognition of signs and symptoms provides data for early intervention.

• Assist client and family in identifying lifestyle changes that may be required:
  ○ Avoid standing or sitting for long periods of time; elevate edematous limbs.
  ○ Avoid crossing legs.
  ○ Avoid constrictive clothing (girdles, garters, knee-highs, rubber bands to hold up stocking, and so on).
  ○ Consider wearing antiembolism stockings.
  ○ Avoid excess salt. Teach family and patient to read labels for sodium content. Avoid canned and fast foods.
  ○ Use spices other than salt in cooking.
  ○ Avoid lying in one position for longer than 2 hours.
  ○ Raise head of bed or sit in chair if having difficulty breathing.
  ○ Restrict fluid intake as necessary (for example, usual in kidney and liver disease).
  ○ Weigh daily wearing the same clothes, using the same scale, and at the same time of the day.
	Knowledge and support provide motivation for change and increase potential for positive outcome.

• Teach purposes and side effects of medication, for example, diuretics or cardiac medications.	Promotes appropriate use of medication and reduction of side effects.

FLOW CHART EVALUATION
Flow Chart Expected Outcome 1

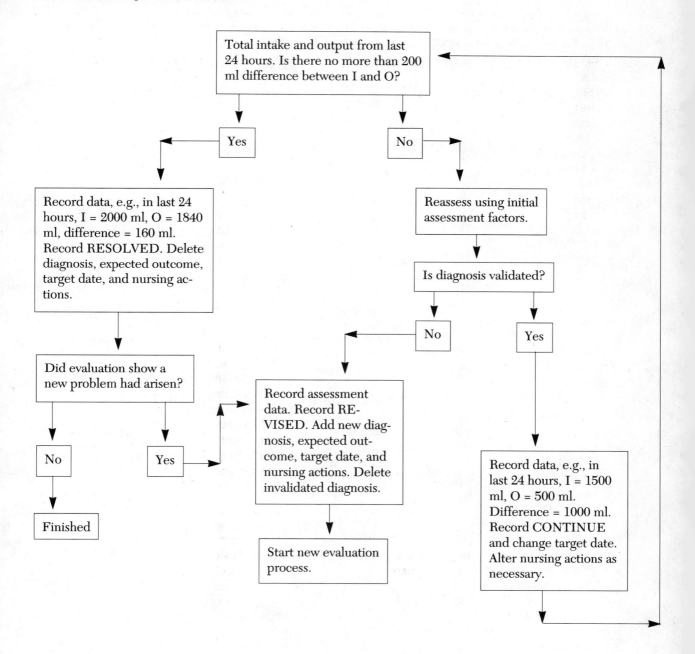

Flow Chart Expected Outcome 2

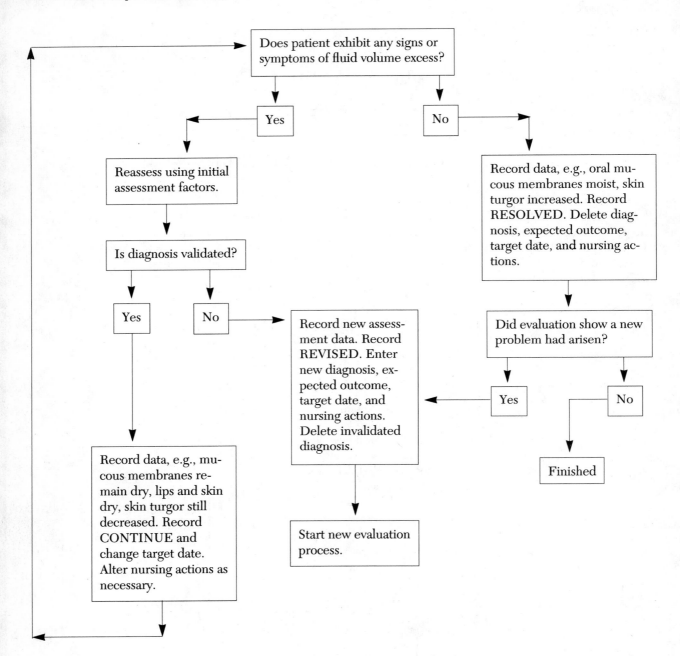

Hyperthermia

DEFINITION

A state in which an individual's body temperature is elevated above his or her normal range

NANDA TAXONOMY: EXCHANGING 1.2.2.3

DEFINING CHARACTERISTICS

1. Major defining characteristics:
   Increase in body temperature above normal range
2. Minor defining characteristics:
   a. Flushed skin
   b. Warm to touch
   c. Increased respiratory rate
   d. Tachycardia
   e. Seizures or convulsion

RELATED FACTORS

1. Exposure to hot environment
2. Vigorous activity
3. Medications or anesthesia
4. Inappropriate clothing
5. Increased metabolic rate
6. Illness or trauma
7. Dehydration
8. Inability or decreased ability to perspire

RELATED CLINICAL CONCERNS

1. Any infectious process
2. Septicemia
3. Hyperthyroidism
4. Any disease leading to dehydration, for example, diarrhea, vomiting, hemorrhage
5. Any condition causing pressure on the brainstem
6. Heat stroke

HAVE YOU SELECTED THE CORRECT DIAGNOSIS?

High Risk for Altered Body Temperature   This diagnosis indicates that the person is potentially unable to regulate heat production and dissipation within a normal range. In Hyperthermia, the patient's ability to produce heat is not impaired. Heat dissipation is impaired to the degree that Hyperthermia results. (See page 125.)

Continued

HAVE YOU SELECTED THE CORRECT DIAGNOSIS?—*Continued*

Ineffective Thermoregulation   Ineffective Thermoregulation indicates that the patient's body temperature is fluctuating between being elevated and being subnormal. In Hyperthermia the temperature does not fluctuate; it remains elevated until the underlying cause of the elevation is negated or until administration of medications such as Tylenol and aspirin show a definitive effect on the elevation. (See page 234.)

Hypothermia   Hypothermia means the patient's body temperature is subnormal. This indicates the exact opposite measurement from Hyperthermia. (See page 186.)

EXPECTED OUTCOMES

1. Will return to normal body temperature (range between 97.3 and 98.8°F) by (date) and/or
2. Will identify at least (number) measures to use in correcting hyperthermia by (date)

TARGET DATE

Because hyperthermia can be life-threatening, initial target dates should be in terms of hours. After the patient has demonstrated some stability toward a normal range, the target date can be increased to 2 to 4 days.

NURSING ACTIONS/INTERVENTIONS WITH RATIONALES

Adult Health

Actions/Interventions	Rationales
• Monitor temperature every hour on the (hour/half hour) while awake and temperature remains elevated. Measure temperature every 2 hours during night (note times here). After temperature begins to decrease, lengthen time between temperature measurements.	Hyperthermia is incompatible with cellular life.
• Sponge patient with cool water or rubbing alcohol, or apply continuous cold packs, or place patient in a tub of tepid water until temperature is lowered to at least 102°F. (Be careful not to overchill the patient.) Dry patient well, and keep him or her dry and clean.	Basic measures to assist in temperature reduction via heat dissipation. Overchilling could cause shivering, which increases heat production.
• Use a fan or place patient in front of an air conditioner. Cool environment to no more than 70°F.	Promotes cooling via heat dissipation.

- Monitor and use equipment according to manufacturer's guidelines and policies of unit, for example, cooling blanket.
- Give antipyretic drugs as ordered. Closely monitor effects, and document effects within 30 minutes after medications have been given.

Antipyretics assist in temperature reduction. Monitoring ensures that patient is not changed to a condition of hypothermia; plus monitoring allows the health care team to assess the effectiveness of the antipyretic. Ineffectiveness would require changing to a different antipyretic.

- Maintain seizure precautions until temperature stabilizes.
- Give sips of salt water every 30 minutes if patient is conscious and not vomiting.
- Encourage fluids up to 3000 ml every 24 hours.

Hyperthermia can lead to febrile seizures due to overstimulation of the nervous system.
Assists in maintaining fluid and electrolyte balance.
Helps maintain fluid and electrolyte balance and assists in replacing fluid lost through perspiration.

- Give skin, mouth, and nasal care at least every 4 hours while awake (note times here). Change bed linens and pajamas as often as necessary.

Hyperthermia promotes mouth breathing in an effort to dissipate heat. Mouth breathing is drying to the oral mucous membrane. Keeping bed linens and pajamas dry helps avoid shivering.

- Do not give stimulants.

Causes vasoconstriction, which could increase hyperthermia.

- Gather data relevant to underlying contributing factors at least once per shift.
- Provide health care teaching, beginning on admission, regarding:
  - Need for frequent temperature checks
  - Related medical or nursing care
  - Safety needs when using ice packs or electric cooling blanket
  - How family can assist in care
  - Importance of hydration
  - Possible fear or altered comfort of patient with fever due to discomfort, fast heart rate, dizziness, and general feeling of illness
  - Possible seizure activity

Control of underlying factors helps prevent occurrence of hyperthermia.
Relieves anxiety and allows patient and family to participate in care. Initiates home care planning.

- Carry out appropriate infection control in the event or potential event of infectious disease process according to actual or suspected organisms.

Prevents spread of infection.

- Assist in promoting a quiet environment.

Allows for essential sleep and rest needs. Hyperthermia causes increased metabolic rate.

Child Health

Actions/Interventions	Rationales
• Monitor temperature every 30 minutes until temperature stabilizes.	Frequent assessment per tympanic (aural) thermometer, or as specified, will provide cues to evaluate efficacy of treatment and monitor underlying pathology.

• Administer antipyretics, antiseizure or antibiotic medications as ordered with precaution for:
  ○ Maintenance of IV line
  ○ Drug safe range for child's age and weight
  ○ Potential untoward response
  ○ IV compatibility
  ○ Infant's or child's renal, hepatic, and GI status
	Unique components for each individual patient must be considered within usual treatment modalities to help bring safe and timely return of temperature while avoiding iatrogenic complications.

• Provide padding to siderails of crib or bed to prevent injury in event of possible seizures.	Protection from injury in likelihood of uncontrolled sudden bodily movement serves to protect patient from further problems. Uses universal seizure precautions.
• Ensure that airway maintenance is addressed by appropriate suctioning and airway equipment according to age.	As a part of seizure activity, there is always the potential of loss of consciousness with respiratory involvement.

Women's Health

NOTE: Newborn is included with Women's Health because newborn care is administered by nurses on either a maternity, obstetrical, or mother-baby unit.

Actions/Interventions	Rationales
• When under heat source or bililights, monitor the infant every hour for increased redness and sweating. Check heat source at least every 30 minutes (overhead, isolettes, or bililights).	Provides safe environment for infant.
• Monitor infant's temperature, skin turgor, and fontanels (bulging or sunken) for signs and symptoms of dehydration every 30 minutes while under heat source. First temperature measurement should be rectal; thereafter can be axillary.	Provides essential information as to infant's current status and promotes a safe environment for infant.
• Check for urination; infant should wet at least six diapers every 24 hours.	Basic monitoring of infant's physiologic functioning.
• Replace lost fluids by offering the infant breast, water, or formula at least every 2 hours on the (odd/even) hour.	Decreases insensible fluid loss and maintains body temperature within normal range. This action will decrease the infant's needs for IV glucose.

- Pregnancy:
  - Teach patient to avoid use of hot tubs or saunas:
    (1) During first trimester, concerns about possible CNS defects in fetus and failure of neural tube closure[43]
    (2) During second and third trimesters, concerns about cardiac load for mother[43]
  - Provide cooling fans for mothers during labor and for patients on $MgSO_4$ therapy
  - Keep labor room cool for mother's comfort.

Provides safe environment for mother and prevents injury to fetus.

Mental Health

Actions/Interventions	Rationales

• Monitor clients receiving neuroleptic drugs for decreased ability to sweat by observing for decreased perspiration and an increase in body temperature with activity, especially in warm weather. Monitor these clients for hyperpyrexia (up to 107°F). Notify physician of alterations in temperature. Note alteration in the client's plan of care and initiate the following actions:
  ○ Client should not go outside in the warmest part of the day during warm weather.
  ○ Maintain client's fluid intake up to 3000 ml every 24 hours by (this is especially important for clients who are also receiving lithium carbonate; lithium levels should be carefully evaluated):
    (1) Having client's favorite fluids on the unit.
    (2) Having client drink 240 ml (8-oz glass) of fluids every hour while awake and 240 ml with each meal. If necessary the nurse will sit with the client while the fluid is consumed.
    (3) Maintaining record of client's intake and output.
  ○ Dress client in light, loose clothing.
  ○ If client is disoriented or confused, provide one-on-one observation.
	Clients who are receiving neuroleptic medications are at risk for developing neuroleptic malignant syndrome, which can be life-threatening.[33]
	
	High fevers can alter mental status and thus decrease the client's ability to make proper judgments.

Continued

Actions/Interventions	Rationales
• Decrease client's activity level by: ○ Decreasing stimuli ○ Sitting with client and talking quietly or involving client in a table game or activity that requires little large-muscle movement (note activities that client enjoys here) ○ Assigning room near nurse's station and dayroom areas • Monitor client's mental status every hour. • Do not provide client with alteration in mental status with small electrical cooling devices unless he or she receives constant supervision. • Give client as much information as possible about his or her condition and about measures that are implemented to decrease temperature. • Teach client and family about measures to decrease or eliminate risk for hyperthermia. (See Home Health for teaching information.) • Consult with appropriate assistive resources as indicated. (See Appendix B.)	Increased physical activity increases body temperature, and the decreased ability to sweat, secondary to medications, inhibits the body's normal adaptive response.[39]

Gerontic Health

Nursing actions for the gerontic patient with this diagnosis are the same as the adult health and home health nursing actions.

Home Health

Actions/Interventions	Rationales
• Monitor for factors contributing to hyperthermia (see Defining Characteristics).	Identification of risk factors provides for intervention to reduce or prevent negative outcomes.
• Teach client and family signs and symptoms of hyperthermia: ○ Flushed skin ○ Increased respiratory rate ○ Increased heart rate ○ Increase in body temperature ○ Seizure precautions and care	Provides data for early intervention.
• Teach measures to decrease or eliminate the risk of hyperthermia: ○ Wearing appropriate clothing	Provides basic knowledge that increases the probability of successful self-care.

- ○ Taking appropriate care of underlying disease
- ○ Avoiding exposure to hot environments
- ○ Preventing dehydration
- ○ Using antipyretics
- ○ Performing early intervention with gradual cooling
- Involve client and family in planning, implementing, and promoting reduction or elimination of the risk for hyperthermia.
- Assist client and family to identify lifestyle changes that may be required.

- Measure temperature using appropriate method for developmental age of person.
- Teach survival techniques if client works or plays outdoors.
- Ensure proper hydration.
- Transport to health care facility.
- Use emergency transport system.

Involvement provides opportunity for increased motivation and ability to appropriately intervene.

Knowledge and support provide motivation for change and increase potential for a positive outcome.

FLOW CHART EVALUATION
Flow Chart Expected Outcome 1

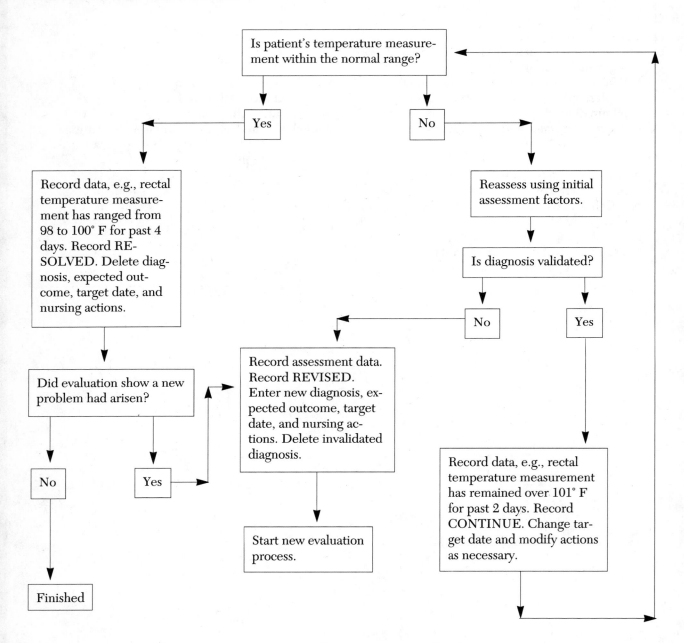

Flow Chart Expected Outcome 2

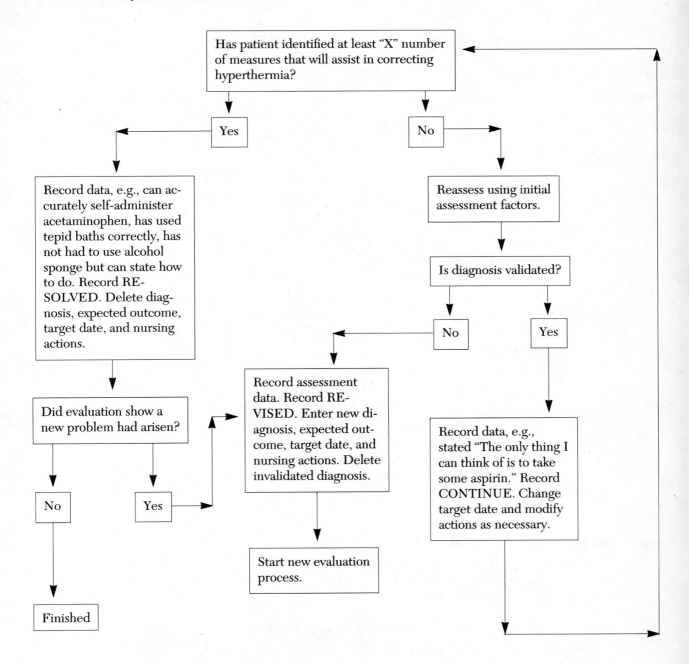

Hypothermia

DEFINITION

The state in which an individual's body temperature is reduced below normal range.

NANDA TAXONOMY: EXCHANGING 1.2.2.2

DEFINING CHARACTERISTICS

1. Major defining characteristics:
   a. Reduction in body temperature below normal range
   b. Shivering (mild)
   c. Cool skin
   d. Pallor (moderate)
2. Minor defining characteristics:
   a. Slow capillary refill
   b. Tachycardia
   c. Cyanotic nail beds
   d. Hypertension
   e. Piloerection

RELATED FACTORS

1. Exposure to cool or cold environment
2. Illness or trauma
3. Damage to hypothalamus
4. Inability or decreased ability to shiver
5. Malnutrition
6. Inadequate clothing
7. Consumption of alcohol
8. Medications causing vasodilation
9. Evaporation from skin in cool environment
10. Decreased metabolic rate
11. Inactivity
12. Aging

RELATED CLINICAL CONCERNS

1. Hypothyroidism
2. Anorexia nervosa
3. Any injury to the brainstem

HAVE YOU SELECTED THE CORRECT DIAGNOSIS?

High Risk for Altered Body Temperature This diagnosis indicates that the person is potentially unable to regulate heat production and heat dissipation within a normal range. In Hypothermia, the patient's ability to dissipate heat is not impaired. Heat production is impaired to the degree that Hypothermia results. (See page 125.)

Ineffective Thermoregulation The body temperature fluctuates between being too high and too low. In Hypothermia, the temperature does not fluctuate; it remains low. (See page 234.)

Hyperthermia The patient's temperature is above normal, not below normal. (See page 177.)

EXPECTED OUTCOMES

1. Will return to normal body temperature range (between 97.3 and 98.8°F) by (date) and/or
2. Will identify at least (number) measures to use in correcting hypothermia by (date)

TARGET DATE

Hypothermia can be life-threatening; therefore, initial target dates should be in terms of hours. After the patient has demonstrated some stability toward a normal range, target dates can be increased from 2 to 4 days.

NURSING ACTIONS/INTERVENTIONS WITH RATIONALES

Adult Health

Actions/Interventions	Rationales
• Warm the patient quickly. Use blankets, warming blankets, warm water (102 to 105°F), extra clothing, warm drinks, and/or warm room. Do not use a heat lamp or hot-water bottles. Prevent air drafts in room. Monitor safe functioning of equipment used in thermoregulation.	Basic measures that assist in increasing core temperature and prevent excess heat dissipation. Heat lamps and hot-water bottles warm only a limited area and increase the likelihood of local tissue damage.
• Monitor temperature measurement every hour until temperature returns to normal levels and stabilizes.	Assesses effectiveness of therapy.
• Prevent injury. Gently massage body; however, *do not* rub a body part if frostbite is evident.	Massage helps stimulate circulation; however, massage of a frostbitten area will promote tissue death and gangrene. In frostbite, circulation has to be gradually reestablished through warming.
• Address skin protective needs by frequent monitoring for breakdown or altered circulation.	Hypothermia causes peripheral vasoconstriction, which leads to a high risk for impaired skin integrity.
• Give fluids such as salt and soda solution. Have patient sip slowly (if conscious and not vomiting). *Do not* give alcohol.	Assists in maintaining fluid and electrolyte balance. Alcohol would promote vasoconstriction.

Continued

Actions/Interventions	Rationales
• Monitor respiratory rate and depth and breath sounds every hour. Provide for airway suctioning and positioning as needed.	Hypothermia and its related factors promote the development of respiratory complications.
• Bathe with appropriate protection and covering.	Prevents heat loss.
• Devote appropriate attention to prevention of major complications such as shock, cardiac failure, tissue necrosis, infection, fluid and electrolyte imbalance, convulsions or loss of consciousness, respiratory failure, and renal failure.	Awareness of the complications of hypothermia will help prevent the complications.
• Administer medications as ordered.	
• Monitor effects and record within 30 minutes after administration.	Assists in monitoring effectiveness of therapy
• Obtain a detailed history regarding: ○ Onset ○ Related trauma and causative factors ○ Duration of hypothermia	
• Provide opportunities for patient and family to ask questions and relay concerns by including 30 minutes for this every shift. (Note times here.)	Decreases anxiety and facilitates home care teaching.
• Allow for appropriate attention to resolution of psychological trauma, especially in instances of severe exposure to cold, at least once per shift. (Note times here.)	Helps in reducing patient's anxiety and facilitates patient's resolving lingering effects of trauma.
• Teach patient and family measures to decrease or eliminate the risk for hypothermia, to include: ○ Wearing appropriate clothing when outdoors ○ Maintaining room temperature at minimum of 65°F ○ Wearing clothing in layers ○ Covering the head, hands, and feet when outdoors (especially the head) ○ Removing wet clothing	Permits patient to participate in self-care and promotes compliance to prevent future episodes.
• Teach patient about the kinds of behavior that increase the risk for hypothermia: ○ Drug and alcohol abuse ○ Working, living, or playing outdoors ○ Poor nutrition, especially when body fat is reduced below normal levels as in anorexia nervosa	
• Teach patient and family signs and symptoms of early hypothermia: ○ Confusion, disorientation ○ Slurred speech	

○ Low blood pressure
○ Difficulty in awakening
○ Weak pulse
○ Cold stomach
○ Impaired coordination

Actions/Interventions	Rationales
• Make appropriate arrangements for follow-up after discharge from hospital. Identify support groups in the community for the patient and family.	Fosters resources for long-term management in terms of adequate housing, financial resources, and social habits. (See Appendix B.)
• Consult with appropriate assistive resources as indicated: ○ Energy audit by public service company to identify possible sources ○ Social services to provide information on emergency shelters, clothing, and food banks ○ Financial counseling if heating the home is financially difficult	Promotes effective long-term management and prevention of future episode.

Child Health

Actions/Interventions	Rationales
• Provide for maintenance of body temperature by hat (stockinette for infant), open radiant warmer, isolette, or heating blanket.	Heat loss is greatest via the head in young infants as well as by convection and evaporation. Suitable maintenance of temperature by appropriate equipment will help to maintain neutral body core temperature.
• Incorporate other health care team members to address collaborative needs. (See Appendix B.)	Provision of support for long-term follow-up will place value on the need for care and the importance of compliance. Assists in reducing anxiety.
• Provide teaching to address unknown and necessary information for child and family in terms they can relate to (for example, temperature measurement).	Serves to establish foundation of trust and provides essential basis for follow-up care.
• Anticipate safety needs according to patient's age and development status.	Each opportunity for reinforcing the importance of safety as a part of well-child follow-up should not be overlooked. As related to the use of the thermometer, emphasize caution with rectal thermometer to prevent trauma to anal sphincter and tissue, and caution family regarding the use of mercury-glass thermometer and breakage. In the event of use of electronic equipment, emphasize the importance of protection to skin, constant surveillance, and unique safety needs per manufacturer.

Women's Health

NOTE: This nursing diagnosis will pertain to the woman the same as to any other adult. The reader is referred to the other sections for specific nursing actions pertaining to women and hypothermia. Infants control their body temperature with nonshivering thermogenesis. This process is accompanied by an increase in oxygen and calorie consumption. Therefore, use of a radiant warmer or pre-warmed mattress for initial care provides environmental heat generation rather than heat loss. However, it is important to note that hypothermia and cold stress in the neonate are related to the amount of oxygen needed by the infant to control apnea and acid-base balance. It is estimated that to replace a heat loss during a temperature drop of 3.5°C (6.3°F), the infant will require a 100 percent increase in oxygen consumption for more than 1½ hours. Metabolic acidosis can occur quickly if the infant becomes hypothermic.[27]

Newborn

Actions/Interventions	Rationales

• To prevent hypothermia in the newborn:
  ○ Dry new infant thoroughly.
  ○ Cover with blanket.
  ○ Lay next to mother's body (cover mother and infant by placing blanket over them).
  ○ Place infant under radiant heat source.
  ○ Keep out of drafts.
• Observe infant for hypoglycemia. Check temperature every hour until stable, then every 4 hours for 24 hours. May be taken rectally, by axilla, or by skin (continuous probe).
	Prevention of heat loss in the infant will reduce oxygen and calorie consumption and prevent metabolic acidosis.

Mental Health

Actions/Interventions	Rationales
• Monitor client's mental status every 2 hours (note times here); report alterations to physician. • If client is receiving antipsychotics or antidepressants, report this to the physician when alteration is first noted. • Protect client from contact with uncontrolled hot objects such as space heaters and radiators by teaching clients and family to remove these from the environment.	Antipsychotic and antidepressant medications can alter thermoregulation, which results in hypothermia.[39]

| • Allow client to use heating pads and electric blankets *only* with supervision. | Basic safety measures. |
| • Teach client the potential for medication to affect body temperature regulation, especially in the elderly. | |

Gerontic Health

Nursing actions for the gerontic patient with this diagnosis are the same as those given in Adult Health and Mental Health.

Home Health

Actions/Interventions	Rationales
• Involve client and family in planning, implementing, and promoting reduction or elimination of the risk for hypothermia.	Involvement provides likelihood of increased motivation and ability to appropriately intervene.
• Assist client and family to identify life-style changes that may be required:	Knowledge and support provides motivation for change and increases the potential for a positive outcome.
○ Avoiding drug and alcohol abuse	
○ Learning survival techniques if client works or plays outdoors (for example, camping, hiking, or skiing)	
○ Keeping person dry	
○ Transporting to health care facility	
○ Using emergency transport system	

FLOW CHART EVALUATION
Flow Chart Expected Outcome 1

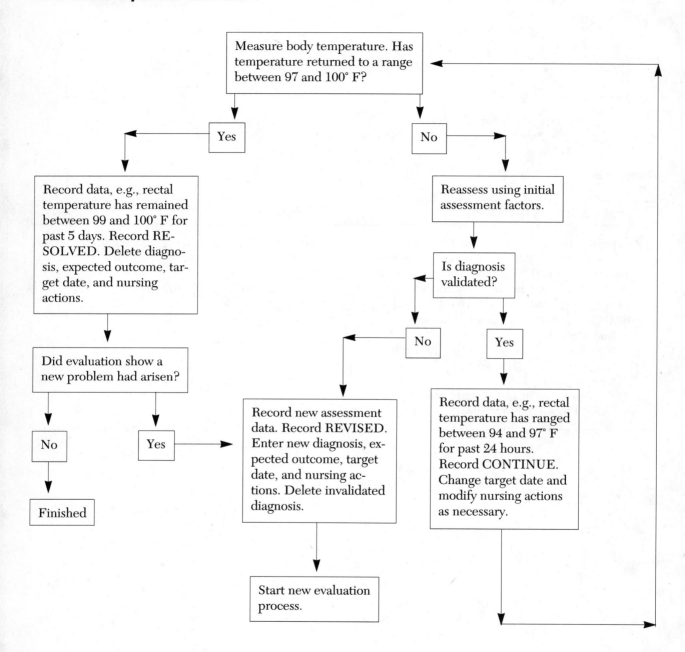

Flow Chart Expected Outcome 2

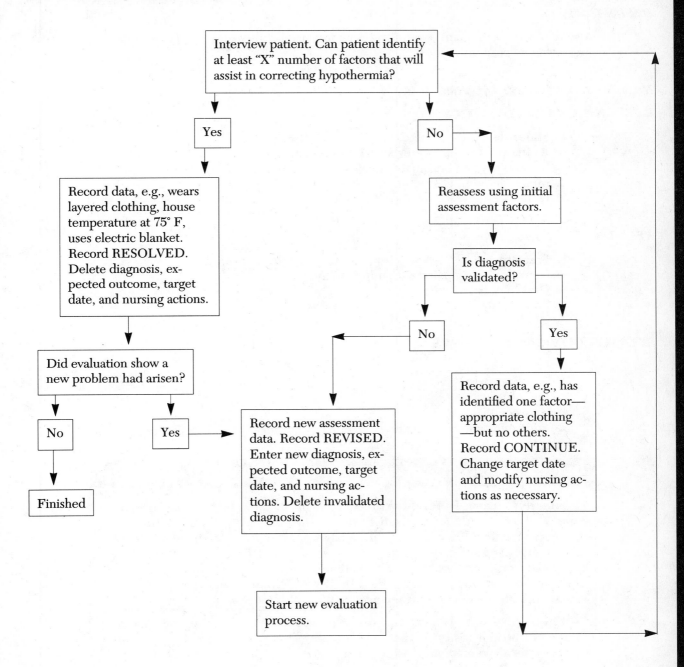

Infant Feeding Pattern, Ineffective

DEFINITION

A state in which an infant demonstrates an impaired ability to suck or coordinate the suck-swallow response.

NANDA TAXONOMY: MOVING 6.5.1.4

DEFINING CHARACTERISTICS

1. Major defining characteristics:
   a. Inability to initiate or sustain an effective suck
   b. Inability to coordinate sucking, swallowing, and breathing
2. Minor defining characteristics:
   None

RELATED FACTORS

1. Prematurity
2. Neurological impairment and/or delay
3. Oral hypersensitivity
4. Prolonged NPO

RELATED CLINICAL CONCERNS

1. Prematurity
2. Cerebral palsy
3. Thrush
4. Hydrocephalus
5. Any condition that would require major surgery immediately after birth

HAVE YOU SELECTED THE CORRECT DIAGNOSIS?

Ineffective Breast-Feeding   With this diagnosis the infant is able to suckle and swallow, but there is dissatisfaction or difficulty with the breast-feeding process. The key difference would be based on the defining characteristics of Ineffective Breast-Feeding versus Ineffective Infant Feeding Pattern. If the infant demonstrates problems with initiating, sustaining, or coordinating sucking, swallowing, and breathing, then Ineffective Infant Feeding Pattern is the most appropriate diagnosis. (See page 140.)

Altered Nutrition: Less than Body Requirements   Certainly this diagnosis could be the result of Ineffective Infant Feeding Pattern if the feeding problem is not remedied. However, correction of the primary problems would prevent the development of this diagnosis. (See page 200.)

EXPECTED OUTCOMES

1. Will demonstrate normal ability to suck-swallow by (date) and/or
2. Will gain at least (number) ounces by (date)

TARGET DATE

This diagnosis would be life-threatening; therefore, progress should initially be evaluated every few hours. After the infant has begun to exhibit at least some sucking-swallowing, then the target date can be moved to every 2 days.

NURSING ACTIONS/INTERVENTIONS WITH RATIONALES

Adult Health

For this diagnosis, Child Health and Women's Health (Newborn) serve as the generic actions. This diagnosis would not be used in Adult Health.

Child Health

Actions/Interventions	Rationales

• Monitor for all possible contributory factors:
  ○ Actual physiologic sucking potential
  ○ Other objective concerns, for example, swallowing or respiratory
  ○ Objective history data, for example, prematurity or congenital anomalies
  ○ Maternal-infant reciprocity
  ○ Subjective data per caregivers or parents
	A thorough assessment and monitoring will serve as the critical basis for appropriate individualizing and prioritizing of a plan of health care.

• Provide anticipatory support to infant for respiratory difficulties that could increase the probability of aspiration.
 	
• Ascertain the most appropriate feeding protocol for the infant, with attention to:
  ○ Nutritional needs according to desired weight gain
  ○ Actual feeding mode, for example, modified nipple, larger-hole nipple, syringe adapted for feeding, position for feeding, or gastric tube
  ○ Health status and prognosis
  ○ Compliance factors
  ○ Socioeconomic factors
  ○ Maternal-infant concerns
	Airway maintenance is a basic safety precaution for this infant. Airway and suctioning equipment will be standard. (See nursing actions for High Risk for Aspiration.) A realistic yet holistic approach will provide a foundation for multidisciplinary management with best likelihood for success. Specific criteria will provide measurable progress parameters.

• Explore the feelings caregivers or parents have related to the ineffective feeding pattern.	Often the expression of feelings will reduce anxiety and may allow further potential alterations to be minimized by early intervention.
• Strictly monitor and calculate intake, output, and caloric count on each shift, and total each 24 hours.	Caloric intake and hydration status are indirectly and directly used to monitor the infant's progress in tolerance of feeding and feeding efficacy.

Continued

Actions/Interventions	Rationales
• Weigh infant daily or more often as indicated.	Weight gain would serve as a major indicator of effective feeding and assist in assessment of hydration.
• Collaborate with other health care professionals to better meet the infant's needs. (See Appendix B.)	A multidisciplinary approach is most effective in level and cost of care.
• Allow for appropriate time to prepare infant for feeding, and provide a calm, soothing milieu.	A nonhurried, nonstressful milieu will promote the infant's relaxation and allow the infant to perceive feeding as a pleasant experience.
• Encourage family to participate in feeding and plans for feeding.	Inclusion of family empowers the family and augments their self-confidence and coping.
• Provide teaching based on an assessment of parental knowledge needs and/or deficits.	Knowledge provides a means of decreasing anxiety. When based on assessed needs, it will reflect the individualized needs and more likely meet the parents' learning needs.
• Allow for time to clarify feeding protocols, questions, and discharge planning.	Appropriate attention to questions and concerns parents may have will assist in reducing anxiety, thereby allowing for learning and a greater likelihood of adherence to the therapeutic regimen.

Women's Health

Actions/Interventions	Rationales
• Provide support and information to mother and significant other. Explain the infant's inability to suck, and provide suggestions and options (based on etiology of sucking problem) to correct or reduce problem.[30,45,46]	The basic rationale for all the nursing actions in this diagnosis is to provide nutrition to the infant in the most appropriate, cost-effective, and successful manner.
• Describe the anatomy and physiology of sucking to the mother.	Assists in decreasing anxiety, provides a base for teaching, and permits long-range planning. Encourages proper suckling by the infant.
• Explain importance of positioning for both bottle- and breast-feeding.[46,47,48]	
• Provide support and supervision to assist mother in encouraging infant to suck properly.	
• If necessary, provide supplemental nutrition system while teaching infant to suck, for example, dropper, syringe, spoon, cup, or supplementation device.[49,50]	Pays attention to basic nutrition while also attending to problem with sucking.
• Refer to lactation consultant or clinical nurse specialist for assistance and support in teaching infant to suck.	

- Assist mother and significant others to choose feeding system for infant (breast, bottle, or tube) that will supply best nutrition.

Provides basic support to encourage essential nutrition.

Mental Health

This diagnosis would not be used in Mental Health.

Gerontic Health

This diagnosis is not appropriate for the gerontic patient.

Home Health

The nursing actions for home health would be the same as for women's health.

FLOW CHART EVALUATION
Flow Chart Expected Outcome 1

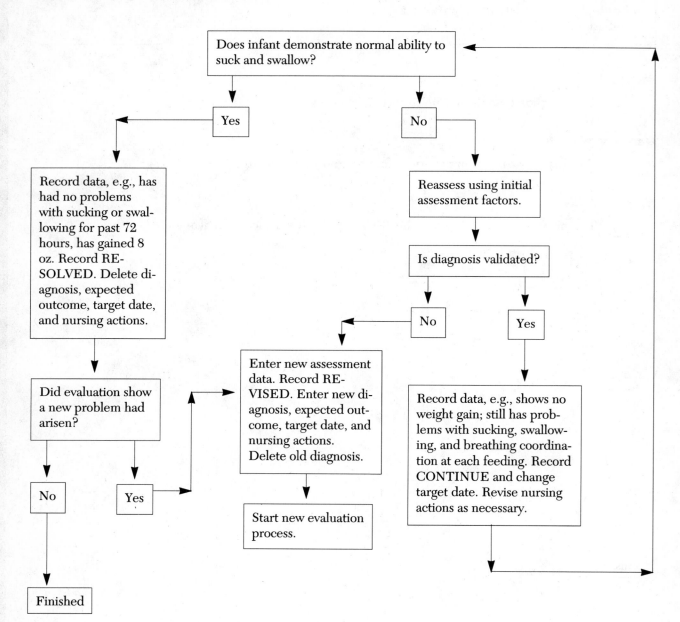

Flow Chart Expected Outcome 2

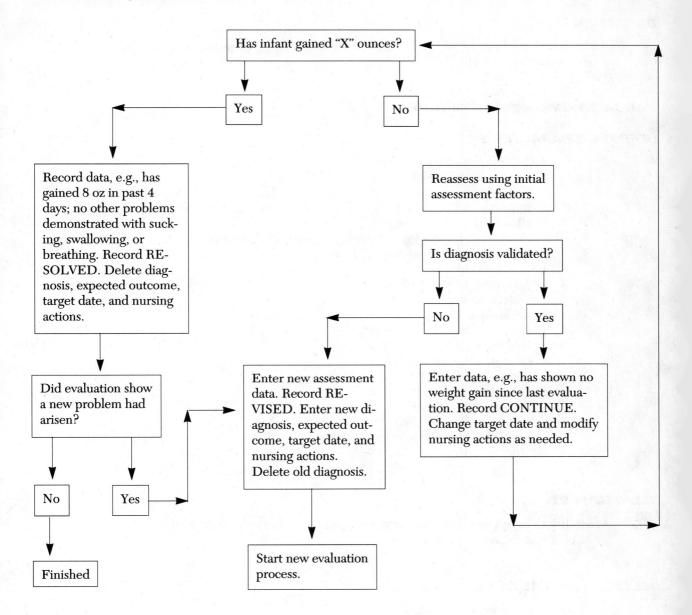

Nutrition, Altered: Less than Body Requirements

DEFINITION

The state in which an individual experiences an intake of nutrients insufficient to meet metabolic needs.

NANDA TAXONOMY: EXCHANGING 1.1.2.2

DEFINING CHARACTERISTICS

1. Major defining characteristics:
   a. Loss of weight with adequate food intake
   b. Body weight 20 percent or more under ideal
   c. Reported inadequate food intake less than the RDA (recommended daily allowance)
   d. Weakness of muscles required for swallowing or mastication
   e. Reported or evident lack of food
   f. Aversion to eating
   g. Reported altered taste sensation
   h. Satiety immediately after ingesting food
   i. Abdominal cramping
   j. Diarrhea and/or steatorrhea
   k. Hyperactive bowel sounds
   l. Lack of interest in food
   m. Perceived inability to ingest food
   n. Pale conjunctival and mucous membranes
   o. Poor muscle tone
   p. Excessive loss of hair
   q. Lack of information, misinformation
   r. Misconception

RELATED FACTORS

Inability to ingest or digest food or absorb nutrients due to biological, psychological, or economic factors.

RELATED CLINICAL CONCERNS

1. Anorexia nervosa/bulemia
2. Cancer
3. AIDS
4. Alzheimer's disease
5. Anemia
6. Ostomies
7. Schizophrenia, paranoid

HAVE YOU SELECTED THE CORRECT DIAGNOSIS?

Altered Oral Mucous Membranes If the oral mucous membranes are severely inflamed or damaged, food intake could be so painful that the person ceases intake to avoid the pain. While the end result might be Altered Nutrition: Less than Body Requirements, initial intervention would have to be aimed at handling the oral mucosal problem. (See page 239.)

Altered Bowel Elimination: Diarrhea In this instance the body cannot absorb the necessary nutrients because the food material passes through the gastrointestinal tract too rapidly. (See page 285.)

Altered Tissue Perfusion Once the food has been ingested, digested, and absorbed, its components must get to the cells. If there is Altered Tissue Perfusion, the nutrients may not be able to get to the cells in sufficient quantities to do any good. (See page 484.)

Self-Care Deficit: Feeding, or Altered Sensory Perception Visual, Olfactory, and/or Gustatory, or Altered Health Maintenance may be the primary problem(s). If the person does not sense hunger through the usual means—seeing, smelling, or tasting—or if the person thinks he or she has already eaten, then the desire to eat may not exist. Even if the person senses hunger, the inability to feed oneself, to shop for food, or to prepare food could result in less-than-adequate nutrition. (See pages 472 and 562.)

Pain If the preparation or actual eating of food increases pain level, then the patient might elect to avoid eating to assist in pain control. (See page 246.)

Fear, Dysfunctional Grieving, Social Isolation, Body Image Disturbance, Self-Esteem Disturbance, and Spiritual Distress These are psychosocial problems that can impact nutrition. Each of these may create a decreased desire to eat, or even if food is eaten, the person may vomit because the stomach will not accept the food. Additionally, if the person eats, he or she may only pick at the food and not ingest enough to maintain the body's need for nutrients. (See pages 618, 628, 668, 732, 781 and 923.)

Knowledge Deficit The person may not really know how much or what kind of food is more beneficial to his or her body. (See page 536.)

EXPECTED OUTCOMES

1. Will gain (number) of pounds by (date) and/or
2. Will design and implement a personal nutritional improvement plan by (date) that is accurate, achievable, and realistic

TARGET DATE

This diagnosis reflects a long-term care problem; therefore, a target date of 5 days or more from the date of admission would be acceptable.

NURSING ACTIONS/INTERVENTIONS WITH RATIONALES

Adult Health

Actions/Interventions	Rationales
• Increase food and fluid intake at each meal or feeding: 　○ Reduce noxious stimuli. 　○ Open all food containers and release odors outside patient's room. 　○ According to individual needs, either provide privacy for eating or provide communal dining. 　○ Administer appropriate medications 30 minutes before meals (for example, analgesics or antiemetics). Record effects of medications within 30 minutes of administration.	Basic methods and procedures that enhance appetite.
○ If patient requires suctioning, do so at least 15 minutes before mealtime. Keep suctioning equipment available but out of immediate eating site.	Suctioning removes secretions that may cause nausea. Timing of activities promotes rest prior to meals.
• Provide at least a 30-minute rest period prior to meal.	Conserves energy for feeding self and digestion.
• Give oral hygiene 30 minutes before meals and as required.	Moistens and cleanses oral mucous membranes, which promotes eating.
• When assisting patient to eat or feeding patient: 　○ Raise head of bed. 　○ Help wash hands. 　○ Open carton and packages. 　○ Cut food into small, bite-size pieces. 　○ Provide assistive devices (for example, large-handled spoon or fork, all-in-one utensil, or plate guard).	
• Offer small, frequent feedings every 2 to 3 hours rather than just three meals per day. Allow patient to assist with food choices and feeding schedules.	Three large meals a day give a sense of fullness, and size of servings may be overwhelming to patient. Smaller meals facilitate gastric emptying, thus promoting an overall larger food intake.
• Focus fluid intake between meals: 　○ Limit fluid intake at meals. 　○ Offer wine at meals or immediately prior to meals.	Alcohol stimulates gastric secretions and stimulates the appetite.
• Encourage patient to eat slowly.	Allows the patient to savor the taste of food. Facilitates the digestion process.
• Have patient chew gum before meals, or have patient visualize lemons or sour pickles.	Stimulates salivation.

- Offer between-meal supplements. Focus on high-protein diet and liquids.

- Avoid gas-producing foods and carbonated beverages.
- Avoid very hot or very cold foods.

- Encourage significant others to bring special food from home.

- Allow for 30-minute (minimum) rest periods after eating.
- Measure and total intake and output every 8 hours. Total every 24 hours.
- Make sure intake and output is balancing at least every 72 hours.

- Weigh daily at (state time) and in same-weight clothing. Have patient empty bladder before weighing. Teach patient this routine for continued weighing at home.
- Encourage exercise at least twice per shift to the extent possible without tiring. If exercise capacity is limited, do passive or active range of motion every 4 hours at (state times here) while awake.
- Monitor:
  ○ Vital signs every 4 hours while awake at (state times here) and as required based on measurement results
  ○ Airway, sensorium, chest sounds, bowel sounds, skin turgor, mucous membranes, bowel function, urine specific gravity, and glucose level at least once per shift.
  ○ Laboratory values (for example, electrolyte levels, hematocrit, hemoglobin, blood glucose, serum albumin, and/or total protein)
- Provide frequent positive reinforcement for:
  ○ Weight gain
  ○ Increased intake
  ○ Ignoring weight loss
  ○ Using consistent approach
  ○ Indications of successful learning of items in next nursing action.
- Teach patient and significant others:
  ○ Balanced diet based on the basic four food groups

Provides additional caloric intake. Providing high-protein foods and fluids helps prevent muscle-tissue loss.
Gas-producing foods promote nausea and a feeling of fullness.
Extremes in temperature lead to a decrease in appetite and promote irritation of oral mucous membranes.
Familiar food promotes appetite and empowers patient and family in regard to diet. Allows an opportunity for teaching about diet.
Facilitates digestion and reduces stress.

Allows monitoring of renal function and ensures weight gain is not due to fluid retention.
Assesses effectiveness of therapy and interventions. Promotes patient's control of weight after discharge.

Stimulates appetite and prevents complications from immobility.

Allows early detection of complications and assists in monitoring effectiveness of therapy.

Provides essential information needed to prevent future episodes.

Continued

Actions/Interventions	Rationales
○ Role of diet in health (for example, healing, energy, and normal body functioning) ○ How to keep food diary with calorie count ○ How to add spices to food to improve taste and aroma ○ Use of exchange lists ○ Relaxation techniques • Refer, as necessary, to other health care providers. (See Appendix B.)	Provides ongoing support for long-term care.

ADDITIONAL INFORMATION

There will be situations in which the patient's nutritional condition has progressed to the point that tube feedings, intravenous therapy, or total parenteral nutrition will become necessary. In addition to the nursing actions for the overall nursing diagnosis of Altered Nutrition: Less than Body Requirements, the following actions should be added:

Tube Feedings

Actions/Interventions	Rationales
• Check placement and patency prior to each feeding. Initial placement should be checked using radiographic verification since ausculatory methods are not always accurate. Check gastric aspiration for acidic pH.[51,52]	Prevents aspiration and monitors for complication of stress ulcer.
• Aspirate tube prior to each feeding. Measure amount of residual from previous feeding. If 150 ml or more remains, delay feeding and notify physician.	Prevents overloading of stomach and initiates assessment for reason stomach is not emptying.
• Check temperature of feeding before administering. Temperature should be slightly below room temperature.	Prevents abdominal cramping and reflux.
• Measure amount of feeding exactly. Flush tube with water immediately after feeding.	Avoid overloading stomach. Flushing ensures that all feeding has entered stomach and prevents clogging of tube.
• Crush medications in water or dissolve in water before giving. Flush tube with water immediately after administering medication.	Permits maintenance of therapeutic regimen and prevents clogging of tube by medication.
• Keep patient in semi-Fowler's position for at least 30 minutes following feeding.	Prevents reflux and aspiration of feeding.
• Cleanse and lubricate nares after each feeding.	Helps prevent breakdown of nasal mucosa. Promotes comfort.

• Check taping of tube following each feeding.	Ensures security of tube and promotes comfort.
• If feeding is to be administered by gravity method (preferred), make sure all air is out of tubing.	Air in stomach is uncomfortable, creates feeling of fullness, promotes nausea, and displaces space needed for nutritional feeding. Decreases the risk of aspiration and lets gravity assist in fluid flow through stomach.

Continuous Tube Feeding

In certain situations, such as severe dysphagia, clients may be placed on continuous feeding via a pump. When continuous feeding is in effect, the following additional actions should be implemented.

Actions/Interventions	Rationales
• Maintain the head of the bed at a 30-degree angle at all times.	
• Monitor infusion rate at least every 4 hours around the clock at (times).	Ensures that correct flow rate is being maintained.
• Monitor respiratory rate, effort, and lung sounds at least every 4 hours around the clock at (times).	Allows monitoring for possible aspiration.
• Request medication in liquid form whenever possible.	Decreases the potential blocking off of feeding tube with particulate matter.
• Check for security of tube placement at least every 4 hours around the clock at (times).	Guards against tube displacement.
• Provide oral care every 4 hours while awake at (times). Oral care is especially important when the nasogastric route is used.	An increase in mouth breathing leads to drying of the oral cavity and to accumulation of debris in the mouth.

Intravenous

Actions/Interventions	Rationales
• Check insertion site for warmth, redness, swelling, leakage, and pain at least every 4 hours at (state times here).	Basic monitoring for infiltration and venous irritation.
• Check flow rate at a maximum of every hour on the (hour, half-hour).	Prevents fluid overload.
• Check for signs and symptoms of circulatory overload at least every 2 hours (state times here) (for example, headache, neck vein distention, tachycardia, increased blood pressure, or respiratory changes).	
• Change tubing according to agency's stated standard or policy.	Implementation of Centers for Disease Control (CDC) guidelines. Prevention of complications from tubing.

Total Parenteral Nutrition

Actions/Interventions	Rationales

• Do not administer without pump.
• Change tubing and filter daily at (state time here).
• Change dressing every other day beginning (date):
  ○ Use aseptic technique.
  ○ Gently cleanse area around catheter (state specifically how here — most agencies have specific policy).
  ○ Use a bacteriostatic, not antibiotic, ointment.
  ○ Apply a dry, airtight dressing.
• Check insertion site for warmth, redness, swelling, leakage, and pain at least every 4 hours at (state times here).
	The pump allows for accurate flow rate. Ensures proper flow of parental nutrition and avoids complications.
	Basic infection preventive measures.
	
	Basic monitoring for infiltration and venous irritation.

Child Health

> NOTE: This diagnosis represents a long-term care issue. Therefore, a series of subgoals of smaller amounts of weight to be gained in a lesser period of time may be necessary. Long-term goals are still to be formulated and revised as the patient's status demands. Also, there will undoubtedly be instances in which overlap may exist for other nursing diagnoses. Specifically, as an example, in the instance of an alteration in nutrition related to actual failure to thrive, one must refer to appropriate role performance on the part of the mother with consideration for holistic nursing management. It would be most critical to include a few specific nursing process components to reflect the critical needs for the mother-infant dyad.

Actions/Interventions	Rationales
• Feed the infant on a regular schedule that offers nutrients appropriate to metabolic needs. For example, an infant of less than 5 lb will eat more often but in lesser amounts (2 to 3 oz every 2 to 3 hours) than an infant of 15 lb (4 to 5 oz every 3 to 4 hours). • Assist or feed patient: ○ Elevate head of bed, or place infant in infant seat and older infant or toddler in highchair with safety belt in place. If necessary, hold infant. (This will be dictated in part by patient's status and presence of various tubes and equipment.)	The stomach capacity and digestive concerns for each patient must be considered to realistically plan for weight gain over a slow, steady, incremental time frame. Appropriate attention to aesthetic, physical, and emotional details related to feeding will help to provide the optimal potential for pleasant, long-lasting eating patterns. The limitation of psychological, emotional duress cannot be overemphasized and must be considered in each parent-child unit.

- ○ Help patient wash hands. For infants and toddlers, administer diaper change as needed.
- ○ Warm foods and formula as needed, and test on wrist before feeding infant or child.
- ○ Provide aids appropriate for age and physical capacity as needed, such as two-handed cups for toddlers, favorite spoon, or Velcro strap for utensils for child with cerebral palsy.
- ○ Offer small, age-appropriate feedings with input from family members regarding child's preferences.
- ○ Encourage patient to eat slowly and to chew food thoroughly. For infant, bubble before, during, and after feeding.
- • Provide role-modeling opportunities in a nonthreatening, nonjudgmental manner to assist parents in learning about feeding an infant or child.

Nonthreatening role modeling and personal encouragement fosters compliance and lessens anxiety.

- • Weigh patient on same scale and at same time (state time here) daily. Weigh infants without clothes and older children in underwear.

Weight gain serves as a critical indicator of efficacy of treatment. Maintaining consistency in weighing lessens the number of potential intervening variables that would result in an inaccurate weight.

- • Teach patient and family:
- ○ Balanced diet appropriate for age using basic four food groups.
- ○ Role of diet in health (for example, healing, energy, and normal body functioning). If infant is medically diagnosed as Failure to Thrive, offer appropriate emotional support, and allow at least 30 minutes three times a day (state times here) for exploring dyad relationships.
- ○ How to use spices and child-oriented approach in encouraging child to eat (for example, peach fruit salad, with peach as a face, garnished with cherries and raisins for eyes and nose, half of a pineapple round for mouth).
- ○ How to monitor for possible food allergies, especially in toddlers with history of allergies.
- ○ How to weigh self appropriately if applicable, or for parents to weigh child.
- • Provide positive reinforcement as often as appropriate for parents and child demonstrating critical behavior.

Reinforcement of desired behaviors fosters long-term compliance, thereby empowering the family with satisfaction and confidence for ultimate self-care management with minimal intervention by others.

Women's Health

NOTE: Poverty and substance abuse are often associated with nutritional deficits. Remember that underweight women who are pregnant will exhibit a different pattern of weight gain than normal-weight women. This difference exhibits a rapid weight gain at the beginning of the first trimester of about 1 pound per week by 20 weeks, in the underweight woman, weight gain can be as much as 18 to 20 pounds. Remember to teach the parents signs and symptoms of weight loss in the neonate.[27]

Actions/Interventions	Rationales

• Collaborate with dietitian in planning and teaching diet:
    ○ Emphasize high-quality calories (cottage cheese, lean meats, fish, tofu, whole grains, fruits, vegetables).
    ○ Avoid excess intake of fats and sugar.
    ○ Assist patient in identifying methods to keep caloric intake within the recommended limit.
 • Verify prepregnant weight.
	Gives baseline from which to plan better nutrition.
	
	 Assists in planning realistic diet changes within the patient's means and according to the patient's particular needs and habits.

• Determine if weight loss during first trimester is due to nausea and vomiting.
 • Check activity level against daily dietary intake.
 • Check for food intolerances.
 • Check environmental influences:
    ○ Hot weather
    ○ Cultural practices
    ○ Pica eating
    ○ Economic situation
    ○ Ascertain economic status and ability to buy food
    ○ Monitor woman's emotional response to the pregnancy and to additional weight gain	

NOTE: Dieting is never recommended during pregnancy because it deprives mother and fetus of nutrients needed for tissue growth and because weight loss is accompanied by maternal ketosis, a direct threat to fetal well-being.[5,43]

• Identify additional caloric needs and sources of those calories for the nursing mother:[53,54]
   ○ Additional 500 cal per day above normal dietary intake is needed to produce adequate milk (depending on the individual, a total of 2500 to 3000 cal per day).

- ○ Additional fluids are necessary to produce adequate milk.
- Collaborate with nutritionist to provide a healthy dietary pattern for the lactating mother.
- Monitor mother's energy levels and health maintenance:
  - ○ Does she complain of fatigue?
  - ○ Does she have sufficient energy to complete her daily activities?
  - ○ Does the dietary assessment show irregular dietary intake?
  - ○ Is she more than 10 percent below the ideal weight for her body stature?
- For breast-feeding the newborn or neonate during the first 6 months, teach the mother:
  - ○ The major source of nourishment is human milk.
  - ○ Vitamin supplements can be used as recommended by physician:
    - (1) Vitamin D
    - (2) Fluoride
    - (3) If indicated, iron
- Infant should be taking in approximately 420 ml daily soon after birth and building to 1200 ml daily at the end of 3 months.
- Monitor for fluid deficit at least daily:
  - ○ "Fussy baby," especially if immediately after feeding
  - ○ Constipation (remember, breast-fed babies have fewer stools than formula-fed babies).
- Weight loss or slow weight gain: Closely monitor baby, mother, and nursing routine.
  - ○ Is baby getting empty calories (for example, a lot of water between feedings)?
  - ○ Avoid nipple confusion, which results from switching baby from breast to bottle and vice versa many times.
  - ○ Count number of diapers per day (should have 6 to 8 really wet diapers per day).
  - ○ Is there intolerance to mother's milk or bottle formula?
  - ○ Is there illness or lactose intolerance?
  - ○ Is nursing infrequent? (Infrequent nursing can cause slow weight gain.)

Provides basis for ensuring good nutrition and assists in successful breast-feeding.

Provides for good nutritional status of the newborn.

Allows early intervention for this problem.

Mental Health

> NOTE: Due to long-term care requirements for these clients, target dates should be determined in weeks or months, not hours or days.

Actions/Interventions	Rationales
• Do not attempt teaching or long-term goal setting with client until concentration has improved (symptom of starvation).	Starvation can impact cognitive functioning.[55]
• Establish contract with client to remain on prescribed diet and not to perform maladaptive behavior (that is, vomiting or use of laxatives). State specific behavior for client here.	Provides client with sense of control and clearly establishes the consequences and rewards for behavior.
• Place client on 24-hour constant observation (this will be discontinued when client ends maladaptive behavior or at specific times that nursing staff assess are low risk).	Provides consistency and structure during the stressful early period of treatment.
• Place client on constant observation during meals and at high-risk times for maladaptive behavior (such as 1 hour after meals or while using the bathroom). This action will take effect when the preceding action is discontinued.	Provides support for client during stressful period.
• Do not allow client to discuss weight or calories. Excessive discussion of food is also discouraged.	Decreases client's abnormal focus on food and promotes normal eating patterns. This behavior is more indicative of starvation than an eating disorder.[55]
• Require client to eat prescribed diet (all food on tray each meal except for those three or four foods client was allowed to omit in the admission contract). List client's omitted food here.	Promotes client's sense of control and participation in decision making within appropriate limits.
• Sit with client during meals and provide positive support and encouragement for the feelings and concerns the client may have.	Provides a positive supportive context for client.[55]
• Do not threaten client with punishment (tube feeding or IVs).	
• Report all maladaptive behavior to the client's primary nurse or physician for confrontation in individual therapy sessions.	
• Spend (number) minutes with client every (number) minutes to establish relationship.	
• Respond to queries related to fears of being required to gain too much weight with reassurance that the goal of treatment is to return client to health and that he or she will not be allowed to become overweight.	

• If client vomits, have him or her assist with the cleanup, and require him or her to drink an equal amount of a nutritional replacement drink.	Provides natural consequences for behavior.
• Encourage client to attend group therapy (specific encouraging behavior should be listed here, such as assisting client to complete morning care on time or other interventions that are useful for this client).	Provides support from peers and a source of honest feedback.[55]
• Encourage client's family by (list specific encouraging behaviors for this family) to attend family therapy sessions.	Provides support for the family and an opportunity for the family to work through their concerns together.[55]
• Assist client with clothing selection: Clothes should not be too loose (hiding weight loss) or too tight (assisting client to feel overweight even though appropriate weight is achieved).	Altered body image makes it difficult for clients to make appropriate choices. Honest feedback and support from the nursing staff makes the transition to "healthy" choices easier.
• When maintenance weight is achieved, assist client with selection of appropriate foods from hospital menu.	As symptoms of starvation are resolved, clients are better able to make appropriate choices, and gradual returning of control prepares the client to accept responsibility at discharge.[55]

Gerontic Health

Nursing actions for the gerontic patient with this diagnosis are the same as those for adult health.

Home Health

NOTE: Due to long-term care requirements for these clients, target dates should be determined in weeks or months, not hours or days.

Actions/Interventions	Rationales
• Reduce associated factors, for example: ○ Minimize noxious odors by using foods that require minimal cooking; or if someone else is cooking for client, arrange for client to be away from cooking area. ○ Provide social atmosphere desired by client. ○ Plan medications to decrease pain and nausea around mealtime. ○ Plan meals away from area where treatments are performed.	Provides positive environment to promote nutritional intake.

Continued

Actions/Interventions	Rationales
○ Maintain oral hygiene before and after meals; instruct client and family in proper brushing, flossing, and use of water pick. ○ Encourage client to prepare favorite foods. ○ Avoid foods that contribute to noxious symptoms such as gas, nausea, or GI distress. ○ Discourage fasting. ○ Teach stress-reduction exercises. ○ Maintain exercise program as tolerated. • Teach to add high-calorie, high-protein, and high-fat items to meal preparation activities; for example, use milk in soups, add cheese to food, and use butter or margarine in soups and on vegetables.	Promotes weight gain and prevents loss of muscle mass.
• Teach or provide assistance to patient to rest before meals. If client is doing the meal preparation, teach him or her to cook large quantities and freeze several meals at a time and to seek assistance in meal preparation when fatigued.	Provides optimal conditions to avoid overfatigue.

FLOW CHART EVALUATION
Flow Chart Expected Outcome 1

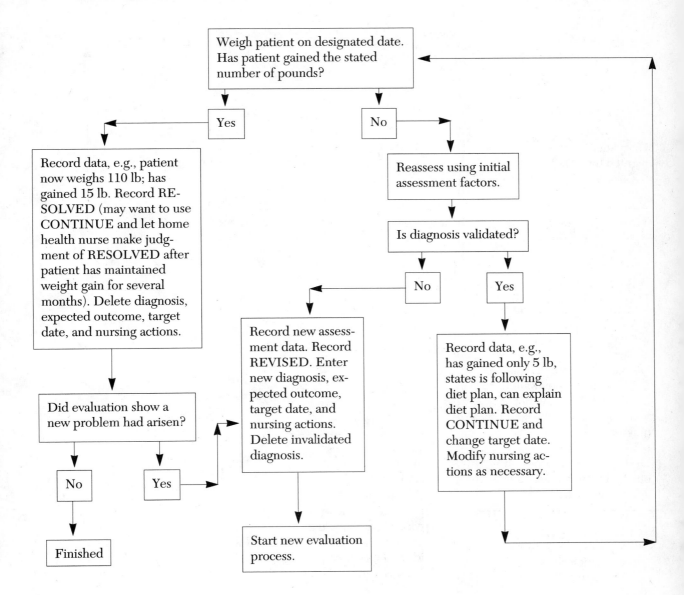

Flow Chart Expected Outcome 2

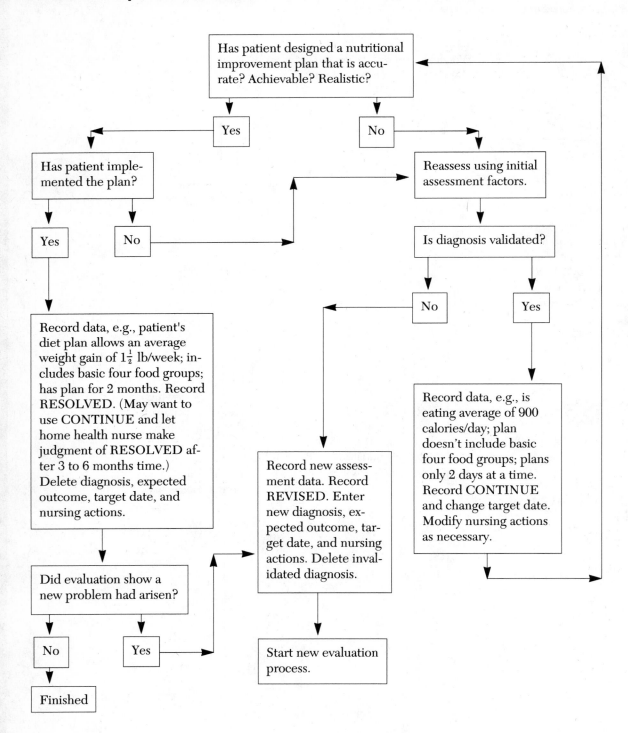

Nutrition, Altered: High Risk for, or More than Body Requirements

DEFINITION

High Risk for: The state in which an individual is at risk of experiencing an intake of nutrients that exceeds metabolic needs.

Actual: The state in which an individual is experiencing an intake of nutrients that exceeds metabolic needs.

NANDA TAXONOMY: EXCHANGING 1.1.2.1 AND 1.1.2.3

DEFINING CHARACTERISTICS

1. High Risk for (presence of risk factors):
   a. Reported or observed obesity in one or both parents*
   b. Rapid transition across growth percentiles in infants or children*
   c. Reported use of solid food as major food source before 5 months of age
   d. Observed use of food as reward or comfort measure
   e. Reported or observed higher baseline weight at beginning of each pregnancy
   f. Dysfunctional eating patterns:
      (1) Pairing food with other activities
      (2) Concentrating food intake at end of day
      (3) Eating in response to external cues such as time of day or social situation
      (4) Eating in response to internal cues other than hunger, such as anxiety.
2. More than Body Requirements:
   a. Major defining characteristics:
      (1) Weight 10 percent over ideal for height and frame
      (2) Weight 20 percent over ideal for height and frame*
      (3) Triceps skin fold greater than 15 mm in men, 25 mm in women*
      (4) Sedentary activity level
      (5) Reported or observed dysfunctional eating pattern:
         (a) Pairing food with other activities
         (b) Concentrating food intake at end of day
         (c) Eating in response to external cues such as time of day or social situation
         (d) Eating in response to internal cues other than hunger, for example, anxiety
   b. Minor defining characteristics:
      None given

RELATED FACTORS

1. *High risk for*: The risk factors also serve as the related factors.
2. *More than body requirements*: Excessive intake in relation to metabolic needs.

---

*Critical

RELATED CLINICAL CONCERNS

1. Alzheimer's disease
2. Morbid obesity
3. Hypothyroidism
4. Disorders requiring medicating with corticosteroids
5. Any disorder resulting in prolonged immobility

HAVE YOU SELECTED THE CORRECT DIAGNOSIS?

Knowledge Deficit The patient, because of cultural background, may not know the appropriate food groups and the nutritional value of the foods. Additionally, the cultural beliefs held by a patient may not value thinness. Therefore, the people of a particular culture may actually promote obesity. (See page 536.)

Altered Health Maintenance Due to other problems, the patient may not be able or willing to modify nutritional intake even though he or she has information about good nutritional patterns. (See page 38.)

Other Possible Diagnoses Several diagnoses from the psychosocial realm may be the underlying problem that has resulted in High Risk for or More than Body Requirements. Powerlessness, Self-Esteem Disturbance, Social Isolation, Body Image Disturbance, or Ineffective Individual Coping may also need to be dealt with in the patient who is at high risk for or actually has Altered Nutrition: More than Body Requirements.

EXPECTED OUTCOMES

1. Will lose (number) of pounds by (date) and/or
2. Will have (percentage) decrease in body fat by (date)

NOTE: Goal is 22 percent fat for women and 15 percent fat for men.[44]

TARGET DATE

Because this diagnosis reflects long-term care in terms of both cause and correction, a target date of 5 days or more would not be unreasonable.

NURSING ACTIONS/INTENTIONS WITH RATIONALES

Adult Health

Actions/Interventions	Rationales
• Assist patient to identify dysfunctional eating habits during first day of hospitalization by: ○ Reviewing 1 week's dietary intake	Provides basic information needed to plan changes in dysfunctional habits to begin weight-loss program.

- ○ Associating times of eating and types of food with corresponding events, for example, in response to internal cues or in response to external cues.
  - ○ Reviewing 1 week's exercise pattern
- Check activity level against daily dietary intake.
- Discuss with patient potential or real motivation for desiring to lose weight at this time.

Assists in understanding the patient's rewards for goals and assists in establishment of goals and rewards.

- Discuss with patient past attempts at weight loss and factors that contributed to his or her success or failure.

Provides increased individualization and continuity of care, which facilitate the development of a therapeutic relationship.[56]

- Limit patient's intake to number of calories recommended by physician and/or nutritionist.

Reduces calories to promote weight loss yet maintain body's nutritional status.

- Weigh patient daily at (state time). Teach patient to weigh self at the same time each morning in same clothing. Help patient to establish a graphic to allow visualization of progress, for example, bar chart or chart with gold star for each weight-loss day.

Provides a visible means of ascertaining weight-loss progress.

- Provide good skin care and monitor skin daily, especially skin folds and areas where skin meets skin.

These areas are especially prone to impaired skin integrity due to the collection of moisture and continuous friction.

- Measure total intake and output every 8 hours. Encourage intake of low-calorie, caffeine-free drinks.

Ensure renal functioning and maintenance of fluid balance. A significant amount of weight loss in the first few days is due to fluid excretion. Low-calorie, caffeine-free drinks help offset "hunger pains."

- Collaborate with physical therapist in establishing an exercise program.

Exercise burns calories and tones muscles.

- Assist patient in selecting an exercise program by providing patient with a broad range of options and have patient select one he or she will enjoy.

Will assist in narrowing the range between calories consumed and calories burned.
Facilitates development of adaptive coping behaviors.

- Develop a schedule and goals for implementing the exercise plan (set goals that are achievable; usually this is 50 percent of what the patient estimates is achievable). Develop a reward schedule for achievement of exercise goals, and record this plan here.

Promotes patient self-esteem when goals can be accomplished, and provides motivation for continued efforts.

- Teach stress reduction techniques — for example, progressive relaxation, scheduled quiet time, and time management — and have patient return-demonstrate for a minimum of 30 minutes at least twice a day at (times).

Helps to alleviate eating associated with stress. Facilitates patient's development of alternative coping behaviors.

Continued

Actions/Interventions	Rationales

• Assist patient to establish a food diary beginning on the first day of hospitalization. This diary should be maintained until weight has stabilized within normal limits. The diary should be a record of:
  ○ What eating, that is, caloric intake
  ○ Where eating, that is, all actual sites
  ○ When eating, that is, time of day, length of time spent eating, and circumstances leading to deciding to eat
  ○ Activity during this time
  ○ Feelings and emotions before, during, and after eating
  ○ All physical activity, for example, "Walked $1\frac{1}{2}$ blocks from car to office"
	Helps patient to identify real intake and to identify behavioral and emotional antecedents to dysfunctional eating behavior.[58,59]

• Review diary with patient on a daily basis and list those factors that will assist with a weight-loss plan and those that will hinder a weight-loss plan.	

• Teach patient principles of balanced diet or refer to dietitian for instructions, at least 3 days prior to discharge:
  ○ Basic four food groups
  ○ Recommended daily allowances
  ○ Weighing and measuring foods
  ○ Exchange lists
	Provides basic knowledge needed to control weight at home. Promotes self-care. Promotes patient's perception of control.

• Instruct patient to grocery shop from a list and soon after eating.	
• Discuss with patient those foods that provide the greatest risk of decreasing self-control, and develop a plan for eliminating them from the diet.	
• Use visual aids to increase effectiveness of diet teaching.	
• Schedule adequate time for teaching — convey positive attitude and reinforce information about food groups.	
• Spend 30 minutes at least twice a day at (times) with the patient reviewing the benefits of weight loss and the progress made to this point. Do not focus on the concept of loss when talking with the patient; use terms such as "reduction" and "gains in self-concept" to provide positive ideas.	Promotes a positive orientation and sense of control for the patient.[56]
• Discuss with the patient other life achievements and strategies that assisted in attaining these achievements. Focus on the	Promotes positive orientation and focuses on strengths patient already possesses.

concept of perseverance in attaining the achievement, or discuss with the patient the last long trip taken and apply the concept of persevering and planning that allowed the trip to be taken. Relate the ideas of persevering and planning to the task of weight loss.

- Present the concept of approaching goals one day at a time rather than attempting or reflecting on all of the task.

Promotes positive orientation by setting readily achievable goals.

- Review pros and cons of alternate weight-loss options with patient:
  ○ Fad diets
  ○ Diet pills
  ○ Liquid diet preparations
  ○ Surgery
  ○ Diuretics
  ○ Laxatives
  ○ Binging and purging

Promotes safety in weight-loss plan. Avoids serious complications such as heart failure due to questionable weight-loss ideas.

- Demonstrate adaptations in eating that could promote weight loss:
  ○ Smaller plate
  ○ One-half of usual serving
  ○ No second servings
  ○ Laying fork down between bites
  ○ Chewing each bite at least "X" number of times

Assists in behavior modification needed to lose weight.

- Teach alternative food preparation habits that will reduce calories while increasing nutritional content of diet:
  ○ Boil or broil instead of frying food.
  ○ Use nonstick spray for pans instead of butter, margarine, or fat.
  ○ Use fruits and vegetables.
  ○ Increase use of fish or poultry over beef or pork.
  ○ Drink water or herbal tea for thirst; do not confuse thirst with hunger.
  ○ Reduce or eliminate fat and sugar from recipes.
  ○ Use fresh ingredients whenever possible for increased flavor.
  ○ Use fresh fruit canned in its own juice for sweetening instead of sugar.
  ○ Use plain yogurt or blended and seasoned tofu as substitutes for sour cream.

Reduction of fat in meal preparation assists in calorie reduction and weight loss. Often excess food is consumed for water content when water would satisfy the need. Facilitates development of adaptive eating behaviors.

- Provide patient with a calorie list of fast-food items and plan for maintaining desired goals by:

Promotes patient's perception of control. Provides planned strategies for coping before entering potentially difficult situations.

Continued

Actions/Interventions	Rationales
○ Developing a list of those fast-food items that provide the best food value for the calories. ○ Assisting the patient with developing recipes to use at home that are calorie-wise and easily prepared to decrease the temptation to use fast food. ○ Developing a list of those restaurants that provide options for reducing calorie intake, such as those with salad bars or those that allow customers to eliminate certain items from a serving such as high-calorie condiments.	
• Have patient design own weight-loss plan at least 3 days prior to discharge to allow practice and revision as necessary: ○ Caloric intake ○ Activity ○ Behavioral or life-style changes, that is, those behaviors that will replace factors that inhibit weight loss	Allows patient to assume control for long-term therapy. The more the patient is involved in planning care, the higher the probability for compliance.
• Encourage patient to increase activity by: ○ Walking up stairs instead of riding elevators at work ○ Taking walks in the evening before retiring	
• Consult with family and visitors regarding importance of patient's adhering to diet. Caution against bringing food and so on from home.	Involves others in supporting patient in weight-loss effort.
• Discuss with patient and significant others the necessary alterations in eating behavior, and develop a list of ways the significant others can be supportive of these alterations.	
• Use appropriate behavior modification techniques to reinforce teaching. Refer patient and family to psychiatric nurse practitioner for appropriate techniques to use at home as well as assistance with guilt, anxiety, and so on over being obese.	Reinforcement supports change.
• Plan for times when patient will indulge in high-calorie meals or snacks, such as holidays, by developing an attitude of nonfailure and regained control or coping. Time may be planned for the patient to "break" the diet.	Promotes patient's perception of control.
• If binging has been a problem and other techniques have not effectively eliminated	If patient does not follow up with planned binge, this will demonstrate patient control

it, then assist the patient in planning the next binge to the final detail.

over binges and the patient's strength can be promoted. If the patient engages in the planned binge, this can also demonstrate control, and the patient regains power and can then proceed to schedule and plan binges, altering the frequency and amount consumed gradually. Either option should be positively received by the nurse with appropriate follow-up to promote the patient's positive orientation.[56,59]

- Suggest patient contract with a significant other or home health nurse prior to discharge.

Provides added reinforcement and support for continued weight loss.

- Develop a list of rewards for positive changes. These rewards should be ones the patient will give himself or herself or that can be given by the health care team or patient support system and should not be related to food. The patient's reward schedule should be listed here.

Many patients will have difficulty identifying nonfood rewards, and a great deal of support may be needed. Rewards should initially be scheduled on a daily basis for successful achievement of behavior related to weight loss and can then be gradually expanded to weekly or monthly rewards. Rewards promote the patient's self-esteem and provide motivation for continued efforts.

- Instruct patient to postpone desires to eat between meals by doing 5 minutes of slow deep-breathing and reviewing three of the identified positive motivating factors for weight loss for this patient. If the desire to eat remains, have the patient drink a glass of water or cup of herb tea and spend 10 minutes engaged in an activity such as writing a letter, working on a hobby, reading, sewing, playing with children or spouse or significant other—anything but watching television (this activity generally contains too many food cues).

Provides patient time to substitute positive coping behaviors for dysfunctional eating behavior.[57]

- Refer to community resources at least 3 days prior to discharge from hospital. (See Appendix B.)

Provides long-range support for continued success with weight loss.

Child Health

Orders are the same as for the adult. Make actions specific to the child according to the child's developmental level.

Women's Health

Actions/Interventions	Rationales
• Verify the prepregnancy weight.	Provides basis for planning diet with patient.
• Obtain a 24-hour diet history. Ask patient to select a typical day.	
• Calculate the woman's calorie and protein intake.	
• Rule out excessive edema and hypertension. Measure ankles and abdominal girth and record. Remeasure each day. Measure BP every 4 hours while awake at (state times here).	
• Encourage patient to increase her activity by: ○ Joining exercise groups for pregnancy (usually found in childbirth classes in community) ○ Joining swim exercise groups for pregnancy (usually found at YWCAs or community centers)	Assists in maintaining desired weight gain; improves muscle tone and circulation.
• Refer to appropriate support groups for assistance in exercise programs for pregnant women (for example, physical therapist, local groups who have swimming classes for pregnant women, and childbirth classes).	
• If recommended intake is 2400 cal per day but 24-hour diet recall reveals a higher caloric intake: ○ Recommend reduction of fat in diet (for example, decrease amount of cooking oil used, use less salad dressing and margarine, cut excess fat off meat, and take skin off chicken before preparing). ○ Check out size of food portions. ○ Stress appetite control with high-quality sources of energy and protein.	Basic measures and teaching factors to assist in weight control.
• Assist mothers with cultural or economic restrictions to introduce more variety into their diets.	
• Stress that weight gain is the only way the fetus can be supplied with nourishment.	
• Point out that added body fat will be burned and will provide necessary energy during lactation (breast-feeding).	
• Assist pregnant adolescents within 3 years of menarche to plan diets that have needed additional nutrients.	Diet has to be planned to meet the growth needs of the adolescent as well as those of the fetus.
• Discourage any attempts at weight reduction or dieting.	

NOTE: Dieting is never recommended during pregnancy because it deprives mother and fetus of nutrients needed for tissue growth and because weight loss is accompanied by maternal ketosis, a direct threat to fetal well-being.[22,41]

ADDITIONAL INFORMATION A satisfactory pattern of weight gain for the average woman is:[5]

10 weeks of gestation	650 g (approximately 1.5 pounds)
20 weeks of gestation	4000 g (approximately 9.0 pounds)
30 weeks of gestation	8500 g (approximately 19.0 pounds)
40 weeks of gestation	12,500 g (approximately 27.5 pounds)

Over the course of the pregnancy, a total weight gain of 25 to 35 pounds is recommended for both nonobese and obese pregnant women. During the second and third trimesters, a gain of about 1 pound per week is considered desirable.

Mental Health

Nursing actions for the mental health client with this diagnosis are the same as those actions for adult health.

Gerontic Health

Nursing actions for the gerontic patient with this diagnosis are the same as those actions in Adult Health and Home Health.

Home Health

Actions/Interventions	Rationales
• Assist client in identifying lifestyle changes that may be required: ○ Regular exercise should be scheduled at least three times per week and should include stretching, flexibility, and aerobic activity (20 minutes) at target training rate. ○ Nutritional habits should include decreasing fat and simple carbohydrates and increasing complex carbohydrates.	Knowledge and support provides motivation for change and increases the potential for positive outcomes.
• Assist client and family in identifying cues other than weight and calories; instead, client and family should focus on patient's feeling of well-being, percent of body fat, increased exercise endurance, better-fitting clothes, and so on. • Have client and family design a personalized plan: ○ Menu planning ○ Decreased fats and simple carbohydrates and increased complex carbohydrates ○ Regular, balanced exercise ○ Life-style changes	Excess focus on the weight as measured by the scale and on calorie counting may increase the probability of failure and encourage the pattern of repeated weight loss followed by weight gain. This pattern results in increased percentage of body fat. A personalized plan improves the probability of adherence to the plan.

FLOW CHART EVALUATION
Flow Chart Expected Outcome 1

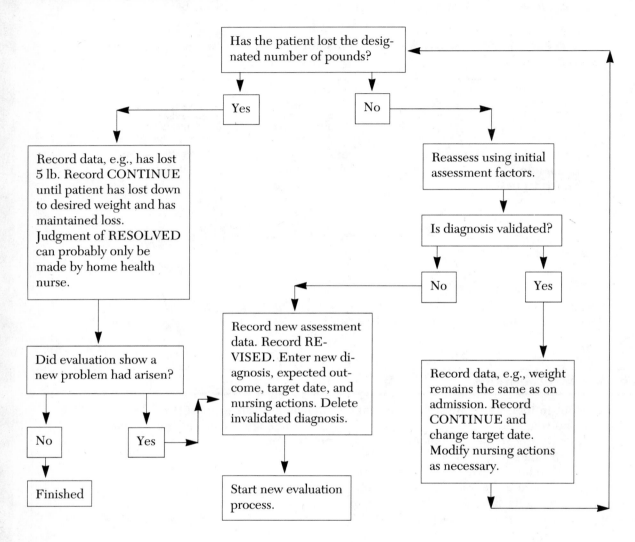

Flow Chart Expected Outcome 2

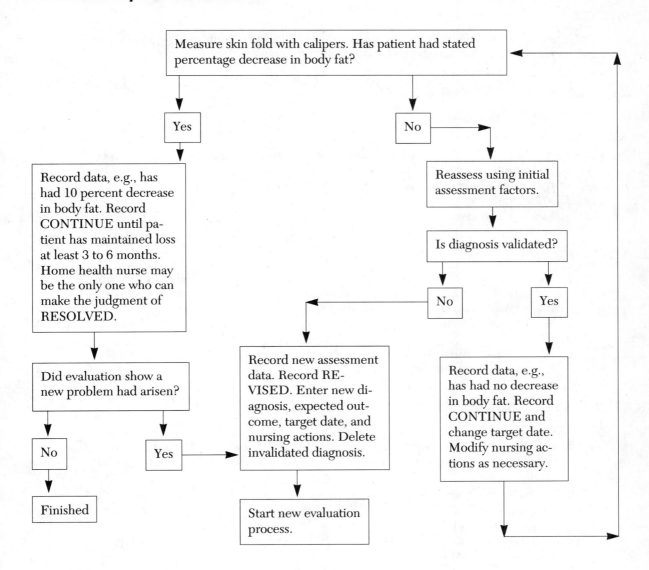

Swallowing, Impaired

DEFINITION

The state in which an individual has decreased ability to voluntarily pass fluids and/or solids from the mouth to the stomach.

NANDA TAXONOMY: MOVING 6.5.1.1

DEFINING CHARACTERISTICS

1. Major defining characteristics:
   a. Observed evidence of difficulty in swallowing, for example, stasis of food in oral cavity
   b. Coughing or choking
2. Minor defining characteristics:
   Evidence of aspiration

RELATED FACTORS

1. Neuromuscular impairment (for example, decreased or absent gag reflex, decreased strength or excursion of muscles involved in mastication, perceptual impairment, or facial paralysis)
2. Mechanical obstruction (for example, edema, tracheostomy tube, or tumor)
3. Fatigue
4. Limited awareness
5. Reddened, irritated oropharyngeal cavity

RELATED CLINICAL CONCERNS

1. Cerebrovascular accident
2. Any neuromuscular diagnosis, for example, myasthenia gravis, muscular dystrophy, cerebral palsy, Parkinson's disease, Alzheimer's disease, poliomyelitis
3. Hyperthyroidism
4. Any medical diagnosis related to decreased level of consciousness, for example, seizures, concussions, or increased intracranial pressure
5. Tracheoesophageal problems, for example, fistula, tumor, edema, or presence of tracheostomy tube
6. Anxiety

HAVE YOU SELECTED THE CORRECT DIAGNOSIS?

Altered Oral Mucous Membrane Impaired Swallowing implies that there is a mechanical or physiologic obstruction between the oropharynx and the esophagus. An Altered Oral Mucous Membrane indicates that only the oral cavity is involved. Structures below the oral cavity per se are not affected. If liquids or solids are able to pass through the oral cavity, even though pain or difficulty might be present, there will be nothing obstructing its passage through the esophagus to the stomach. Therefore, if solids or liquids are able to pass into the stomach without crowing, coughing, or choking, the appropriate nursing diagnosis is *not* Impaired Swallowing. (See page 239.)

Altered Nutrition: Less than Body Requirements Certainly Altered Nutrition: Less than Body Requirements would be a consideration and probably a secondary problem to Impaired Swallowing. Choosing between the two diagnoses would be based on the related factors, with Impaired Swallowing taking priority over the Altered Nutrition initially. (See page 200.)

EXPECTED OUTCOMES

1. Will be able to freely swallow (solids) (liquids) by (date) and/or
2. Will not have any aspiration problems by (date)

TARGET DATE

Since Impaired Swallowing can be life-threatening, the patient should be checked for progress daily. After the condition has improved, progress could be checked at 3-day intervals.

NURSING ACTIONS/INTERVENTIONS WITH RATIONALES

Adult Health

Actions/Interventions	Rationales
• Monitor for lesions or infectious processes of the mouth and oropharynx at least once per shift.	Lesions or ulcers in the mouth promote difficulty in swallowing.
• Test, prior to every offering of food, fluid, and so on, for presence of gag reflex.	To prevent choking and aspiration.
• Test swallowing capacity with clear, sterile water *only*, prior to offering food or fluids. Have suctioning equipment and tracheostomy tray on standby in patient's room.	Provides equipment needed in case of aspiration or respiratory obstruction emergency.
• Support hydration and caloric intake. Collaborate with physician regarding the need for IVs, hyperalimentation, and so on.	Maintains fluid and electrolytes even though patient may not be able to swallow.
• Maintain appropriate upright position during feeding.	Gravity assists in facilitation of swallowing.
• Warm fluids before offering them to patient.	Warm fluids assist swallowing through mild relaxation of esophageal muscles.
• Stay with the patient while he or she tries to eat.	Basic safety measure for patient who has difficulty in swallowing.
• Be supportive to patient during swallowing efforts.	Swallowing difficulty is very frustrating for the patient.
• Consult with nutritionist about patient's preferred food list and about enhancing the	

Continued

Actions/Interventions	Rationales
nutritional value of those foods that are easier for the patient to swallow (for example, adding vitamins to warm liquids).	
• Provide for rest periods before and after eating.	Coughing episodes are frequent with impaired swallowing and coughing is very tiring.
• Measure and document intake and output each shift. Total each 24 hours.	Basic monitoring of patient's condition. Permits a consistent and more accurate comparison.
• Weigh patient each day at the same time (note time here) and in same-weight clothing.	
• Advance diet as tolerated.	
• Teach the patient who has had supraglottic surgery an alternate method of swallowing:	Facilitates active swallowing and support for patient as he or she begins to adapt to impaired swallowing.
○ Have the patient clear his or her throat by coughing and expectorating. If patient unable to expectorate, suction the secretions.	
○ Have the patient inhale as food in put in the mouth.	
○ Have the patient then perform a Valsalva maneuver as he or she is swallowing.	
○ Have the patient cough, swallow again, and exhale deeply.	
○ Start with soft, nonacidic, noncrumbly foods rather than liquids. Liquids are more difficult to control.	
○ Provide privacy for the patient as he or she learns alternate swallowing.	
○ Teach at least one family member or significant other how to support the patient in alternate swallowing, suctioning, Heimlich maneuver, and so on.	
• Refer as needed to other health care team members. (See Appendix B.)	Collaboration supports a holistic approach to patient care.

Child Health

Actions/Interventions	Rationales
• Monitor for contributory factors, especially palate formation, possible tracheoesophageal fistula, or other congenital anomalies.	A thorough assessment will best identify those patients who have greater than usual likelihood of swallowing difficulties due to structural, acquired, or circumstantial conditions.
• Maintain infant in upright position after feedings for at least 1½ hours.	An upright position will favor, by gravity, the digestion and absorption of nutrients, thereby

- Address anticipatory safety needs for possible choking:
  - Have appropriate suctioning equipment available.
  - Teach parents CPR.
  - Provide parenting support for CPR and suctioning.
  - Assist family to identify ways to cope with swallowing disorder, for example, extra help in feeding.
- Administer medications as ordered. Avoid powder or pill forms. Use elixirs, or mix as needed.

decreasing the likelihood of reflux and resultant potential for choking.
Usual anticipatory airway management is appropriate in long-term patient management while education and teaching concerns can be addressed in a supportive environment, thereby reducing anxiety in event of cardiopulmonary arrest secondary to impaired swallowing.

Pills or powders may increase the likelihood of impaired swallowing in young children or infants. Appropriate mixing with fruit syrups or using manufacturer's elixir or suspension form of the drug lessens the likelihood of impaired swallowing.

Women's Health

The nursing actions for a woman with the nursing diagnosis of Impaired Swallowing are the same as those for adult health.

Mental Health

NOTE: The following nursing actions are specific considerations for the mental health client who has Impaired Swallowing that is caused or increased by anxiety. Refer to mental health nursing actions for the diagnosis of Anxiety for interventions related to decreasing and resolving the client's anxiety. If swallowing problems are related to an eating disorder, refer to mental health nursing actions for Altered Nutrition: Less than Body Requirements.

Actions/Interventions	Rationales
• Provide a quiet, relaxed environment during meals by discussing with client the situations that increase anxiety and excluding those factors from the situation. Provide things such as favorite music and friends or family that increase relaxation. (Note information provided by client here, especially those things that need to be provided by the nursing staff.)	Promotes client's control and facilitates relaxation response, thus inhibiting the sympathetic nervous system response.[56,58]
• Provide medications in liquid or injectable form. (Note any special preference client may have in presentation of medications here.)	Liquids are easier to swallow than tablets. Providing medications by injection would avoid any swallowing problems.

Continued

Actions/Interventions	Rationales
• Teach client deep muscle relaxation. (Refer to the mental health nursing actions for Anxiety for actions related to decreasing anxiety.)	Promotes client control and inhibits the sympathetic nervous system response.
• Discuss with client foods that are the easiest and the most difficult to swallow. Note information from this discusson here. (Note time and person responsible for this discussion here.)	Promotes client control.
• Plan client's most nutritious meals for the time of day client is most relaxed, and note that time here.	
• Provide client with high-energy snacks several times during the day. (Note snacks preferred by client and times they are to be offered here.)	Provides additional calories in frequent small amounts.
• Assign primary nurse to sit with client 30 minutes (this can be increased to an hour as client tolerates interaction time better) two times a day to discuss concerns related to swallowing. (This can be included in the time described under the nursing actions for Anxiety.) As the nurse-client relationship moves to a working phase, discussion can include those factors that precipitated client's focus on swallowing. These factors could be a trauma directly related to swallowing, such as an attack in which the client was choked or in which oral sex was forced.	Provides increased individuation and continuity of care, facilitating the development of a therapeutic relationship. The nursing process requires that a trusting and functional relationship exist between nurse and client.[56]
• Teach client and client's support system nutrition factors that will improve swallowing and maintain adequate nutrition. Note here the names of those persons client would like included in this teaching. Note time arranged and person responsible for this teaching here.	Promotes long-term support for assistance with problem.

Gerontic Health

Nursing actions for the gerontic patient with this diagnosis are the same as those for adult health and home health.

Home Health

Actions/Interventions	Rationales
• Teach measures to decrease or eliminate Impaired Swallowing:	Prevents or diminishes problems. Promotes self-care and provides database for early intervention.
○ Principles of oral hygiene	
○ Small pieces of food or pureed food as necessary	
○ Aspiration precautions, for example, eat and drink sitting up, do not force-feed or fill mouth too full, or CPR	
○ Proper nutrition and hydration	
○ Use of adaptive equipment as required	
• Teach to monitor, on at least a daily basis, for factors contributing to Impaired Swallowing, for example, fatigue, obstruction, neuromuscular impairment, or irritated oropharyngeal cavity.	
• Involve client and family in planning, implementing, and promoting reduction or elimination of Impaired Swallowing by establishing regular family conferences to provide for mutual goal setting and to improve communication.	Goal setting and communication promote positive outcomes.
• Assist client and family in life-style changes that may be required:	Knowledge and support provide motivation for change and increase the potential for a positive outcome.
○ Client may need to be fed.	
○ Mealtimes should be quiet and uninterrupted, and they should be scheduled at consistent times on a daily basis.	
○ Client may require special diet and special utensils.	

FLOW CHART EVALUATION
Flow Chart Expected Outcome 1

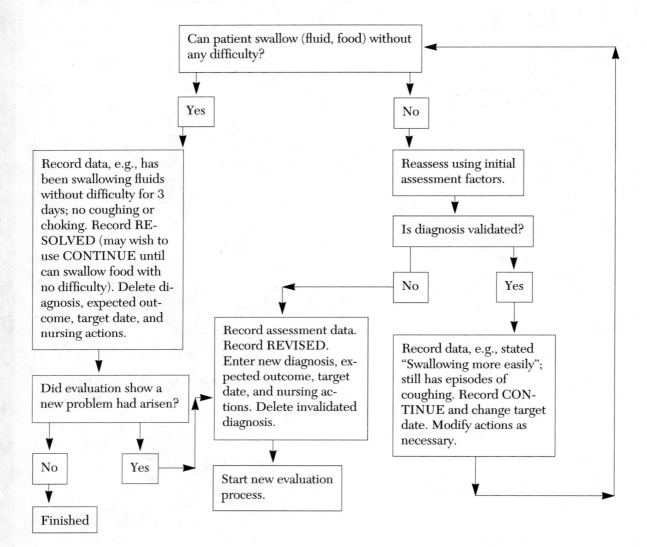

Can patient swallow (fluid, food) without any difficulty?

Yes

No

Record data, e.g., has been swallowing fluids without difficulty for 3 days; no coughing or choking. Record RE-SOLVED (may wish to use CONTINUE until can swallow food with no difficulty). Delete diagnosis, expected outcome, target date, and nursing actions.

Reassess using initial assessment factors.

Is diagnosis validated?

No

Yes

Did evaluation show a new problem had arisen?

Record assessment data. Record REVISED. Enter new diagnosis, expected outcome, target date, and nursing actions. Delete invalidated diagnosis.

Record data, e.g., stated "Swallowing more easily"; still has episodes of coughing. Record CON-TINUE and change target date. Modify actions as necessary.

No

Yes

Finished

Start new evaluation process.

Nutritional-Metabolic Pattern

Flow Chart Expected Outcome 2

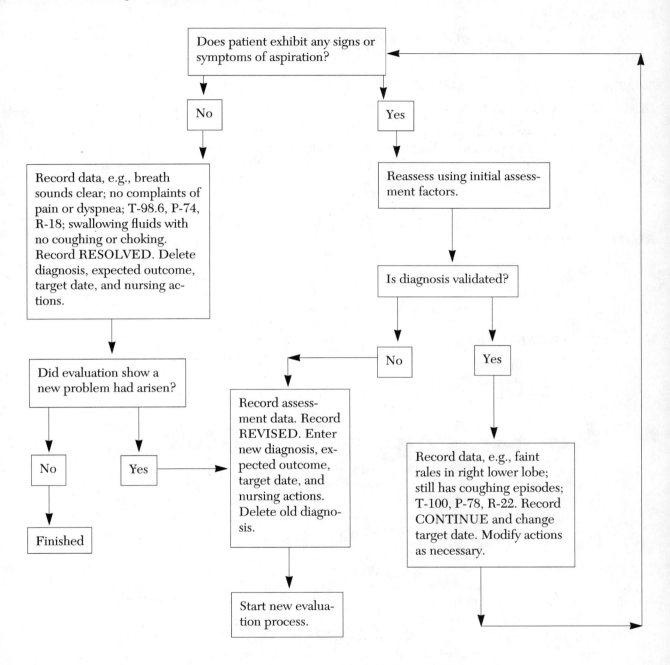

Thermoregulation, Ineffective

DEFINITION

The state in which the individual's temperature fluctuates between hypothermia and hyperthermia.

NANDA TAXONOMY: EXCHANGING 1.2.2.4

DEFINING CHARACTERISTICS

1. Major defining characteristics:
   a. Fluctuations in body temperature above or below the normal range
   b. See also major and minor characteristics present in hypothermia and hyperthermia
2. Minor defining characteristics:
   None given

RELATED FACTORS

1. Trauma or illness
2. Immaturity
3. Aging
4. Fluctuating environmental temperature

RELATED CLINICAL CONCERNS

1. Any infection
2. Any surgery
3. Septicemia

HAVE YOU SELECTED THE CORRECT DIAGNOSIS?

Hyperthermia   Hyperthermia means that a person maintains a body temperature greater than normal for himself or herself. In Ineffective Thermoregulation, the client's temperature is changing between hyperthermia and hypothermia. If the temperature measurement is remaining above normal, the correct diagnosis is Hyperthermia, not Ineffective Thermoregulation. (See page 177.)

Hypothermia   Hypothermia means that a person maintains a body temperature below normal for himself or herself. If the temperature is consistently remaining below normal, the correct diagnosis is Hypothermia, not Ineffective Thermoregulation. (See page 186.)

High Risk for Altered Body Temperature   With this diagnosis the patient has a potential inability to regulate heat production and heat dissipation within a normal range. With this diagnosis, the key point to remember is that a temperature abnormality does not exist yet, but the risk factors present indicate that such a problem could develop. If the temperature measurements are fluctuating between hypothermia and hyperthermia, the correct diagnosis is Ineffective Thermoregulation. (See page 125.)

EXPECTED OUTCOMES

1. Will maintain a body temperature between 97 and 99° F by (date) and/or
2. Will identify at least (number) measures to use in correcting Ineffective Thermoregulation by (date)

TARGET DATE

Initial target dates will be stated in terms of hours. After stabilization, an appropriate target date would be 3 days.

NURSING ACTIONS/INTERVENTIONS AND RATIONALES

Adult Health

Actions/Interventions	Rationales
• Monitor vital signs at least every hour on the (hour or half-hour).	Monitors basic trends in temperature fluctuations. Permits early recognition of ineffective thermoregulation.
• Maintain room temperature at all times at 72° F. Provide warmth or cooling as needed to maintain temperature in desired range; avoid drafts and chilling for the patient.	Offsets environmental impact on thermoregulation.
• Reduce stress for patient. Provide quiet, nonstimulating environment.	Assists body to maintain homeostasis. Stress could contribute to problems with thermoregulation due to increased basal metabolic rate.
• If the patient is hypothermic, see nursing actions for Hypothermia on page 186. • If patient is hyperthermic, see nursing actions for Hyperthermia on page 177.	Thermoregulation problems may vary from Hypothermia to hyperthermia.
• Make referrals for appropriate follow-up before dismissal from hospital. (See Appendix B.)	Provides long-range, cost-effective support.

Child Health

Actions/Interventions	Rationales
• Protect child from excessive chilling during bathing or procedures.	Evaporation and significant change of temperature for even short periods of time will contribute to heat loss for the young child or infant, and contribute even more so during illness.
• Assist in answering parent's or child's questions regarding monitoring temperature	Appropriate teaching fosters compliance and reduces anxiety.

Continued

Actions/Interventions	Rationales
procedures, or other educational needs such as administration of medications.	
• Assist parents in dealing with anxiety in times of unknown causes or prognosis by allowing 30 minutes per shift for venting anxiety (state times here). Specifically interview parents to ascertain anxiety.	Because the emphasis on monitoring and treating altered thermoregulation is so great, it can be easy to overlook the parents and their concerns. Specific attention must be given to ascertaining how the patient and family are feeling about all the many concerns generated.
• Involve parents and family in child's care whenever appropriate, especially for comforting child.	Parental involvement fosters empowerment and regaining of self-care, thereby re-establishing the likelihood of effective family coping.

Women's Health

This nursing diagnosis will pertain to women the same as any other adult. The reader is referred to the adult health, and home health nursing actions for this diagnosis.

Mental Health

The nursing actions for this diagnosis in the mental health client are the same as those in Adult Health.

Gerontic Health

Nursing actions for the gerontic patient with this diagnosis are the same as those actions in Adult Health and Home Health.

Home Health

Actions/Interventions	Rationales
• Monitor for factors contributing to Ineffective Thermoregulation (illness, trauma, immaturity, aging, or fluctuating environmental temperature).	Allows early recognition and early implementation of therapy.
• Involve client and family in planning, implementing, and promoting reduction or elimination of Ineffective Thermoregulation.	Personal involvement and input increase likelihood of maintenance of plan.
• Teach client and family early signs and symptoms of Ineffective Thermoregulation (see Hyperthermia and Hypothermia).	
• Teach client and family measures to decrease or eliminate Ineffective Thermoregulation (see Hyperthermia and Hypothermia).	
• Assist client and family to identify life-style changes that may be required (see Hyperthermia and Hypothermia).	Provides basic information and planning to successfully manage condition at home.

FLOW CHART EVALUATION
Flow Chart Expected Outcome 1

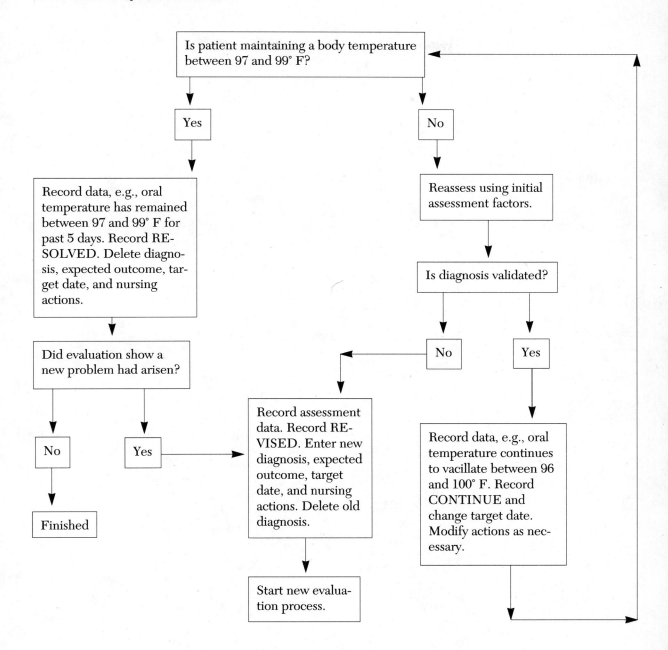

Flow Chart Expected Outcome 2

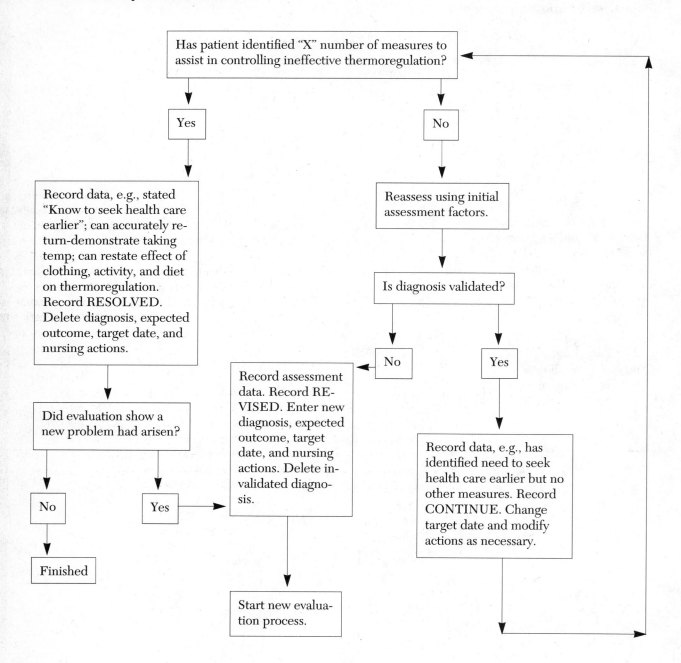

Tissue Integrity, Impaired

DEFINITION

Tissue Integrity, Impaired: A state in which an individual experiences damage to mucous membrane, corneal, integumentary, or subcutaneous tissue.

High Risk for Impaired Skin Integrity: A state in which the individual's skin is at risk of being adversely altered.

Impaired Skin Integrity: A state in which the individual's skin is adversely altered.

Altered Oral Mucous Membrane: The state in which an individual experiences disruptions in the tissue layers of the oral cavity.

NANDA TAXONOMY: EXCHANGING 1.6.2.1, 1.6.2.1.2.2, 1.6.2.1.2.1, AND 1.6.2.1.1

DEFINING CHARACTERISTICS

1. Impaired Tissue Integrity:
   a. Major defining characteristics:
      Damaged or destroyed tissue (cornea, mucous membrane, integumentary, or subcutaneous)
   b. Minor defining characteristics:
      None given
2. High Risk for Impaired Skin Integrity:
   a. External (environmental):
      (1) Hypo- or hyperthermia
      (2) Chemical substance
      (3) Mechanical factors:
         (a) Shearing forces
         (b) Pressure
         (c) Restraint
      (4) Radiation
      (5) Physical immobilization
      (6) Excretions or secretions
      (7) Humidity
   b. Internal (somatic):
      (1) Medication
      (2) Alterations in nutritional state:
         (a) Obesity
         (b) Emaciation
      (3) Altered metabolic state
      (4) Altered circulation
      (5) Altered sensation
      (6) Altered pigmentation
      (7) Skeletal prominence
      (8) Developmental factors
      (9) Alterations in skin turgor (change in elasticity)
      (10) Psychogenic
      (11) Immunologic

3. Impaired Skin Integrity:
   a. Major defining characteristics:
      (1) Disruption of skin surfaces
      (2) Destruction of skin layers
      (3) Invasion of body structures
   b. Minor defining characteristics:
      None given

4. Altered Oral Mucous Membranes:
   a. Major defining characteristics:
      (1) Oral pain or discomfort
      (2) Coated tongue
      (3) Xertostomia (dry mouth)
      (4) Stomatitis
      (5) Oral lesions or ulcers
      (6) Lack of or decreased salivation
      (7) Leukoplakia
      (8) Edema
      (9) Hyperemia
      (10) Oral plaque
      (11) Desquamation
      (12) Vesicles
      (13) Hemorrhagic gingivitis
      (14) Carious teeth
      (15) Halitosis
   b. Minor defining characteristics:
      None given

RELATED FACTORS

1. Impaired Tissue Integrity:
   a. Altered circulation
   b. Nutritional deficit or excess
   c. Fluid deficit or excess
   d. Knowledge deficit
   e. Impaired physical mobility
   f. Irritants:
      (1) Chemical (including body excretions, secretions, and medications)
      (2) Thermal (temperature extremes)
      (3) Mechanical (pressure, shear, or friction)
      (4) Radiation (including therapeutic radiation)
2. High Risk for Impaired Skin Integrity:
   The risk factors also serve as the related factors.
3. Impaired Skin Integrity:
   a. External (environmental):
      (1) Hypo- or hyperthermia
      (2) Chemical substance
      (3) Mechanical factors:
         (a) Shearing forces
         (b) Pressure
         (c) Restraint

      (4) Radiation

      (5) Physical immobilization

      (6) Excretions or secretions

      (7) Humidity

    b. Internal (somatic):

      (1) Medication

      (2) Alterations in nutritional state:

        (a) Obesity

        (b) Emaciation

      (3) Altered metabolic state

      (4) Altered circulation

      (5) Altered sensation

      (6) Altered pigmentation

      (7) Skeletal prominence

      (8) Developmental factors

      (9) Alterations in skin turgor (change in elasticity)

     (10) Psychogenic

     (11) Immunologic

4. Altered Oral Mucous Membrane:

    a. Pathological conditions—oral cavity (radiation to head or neck)

    b. Dehydration

    c. Trauma:

      (1) Chemical, for example, acidic foods, drugs, noxious agents, or alcohol

      (2) Mechanical, for example, ill-fitting dentures, braces, tubes (endotracheal/nasogastric), or surgery in oral cavity

    d. NPO for more than 24 hours

    e. Ineffective oral hygiene

    f. Mouth breathing

    g. Malnutrition

    h. Infection

    i. Lack of or decreased salivation

    j. Medication

RELATED CLINICAL CONCERNS

1. Any condition requiring immobilization of patient
2. Burns—chemical, thermal, or radiation
3. Accidents—motor vehicle, farm equipment, motorcycles, and so on
4. AIDS
5. Congestive heart failure
6. Diabetes mellitus

HAVE YOU SELECTED THE CORRECT DIAGNOSIS?

Impaired Skin Integrity   If the tissue damage involves only the skin and its subcutaneous tissues, then the most correct diagnosis is Impaired Skin Integrity. High Risk for Impaired Skin Integrity would be the most appropriate diagnosis if the patient were presenting a majority of risk factors for a skin integrity problem but the problem had not yet developed. (See page 239.)

Continued

HAVE YOU SELECTED THE CORRECT DIAGNOSIS?—*Continued*

Altered Oral Mucous Membranes   If the tissue damage involves only the oral mucous membranes, then the best diagnosis is Altered Oral Mucous Membrane. Impaired Tissue Integrity is a higher-level diagnosis and would cover a wider range of tissue types. Altered Oral Mucous Membranes and the two diagnoses related to Skin Integrity are more specific and exact diagnoses and should be used before Impaired Tissue Integrity *if* the problem can be definitively isolated to either the oral mucous membrane or the skin. (See page 239.)

EXPECTED OUTCOMES

1. Will exhibit no signs or symptoms of increased tissue integrity problems (for example, increased size or infection) by (date) and/or
2. Will implement plan to avoid future episodes of Impaired Tissue Integrity by (date)

TARGET DATE

Tissue integrity problems can begin developing within hours of a patient's admission if caution is not taken regarding turning, cleaning, and so on. Therefore, an initial target date of 2 days after admission would be most appropriate.

NURSING ACTIONS/INTERVENTIONS WITH RATIONALES

Adult Health

Actions/Interventions	Rationales
• Perform active or passive range-of-motion exercises at least once per shift at (state times here).	Stimulates circulation, which provides nourishment and carries away waste, thus reducing the likelihood of tissue breakdown.
• Ambulate to extent possible.	
• Change position at least hourly, and teach patient to change position at least every 30 minutes. Do not position on affected area.	
• If patient is unable to turn self, have several persons available to help lift, then turn.	
• Gently massage pressure points and bony prominences following each position change.	
• Teach patient and significant others how to turn patient without shearing force being involved. Be sure bed has siderails and a trapeze (overhead) bar for assistance with turning. Move slowly.	
• Use soft, wrinkle-free linen only.	
• Place cornstarch or powder on linens.	

- Make sure footboard is in place for patient to use for bracing.
- Avoid use of rubber or plastic in direct contact with patient.
- Reduce pressure on affected skin surface by using:
  - Egg crate
  - Alternating air mattress
  - Sheepskin
  - Commercial wafer barriers
  - Thick dressing used as pad on bony prominences
  - Bed cradle

Pressure predisposes tissue breakdown.

- Collaborate with dietitian regarding well-balanced diet. Assist patient to eat as necessary.

Prevents tissue breakdown due to negative nitrogen balance.

- Monitor dietary intake, and avoid irritant food and fluid intake (for example, highly spiced food or extremes of temperature).

These factors would increase probability of oral mucous membrane problems.

- Encourage fluid intake to at least 2000 ml per 24 hours.

Maintains fluid and electrolyte balance, which is necessary for tissue repair and normal functioning.

- Measure and total intake and output every 8 hours.
- Cleanse perineal area carefully after each urination or bowel movement. Monitor closely for any urinary or fecal incontinence.

Allowing body wastes to remain on skin promotes tissue breakdown. Incontinence would increase probability of such an event.

- Teach patient principles of good skin hygiene.

Promotes self-care and self-management to prevent problem.

- Have patient cough and deep-breathe every 2 hours on the (odd/even) hour.

Basic care measures to offset other complications that develop in tandem with impaired tissue integrity.

- Administer oral hygiene at least three times a day after each meal and prn:

Basic care measures to maintain oral mucosa.

  - Brush teeth, gums, and tongue with soft-bristled brush, sponge stick, or gauze-wrapped finger.
  - Floss teeth.
  - Rinse mouth thoroughly after brushing: Avoid commercial mouthwashes and preparations with alcohol, lemon, or glycerin. Use normal saline or oxidizing agent (mild hydrogen peroxide solution, Gly-oxide, or sodium bicarbonate solution).
  - If patient is unable to rinse, turn on side and do oral irrigation.
  - Teach patient how to use water pick.
  - Teach patient and significant others proper oral hygiene.

Continued

Actions/Interventions	Rationales
○ If patient has dentures, cleanse with equal parts of hydrogen peroxide and water. ○ Apply lubricant to lips at least every 2 hours on the (odd/even) hour. • Maintain good body hygiene. Be sure patient has at least a sponge bath every day *unless* skin is too dry. • Monitor for signs of infection at least daily.	Infection, through production of toxins, wastes, and so on increases the probability of tissue damage.
• Keep room temperature and humidity constant. Room temperature should be kept close to 72° F and humidity at a low level unless otherwise ordered. • Darken room, as necessary, to protect eyes. • Encourage patient to chew sugar-free gum to stimulate salivation. • Administer medications as ordered, and record response (for example, topical oral antibiotics or analgesic mouthwashes). Record response within 30 minutes of administration. • Encourage patient to avoid smoking. • Provide between-meal food or fluids that patient has identified as soothing, for example, warm or cool. • *If lesions develop:* Cleanse area daily at (time) according to prescribed regimen. • Collaborate with an enterstomal therapist and the physician regarding care specific to the patient. • Protect open surface with such products as: ○ Karaya powder ○ Skin gel ○ Wafer barrier ○ Other commercial skin preparations • Change dressings when needed, using aseptic technique. Collaborate with physician regarding dressing type and use of topical agents. • Teach patient and significant others care of the wound prior to discharge. • Avoid use of adhesive tape. If tape must be applied, use nonallergic tape. • Avoid use of doughnut ring. • Use mild, unscented soap (or soap substitute) and cool or lukewarm water.	Keeps skin cool and dry to prevent perspiration. Highly irritating to mucous membranes. Basic care measures for impaired skin integrity.

- Avoid vigorous rubbing, but do massage gently using a lanolin-based unscented lotion.
- Pat area dry. Be sure area is thoroughly dry.
- Expose to air, sunlight, or heat lamp at least four times a day at (state times here). Check patient at least every 5 minutes if using heat lamp.
- Monitor:
  - Skin surface and pressure areas at least every 4 hours at (state times here) for blanching, erythema, temperature difference (for example, increased warmth), or moisture
  - Size and color of lesion at least every 4 hours at (state times here)
  - Fluid and electrolyte balance
- Particularly watch for signs or symptoms of edema. Collaborate with physician regarding frequency of measurement of electrolyte levels.
- Caution patient and assist to avoid scratching irritated areas:
  - Trim and file nails.
  - Apply cool compresses.
- Collaborate with physician regarding medicated baths (for example, oatmeal) and topical ointments.
- Teach patient to press, rather than scratch, area that is itching.
- Refer to community health agencies and other health care providers as appropriate. (See Appendix B.)

These measures would allow early detection of any complications.

Avoids further irritation of already damaged tissue.

Provides ongoing support. Cost-effective use of available resources.

Child Health

Actions/Interventions	Rationales
• Handle infant gently; especially caution paramedical personnel regarding need for gentle handling.	The epidermis of infants and young children is thin and lacking in subcutaneous depth. Others, such as x-ray technicians, may not realize the fragile nature of skin as they carry out necessary procedures.
• Place patient on sheepskin or flotation pad, or, if parents choose, allow infant or child to be held frequently.	Alternating surface contact and position favors circulatory return to central venous system.

Continued

Actions/Interventions	Rationales

• Caution patient and parents to avoid scratching irritated area:
  ○ Trim nails with appropriate scissors; receive parental permission if necessary.
  ○ Make small mitts if necessary from cotton stockinette used for precasting.
	Anticipates potential injury of delicate epidermis, especially when irritation may prompt itching.

• Monitor perineal area for possible allergy to diapers.	Various synthetics in diapers may evoke allergenic responses and either cause or worsen existent skin irritation.

• Encourage fluids:
  ○ *Infant:* 250 to 300 ml per 24 hours
  ○ *Toddler:* 1150 to 1300 ml per 24 hours
  ○ *Preschooler:* 1600 ml per 24 hours
(These are approximate ranges. The physician may order specific amounts according to the child's age and condition.)
	Adequate hydration will assist in normal homeostatic mechanisms, which will affect the skin's integrity.

• Provide protection such as bandage or padding to tissue site involved.	Anticipation and protection from injury serve to limit the depth and/or degree of altered skin integrity.

• Monitor and document circulation to affected tissue via:
  ○ Peripheral arterial pulses
  ○ Blanching or capillary refill
  ○ Tissue color
  ○ Sensation to touch or temperature
  ○ Tissue general condition, for example, bruising or lacerations
  ○ Drainage, for example, amount, odor, or color
  ○ Range-of-motion limitations
	These factors represent basic appropriate criteria for circulatory checks. They may be added to in instances of specific concerns such as compartmental syndrome associated with hand trauma.

• Administer oral hygiene according to needs and status:
  ○ Glycerin and lemon swabs for NPO infant
  ○ Special orders for postoperative cleft palate or cleft lip repair
	Appropriate oral hygiene will decrease the likelihood of altered integrity of surrounding tissues and is critical for care of altered associated oral disorders.

• Teach parents to limit time infant sucks bottle in reclining position to best prevent "bottle syndrome" and decayed teeth.	Evidence suggests that bottle syndrome is prevented by not having infant go to sleep with bottle. Rather, completion of feeding and removal of bottle is suggested before placing infant in crib.
• Protect the altered tissue site as needed during movement by providing support to the limb.	Provision of support and usual use of body parts will favor adequate circulation and prevent further injury.
• Provide range of motion and ambulation as permitted to encourage vascular return.	
• Position patient while in bed so that the head of the bed is elevated slightly and involved limb is elevated approximately 20 degrees.	Appropriate venous return is favored by resultant gravity with limb higher than heart.

- Address altered thermoregulation, and especially protect patient from chilling or shock due to dehydration or sepsis.

In severe instances of altered thermoregulation or related pathology, there may not be the usual manifestations of deviations from normals. It may also be difficult to assess sensation in the young infant due to the infant's inability to provide verbal feedback.

- Use restraints judiciously for involved limb or body site.

Any undue constriction or threat to circulation must be weighed appropriately in making decisions whether or not to restrain the child.

- Monitor intravenous infusion and administration of medications cautiously; avoid use of sites in close proximity to area of altered tissue integrity.

This is usual protocol for IV therapy and must be considered paramount as IV medications or solutions pose serious threats to the veins and surrounding tissues.

- Allow patient and family time to express concerns by providing at least 30 minutes per shift for family counseling. (State times here.)

Reduces anxiety since their concerns can be made known and their feelings valued.

- Teach patient and family:
  - Need for follow-up care
  - Signs and symptoms to be reported:
    (1) Increased temperature (101° F or above)
    (2) Foul odors or drainage
    (3) Delayed healing or increase in damage site size
    (4) Loss of sensation or pulsation in limb or site
    (5) Any increase in pain
  - Prosthetic device if indicated
  - Aids in mobility, such as crutches or walker
  - Need to avoid constrictive clothing
  - Appropriate dietary restriction or needs

Appropriate education serves to build self-confidence and effects long-term compliance with treatment and health management.

Women's Health

Actions/Interventions	Rationales
• Monitor perineum and rectum after childbirth for injury or healing at least once per shift at (state times here). Monitor episiotomy site for redness, edema, and hematomas each 15 minutes immediately after delivery for 1 hour, then once each shift thereafter.	Assesses basic physical condition as a basis for providing care and preventing complications.
• Collaborate with physician regarding:	Provides comfort and promotes healing.

Continued

Actions/Interventions	Rationales
○ Applying ice packs or cold pads to perineum for the first 8 to 12 hours after delivery to reduce edema and increase comfort	
○ Sitz baths twice a day at (state times here) and as necessary for pain and discomfort	
○ Analgesics and topical anesthetics as necessary for pain and discomfort	
• Teach good perineal hygiene and self-care:	Promotes healing and encourages self-care.
○ Rinse perineal area with warm water after each voiding.	
○ Pat dry gently from front to back to prevent contamination.	
○ Apply perineal pad from front to back to prevent contamination.	
○ Change pads frequently to prevent infection and irritation.	
• Provide factual information on resumption of sexual activities after childbirth:	Provides basic information to promote safe self-care.
○ First intercourse should be after adequate healing period (usually 3 to 4 weeks).	
○ Intercourse should be slow and easy (woman on top can better control angle, depth, and penetration).	
• Teach postmenopausal women the signs and symptoms of atrophic vaginitis:	Provides basic information that promotes self-care and health maintenance.
○ Watery discharge	
○ Burning and itching of vagina or vulva	
• Encourage examinations (Pap smears) for estrogen levels at least annually.	
• In collaboration with physician, encourage use as needed of:	
○ Estrogen replacement creams or vaginal suppositories	
○ Extra lubrication during intercourse	
• Teach breast-feeding mothers about breast care:	Provides basic information that assists in preventing skin breakdown, and promotes self-care as well as promoting successful lactation.
○ Inspect for cracks or fissures in nipples.	
○ Wear supportive bra (breast binder) to relieve engorgement.	
○ Shower daily. Do not use soap on breasts, and allow to air dry.	
○ Use lanolin-based cream (Vitamin E cream, Massé, or A&D) to prevent drying and cracking of nipples.	

- Enhance let-down reflex:
  - Early, frequent feedings. Ten minutes on each side is easier on sore nipples than nursing less frequently.
  - Nurse at both breasts each feeding. Switch sides to begin nursing each time; for example, if baby nursed first on left side at last feeding, begin on right side this time. A safety pin or small ribbon on bra strap will remind mother which side she used first the last time.
  - Change positions from one feeding to next (distributes sucking pressure).
  - Check baby's position on breast; be certain areola is in mouth, not just nipple.
  - Begin nursing on least-sore side first, if possible; then switch baby to other side.
  - Apply ice to nipple just before nursing to decrease pain. (Fold squares, put them in the freezer, and apply as needed.)
- Collaborate with physician regarding analgesics as needed. Caution patient not to take over-the-counter medication since some medications are passed to the baby via breast milk.

Promotes let-down reflex and successful breast-feeding.

NOTE: Between the third and sixth months of pregnancy, the process of tooth calcification (hardening) begins in the fetus. What the mother consumes in her diet will affect the development of the unborn child's teeth. A well-balanced diet will usually provide correct amounts of nutrients for both mother and child.

- Teach patient to practice good oral hygiene at least twice a day as well as prn:
  - Each time patient eats and, if nauseated and vomiting, after each attack of vomiting.
  - If the smell of toothpaste or mouth rinse makes patient nauseated, use baking soda.
- Reduce the number of times sugar-rich foods are eaten between meals.
- Teach patient to snack on fruits, vegetables, cheese, cottage cheese, whole grains, or milk.

Promotes sense of well-being, assists in promoting proper growth and development of fetus, and encourages health maintenance.

Provides basic information to patient that promotes health maintenance and increases awareness of need for self-care.

- Have patient increase daily calcium intake by at least a total of 1.2 g per day.
- Collaborate with obstetrician and dentist to plan needed dental care during pregnancy.
- Assist in planning best time in pregnancy for dental visits:
  - Not during the first 3 months if:
    (1) Previous obstetric history includes miscarriage

Continued

Actions/Interventions	Rationales

(2) Threatened miscarriage
    (3) Other medical indications
    (4) Hypersensitive to gagging (will increase nausea and vomiting)
  ○ Not during the last 3 months if:
    (1) Not able to sit in dental chair for long periods of time
    (2) Obstetric history of premature labor
• Emphasize having only needed x-rays. Caution patient to request a lead apron.
	Prevents x-ray exposure to fetus.

ADDITIONAL INFORMATION

NOTE: Nursing actions for newborn health immediately follows the women's health nursing actions. As previously mentioned, newborn actions are included in this section because newborn care is most often administered by nurses in the obstetrical or women's health area. Focus needs to be made on the newborn simply because the newborn's oral mucous membrane problems can be easily overlooked.

• In collaboration with dentist, teach parents the oral and dental needs of the neonate:
  ○ Use of fluoride.
  ○ Proper use of pacifiers.
  ○ Do not use homemade pacifiers.
  ○ Use pacifiers recommended by dentist.
  ○ Allow infant who is teething to chew on soft toothbrush (will encourage later brushing of teeth since allows infant to become familiar with toothbrush in mouth):
  Hold on to brush.
  Give to infant only when adult is present.
• Administering oral hygiene:
  ○ Massage and rub infant's gums with finger daily.
  ○ Inspect oral cavity daily for hygiene and problems.
• Take infant for first dental visit between 18 months and 2 years of age.
• Dental caries (decay) can be a result of prolonged nursing or delayed weaning:
  ○ Do not allow infant to nurse at breast or bottle beyond required feeding time.
  ○ Do not allow infant to sleep habitually at the breast or with a bottle in the mouth.
  ○ Teach the neonate's parents to:
    (1) Avoid giving sweet liquids (soft drinks) or fruit juices in bottle.
    (2) Wean child from bottle to cup soon after first birthday.
	Promotes good health and provides information as a basis for parental care of infant. Assists in preventing infection.

(3) When continuing to nurse infant, give water in cup soon after first birthday.

(4) Use good handwashing techniques to prevent infection with or reinfection of thrush.

(5) Do not place infant on sheets where mother has been sitting.

(6) Thoroughly clean breast or bottle-feeding equipment.

Mental Health

Actions/Interventions	Rationales
• Refer to Chapter 8 for stress reduction measures and interventions for the stressors that produce psychogenic skin reactions.	
• If client is placed in restraints:	
○ Monitor the integrity of skin under restraints every hour.	
• Apply lanolin-based lotion and cornstarch or powder to area under restraint at least every 2 hours on the (odd/even) hour and PRN.	Lubricates skin and decreases risk for breakdown.
○ Pad restraints with nonabrasive materials such as sheepskin.	Decreases mechanical friction against the skin and decreases risk for breakdown.
○ Keep area of restraint next to the skin clean and dry.	
○ Release restraints one at a time every 2 hours on (odd/even) hour and PRN. Remove restraints as soon as the client will tolerate one-to-one care without risk to self or others.	
○ Maintain proper movement and alignment of affected body parts.	Decreases mechanical friction on specific areas for long periods of time, thus decreasing risk for breakdown.
○ Change client's position every 2 hours on (odd/even) hour.	
○ Offer client fluids every 15 minutes. List preferred fluids here.	Hydration improves skin condition.
○ While client is very agitated and physically active, provide constant one-to-one observation.	
○ While limb is out of restraints, have client move limb through range of motion.	Promotes circulation and assists in preventing the consequences of immobility.
○ If client is in four-point restraints, place him or her on side or stomach and change this position every 2 hours on (odd/even) hour.	Client safety is of primary importance. This positioning prevents aspiration by facilitating drainage of fluids away from the airway.

Continued

Actions/Interventions	Rationales
○ Monitor skin condition of pressure areas. ○ If client is in four-point restraints, provide one-on-one observation. ○ Continually remind client of reason for restraint and conditions for having the restraints removed. ○ Talk with client in calm, quiet voice and use client's name. ○ Use restraints that are wide and have padding. Make sure padding is kept clean and dry and free of wrinkles.	Provides supportive environment to client.
• If Impaired Tissue Integrity is the result of self-harm, place client on one-on-one observation until the risk of future harm has diminished. • Monitor self-inflicted injuries hourly for the first 24 hours for signs of infection and further damage. Note information on a flow sheet. After the first 24 hours, monitor on a daily basis.	Client safety is of primary importance. Provides ongoing supervision to inhibit impulsive behavior and encourages use of alternative coping behaviors. Early identification and treatment of infection can prevent more serious damage.
• Provide equipment and time for the client to practice oral hygiene at least after each meal.	Removes debris and food particles, thus reducing the risk of tissue injury.
• Discuss with client life-style changes to improve condition of mucous membranes, including nutritional habits, use of tobacco product, use of alcohol, maintenance of proper hydration, and effects of frequent vomiting. • Discuss with client side effects of medications that contribute to alterations in oral mucous membranes, such as antibiotics, antihistamines, phenytoin, antidepressants, and antipsychotics.	Alerts client to life-style patterns that increase risk for injury to oral mucous membranes. If risk factors are present, frequent assessment and increased attention to oral hygiene can decrease the risk of membrane breakdown.
• Teach client to use nonsucrose candy or gum to stimulate flow of saliva. • Teach client to avoid excessive wind and sun exposure, especially with antipsychotic drugs. • If client is taking antipsychotic drugs, suggest the use of a sunscreen containing **PABA.**	Maintains hydration of membranes and decreases chance of breakdown. These medications can cause photosensitivity.[25]

Gerontic Health

Actions/Interventions	Rationales
• Nursing actions for this diagnosis in the gerontic patient are essentially the same as those for adult health and home health, with the following special notations: Use only superfatted, nonperfumed, mild, nondetergent, and hexaclorophine-free soap in bathing the patient.[60]	The incidence of dry skin in the older adult is increased due to decreased production of natural skin oils.
• When drying the skin after bathing, pat the skin dry rather than rubbing, and apply lubricating lotion while the skin is still damp.	Increases the moisture level of the patient's skin. Careful attention to dry skin conditions in the older adult will assist in maintaining tissue integrity for the older adult.

Home Health

Actions/Interventions	Rationales

• Teach self-monitoring techniques to prevent tissue breakdown and to initiate early treatment:
  ○ Inspect the skin at least daily. Change position at least every 2 hours.
  ○ Massage pressure points and bony prominences gently at least three times a day.
  ○ Avoid rubber or plastic mattress covers or sheets.
  ○ Use proper body alignment and padding to reduce pressure on affected areas.
  ○ At least once per day engage in physical activity (active or passive) that will develop a full range of motion of all joints and relieve pressure on risk area.
  ○ Consult health care provider for treatment of actual skin lesions.
  ○ Avoid scratching lesions.
	Promotes self-care.

• Teach signs and symptoms of tissue breakdown, for example, redness over bony prominences, pain or discomfort in localized area, skin lesions, or itching.	Provides data for early intervention.
• Teach measures to promote tissue integrity: ○ Keep skin clean and dry. Wash urine and feces off of skin immediately.	Provides knowledge and skills that will prevent or minimize skin breakdown.

Continued

Actions/Interventions	Rationales
○ Maintain adequate hydration, for example, oral fluids, mild soap for bathing, or place nonscented lotion or petroleum jelly on skin after bathing to moisturize. ○ Maintain adequate protein intake. ○ Use mild laundry detergent on clothes; double-rinse clothes, linens, and diapers if skin is sensitive. ○ Change position at least every 2 hours on (odd/even) hour. Avoid prolonged sitting, standing, or lying in one position for extended periods. ○ Use sunscreen to prevent sun damage. ○ Avoid excessive wind and sun exposure. ○ Wear properly fitting shoes. ○ Avoid shearing force when moving in bed or chair.	

FLOW CHART EVALUATION
Flow Chart Expected Outcome 1

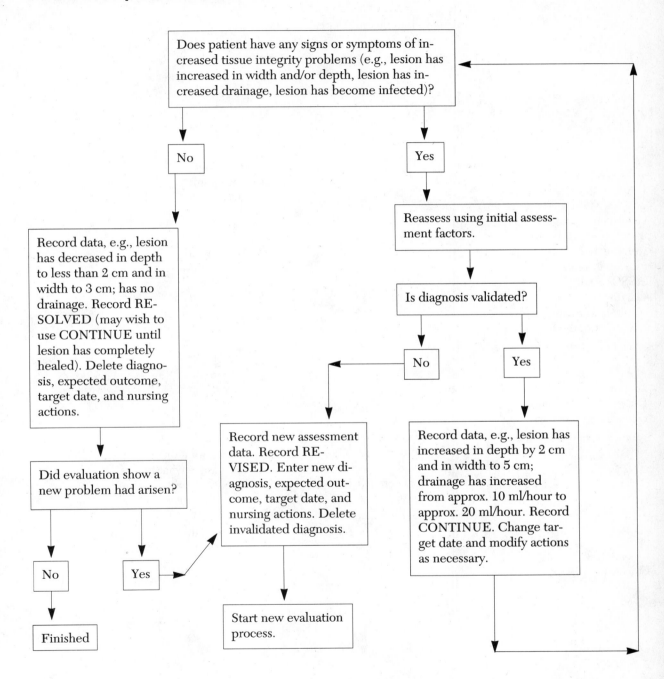

Flow Chart Expected Outcome 2

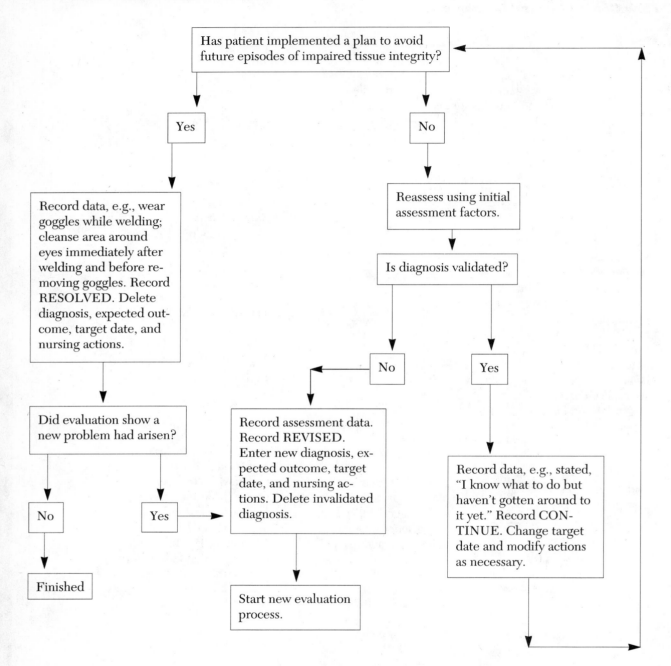

Has patient implemented a plan to avoid future episodes of impaired tissue integrity?

Yes

No

Record data, e.g., wear goggles while welding; cleanse area around eyes immediately after welding and before removing goggles. Record RESOLVED. Delete diagnosis, expected outcome, target date, and nursing actions.

Reassess using initial assessment factors.

Is diagnosis validated?

No

Yes

Did evaluation show a new problem had arisen?

Record assessment data. Record REVISED. Enter new diagnosis, expected outcome, target date, and nursing actions. Delete invalidated diagnosis.

Record data, e.g., stated, "I know what to do but haven't gotten around to it yet." Record CONTINUE. Change target date and modify actions as necessary.

No

Yes

Finished

Start new evaluation process.

References

1. Potter, PA and Perry, AG: Instructors' Manual for Fundamentals of Nursing: Concepts, Process and Practice, ed 2. CV Mosby, St. Louis, 1989.
2. Flynn, JM and Heffron, PB: Nursing: From Concept to Practice, ed 2. Appleton-Lange, Norwalk, CT, 1988.
3. Mitchell, PH and Loustau, A: Concepts Basic to Nursing Practice. McGraw-Hill, New York, 1981.
4. Murray, RB and Zentner, J: Nursing Assessment and Health Promotion Strategies Through the Life Span, ed 4. Appleton-Lange, Norwalk, CT, 1989.
5. Neeson, JD and May, KA: Comprehensive Maternity Nursing: Nursing Process and the Childbearing Family. JB Lippincott, Philadelphia, 1986.
6. Frigerio, C, Schutz, Y, Whitehead, R, and Jdequien, E: A new procedure to assess the energy requirements of lactation in Gambian women. Am J Clin Nutr 54:526–533.
7. Kemp, M., et al: Factors that contribute to pressure sores in surgical patients. Res Nurs Health 13:293, 1990.
8. Guyton, A: Textbook of Medical Physiology, ed 8. WB Saunders, Philadelphia, 1991.
9. Schuster, CS and Ashburn, SS: The Process of Human Development: A Holistic Life-Span Approach, ed 3. JB Lippincott, New York, 1992.
10. Korones, SB: High-Risk Newborn Infants: The Basis for Intensive Nursing Care, ed 4. CV Mosby, St. Louis, 1986.
11. Driscoll, J and Heird, W: Maintenance fluid therapy during the neonatal period. In Winters, RW (ed): Principles of Pediatric Fluid Therapy, ed 2. Little, Brown & Co, Boston, 1982.
12. Brandt, PA, Chinn, PE, and Smith, ME: Current Practice in Pediatric Nursing. CV Mosby, St. Louis, 1980.
13. McCrory, WW: Developmental Nephrology. Harvard University Press, Cambridge, MA, 1972.
14. Masiak, MJ, Naylor, MD, and Hayman, LL: Fluids and Electrolytes Through the Life Cycle. Appleton-Century-Crofts, East Norwalk, CT, 1985.
15. Stone, L and Church, J: Childhood and Adolescence: A Psychology of the Growing Person. Random House, New York, 1968.
16. Young, C, et al: Body composition of pre-adolescent and adolescent girls. J Am Diab Assoc 53:579, 1968.
17. Chinn, P and Leitch, C: Child Health Maintenance: A Guide to Clinical Assessment, ed 2. CV Mosby, St. Louis, 1979.
18. Mitchell, HS, et al: Nutrition in Health and Disease, ed 17. JB Lippincott, New York, 1982.
19. Shafer, J: Dysgeusia in the elderly. Lancet, 1:35, 1965.
20. Kopak, C: Sensory loss in the aged: The role of the nurse and the family. Nurs Clin North Am 18:373, 1983.
21. Cugini, P, et al: Methodologically critical interaction of circadian rhythm, sex and aging characterize serum aldosterone and female adenopause. J Gerontol 37:403, 1982.
22. Carnevali, DL and Patrick, M: Nursing Management for the Elderly, ed 2. JB Lippincott, Philadelphia, 1986.
23. North American Nursing Diagnosis Association: Taxonomy I: Revised 1990. Author, St. Louis, 1990.
24. Bassuk, E and Schoonover, S: The Practitioner's Guide to Psychoactive Drugs. Plenum Medical Book Company, New York, 1977.
25. Townsend, M: Drug Guide for Psychiatric Nursing. FA Davis, Philadelphia, 1990.
26. North American Nursing Diagnosis Association: Proposed New Nursing Diagnoses: NANDA 10th Conference. Author, St. Louis, 1992.
27. Reeder, SJ, Martin, LL, and Koniak, D: Maternity Nursing: Family, Newborn and Women's Health Care, ed 17. JB Lippincott, Philadelphia, 1992.
28. Barger, J and Bull, P: A comparison of the bacterial composition of breast milk stored at room temperature and stored in the refrigerator. International Journal of Childbirth Education 5:29, 1987.
29. Cunningham, AS, Jelliffe, DB, and Jelliffe, EF: Breastfeeding and health in the 1980s: A global epidemiologic review. J Pediatr 118:1, 1991.
30. Lawrence, RA: Breastfeeding: A Guide for the Medical Profession, ed 3. CV Mosby, St. Louis, 1989.
31. Newman, J: Breastfeeding problems associated with early introduction of bottles and pacifiers. J Hum Lact 6:59, 1990.
32. Walker, M: Breastfeeding Premature Babies: Lactation Consultant Series. La Leche League International, Franklin Park, IL, 1990.
33. Mead, LJ, et al: Breastfeeding success with preterm quadruplets. J Obstet Gynecol Neonatal Nurs 21:221, 1992.
34. McCoy, R, et al: Nursing management of breastfeeding for preterm infants. J Perinat Neonatal Nurs 2:42, 1988.
35. Meier, P and Anderson, GC: Responses of small preterm infants to bottle and breastfeeding. MCN Am J Matern Child Nurs 12:97, 1987.
36. Wilks, S and Meier, P: Helping mothers express milk suitable for preterm and high-risk infant feeding. MCN Am J Matern Child Nurs 13:121, 1988.

37. Whaley, LF and Wong, DL: Nursing Care of Infants and Children, ed 4. CV Mosby, St. Louis, 1991.
38. Mandeville, LK and Troiano, NH: High Risk Intrapartum Nursing. JB Lippincott, Philadelphia, 1992.
39. Beland, I and Passos, J: Clinical Nursing: Pathophysiological and Psychosocial Approaches, ed 4. Macmillan, New York, 1981.
40. Cosgray, RE, et al: The water-intoxicated patient. Arch Psychiatr Nsg 5:308, 1990.
41. Lapierre, E, et al: Polydipsia and hyponatremia in psychiatric patients: Challenge to creative nursing care. Arch Psychiatr Nsg 2:87, 1990.
42. Boyd, MA: Polydipsia in the chronically mentally ill: A review. Arch Psychiatr Nsg 3:166, 1990.
43. Olds, SB, London, ML, and Ladewig, PA: Maternal Newborn Nursing: A Family-Centered Approach. Addison-Wesley, Menlo Park, CA, 1988.
44. Bailey, C: Fit or Fat? Houghton Mifflin, Boston, 1978.
45. Meier, P and Pugh, EJ: Breastfeeding behavior of small preterm infants. MCN Am J Matern Child Nurs 10:396, 1985.
46. Niefert, MR and Secat, JM: Milk yield and prolactin rise with simultaneous breast pump. Ambulatory Pediatric Assocation Meeting Abstracts, Washington, DC, May, 1985.
47. Frantz, KB: Managing Nipple Problems (Reprint No. 11). La Leche League International, Franklin Park, IL, 1982.
48. Neifert, MR and Secat, JM: Lactation insufficiency: A rational approach. Birth 16:182, 1989.
49. Walker, M: Management of selected early breastfeeding problems seen in clinical practice. Birth 16:148, 1989.
50. Anderson, GC, et al: Development of sucking in term infants from birth to four hours postbirth. Res Nurs Health 5:21, 1982
51. Metheney, N, et al: Detection of Inadvertent Respiratory Placement of Small-Bore Feeding Tubes. Heart Lung 19:631, 1990.
52. Metheney, N, et al.: Effectiveness of Ausculatory Method in Predicting Feeding Tube Location. Nurs Res 39:266, 1990.
53. Nursing Mothers' Council of the Boston Association for Childbirth Education: Breastfeeding Your Baby. Avery, Garden City, NY, 1989.
54. Grams, M: Breastfeeding Source Book. Achievement Press, Sheridan, WY, 1990.
55. Garner, D and Garfinkel, P (eds): Handbook of Psychotherapy for Anorexia Nervosa and Bulimia. Guilford, New York, 1985.
56. Erickson, HC, Tomlin, EM, and Swain, MP: Modeling and Role-Modeling: A Theory and Paradigm for Nursing. Prentice-Hall, Englewood Cliffs, NJ, 1983.
57. Haber, J, et al: Comprehensive Psychiatric Nursing, ed 4. Mosby Year Book, St. Louis, 1992.
58. Wilson, HS and Kneisl, CR: Psychiatric Nursing, ed 4. Addison-Wesley, Redwood City, CA, 1992.
59. Watzlawick, P, Weakland, J, and Fisch, R: Change: Principles of Problem Formation and Problem Resolution. WW Norton, New York, 1974.
60. Maas, M, Buckealter, K, and Hardy, M: Nursing Diagnoses and Interventions for the Elderly. Addison-Wesley Nursing, Fort Collins, CO, 1991.

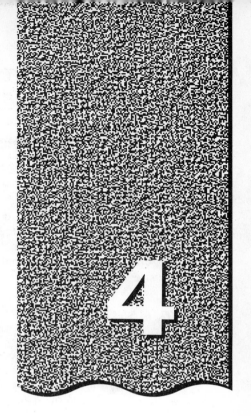

4

Elimination Pattern

PATTERN INTRODUCTION
Pattern Description

The Elimination Pattern focuses on bowel and bladder functioning. While excretion also occurs through the skin and the lungs, the primary mechanisms of waste excretion are the bowel and bladder.

A problem within the Elimination Pattern may be the primary reason for seeking health care or may arise secondary to another health problem such as impaired mobility. There are very few of the other patterns or nursing diagnoses that will not have an ultimate impact on the elimination pattern from either a physiologic, psychologic, or sociologic direction.

Included in the Elimination Pattern are the person's habits in terms of excretory regularity as well as aids that the person uses to maintain regularity or any devices he or she uses to control either bowel or bladder incontinence.

Pattern Assessment

1. Is there stool leakage when the patient coughs, sneezes, or laughs?
   a. Yes (Bowel Incontinence)
   b. No
2. Is there involuntary passage of stool?
   a. Yes (Bowel Incontinence)
   b. No
3. Does the patient take laxatives on a routine basis?
   a. Yes (Colonic Constipation; Perceived Constipation)
   b. No
4. Have number of bowel movements decreased?
   a. Yes (Constipation; Colonic Constipation)
   b. No
5. Are stools hard-formed?
   a. Yes (Constipation; Colonic Constipation)
   b. No
6. Does the patient have to strain to have bowel movement?
   a. Yes (Constipation; Colonic Constipation)
   b. No
7. Does the patient believe he or she is frequently constipated?
   a. Yes (Perceived Constipation)
   b. No
8. Does the patient expect to have a bowel movement at the same time each day?
   a. Yes (Perceived Constipation)
   b. No
9. Are bowel sounds increased?
   a. Yes (Diarrhea)
   b. No
10. Have number of bowel movements increased?
    a. Yes (Diarrhea)
    b. No
11. Does the patient complain of loose, liquid stools?
    a. Yes (Diarrhea)
    b. No

12. Is there increased frequency of voiding?
    a. Yes (Altered Urinary Elimination; Stress Incontinence; Urge Incontinence)
    b. No
13. Is there dribbling of urine when the patient laughs, coughs, or sneezes?
    a. Yes (Stress Incontinence)
    b. No
14. Once need to void is felt, is the patient able to reach toilet in time?
    a. Yes
    b. No (Urge Incontinence; Functional Incontinence)
15. Does the patient complain of bladder spasms?
    a. Yes (Reflex Incontinence; Urge Incontinence)
    b. No
16. Is there a decreased awareness of the need to void?
    a. Yes (Reflex Incontinence; Total Incontinence)
    b. No
17. Is there a decreased urge to void?
    a. Yes (Reflex Incontinence)
    b. No
18. Does the patient void in small amounts?
    a. Yes (Urge Incontinence; Urinary Retention)
    b. No
19. Is there urine flow without bladder distention?
    a. Yes (Total Incontinence)
    b. No
20. Is the bladder distended?
    a. Yes (Urinary Retention)
    b. No
21. Is there decreased urine output?
    a. Yes (Urinary Retention)
    b. No

NURSING DIAGNOSES IN THIS PATTERN

1. Bowel Incontinence (page 268)
2. Constipation (page 275)
   a. Colonic Constipation
   b. Perceived Constipation
3. Diarrhea (page 285)
4. Altered Urinary Elimination: Incontinence (page 293)
   a. Functional Incontinence
   b. Reflex Incontinence
   c. Stress Incontinence
   d. Total Incontinence
   e. Urge Incontinence
5. Urinary Retention (page 304)

Conceptual Information

Elimination, simply defined, refers to the excretion of waste and nondigested products of the metabolic process. Elimination is essential in maintaining fluid, electrolyte, and nutritional balance of the body. A disruption in an individual's usual elimination pattern can be life-threatening since a person cannot live long without the ability to rid his or her body of waste products.[1,2]

Elimination depends on the interrelated functioning of the gastrointestinal system, urinary system, nervous system, and skin. This chapter will include only the lower urinary tract and gastrointestinal tract since the skin and nervous system are related to nursing diagnoses in other chapters. Also, since the nursing diagnoses related to elimination refer only to elimination and not to the collection and formation of the waste materials, inclusion of other conceptual information would be confusing.

Our society has a dichotomous attitude toward elimination. A great deal of time, effort, and money is expended in designing and advertising bathrooms and aids to elimination, but to discuss elimination is considered rude.[1] Therefore, obtaining a reliable, complete elimination pattern assessment may be difficult. Added to this difficulty is the fact that each person has his or her own normal elimination habit.

Elimination is highly individualized and can be influenced by age, circadian rhythms, culture, diet, activity, stress, and a number of other factors. Elimination has elements of both involuntary and voluntary control. Involuntary control relates primarily to the production of waste materials and the neural signals that the bladder or bowel needs to be emptied. However, each person can usually control both the timing of bowel and bladder evacuation and the use of abdominal and perineal muscles to assist in evacuation.

Food and fluid intake are extremely important in elimination. A fluid intake of 2000 ml per day and a food intake of high-fiber foods would, in the majority of instances, ensure an adequate elimination pattern.[3,4] Alteration in elimination may cause psychosocial problems, such as social isolation due to embarrassment, as well as physiologic problems, such as fluid and/or electrolyte imbalance.

BOWEL ELIMINATION

The lower gastrointestinal tract includes the small and large intestines. The small bowel includes the duodenum, jejunum, and ileum and is about 20 feet in length and 1 inch in diameter. The large bowel includes the cecum, colon, and rectum and terminates at the anus. The large bowel is about 5 feet long and about $2\frac{1}{2}$ inches in diameter. The small bowel and large bowel connect at the ileocecal valve.[2]

The intestines receive partially digested food from the stomach and move the food element through the lower tract, thus assisting in proper absorption of water, nutrients, and electrolytes. The intestines also provide secretory and storage functions. They secrete mucus, potassium, bicarbonate, and enzymes.

The *chyme* (small intestine contents) is moved by peristalsis, and the *feces* (large intestine contents) are propelled by mass movements that are stimulated by the gastrocolic reflex. The gastrocolic reflex occurs in response to food entering the stomach and causing distention, so mass movement occurs only a few times a day. The gastrocolic reflex occurs within 30 minutes after eating and is most predominant after the first meal of the day. Therefore, after the first meal of the day is the most frequent time for bowel elimination. Other reflexes involved in elimination are the duodenocolic reflex and the defecation reflex. The *duodenocolic reflex* is stimulated by the distention of the duodenum as food passes from the stomach to the duodenum. The gastrocolic and duodenocolic reflexes stimulate rectal contraction and, usually, a desire to defecate. The *defecation reflex* occurs in response to feces entering the rectum. This reflex promotes relaxation of the internal anal sphincter, thus also promoting a desire to defecate. Extra fluids upon morning waking potentiate the gastrocolic reflex. If the fluids are warm or contain caffeine, they will also stimulate peristalsis.[1,2]

The secretions of the gastrointestinal tract assist with food passage and further digestion. The passage rate of the contents through the intestines helps determine the absorption amount. The small intestine is responsible for about 90 percent of the absorption of amino acids, sodium, calcium chloride, fatty acids, bile salts, and water. Potassium and bicarbonate are excreted. The usual amount of time for chyme to move from the stomach to the ileocecal valve varies from 3 to 10 hours. It takes about 12 hours for feces to travel from the ileocecal valve to the rectum. One bowel movement may be the result of meals eaten over the past 3 to 4 days, and most of the food residue from any particular meal will have been excreted within 4 days. Passage of contents is primarily influenced by the amount of residue and the motility rate. Feces are normally evacuated on a moderately regular schedule, but the schedule will vary from three times daily to once per week depending on the individual.

When proper absorption does not occur, necessary nutrients and electrolytes are lost for subsequent body use. Small-bowel loss can cause metabolic acidosis and hypokalemia. Large-bowel loss can lead to dehydration and hyponatremia.

The squatting, leaning-forward position is the most supportive position for defecation because it increases intra-abdominal pressure and promotes easier abdominal and perineal muscle contraction and relaxation. Beside positioning, diet, and fluid intake, other aids to elimination include enemas and laxatives.

Enemas assist in evacuation through either promotion of peristalsis, chemical irritation, or lubrication. Volume enemas, 500 to 1000 ml of fluid, cause distention, which increases peristalsis. The addition of heat and soapsuds, for example, adds chemical irritation and increases peristalsis. Straight tap-water enemas should be used cautiously since they are hypotonic and may disturb electrolyte balance. Electrolyte enemas are usually prepackaged and are hypertonic. Hypertonic enemas increase fluid amounts in the bowel through osmosis, thus slightly increasing distention and providing a relatively mild chemical irritation. Both the distention and irritation also result in increased peristalsis. Oil enemas are usually small-volume enemas (100 to 200 ml) and provide lubrication as well as stool softening.[1,5]

Laxatives assist elimination through producing bulk, providing lubrication, causing chemical irritation, or softening stool. The action of laxatives ranges from harsh to mild.

Both laxatives and enemas can be abused. Persistent use of either will diminish normal reflexes so that the individual will begin to require more and more aid. The individual then establishes an aid-dependent habit just as a drug abuser does.

While constipation and diarrhea are the two most common problems with bowel elimination, flatulence may be an associated problem. *Flatus* (intestinal gas) is normal. A problem arises when the individual cannot pass the gas or when abnormally large amounts of gas are produced. Flatus is produced by swallowed air, diffusion of gases from the bloodstream to the gastrointestinal tract, from carbon dioxide formed by the action of bicarbonate with hydrochloric acid or fatty acids, and from bacterial decomposition of food residue. Common causes of gas problems include gas-producing foods (beans, for example), highly irritating foods (pizza, for example), constipating medications (codeine, for example), and inactivity. The problems relate directly to the amount of gas produced and decreased motility. Increased flatus causes distention, which, in turn, can cause pain, respiratory difficulty, and further problems with intestinal motility.[1]

As previously mentioned, any bowel elimination problem can ultimately be life-threatening. Any bowel elimination problem, whether it be constipation, diarrhea, or flatulence, that lasts over 1 to 2 weeks in an adult or over 2 to 3 days for an infant or elderly person requires immediate health care intervention.

URINARY ELIMINATION

The lower urinary tract is composed of the ureters, bladder, and urethra. These anatomical structures serve as storage and excretory pathways for the waste secreted by the kidneys. The ureters extend from the kidney pelvis to the trigone area in the bladder. The ureters are small tubes composed of smooth muscle that propels urine by peristalsis from the kidney to the bladder. The bladder stores the urine until it is excreted through the urethra. Between the base of the bladder and the top of the urethra is the urethral sphincter. The sphincter opens under learned voluntary control. Opening the urethral sphincter allows the urine to pass through the urethra and meatus for elimination. The female urethra is about 3 to 5 cm long, and the male urethra is about 20 cm long.[6]

The desire to void occurs when the bladder (adult) has reached a capacity of 250 to 450 ml of urine. As urine collects to the bladder capacity, the stretch receptors in the bladder muscle are activated. This stretching stimulates the voiding reflex center in the spinal cord (sacral levels 2, 3, and 4), which sends signals to the midbrain and the pons. These stimuli result in inhibition of the spinal reflex center and pudendal nerve, which allows relaxation of the external sphincter and contraction of the bladder, and voiding occurs. The bladder is under parasympathetic control, with the learned voluntary control being guided by the cortex, midbrain, and medulla.[1,6]

The anatomically correct positions for voiding are sitting for the female and standing for the male. It is important to note that in some cultural groups the correct voiding position for the male is squatting. Either standing or squatting is anatomically correct. Difficulties arise if the male is lying down, as, for example, when he is in traction or a body cast. An individual generally voids 200 to 450 ml each voiding time, and it is within normal limits to void 5 to 10 times per day. Common times for urination are upon arising and before retiring. Other times will vary with habits and correspond with work breaks and availability of toilet facilities.[1,6]

Urine volume will vary according to the individual. Urine volume depends on normal kidney functioning, amount of fluid and food intake, environmental temperature, fluid requirements of other organs, presence of open wounds, output by other areas (skin, bowel, and respiration), and medications such as diuretics. The amount of solutes in the urine, an intact neuromuscular system, and the action of the antidiuretic hormone also influence output. A significant impact on urinary output is the opportunity to void at socially acceptable times in private.[1]

Inadequate urinary output may arise from either the kidney's not producing urine (*suppression*) or blockage of urine flow (*retention*) somewhere between the kidney and external urinary meatus. Suppression may result from disease of the kidneys or other body structures and inadequate fluid intake. Retention may be either mechanical or functional in nature. Mechanical retention is due to anatomic blockage such as a stricture or a calculus. *Functional retention* actually refers to any retention that is not mechanical and includes such areas as neurogenic problems.[6]

Urinary control relates to the integrity and strength of the urinary sphincters and perineal musculature. Inability to control urinary output will soon lead to social isolation due to embarrassment over control and odor. Urinary incontinence is more common than most health care professionals realize. Studies[7,8] have indicated that urinary incontinence is quite common among healthy premenopausal middle-aged women, and they have found no relationship between continence status, number of children, history of gynecological surgery, smoking, physical activity, or intake of alcohol and caffeine. The studies found also that very few of these women sought treatment for this incontinence.

Bladder-retraining programs may vary according to individual hospitals and physicians. Consultation with a rehabilitation nurse clinician will provide the most current and reliable information regarding a quality bladder-retraining program.[9] Two measures that may assist with incontinence are Crede's maneuver and the Valsalva maneuver. *Crede's maneuver* involves placing the fingertips together at the midline of the pelvic crest, then massaging deeply and smoothly down to the pubic bone. Check with the physician first since there are contraindications such as ureteral reflux.[5] The *Valsalva maneuver* involves asking the patient to simulate having a bowel movement. Have the patient take a deep breath, hold it, and then bear down as if expelling a bowel movement. Check with the physician first since there are contraindications such as glaucoma, eye surgery, and impaired circulation.[5]

Urine is a waste product formed as a part of body metabolism. Urine is normally produced at a rate of 30 to 50 ml per hour. Under normal circumstances output will balance with intake about every 72 hours. An hourly output under 30 ml, a 24-hour output 500 ml or less, or an intake-output imbalance lasting over 72 hours requires immediate intervention.[1,4]

Developmental Considerations

Elimination depends on the interrelatedness of fluid intake, muscle tone, regularity of habits, culture, state of health, and adequate nutrition.[10]

INFANT

Kidney function does not reach adult levels until 6 months to 1 year of life. Nervous system control is inadequate and renal function does not reach a mature status until approximately 1 year of life.[10] Voiding is stimulated by cold air. The infant usually voids 15 to 60 ml at each voiding during the first 24 hours of life and may void reflexively at birth. If the infant has not voided by 12 hours after birth, there is cause for concern. By the third day, the infant may void 8 to 10 times during each 24 hours, equaling about 100 to 400 ml. Urinary output is affected by the amount of fluid consumed, the amount of activity (increased activity = less urine), and the environmental temperature (increased temperature = less urine).[11] Uric acids crystals may be found in concentrated urine, causing a rusty discoloration to the diaper.[11]

The muscles and elastic tissues of the infant's intestines are poorly developed, and nervous system control is adequate. Water and electrolyte absorption is functional but immature. The intestines are proportionately longer than in the adult. While some digestive enzymes are present, they can only break down simple foods. These digestive enzymes are unable to break down complex carbohydrates or protein.

Meconium is the first waste material that is eliminated by the bowel. This usually occurs during the first 24 hours. After 24 hours, the characteristics of the bowel movement change as it mixes with milk. The characteristics of the stool will depend on whether the infant is breast-fed or bottle-fed. The breast-fed infant will have soft, semiliquid stools that are yellow or golden in color. The bottle-fed infant will have a more formed stool that is light yellow to brown in color.

The infant may have four to eight soft bowel movements a day during the first 4 weeks of life. Flatus often accompanies the passage of stool, and there may be a sour odor to the bowel movement. By the fourth week of life, the number of bowel movements has decreased to two to four a day. By 4 months, there is a predictable interval between bowel movements.

It is common for the infant to push or strain at stool. However, if the stools are very hard or dry, the infant should be assessed for constipation. The bottle-fed infant is more prone to constipation than the breast-fed infant.

Infants sometimes suffer from what is known as colic. *Colic* is described as daily periods of distress caused by rapid, violent peristaltic waves and increased gas pressure in the rectum.[11] The cause is unknown but may have to do with the simple (rather than the complex) digestive enzymes of the infant or a decreased amount of vitamin A, K, or E. Most authorities agree that colic disappears as digestive enzymes become more complex and when normal bacterial flora accumulate.[11]

TODDLER AND PRESCHOOLER

By 2 years of age, the kidneys are able to conserve water and to concentrate urine almost on an adult level, except under stress. The bladder increases in size and is able to hold about 88 ml of urine.

Nervous system and gastrointestinal maturation has occurred during infancy and the beginning of the toddler years. By the time children are 2 to 3 years of age, they are ready to control bowel and bladder functioning. Bowel elimination control is usually attained first; daytime bladder control is second, and nighttime bladder control is third. The child must be able to walk a few steps, control the sphincter, recognize and interpret that the bladder is full, and be able to indicate that he or she wants to go to the bathroom. The child must also value dryness. He or she must recognize that it is more socially acceptable to be dry than to be wet.

Parents should not attempt toilet training, even if the child is ready, if there are family or environmental stressors. Regression is normal during toilet training, and, coupled with undue stress, could cause physical or psychosocial problems.

Bladder training takes time to accomplish. Both the parent and the child must have patience and not get unduly upset when accidents occur. In fact, nighttime bladder control may not be attained until 5 to 8 years of life. Doctors and researchers disagree on the age at which nighttime bed-wetting (*enuresis*) becomes a problem.[11] Parents should limit fluids at night, have the child void before going to bed, and get the child up at least once during the night to assist in attaining nighttime control.

In order to toilet train, the parent should watch for patterns of defecation. Eating stimulates peristaltic activity and evacuation. The child can then be taken to the toilet at the expected time after eating. The child should be told what is expected while on the toilet. Give the child enough time to evacuate the bowel, but do not have the child sit on the toilet too long. The child (and the parent) may then become frustrated.

Children at this age like to give and to please their parents. Evacuation of the bowel is a natural process and should not be approached as if it is a dirty or unnatural process. Children should be rewarded and should feel a pride in accomplishment when they are able to defecate; they should never be punished or be made to feel ashamed or guilty if they are unable to have a bowel movement.

Children usually do not need enemas or laxatives to make them regular. In fact, those artificial aids may be dangerous. Lack of parental understanding of the elimination process and of the developmental aspects of children coupled with harsh punishment for "accidents" may lead a child to an obsessive, meticulous, and rigid personality.

Accidents can and do occur even after a child has been completely toilet trained. These accidents usually occur because the child ignores the defecation urge. Usually this occurs because the child is engrossed in another activity and does not want to take the time to go to the bathroom or because other stressors have a higher priority at the moment.

SCHOOL-AGE CHILD

The urinary system is functioning maturely by this age. The normal output is 500 ml per day. Urinary tract infections are common because of careless hygiene practices in females. The gastrointestinal system attains adult functional maturity during the school years.

ADOLESCENT

There are no noticeable differences in patterns of urinary elimination in this age group. The intestines grow in length and width. The muscles of the intestines become thicker and stronger.

This developmental stage is important in developing bowel habits. The teenager is engaged in developing sexuality. This group may ignore warning signals for elimination because they do not want to leave their activities or because of the close association of the anus to the teenager's developing sexual organs. Additionally, if a problem arises with elimination, adolescents are reluctant to talk about it with either their peers or an adult.

YOUNG ADULT

There is no noticeable difference in patterns of elimination during this developmental period. Total urinary output for 24 hours is 1000 to 2000 ml. The rate of passage of feces is influenced by the nature of the foods consumed and the physical health of the individual. Hemorrhoids are possible in this developmental group, especially females.

ADULT

Adequate daily fluid intake helps to maintain proper elimination functions. There is a gradual decrease in the number of nephrons and therefore decreased renal functioning with age. Additionally, bladder tone diminishes; thus, the adult may urinate more frequently.

Digestive enzymes (gastric acid, pepsin, ptyalin, and pancreatic enzymes) begin to decrease. This may lead to an increasing incidence of intestinal disorders, cancer, and gastrointestinal complaints.

OLDER ADULT

Renal function is slowed by both the structural and functional aging changes, mainly because of decreases in the number of nephrons. Vascular sclerosing also occurs in the renal system, and this combined with fewer nephrons decreases available blood so that the *glomerular filtration rate (GFR)* becomes markedly reduced. While the GFR reduction is still sufficient to handle normal demands, stress or illness can significantly alter the older adult's renal status.[12] Decreased concentrations and dilution ability of the kidneys occur as a result of changes in the renal tubules. Waste products are effectively processed by the kidneys, but over a longer period of time. The decreased efficiency of the kidneys helps make older adults especially vulnerable to medication side effects and problems regarding drug excretion.[13]

The older male adult may have an enlarged prostate gland. Prostatic enlargement can lead to urethritis, incomplete bladder emptying, and difficulty in starting the stream of urine. Bladder changes, resulting from loss of smooth-muscle elasticity, can result in a decreased bladder capacity. Uninhibited bladder contractions may interrupt bladder filling and lead to a premature urge to void. Increased residual urine and incomplete emptying of the bladder result in a higher incidence of urinary tract infections in older adults of both sexes.

Changes in the gastrointestinal tract include a continued decrease in digestive enzymes and questionable changes in absorption in the small intestines. The large intestine may have reduced blood flow secondary to vascular twisting, and there is debate regarding decreased motility in the colon. Problems related to constipation may occur due to increased tolerance for rectal distention rather than decreased motility.[13]

Major factors that effect gastrointestinal (GI) and genitourinary (GU) function in older adults include immobility and medications. Immobility can lead to kidney stones, UTIs secondary to stasis, alterations in food intake, digestion, and elimination.[14] Medications, such as anticholinergics and opiates, can result in delayed motility in the GI tract. Diuretics, hypnotics, and antipsychotics must be considered in light of their effect on GU function.[15]

APPLICABLE NURSING DIAGNOSES
Bowel Incontinence

DEFINITION

A state in which an individual experiences a change in normal bowel habits characterized by involuntary passage of stool.[16]

NANDA TAXONOMY: EXCHANGING 1.3.1.3

DEFINING CHARACTERISTICS[16]

1. Major defining characteristic:
   Involuntary passage of stool
2. Minor defining characteristics:
   None given

RELATED FACTORS[16]

To be developed.

RELATED CLINICAL CONCERNS

1. Alzheimer's disease
2. Guillain-Barré syndrome
3. Spinal cord injury
4. Intestinal surgery
5. Gynecological surgery

HAVE YOU SELECTED THE CORRECT DIAGNOSIS?

Constipation The problem may really be due to constipation with impaction. Incontinence may occur because some feces are leaking around the impaction site and the individual is unable to control their passage and thus appears incontinent. (See page 275.)

Self-Care Deficit: Toileting If the individual is unable to appropriately care for his or her evacuation needs, incontinence may result. (See page 472.)

Diarrhea Diarrhea relates to frequent bowel movements, but the patient is aware of rectal filling and can control the feces until reaching the toilet. With incontinence the patient may not be aware of rectal filling and the stool passage is involuntary. (See page 285.)

EXPECTED OUTCOMES

1. Will have no more than one soft, formed stool per day by (date) and/or
2. Will return to usual bowel elimination habits by (date)

TARGET DATE

Target dates should be based on the individual's usual bowel elimination pattern. Incontinence may require additional retraining time and effort. Therefore, a target date 5 days from admission would be most realistic. Also remember that there must be a realistic potential that bowel continence can be regained by the patient.

NURSING ACTIONS/INTERVENTIONS WITH RATIONALES

Adult Health

Actions/Interventions	Rationales
• Check for fecal impaction on admission, and implement nursing actions for Constipation if impaction is noted.	Impaction may lead to leakage of bowel contents around impacted areas.

Continued

Actions/Interventions	Rationales
• Record each incontinent episode when it occurs as well as the amount, color, and consistency of each stool.	Assists in determining pattern of incontinence.
• Record events associated with incontinent episode, including events both before and after the episode (for example, activity, stress, location, people present, and so on).	Assists in determining pattern of incontinence.
• Monitor anal skin integrity at least once per shift at (times).	Allows early detection of any tissue integrity problems.
• Keep anal area clean and dry.	Bowel contents are damaging to the skin and promote tissue integrity problems.
• Provide room deodorizer and chlorophyll tablets for patient.	Decreases embarrassment due to odors.
• Provide emotional support for patient through teaching, providing time for listening, and so on.	Patient may find incontinence embarrassing and may try to isolate self.
• Initiate bowel training at least 4 days prior to discharge: ○ Administer suppository ½ hour after eating. ○ Toilet ½ hour after suppository insertion. ○ Toilet prior to activity. ○ Stimulate defecation reflex with circular movement in rectum using gloved, lubricated finger.	Establishes consistent pattern and conditions control of elimination.
• Teach patient, beginning as soon after admission as possible: ○ Pelvic floor strengthening exercises (see Constipation) ○ *Diet:* Role of fiber and fluids ○ *Use of assistive devices:* Velcro closings on clothes, or pads ○ Perineal hygiene ○ Appropriate use of suppositories and/or antidiarrheal medications	Basic knowledge promotes understanding of condition and assists patient to change behavior as well as empowering the patient for self-care.
• Refer for home health care assistance.	

Child Health

Nursing actions for Bowel Incontinence in the child are the same as those for adult health. Modifications would be made for child's age and size, for example, medication dosage and fluid amounts.

Women's Health

Bowel incontinence in women caused by uterine prolapse and pelvic relaxation with displacement of pelvic organs (particularly the rectum) is relieved only by surgical repair.[17] Otherwise, nursing actions for Bowel Incontinence in Women's Health are the same as in Adult Health.

Mental Health

Actions/Interventions	Rationales

• If a pattern forms around specific events, develop plan to:
  ○ Encourage person to use bathroom before the event.
  ○ Alter the manner in which specific task is performed to prevent stress (note alterations here).
  ○ Discuss with client alternative ways of coping with stress. (Refer to Chapter 8 for specific nursing actions related to reduction of anxiety and to Chapter 11 for specific nursing actions related to Ineffective Coping.)
	Promotes client's perceived control and increases potential for client's involvement in treatment plan.

• If assessment suggests secondary gains associated with episodes, decrease these by:
  ○ Withdrawing social contact after an episode
  ○ Having client clean himself or herself
  ○ Providing social contact or interactions with the client at times when no incontinence is experienced
	Provides negative consequences for inappropriate coping behavior.

• If not related to secondary gain, spend (number) minutes with client after each episode to allow expression of feelings. • Discuss with client effects this problem has on life-style.	Verbalization of feelings in a nonthreating environment models acceptance of feelings and positive coping behavior. Increases client's awareness of impact inappropriate coping behaviors have on life-style. Provides data for development of alternative coping, promoting client's perceived control.
Refer to home health resources.	

Gerontic Health

Actions/Interventions	Rationales
• Record events associated with incontinent episode.	Assists in determining pattern of incontinence. Older adult may have difficulty in reaching commode or bathroom easily.
• Monitor medication intake for potential to result in bowel incontinence.	Medications with a sedative effect may decrease the ability of the patient to reach toilet facilities in a timely manner.
• Teach toileting skills to caregivers of cognitively impaired older adults. In early dementia, labeling the bathroom and reminding the individual to toilet may result in continence.	Depending on the stage of the disease, a person with dementia may forget to toilet or have difficulty finding a bathroom that is not readily identified.

Home Health

Actions/Interventions	Rationales

• Teach patient and family:
  ○ Appropriate use and frequency of use of prescribed and over-the-counter medications
  ○ To monitor color, frequency, consistency, and pattern of symptoms
  ○ Measures to ensure adequate bowel elimination:
    (1) Proper diet
    (2) Fluid and electrolyte balance
    (3) Pelvic floor and abdominal exercises
  ○ To monitor skin integrity
  ○ To keep bed linens and clothing clean and dry
	These activities assist in preventing constipation and provide data for early recognition of problem.
	
	These measures prevent secondary problems from occurring due to the existing problem.

FLOW CHART EVALUATION
Flow Chart Expected Outcome 1

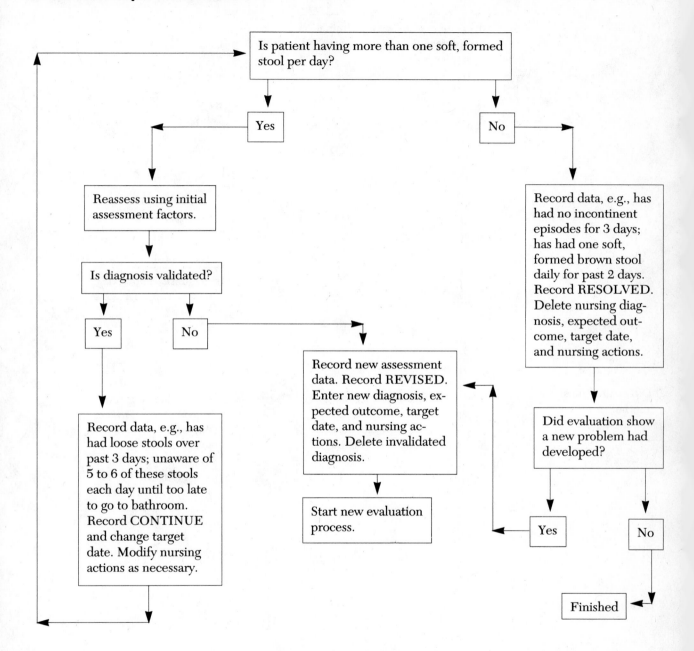

Flow Chart Expected Outcome 2

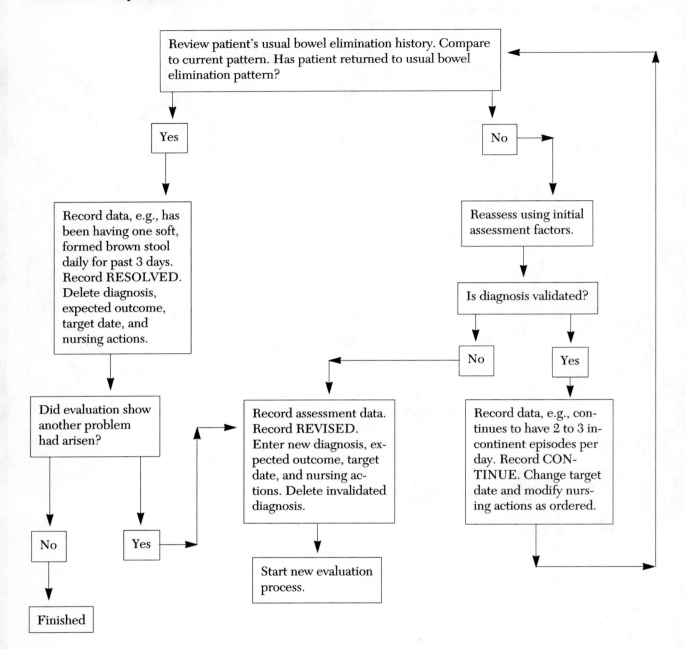

Constipation

DEFINITION

A state in which an individual experiences a change in normal bowel habits characterized by a decrease in frequency and/or passage of hard, dry stools.

Colonic Constipation: The state in which an individual's pattern of elimination is characterized by hard, dry stool that results from a delay in passage of food residue.

Perceived Constipation: The state in which an individual makes a self-diagnosis of constipation and ensures a daily bowel movement through abuse of laxatives, enemas, and suppositories.[16]

NANDA TAXONOMY: EXCHANGING 1.3.1.1, 1.3.1.1.1., 1.3.1.1.2

DEFINING CHARACTERISTICS[16]

1. Constipation:
   a. Major defining characteristics:
      (1) Decreased activity level
      (2) Frequency less than usual pattern
      (3) Hard formed stools
      (4) Palpable mass
      (5) Reported feeling of pressure in rectum
      (6) Reported feeling of rectal fullness
      (7) Straining at stool
   b. Other possible characteristics:
      (1) Abdominal pain
      (2) Appetite impairment
      (3) Back pain
      (4) Headache
      (5) Interference with daily living
      (6) Use of laxative
2. Colonic Constipation:
   a. Major defining characteristics:
      (1) Decreased frequency
      (2) Hard, dry stool
      (3) Straining at stool
      (4) Painful defecation
      (5) Abdominal distention
      (6) Palpable mass
   b. Minor defining characteristics:
      (1) Rectal pressure
      (2) Headache
      (3) Appetite impairment
      (4) Abdominal pain
3. Perceived Constipation:
   a. Major defining characteristics:
      (1) Expectation of a daily bowel movement, with the resulting overuse of laxatives, enemas, and suppositories
      (2) Expected passage of stool at same time each day
   b. Minor defining characteristics:
      None given

RELATED FACTORS[16]

1. Constipation:
   To be developed
2. Colonic Constipation:
   a. Less than adequate fluid intake
   b. Less than adequate dietary intake
   c. Less than adequate fiber
   d. Less than adequate physical activity
   e. Immobility
   f. Lack of privacy
   g. Emotional disturbances
   h. Chronic use of medication and enemas
   i. Stress
   j. Change in daily routine
   k. Metabolic problems, for example, hypothyroidism, hypocalcemia, or hypokalemia
3. Perceived Constipation:
   a. Cultural or family health belief
   b. Faulty appraisal
   c. Impaired thought processes

RELATED CLINICAL CONCERNS

1. Anemias
2. Hypothyroidism
3. Hemorrhoids
4. Renal dialysis
5. Abdominal surgery

HAVE YOU SELECTED THE CORRECT DIAGNOSIS?

Altered Nutrition: Less or More than Body Requirements This might be the primary nursing diagnosis. Either of these diagnoses influences the amount and consistency of the feces. (See pages 200 and 215.)

Fluid Volume Deficit This might also be the primary problem. The feces need adequate lubrication to pass through the gastrointestinal tract. If there is a Fluid Volume Deficit, the feces are harder, more solid, and unable to move through the system. (See page 155.)

Diarrhea or Bowel Incontinence Constipation can be misdiagnosed as Diarrhea or Bowel Incontinence. Diarrhea or incontinence may be a secondary condition to constipation as semiliquid feces may pass around the area of constipation. (See pages 268 and 285.)

Impaired Physical Mobility This diagnosis could be the underlying cause of constipation. Decrease in physical mobility affects every body system. In the GI tract, peristalsis is slowed, which may lead to a backlog of feces and to constipation. (See page 460.)

Self-Care Deficit: Toileting This diagnosis may also be the primary diagnosis. Difficulty in reaching appropriate toileting facilities and difficulty in cleansing oneself after toileting could lead to a decision to delay bowel movement, with a result of constipation. (See page 472.)

Ineffective Individual Coping and Anxiety These diagnoses are two psychosocial nursing diagnoses from which Constipation needs to be differentiated. Both of these psychosocial diagnoses initiate stress as an autonomic response, and the parasympathetic system stimuli (which controls motility of the GI tract) is reduced. This reduced motility may lead to constipation. (See pages 605 and 892.)

EXPECTED OUTCOMES

1. Will return, as nearly as possible, to usual bowel elimination habits by (date) and/or
2. Will design and carry out a plan to avoid constipation by (date)

TARGET DATE

Target dates should be based on the individual's usual bowel elimination habits. A target date 3 to 5 days from admission would be reasonable for the majority of patients.

NURSING ACTIONS/INTERVENTIONS WITH RATIONALES

Adult Health

Actions/Interventions	Rationales
• Record amount, color, and consistency of bowel movement following each bowel movement. Question patient regarding bowel movements at least once per shift. Also record if no bowel movement on each shift.	Basic assessment of problem severity as well as monitoring effectiveness of therapy.
• Monitor and record symptoms associated with passage of bowel movement: ○ Any straining, pain, or headache ○ Any rectal bleeding or fissures	Allows early detection of additional problems.
• If fecal impaction: ○ Attempt digital removal using gloves and lubrication. ○ Administer oil retention enema of small volume. Have patient retain for at least 1 hour. Use small-volume saline enema if oil retention does not relieve impaction.	Prioritization of methods used to break up and remove impaction.
• Collaborate with physician regarding use of glycerin or other types of suppositories.	

Continued

Actions/Interventions	Rationales
• Measure and total intake and output every shift. Be sure to include estimation of loss by perspiration.	Allows monitoring of fluid balance.
• Force fluids, of patient's choice, to at least 2000 ml daily. Encourage 8 ounces of fluid every 2 hours on the (odd/even) hour beginning at awakening each morning.	Increases moisture and water content of feces for easier movement through intestines and anus.
• Increase patient's activity to extent possible through ambulation at least three times per shift while awake.	Activity promotes stimulation of bowel and will assist in elimination.
• Assist patient with exercises, every 4 hours while awake: ○ Bent-knee situps. ○ Straight- or bent-leg lifts. ○ Alternating contraction and relaxation of perineal muscles while sitting in a chair and with feet placed apart on floor. Have patient repeat each exercise at least five times.	Strengthens pelvic floor and abdominal muscles.
• Assist patient with implementation of stress reduction techniques at least once per shift.	Promotes relaxation and can increase feces passage through the intestines. Stimulates defecation reflex and urge.
• Digitally stimulate anal sphincter at scheduled times (usually after meals—state times here).	
• Provide privacy and sufficient time for bowel elimination.	Decreases stress and promotes relaxation, which increases likelihood of bowel movement.
• Help patient assume anatomically correct position for bowel movements.	Promotes effective use of abdominal muscles and allows gravity to assist in defecation.
• Use rectal tube, heat, activity, and change of position every 2 hours on the (odd/even) hour for problems with flatulence.	Promotes passage of flatus.
• Monitor anal skin integrity at least once per shift.	Straining at stool can cause splits and tears of the anal tissue.
• Provide room deodorizer for patient as needed.	Helps to eliminate odors; decreases embarrassment.
• Use cool compresses to anus every 2 hours as needed.	Alleviates anal itching.
• Teach patient, starting as soon after admission as possible: ○ The importance of a bowel routine and the need to respond to the urge to defecate as soon as possible ○ To stimulate gastrocolic reflex through drinking prune juice or hot liquid upon arising ○ To allow sufficient time for bowel movement and plan time for elimination	Promotes understanding of self-care needs prior to discharge.

○ To include high-fiber foods and extra liquid in daily diet

○ To avoid prolonged use of elimination aids such as laxatives and enemas

○ To avoid straining

○ To use proper perineal hygiene

○ To describe the relationship of diet and activity to bowel elimination

- Collaborate, as soon as possible after admission:

  ○ With dietitian regarding a high-fiber, high-roughage diet (the more food a patient eats, the fewer laxatives the patient will require[18])

  ○ With physical therapist regarding exercise program

  ○ With physician regarding mild analgesics and ointments for control of pain associated with bowel movements

  ○ With physician regarding use of stool softeners, laxatives, suppositories, and enemas

  ○ With enterstomal therapist regarding ostomy care (that is, irrigations, stoma and skin care, and appliances)

  ○ With psychiatric nurse clinician regarding counseling for patient and family regarding possible underlying emotional components

  ○ With home health nurse regarding follow-up planning for home and usual daily activities of living with emphasis on stress, and so on

Provides basic resources and information needed; promotes holistic approach to treatment.

Child Health

Nursing actions for Constipation in the child are the same as those for adult health. Modifications would be made for child's age and size, for example, medication dosage or fluid amounts.

Women's Health

Actions/Interventions	Rationales
- Assist patient in identifying life-style adjustments that may be needed due to changes in physiologic function or needs during experiential phases of life (for example, pregnancy, postpartum, and after gynecologic surgery).	Provides information needed as basis for planning care and health maintenance.

Continued

Actions/Interventions	Rationales

• Teach client changes that occur during pregnancy that contribute to decreased gastric motility and potential constipation, for example:
  ○ Nausea and vomiting in early pregnancy can lead to decreased fluid intake.
  ○ Increased use of mother's body fluid intake to produce lactation can lead to decrease in overall fluid intake.
  ○ Supplemental iron during pregnancy can lead to severe constipation.
  ○ Fear of injury or pain upon defecation after birth can lead to constipation.
	Provides basic information for self-care during pregnancy, birthing process, and postpartum.

• Teach anatomic shifting of abdominal contents due to fetal growth.
• Teach hormonal influences (for example, increased progesterone) on bodily functions:
  ○ Decreased stomach emptying time
  ○ Decreased peristalsis
  ○ Increase in water reabsorption
  ○ Relaxation of abdominal muscles
  ○ Increase in flatulence
	Provides information as a basis for nutrition plan during pregnancy. Promotes self-care.

• Teach the effects of the increase in oral iron or calcium supplements on the gastrointestinal tract, for example, constipation. Describe the physical changes present in the immediate postpartum period that affect the gastrointestinal tract:
  ○ Lax abdominal muscles
  ○ Fluid loss (perspiration, urine, lochia, or dehydration during labor and delivery)
  ○ Hunger
	Provides basis for teaching patient plan of self-care at home and promotes healing process.

• Assist patient in planning a diet that will promote healing, replace lost fluids, and help with return to normal bowel evacuation.
• Instruct patient in the use of ointments, anesthetic sprays, sitz baths, and witch hazel compresses to relieve episiotomy pain and reduce hemorrhoids.
• Instruct patient in how to do pelvic floor exercises (Kegel exercises) to assist in healing and in reducing pain.
• Teach nursing mothers alternate methods of assistance with bowel evacuation other than cathartics (cathartics are expressed in breast milk):
  ○ Prune juice
  ○ Hot liquids
	Promotes successful lactation, good self-care, and good nutrition and provides basis for teaching care.

- ○ High-fiber, high-roughage diet
- ○ Daily exercise
- Describe the physical changes present in the immediate postoperative period (C-section and gynecological surgery) that affect the gastrointestinal tract:
  - ○ Fluid loss (blood loss or dehydration as a result of being NPO and undergoing surgery)
  - ○ Decreased peristalsis
  - ○ Bowel manipulation during surgery
  - ○ Increased use of analgesics and anesthesia

Provides basis for teaching and planning of care. Promotes and encourages self-care.

Mental Health

The nursing actions for this diagnosis in Mental Health are the same as those for adult health. Please refer to those recommended actions.

Gerontic Health

Actions/Interventions	Rationales
• Review medication record for drugs that may have constipation as a side effect.	Older adults receiving antidepressants, anticholinergics, tranquilizers, or certain antacids may experience constipation due to the drug-delayed motility of waste matter through the intestine. Older adults are more likely to be on multiple medications that can result in constipation.
• Collaborate with physician regarding changes in medication to avoid the side effect of constipation.	

Home Health

NOTE: Adult health actions are appropriate for home health. The locus of control shifts from the nurse to the client, family, or caregiver.

Actions/Interventions	Rationales
• The nurse will teach others to complete activities.	Client and members of family may have different ideas regarding appropriate elimination patterns.
• Teach client and family the definition of constipation. Determine if problem is perceived by client and family as being due to incorrect definition or is based on physiologic dysfunction.	Nursing interventions for physiologic definition are outlined in the Adult Health nursing action. Nursing interventions for varying definitions will require family involvement.

Continued

Actions/Interventions	Rationales

• Assist client and family in identifying life-style changes that may be required:
  ○ Establishment of a regular elimination routine based on cultural and individual variations
  ○ Stress management techniques
  ○ Decrease in concentrated, refined foods
  ○ Identification of any food intolerances or allergies and avoidance of those foods
  ○ Appropriate use and frequency of use of prescribed and over-the-counter medications
  ○ Physiologic parameters of constipation
	Home-based care requires involvement of family. Bowel elimination problems may require adjustments in family activities.

FLOW CHART EVALUATION
Flow Chart Expected Outcome 1

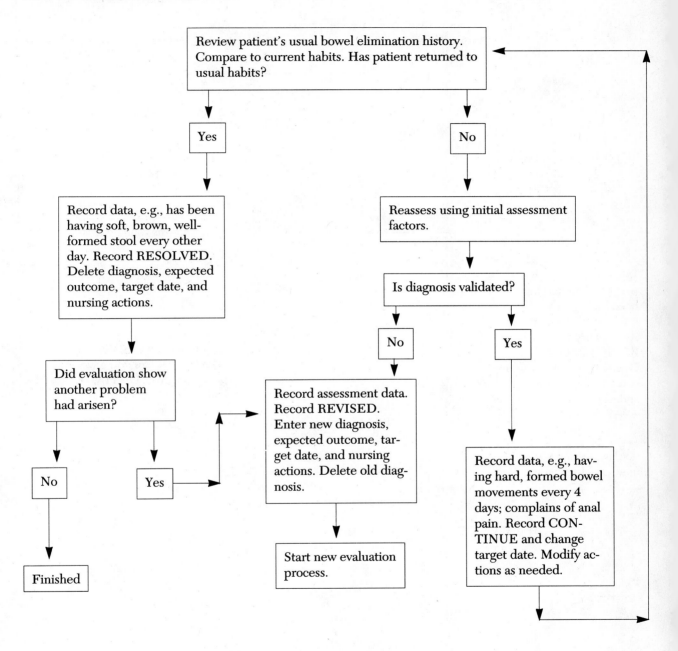

Flow Chart Expected Outcome 2

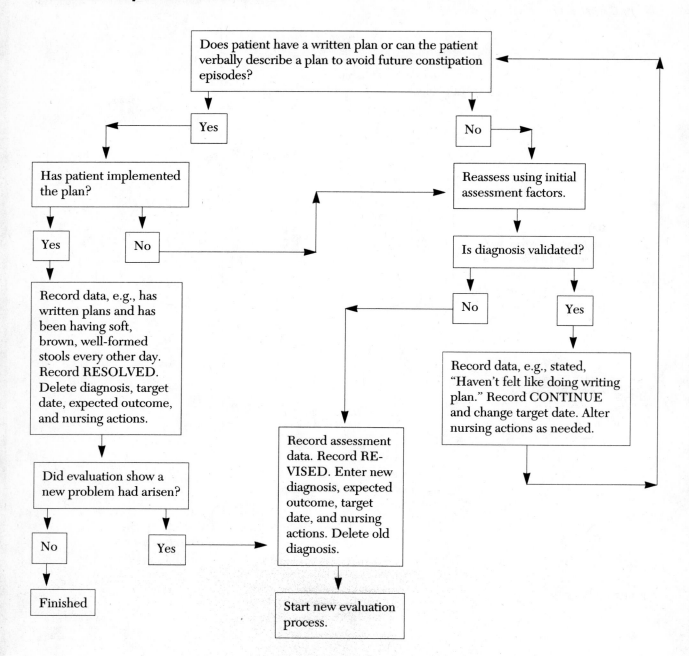

Diarrhea

DEFINITION

A state in which an individual experiences a change in normal bowel habits characterized by the frequent passage of loose, fluid, unformed stools.

NANDA TAXONOMY: EXCHANGING 1.3.1.2

DEFINING CHARACTERISTICS[16]

1. Major defining characteristics:
   a. Abdominal pain
   b. Cramping
   c. Increased frequency of bowel sounds
   d. Loose, liquid stools
   e. Urgency
2. Other possible characteristic:
   Change in color

RELATED FACTORS[16]

To be developed.

RELATED CLINICAL CONCERNS

1. Inflammatory Bowel Disease (Ulcerative Colitis, Crohn's Disease, Enteritis)
2. Anemias
3. Gastric Bypass or Gastric Partitioning Surgery
4. Gastritis

HAVE YOU SELECTED THE CORRECT DIAGNOSIS?

Constipation   Diarrhea may be secondary to constipation. In instances of severe constipation or impaction, semiliquid feces can leak around the areas of immotility and will appear to be diarrhea. (See page 275.)

Altered Nutrition: Less than Body Requirements   If the individual is not ingesting enough food or sufficient bulk to allow feces to be well formed, diarrhea may well result. (See page 200.)

Fluid Volume Deficit or Fluid Volume Excess   While research has not definitely supported the impact of fluid volume on bowel elimination, it is a common practice to pay attention to these diagnoses when either constipation or diarrhea is present. The basic idea appears to be that the amount of fluid ingested or absorbed by the body can affect the consistency of the fecal material. (See pages 155 and 166.)

Anxiety, Self-Esteem Disturbance, or Ineffective Individual Coping   Any of these psychosocial diagnoses precipitate a stress response. Indices of stress include gastrointestinal signs and symptoms, including diarrhea, vomiting, and "butterflies" in the stomach. (See pages 605, 668 and 892.)

Continued

> ## HAVE YOU SELECTED THE CORRECT DIAGNOSIS?—*Continued*
>
> **Sleep Pattern Disturbance**   If a person's biologic clock is changed because of altered sleep-wake patterns, body responses attuned to the biologic clock will also be altered. This includes usual elimination patterns, and diarrhea may result. (See page 507.)

EXPECTED OUTCOMES

1. Will have no more than one soft, formed bowel movement per day by (date) and/or
2. Will return to usual bowel elimination habits by (date)

TARGET DATE

Target dates should be based on the individual's usual bowel elimination habits. Thus, a target date 3 days from the day of admission would be reasonable for the majority of patients. Since diarrhea can be life-threatening for infants and older adults, a target date of 2 days would not be too soon.

NURSING ACTIONS/INTERVENTIONS WITH RATIONALES

Adult Health

Actions/Interventions	Rationales
• Record amount, color, consistency, and odor following each bowel movement.	Basic monitoring of condition as well as monitoring of effectiveness of therapy.
• Monitor weight and electrolytes at least every 2 days while diarrhea persists (state dates here).	Monitors hydration status.
• Measure and total intake and output every shift.	Monitors hydration status.
• Decrease bowel stimulation through placing patient on NPO status or clear liquid diet and intravenous (IV) hydration. Slowly reintroduce solid foods.	Rests the bowel while maintaining fluid and electrolyte balance.
• Place patient on enteric precautions until cause of diarrhea is determined.	Some types of diarrhea are infectious and are communicable.
• Make sure bathroom facilities are readily available.	Helps to prevent accidents and prevent embarrassment for patient.
• Administer antidiarrheal medications as ordered, and document results within 1 hour after administration; for example, diarrhea decreased from one stool every 30 minutes to one stool every 2 hours.	Documents effectiveness of medication.

- Increase fluid intake to at least 2500 ml per day.
- Offer fluids high in potassium and sodium at least once per hour, for example, Gatorade or Pedialyte.
- Serve fluids at tepid temperature (avoid temperature extremes such as very hot or very cold).
- List patient's fluid likes and dislikes here.
- Provide perineal skin care after each bowel movement. Monitor anal skin integrity at least once each shift.
- If tube feedings are causal factor, collaborate with physician regarding:
  - Infusion rate
  - Temperature of feeding
  - Dilution of feeding
  - Following feeding with water
  - Administration of Hydrocil at onset of tube feeding (increases stool consistency)[19]
- Provide room deodorizer, chlorophyll tablets, and fresh parsley for patient's use.
- Assist patient with stress reduction exercises at least once per shift; provide quiet, restful atmosphere.
- Collaborate with dietitian regarding low-fiber, low-residue, soft diet.
- List here those foods that patient has described as being irritating.
- Teach patient about:
  - *Diet*: Avoid irritating foods including those within the basic four food groups. Note the influence high-fiber foods and fruits have on diarrhea.
  - *Fluids*: Maintain an intake and output balance. Note the influence environmental temperature, level of activity, and consumption of caffeine and milk have on diarrhea.
  - *Medications*: Exercise caution with over-the-counter medications. Note that some of these medications are antidiarrheal, while some promote diarrhea, such as antacids.

Maintains hydration status.

Dries moisture, prevents skin breakdown, and prevents perineal infection.

Any of these modifications may decrease incidence of diarrhea.

Assists in elimination of odor; promotes pleasant environment.

Promotes relaxation and decreases stimulation of bowel.

Helps to identify foods that stimulate bowel and exacerbate diarrhea.

Increases patient's knowledge of causes, treatment, and complications of diarrhea. Promotes self-care.

Child Health

Actions/Interventions	Rationales
• Weigh diapers for urine and stools; assess specific gravity after each voiding.	A strict assessment of intake and output serves as a basis for monitoring the efficiency of the treatment and may provide a database for treatment protocol. Hydration is monitored via specific gravity as an indication of the renal ability to adjust to fluid and electrolyte imbalance.
• Monitor for signs and symptoms of dehydration: ○ Depressed anterior fontanel in infants ○ Poor skin turgor ○ Decreased urinary output	Dehydration is extremely dangerous for the infant and requires close monitoring to ensure prompt response and treatment.
• Monitor signs and symptoms associated with bowel movement, including cramping, flatus, and crying.	Associated signs and symptoms serve as supportive data to follow the altered bowel function, with an emphasis on related pain and/or discomfort.
• Provide prompt and gentle cleansing after each diaper change. For older children, offer warm soaks after each diarrheal episode.	Skin breakdown occurs in a short period of time due to frequent bowel movements and the resultant skin irritation.
• Collaborate with physician regarding: ○ Frequent stooling (more than three times per shift) ○ Excessive vomiting ○ Possible dietary alterations for specific formula or diet ○ Monitoring of electrolytes and renal function ○ Maintenance of IV fluids ○ Use of antidiarrheal medications	These nursing measures constitute routine measures to monitor diarrhea and its related problems. Prompt reporting and intervention decrease the likelihood of more serious complications.

Women's Health

> NOTE: Some women experience diarrhea 1 or 2 days before labor begins. It is not certain why this occurs, but it is thought to be due to the irritation of the bowel by the contracting uterus and the decrease in hormonal level (estrogen and progesterone) in late pregnancy. For diarrhea that is a precursor to labor, the following action applies.

Actions/Interventions	Rationales
• Offer oral electrolyte solutions such as: ○ Gatorade ○ Classic Coca-Cola	Provides nutrition, electrolytes, and minerals which support a successful labor process.

- ○ Jell-O
- ○ 10-K
- ○ Pedialyte

Mental Health

Actions/Interventions	Rationales
• Discuss with client the role stress and anxiety play in this problem. • Develop with client stress reduction plan, and practice specific interventions three times a day at (list times here). • Refer to Chapter 8 for specific nursing actions related to the diagnosis of Anxiety.	Diarrhea can be related to autonomic nervous system response to emotions.[20] Promotes client's adaptive response to stress and promotes client's sense of control.

Gerontic Health

Actions/Interventions	Rationales
• Monitor medication intake to assess for potential side effect of diarrhea. • Collaborate with physician regarding possible alterations in medications to decrease the problem of diarrhea.	The older adult may be having diarrhea as a result of antibiotic therapy, use of drugs with a laxative effect such as magnesium-based antacids, or as a sign of drug toxicity secondary to such antiarrhythmics as digitalis, quinidine, or propranolol.

Home Health

Actions/Interventions	Rationales

• Teach client and family:
  ○ How to monitor perianal skin integrity
  ○ Techniques of perianal hygiene
  ○ Techniques of maintaining fluid and electrolyte balance (see Adult Health)
  ○ How to administer antidiarrheal medications
	Similar to adult health. For home health the locus of control is now the client and family, not the nurse.

Continued

Actions/Interventions	Rationales
• Assist client and family to set criteria to help them to determine when a physician or other intervention is required, for example, child having more than three stools in 1 day.	Provides client and family background knowledge to seek appropriate assistance as need arises.

• Assist client and family in identifying life-style changes that may be required:
  ○ Avoid drinking local water when traveling in areas where water supply may be contaminated (foreign countries, streams and lakes when camping).
  ○ Practice stress management.
  ○ Avoid laxative or enema abuse.
  ○ Avoid foods that cause symptoms.
  ○ Avoid binging behavior.
	Behaviors to prevent recurrence of or continuation of the problem.

• Refer to appropriate assistive resources as indicated. (See Appendix B.)	Additional assistance may be required to maintain health. Use of readily available resources is cost-effective.

FLOW CHART EVALUATION
Flow Chart Expected Outcome 1

Is patient having more than one soft, formed stool per day?

Yes

No

Reassess using initial assessment factors.

Record data, e.g., has had one soft, formed brown stool daily for past 2 days. Record RESOLVED. Delete diagnosis, expected outcome, target date, and nursing actions.

Is diagnosis validated?

Yes

No

Record data, e.g., has had loose stools over past 3 days. Record CONTINUE and change target date. Modify nursing actions as necessary.

Record new assessment data. Record REVISED. Enter new diagnosis, expected outcome, target date, and nursing actions. Delete invalidated diagnosis.

Did evaluation show a new problem had developed?

Yes

No

Start new evaluation process.

Finished

Chart Expected Outcome 2

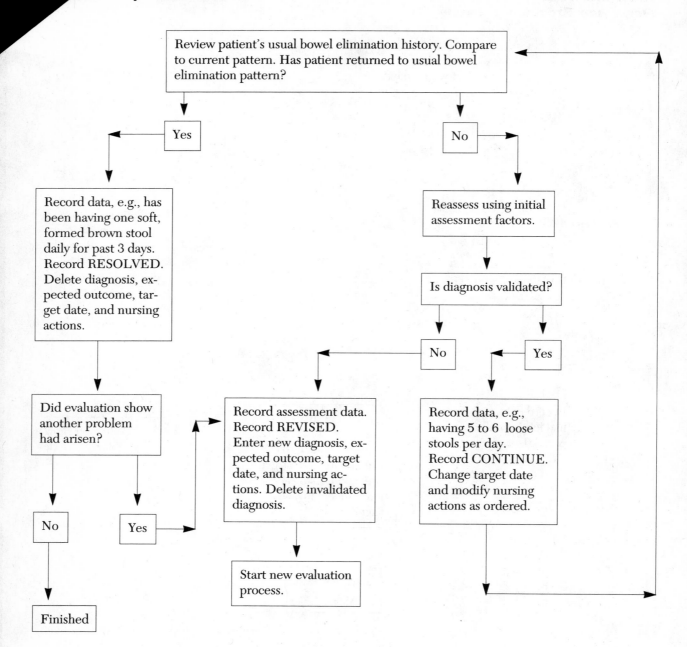

Review patient's usual bowel elimination history. Compare to current pattern. Has patient returned to usual bowel elimination pattern?

Yes

No

Record data, e.g., has been having one soft, formed brown stool daily for past 3 days. Record RESOLVED. Delete diagnosis, expected outcome, target date, and nursing actions.

Reassess using initial assessment factors.

Is diagnosis validated?

No

Yes

Did evaluation show another problem had arisen?

Record assessment data. Record REVISED. Enter new diagnosis, expected outcome, target date, and nursing actions. Delete invalidated diagnosis.

Record data, e.g., having 5 to 6 loose stools per day. Record CONTINUE. Change target date and modify nursing actions as ordered.

No

Yes

Start new evaluation process.

Finished

Urinary Elimination, Altered: Incontinence

DEFINITIONS[16]

Altered Urinary Elimination: The state in which the individual experiences a disturbance in urine elimination.

Functional Incontinence: The state in which an individual experiences an involuntary, unpredictable passage of urine.

Reflex Incontinence: The state in which an individual experiences an involuntary loss of urine, occurring at somewhat predictable intervals when a specific bladder volume is reached.

Stress Incontinence: The state in which an individual experiences a loss of urine of less than 50 ml occurring with increased abdominal pressure.

Total Incontinence: The state in which an individual experiences a continuous and unpredictable loss of urine.

Urge Incontinence: The state in which an individual experiences involuntary passage of urine occurring soon after a strong sense of urgency to void.

NANDA TAXONOMY: EXCHANGING 1.3.2, 1.3.2.1.1, 1.3.2.1.2, 1.3.2.1.3, 1.3.2.1.4, 1.3.2.1.5

DEFINING CHARACTERISTICS[16]

1. Altered Urinary Elimination:
   a. Major defining characteristics:
      (1) Dysuria
      (2) Frequency
      (3) Hesitancy
      (4) Incontinence
      (5) Nocturia
      (6) Retention
      (7) Urgency
   a. Minor defining characteristics:
      None given
2. Functional Incontinence:
   a. Major defining characteristic:
      Urge to void or bladder contractions sufficiently strong to result in loss of urine before reaching an appropriate receptacle.
   b. Minor defining characteristics:
      None given
3. Reflex Incontinence:
   a. Major defining characteristics:
      (1) No awareness of bladder filling
      (2) No urge to void or feelings of bladder fullness
      (3) Uninhibited bladder contraction or spasm at regular intervals
   b. Minor defining characteristics:
      None given
4. Stress Incontinence:
   a. Major defining characteristic:
      Reported or observed dribbling with increased abdominal pressure

b. Minor defining characteristics:
   (1) Urinary urgency
   (2) Urinary frequency (more often than every 2 hours)
5. Total Incontinence:
   a. Major defining characteristics:
      (1) Constant flow of urine occurs at unpredictable times without disten-
          tion or uninhibited bladder contractions or spasms
      (2) Unsuccessful incontinence refractory treatments
      (3) Nocturia
   b. Minor defining characteristics:
      (1) Lack of perineal or bladder-filling awareness
      (2) Unawareness of incontinence
6. Urge Incontinence:
   a. Major defining characteristics:
      (1) Urinary urgency
      (2) Frequency (voiding more often than every 2 hours)
      (3) Bladder contracture or spasm
   b. Minor defining characteristics:
      (1) Nocturia (more than two times per night)
      (2) Voiding in small amounts (less than 100 ml) or in large amounts (more
          than 550 ml)
      (3) Inability to reach toilet in time

RELATED FACTORS[16]

1. Altered Urinary Elimination:
   a. Multiple causality including:
      (1) Anatomical obstruction
      (2) Sensory-motor impairment
      (3) Urinary tract infection
2. Functional Incontinence:
   a. Altered environment
   b. Sensory, cognitive, or mobility deficits
3. Reflex Incontinence:
   Neurological impairment (for example, spinal cord lesion that interferes with
   conduction of cerebral messages above the level of the reflex arc)
4. Stress Incontinence:
   a. Degenerative changes in pelvic muscles and structural supports associated
      with increased age
   b. High intra-abdominal pressure (for example, obesity or gravid uterus)
   c. Incompetent bladder outlet
   d. Overdistension between voidings
   e. Weak pelvic muscles and structural supports
5. Total Incontinence:
   a. Neuropathy preventing transmission of reflex indicating bladder fullness
   b. Neurological dysfunction causing triggering of micturition at unpredict-
      able times
   c. Independent contraction of detrusor reflex due to surgery
   d. Trauma or disease affecting spinal cord nerves
   e. Anatomic (fistula)

6. Urge Incontinence:
   a. Decreased bladder capacity [for example, history of pelvic inflammatory disease (PID), abdominal surgeries, or indwelling urinary catheter]
   b. Irritation of bladder stretch receptors causing spasm (for example, bladder infection)
   c. Alcohol
   d. Caffeine
   e. Increased fluids
   f. Increased urine concentration
   g. Overdistention of bladder

RELATED CLINICAL CONCERNS

1. Spinal cord injury
2. Urinary tract infection
3. Alzheimer's disease
4. Pregnancy
5. Abdominal surgery

HAVE YOU SELECTED THE CORRECT DIAGNOSIS?

Constipation   Anything in the body that creates additional pressure on the bladder or bladder sphincter may precipitate voiding. Constipation can create this additional pressure because of the increased amount of fecal material in the sigmoid colon and rectum. Incontinence may then be a direct result of constipation or fecal impaction. (See page 275.)

Fluid Volume Excess/Fluid Volume Deficit   Since urination depends on input of the stimulus that the bladder is full and since one of the ways the body responds to excess fluid volume is by increasing urinary output, the very fact that there is excess fluid volume may result in the bladder's inability to keep up with the kidney's production of urine. Thus, incontinence may occur. Conversely, Fluid Volume Deficit can result in incontinence by eliminating the sensation of a full bladder and by decreasing the person's awareness of the sensation. (See pages 155 and 166.)

Impaired Physical Mobility   As previously stated, the individual must be able to control the sphincter, walk a few steps, recognize and interpret that the bladder is full, and be able to indicate that he or she wants to go to the bathroom. Even if the person has some control of the sphincter and has correctly recognized and interpreted the cues of a full bladder, if he or she is unable to get to the bathroom or get there in time because of mobility problems, incontinence may result. This may happen especially in a hospital. (See page 460.)

Impaired Verbal Communication   The ability to verbally communicate the need to urinate is important. If the person is unable to tell someone or have someone understand that he or she wants to go to the bathroom, incontinence may occur. (See page 791.)

EXPECTED OUTCOME

1. Will remain continent at least 90 percent of the time by (date) and/or
2. Will design and carry out a personal continence plan by (date)

TARGET DATE

Incontinence will require training time and effort; therefore, a target date 5 days from the date of admission would be reasonable to evaluate the patient's progress toward meeting the expected outcome. Additionally, there must be a realistic potential that urinary continence may be regained by the patient. For this reason, it would need to be qualified for use with handicapped or neurologically deficient clients according to the exact level of continence hoped for.

NURSING ACTIONS/INTERVENTIONS WITH RATIONALES

Adult Health

Actions/Interventions	Rationales

• Record:
  ○ Time and amounts of each voiding
  ○ Whether voiding was continent or incontinent
  ○ Patient's activity before and after incontinent incidence
	Monitors voiding pattern and effectiveness of treatment.

• Monitor, at least every 2 hours on the (odd/even) hour, for continence.
• Monitor:
  ○ Weight at least every 3 days.
  ○ Lab values (for example, electrolytes, white blood cell (WBC), or urinalyses).
  ○ For dependent edema.
  ○ Perineal skin integrity at least once per shift.
	Basic methods to monitor hydration, prevent tissue integrity problems, prevent infection, and promote comfort.

• Record intake and output each shift. • For bladder distention at least every 2 hours on the (odd/even) hour. • Cleanse after each voiding. • Apply medicated ointment as ordered. • Use heat lamp as ordered. • Consult with enterstomal therapist regarding any stoma care. • Give sitz bath.	
• Respond IMMEDIATELY to patient's request for voiding.	Immediate response may prevent an incontinent episode.
• Schedule toileting: ○ Schedule at least 30 minutes before recorded incontinence times.	

- ○ Awaken patient once during night for voiding.

- ○ Encourage patient to consciously hold urine to stretch bladder.
- ○ Teach biofeedback techniques.
- Stimulate voiding at scheduled time by:
  - ○ Assisting patient to maintain normal anatomic position for voiding
  - ○ Having patient lightly brush inner thighs or lower abdomen
  - ○ Running warm water over perineum (measure amount first)
  - ○ Having patient listen to dripping water
  - ○ Placing patient's hands in warm water
  - ○ Using Crede's or Valsalva maneuver
  - ○ Gently tapping over bladder
  - ○ Having patient drink water while trying to void
  - ○ Providing privacy
  - ○ Providing night light and clear path to bathroom
  - ○ Sitting on firm towel roll when incontinence threatens
  - ○ Gradually increasing length of time, by 15 minutes, between voidings
- Schedule fluid intake:
  - ○ Avoid fluids containing caffeine and other fluids that produce a diuretic effect (for example, coffee, grapefruit juice, or alcohol).
  - ○ Encourage 8 ounces of fluid every 2 hours on the (odd/even) hour during the day.
  - ○ Limit fluids after 6 p.m.
- Maintain bowel elimination. Monitor bowel movements and record at least once each shift.
- Beginning on day of admission, teach and have patient return-demonstrate perineal skin care.
- Beginning on day of admission, guard, and teach patient to guard, against nosocomial infection.
- Assist patient with stress reduction and relaxation techniques at least once per shift.
- Collaborate with physician regarding:
  - ○ Intermittent catheterization
  - ○ Medications (for example, urinary antiseptics, analgesics, or anticholinergics)

Voiding at scheduled intervals prevents overdistention and helps to establish a voiding pattern.

Assists in predicting times of voiding. Decreases urge to void at unscheduled times.

Fullness in bowel may exert pressure on bladder, causing bladder incontinence.

Prevents skin irritation, infection, and odor.

Promotes relaxation and self-control of voiding.

Prevents complications related to bladder overdistention.

Actions/Interventions	Rationales
• Collaborate with dietitian regarding food and fluids to acidify urine, for example, cranberry juice or citrus fruits.	Decreases the probability of bladder infections.
• Collaborate with rehabilitation nurse clinician to establish a bladder retraining program.	Allows establishment of a program that is current in content and procedures.
• Teach patient exercises to strengthen pelvic floor muscles (10 times each at least 4 times per day — state times here). ○ Contracting posterior perineal muscles as if trying to stop a bowel movement ○ Contracting anterior perineal muscles as if trying to stop voiding ○ Starting and stopping urine stream ○ Bent-knee situps ○ Bent-leg lifts	Strengthens pelvic floor muscles to better control voiding.
• Teach the patient the importance of maintaining a daily routine: ○ Voiding upon arising ○ Awakening self once during the night ○ Voiding immediately before retiring ○ Not postponing voiding unnecessarily	Helps to establish urinary elimination pattern and prevents overdistention of bladder.
• Encourage patient that he or she can be continent again and encourage to avoid social isolation: ○ Wearing street clothes with protective pads in undergarments ○ Maintaining bladder-retraining program ○ Responding as soon as possible to voiding urge ○ Taking oral chlorophyll tablets ○ Losing weight if necessary	Helps preserve self-concept and body image. Promotes compliance.
• Refer to home health care agency for follow-up.	Provides continuity of care and support system for ongoing care at home.

Child Health

Nursing actions for the child with incontinence are the same as for adult health with appropriate modifications for child's age and weight.

Women's Health

Actions/Interventions	Rationales
• Assist patient in identifying life-style adjustments that may be needed to accommodate changing bladder capacity due to anatomic changes of pregnancy.	Bladder capacity is reduced due to enlarging uterus, displacement of abdominal contents by enlarged uterus, and pressure on bladder by enlarged uterus.
• Teach patient:	
○ To recognize symptoms of urinary tract infection (urgency, burning, or dysuria)	
○ How to take temperature (make sure they know how to read thermometer)	
○ To seek immediate medical care if symptoms of urinary tract infection appear	

Mental Health

NOTE: Clients on hypnotics, antidepressants, and antipsychotics are at risk for this diagnosis. If alteration is related to psychosocial issues and has no physiologic component, initiate the following nursing actions (refer to Adult Health for physiologically produced problems).

Actions/Interventions	Rationales
• Monitor times, places, persons present, and emotional climate around inappropriate voiding episodes.	Identifies target behaviors and establishes a baseline measurement of behavior with possible reinforcers for inappropriate behavior.[21]
• Remind client to void before a high-risk situation or remove secondary gain process from situation.	Removes positive reinforcement for inappropriate behavior.[22]
• Provide the client with supplies necessary to facilitate appropriate voiding behavior (for example, urinal for client in locked seclusion area).	Appropriate behavior cannot be implemented without the appropriate equipment.
• Inform client of acceptable times and places for voiding and of consequences for inappropriate voiding (note consequences here).	Negative reinforcement eliminates or decreases behavior.[22]
• Have client assist with cleaning up any voiding that has occurred in an inappropriate place.	Provides a negative consequence for inappropriate behavior.[22]
• Provide as little interaction with client as possible during cleanup.	Lack of social response acts as negative reinforcement.[21,22]
• Provide client with positive reinforcement for voiding in appropriate place and time (list specific reinforcers for this client here).	Positive reinforcement encourages appropriate behavior.[22]

Continued

Actions/Interventions	Rationales
• Spend (number) minutes with client every hour in an activity the client has identified as enjoyable; do not provide this time or discontinue time if client inappropriately voids during the specified time (list identified activities here).	Interaction with the nurse can provide positive reinforcement. Withdrawing attention for inappropriate behavior provides negative reinforcement.[22]
• If client voids inappropriately (number) times during a shift he or she will spend (number) minutes (no more than 30) in time out. Each inappropriate voiding in time out adds 5 minutes to this time.	Negative consequences decrease or eliminate undesirable behavior.[22]
• As behavior improves add rewards for accumulated times of appropriate voiding (for example, one 2-hour pass for 1 day of appropriate voiding). Record these rewards here.	Intermittent reinforcement can render a response more resistant to extinction once it has been established.[23]
NOTE: Refer to Chapters 8 and 11 for interventions related to the specific alterations that would promote this coping pattern.	

Gerontic Health

Actions/Interventions	Rationales
• Review medication record for drugs such as sedatives, hypnotics, or diuretics that may contribute to urinary incontinence.	Sedatives and hypnotics may result in a delayed response to the urge to void. Diuretic therapy, depending on dosage and time of administration, may result in an inability to reach the bathroom in a timely manner.

Home Health

NOTE: If this nursing diagnosis is made it is imperative that a physician referral be made. Vigorous intervention is required to prevent damage to the urinary tract or systemic infection. If referred to home care under a physician's care, it is important to maintain and evaluate response to prescribed treatments.

Actions/Interventions	Rationales
• Assist client and family in identifying life-style changes that may be required: ○ Using proper perineal hygiene ○ Taking showers instead of tub baths ○ Drinking fluids to cause voiding every 2 to 3 hours to flush out bacteria	Basic measures to prevent recurrence.

- ○ Scheduling fluid intake
- ○ Voiding after intercourse
- ○ Avoiding perfumed soaps, toilet paper, and feminine hygiene sprays
- ○ Wearing cotton underwear
- ○ Using proper handwashing techniques
- ○ Following a daily routine of voiding (see Adult Health actions)
- ○ Establishing a bladder-retraining program
- ○ Doing exercises to strengthen pelvic floor muscles
- ○ Providing an environment conducive to continence
- ○ Wearing street clothes and protective underwear
- ○ Using air purifier
- ○ Participating in activities as tolerated
- ○ Ensuring unobstructed access to bathroom
- ○ Avoiding fluids that produce diuretic effect, for example, caffeine, alcohol, or teas

- • Teach client and family to dilute and acidify the urine:
  - ○ Increasing fluids
  - ○ Introducing cranberry juice, poultry, and so on to increase acid ash

  Bacteria multiply rapidly in alkaline urine.

- • Teach client and family to monitor and maintain skin integrity:
  - ○ Keep skin clean and dry.
  - ○ Keep bed linens and clothing clean and dry.
  - ○ Use proper perineal hygiene.

  Prevents or minimizes problems secondary to incontinence.

- • Assist client and family to set criteria to help them to determine when a physician or other intervention is required, for example, hematuria, fever, or skin breakdown.

  Assists in preventing or minimizing further physiologic damage.

- • Monitor and teach importance of appropriate medications and treatments ordered by physician.

- • Refer to appropriate assistive resources as indicated. (See Appendix B.)

  Additional resources may be needed based upon the underlying problem.

FLOW CHART EVALUATION
Flow Chart Expected Outcome 1

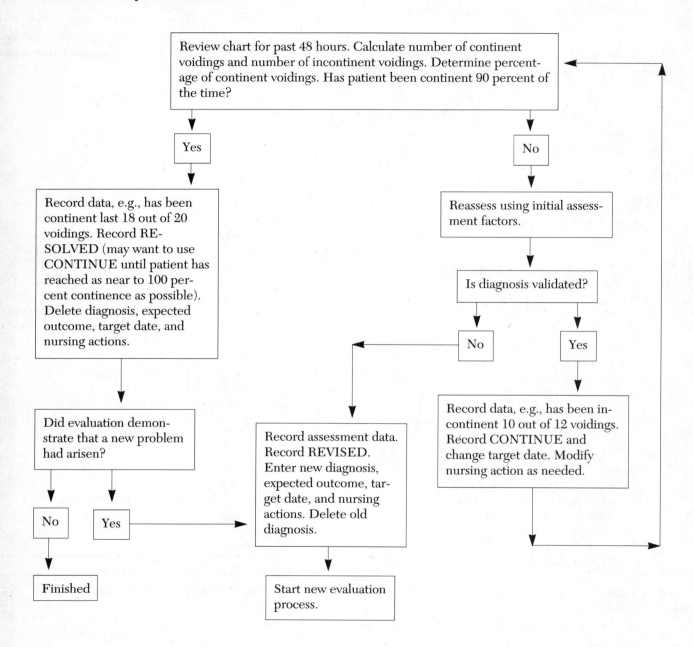

Flow Chart Expected Outcome 2

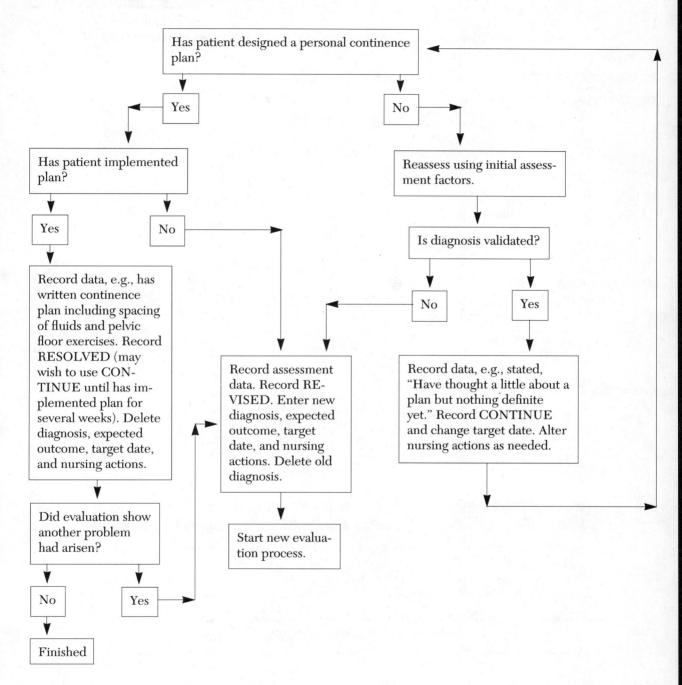

Urinary Retention

DEFINITION

The state in which the individual experiences incomplete emptying of the bladder.

NANDA TAXONOMY: EXCHANGING 1.3.2.2

DEFINING CHARACTERISTICS[16]

1. Major defining characteristics:
   a. Bladder distention
   b. Small, frequent voiding or absence of urine output
2. Minor defining characteristics:
   a. Sensation of bladder fullness
   b. Dribbling
   c. Residual urine
   d. Dysuria
   e. Overflow incontinence

RELATED FACTORS[16]

1. High urethral pressure caused by weak detrusor
2. Inhibition of reflex arc
3. Strong sphincter
4. Blockage

RELATED CLINICAL CONCERNS

1. Benign prostatic hyperplasia
2. Hysterectomy
3. Urinary tract infection
4. Cancer

HAVE YOU SELECTED THE CORRECT DIAGNOSIS?

Incontinence   Overflow incontinence frequently occurs in patients whose primary problem is really retention. The bladder is overdistended in retention, and some urine is passed involuntarily because of the pressure of the retained urine on the bladder sphincter. (See page 293.)

Self-Care Deficit: Toileting   In neurogenic bladder conditions the bladder is chronically overdistended, resulting in urinary retention. (See page 472.)

EXPECTED OUTCOME

1. Will void under voluntary control and empty bladder at least every 4 hours by (date) and/or
2. Will demonstrate no signs or symptoms of urinary retention by (date)

TARGET DATE

Urinary retention poses many dangers to the patient. An acceptable target date to evaluate for lessening of retention would be within 24 to 48 hours after admission.

NURSING ACTIONS/INTERVENTIONS WITH RATIONALES

Adult Health

Actions/Interventions	Rationales
• Monitor bladder for distention at least every 2 hours on the (odd/even) hour.	Monitors pattern and determines effectiveness of treatment; helps prevent complications.
• Measure and record intake and output each shift.	Monitors fluid balance.
• Maintain fluid intake: ○ Encourage fluids to at least 2000 ml per day. ○ Limit fluids after 6 p.m.	Assures sufficient fluid intake, but restricts fluid when activity decreases. Assists in preventing nocturia.
• Monitor: ○ Bowel elimination at least once per shift ○ Urinalyses, electrolytes, and weight at least every 3 days	Constipation may block bladder opening and lead to retention. Empty bowel will facilitate free passage of urine.
• Increase patient activity: ○ Ambulate at least twice per shift while awake at (times). ○ Collaborate with physical therapist, soon after admission, regarding an exercise program.	Strengthens muscles; promotes kidney and bladder functioning.
• Collaborate with rehabilitation nurse clinician to initiate bladder-training program.	Allows establishment of a program that is current in content and procedures.
• Stimulate micturition reflex every 4 hours while awake at (times): ○ Assist patient to assume anatomically correct position for voiding. ○ Remind patient to be conscious of need-to-void sensations.	Helps relax sphincter and strengthens voiding reflex.
• Teach patient to assist bladder contraction: ○ Crede's maneuver ○ Valsalva maneuver ○ Abdominal muscle contraction	
• Beginning on day of admission, teach patient the following exercises: ○ Bent-knee situps ○ Bent-leg lifts ○ Contracting posterior perineal muscles as if trying to stop a bowel movement ○ Contracting anterior perineal muscles as if trying to stop voiding ○ Starting and stopping urine stream	Strengthens pelvic floor muscles.

Continued

Actions/Interventions	Rationales

• Collaborate with physician regarding:
  ○ Intermittent catheterization
  ○ Medications (for example, urinary antiseptics or analgesics)
	Relieves bladder distention, assists to schedule voiding, and prevents infection.

• Refer to home health agency, at least 2 days prior to discharge, for continued monitoring.	Provides continuity of care and a support system for ongoing home care.

Child Health

> NOTE: For infants and children less than 20 pounds, it would be necessary to calculate exact intake and output and fluid requisites according to the etiologic factors present. Attention must be paid to the child's physiological developmental level regarding urinary control.

Actions/Interventions	Rationales
• Provide opportunities for child and parents to verbalize concerns or views related to body image disturbances related to urinary control and retention. Spend at least 30 minutes per shift in privacy with child and parents to permit this verbalization.	Assists in reducing anxiety and attaches value to the patient's and parent's feelings. Promotes the development of a therapeutic relationship.

• Monitor parental (patient as applicable) knowledge of preventive health care for patient:
  ○ Teaching and observation of urinary catheterization
  ○ Maintenance of catheters and supplies
  ○ How to obtain supplies
  ○ How to obtain a sterile culture specimen
  ○ Appropriate restraint of infant
  ○ Potential regarding urinary control
	Parental knowledge will assist in the reduction of anxiety and will provide a greater likelihood for compliance with desired plan of care.

• Provide opportunities for parental participation in the care of the infant or child:
  ○ Feeding
  ○ Bathing
  ○ Monitoring intake and output
  ○ Planning for care to include individual preferences when possible
  ○ Assisting with procedures when appropriate
  ○ Providing for safety needs
  ○ Cautious handwashing to prevent infection
  ○ Appropriate emotional support
	Appropriate parental involvement provides opportunities for trial care and allows parents to practice care in a safe, supportive environment prior to time of total self-care.

- ○ Appropriate diversional activity and relaxation
- ○ Need for pain medication
- Collaborate with other health care professionals as needed. (See Appendix B.)
- Assist family to identify support groups represented in the community for future needs.

Identification of support for the family will best assist them to comply with the desired plan of care while reducing anxiety and promoting self-care.

Women's Health

Actions/Interventions	Rationales
• Collaborate with physician regarding intermittent catheterization.	It is not easy to catheterize a woman postpartum, nor is it desirable to introduce an added risk of infection, so every effort and support should be directed toward helping the woman to void on her own. If, however, she is unable to void or to empty her bladder, an indwelling catheter may be placed for 24 to 48 hours to rest the bladder and allow it to heal, edema to subside, and bladder and urethral tone to return.[24]

Mental Health

NOTE: Clients receiving antipsychotic and antidepressant drugs are at increased risk for this diagnosis. Refer to Adult Health for general actions related to this diagnosis.

Actions/Interventions	Rationales
• Place clients receiving antipsychotic or antidepressant medication on daily assessment for this diagnosis. Elderly clients should be evaluated more frequently if their physical status indicates.	Early intervention and treatment assure better outcome.
• Monitor bladder for distention at least every 4 hours at (times) if verbal reports are unreliable or if they indicate a voiding frequency greater than every 4 hours.	
• Increase client's activity by: ○ Walking with client (number) minutes three times a day at (list times here). ○ Collaborating with physical therapist regarding an exercise program.	Activity maintains muscle strength necessary for maintenance of normal voiding patterns. (See Adult Health for specific exercises to strengthen pelvic floor muscles).

Continued

Actions/Interventions	Rationales
○ Placing client in a room distant from the day area, nursing stations, and other activity if condition does not contraindicate this. ○ Providing physical activities that client indicates are of interest (list those here with the time for each). • Teach deep muscle relaxation, and spend 30 minutes twice a day at (list times here) practicing this with client. Associate relaxation with breathing so that client can eventually relax with deep breathing while attempting to void.	Anxiety can increase muscle tension and therefore contribute to urinary retention.[29]

Gerontic Health

Actions/Interventions	Rationales
• Review medication record for use of antidepressant and antipsychotic medications.	The use of antidepressant and antipsychotic medications can result in urinary retention as a side effect.

Home Health

NOTE: If this nursing diagnosis is made, it is imperative that a physician referral be made. If referred to home care under a physician's care, it is important to maintain and evaluate response to prescribed treatments.

Actions/Interventions	Rationales
• Assist client and family in life-style changes that may be required: ○ Monitor bladder for distention. ○ Record intake and output. ○ Stimulate micturition reflex (see Adult Health). ○ Institute bladder-training program. ○ Perform exercises to strengthen pelvic floor muscles. ○ Use proper position for voiding. ○ Maintain fluid intake. ○ Maintain physical activity as tolerated. ○ Use straight catheterization.	Similar to adult health. Locus of control now is with family and client.

- Assist client and family to set criteria to help them to determine when a physician or other intervention is required, for example, specified intake and output limit, pain, or bladder distention.

  Knowledge will assist client and family to seek timely interventions.

- Monitor and teach importance of appropriate medications and treatments ordered by physician.

  Provides client and family with knowledge to care for problem.

- Refer to appropriate assistive resources as indicated. (See Appendix B.)

  Additional support may be required to help the client and family maintain care at home.

FLOW CHART EVALUATION
Flow Chart Expected Outcome 1

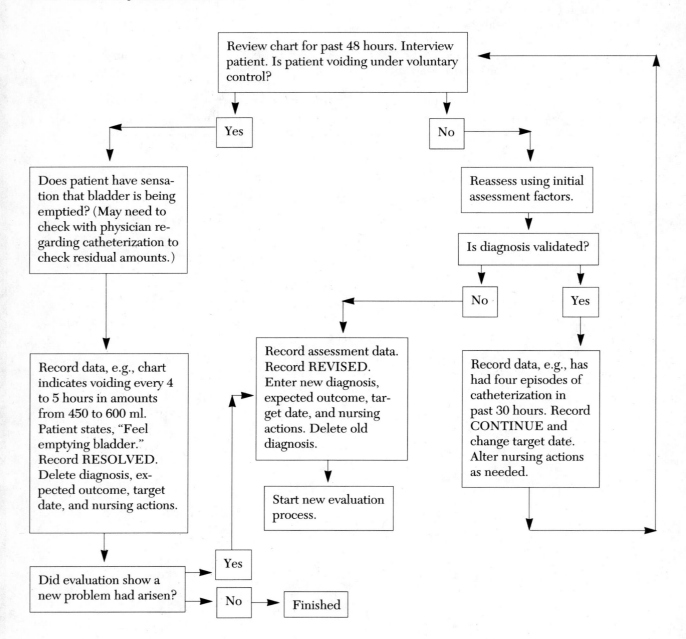

Review chart for past 48 hours. Interview patient. Is patient voiding under voluntary control?

Yes

No

Does patient have sensation that bladder is being emptied? (May need to check with physician regarding catheterization to check residual amounts.)

Reassess using initial assessment factors.

Is diagnosis validated?

No

Yes

Record data, e.g., chart indicates voiding every 4 to 5 hours in amounts from 450 to 600 ml. Patient states, "Feel emptying bladder." Record RESOLVED. Delete diagnosis, expected outcome, target date, and nursing actions.

Record assessment data. Record REVISED. Enter new diagnosis, expected outcome, target date, and nursing actions. Delete old diagnosis.

Record data, e.g., has had four episodes of catheterization in past 30 hours. Record CONTINUE and change target date. Alter nursing actions as needed.

Start new evaluation process.

Did evaluation show a new problem had arisen?

Yes

No

Finished

Flow Chart Expected Outcome 2

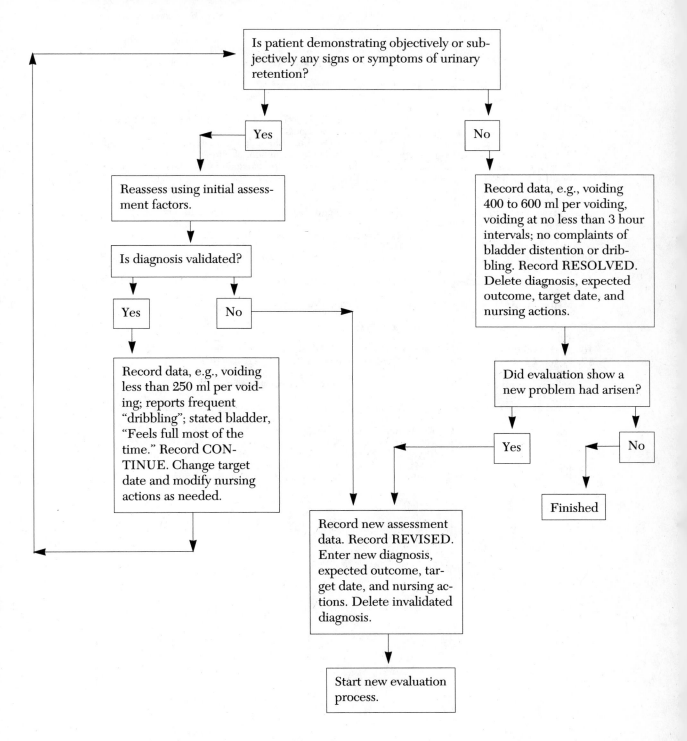

References

1. Bruya, MA: Elimination status. In Mitchell, PH and Loustau, A (eds): Concepts Basic to Nursing, ed 3. McGraw-Hill, New York, 1981.
2. Long, B and Durham, N: Assessment of urinary function. In Phipps, WJ, et al (eds): Medical-Surgical Nursing: Concepts and Clinical Practice, ed 4. CV Mosby, St. Louis, 1991.
3. Flynn, JM and Heffron, PB: Nursing: From Concept to Practice, ed 2. Appleton-Lange, Norwalk, CT, 1988.
4. Kelly, MA: Nursing Diagnosis Source Book. Appleton-Century-Crofts, East Norwalk, CT, 1985.
5. Gettrust, KV and Brabec, PD: Nursing Diagnosis in Clinical Practice: Guides for Care Planning. Delmar Publishers, New York, 1992.
6. Miller, P: Assessment of urinary function. In Phipps, WJ, et al (eds): Medical-Surgical Nursing: Concepts and Clinical Practice, ed 4. CV Mosby, St. Louis, 1991.
7. Sherman, S: Urinary Incontinence in Community Dwelling Elders in Urban and Rural Areas. Unpublished thesis. Texas Tech University Health Sciences Center School of Nursing, Lubbock, TX, 1990.
8. Burgio, K, Mathews, K, and Engel, B: Prevalence, incidence and correlates of urinary incontinence in healthy, middle-aged women. J Urol 196:1255, 1991.
9. Clay, E: Urinary continence/incontinence. Habit retraining: A tested method to regain urinary control. Geriatr Nur 1:252, 1980.
10. Murray, RB and Zentner, JP: Nursing Assessment and Health Promotion through the Life Span, ed 4. Appleton-Lange, Norwalk, CT, 1989.
11. Schuster, CS and Ashburn, SS: The Process of Human Development: A Holistic Life-Span Approach, ed 3. JB Lippincott, Philadelphia, 1992.
12. Carnevali, DL and Patrick, M: Nursing Management for the Elderly, ed 2. JB Lippincott, Philadelphia, 1986.
13. Burggraf, V and Stanley, M: Nursing the Elderly: A Care Plan Approach. JB Lippincott, St. Louis, 1989.
14. Matteson, MA and McConnell, ES: Gerontological Nursing: Concepts and Practices. WB Saunders, Philadelphia, 1988.
15. Mobily, PR and Kelley, LS: Iatrogenesis in the elderly: Factors of immobility. J Gerontol Nurs 17:9, 1991.
16. North American Nursing Diagnosis Association: Taxonomy I, Revised 1990. Author, St. Louis, 1990.
17. Fogel, CI and Wood, NF: Health Care of Women: A Nursing Perspective. CV Mosby, St. Louis, 1981.
18. Schmelzer, M: Effectiveness of wheat bran in preventing constipation of hospitalized orthopaedic surgery patients. Orthop Nurs 9:55, 1990.
19. Heather, C, et al: Effect of bulk forming cathartic on diarrhea in tube fed patients. Heart Lung 20:409, 1991.
20. Luckmann, J and Sorensen, K: Medical-Surgical Nursing. WB Saunders, Philadelphia, 1992.
21. Haber, J, et al: Comprehensive Psychiatric Nursing, ed 4. CV Mosby, St. Louis, 1992
22. Wilson, HS and Kneisl, CR: Psychiatric Nursing, ed 4. Addison-Wesley, Redwood, CA, 1992.
23. Jacobson, N and Margolin, B: Marital Therapy. Brunner/Mazel, New York, 1989.
24. Hawkins, JW and Grovine, B: Postpartum Nursing: Health Care of Women. Springer, New York, 1985.

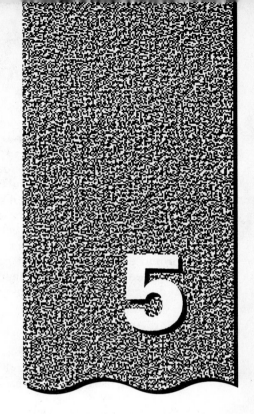

Activity-Exercise Pattern

PATTERN INTRODUCTION
Pattern Description

This pattern focuses on the *activities of daily living (ADL)* and the amount of energy the individual has available to support these activities. The ADL include all aspects of maintaining self-care and incorporate leisure time as well. Because a person's energy level and mobility for ADL are affected by the proper functioning of the neuromuscular, cardiovascular, and respiratory systems, nursing diagnoses related to dysfunctions in these systems are included.

As with the other patterns, a problem in the activity-exercise pattern may be the primary reason for the patient's entering the health care system or may arise secondary to problems in another functional pattern. Any admission to a hospital may promote the development of problems in this area because of the therapeutics required for the medical diagnosis (for example, bed rest) or because of agency rules and regulations (for example, limited visiting hours).

Pattern Assessment

1. Does the patient's heart rate or blood pressure (BP) increase abnormally in response to activity?
   a. Yes (Activity Intolerance)
   b. No
2. Does patient have dyspnea after activity?
   a. Yes (Activity Intolerance)
   b. No
3. Does patient have a medical diagnosis related to the cardiovascular or respiratory system?
   a. Yes (High Risk for Activity Intolerance)
   b. No
4. Does patient have a history of Activity Intolerance?
   a. Yes (High Risk for Activity Intolerance)
   b. No
5. Does patient complain of fatigue or weakness or lack of energy?
   a. Yes (Activity Intolerance or Fatigue)
   b. No
6. Is patient unable to maintain usual routines?
   a. Yes (Fatigue or Self-Care Deficit)
   b. No
7. Does patient report difficulty in concentrating?
   a. Yes (Fatigue)
   b. No
8. Review self-care chart. Does patient have any self-care deficits?
   a. Yes [Self-Care Deficit (specify which area)]
   b. No
9. Can patient engage in usual hobby while in hospital?
   a. Yes
   b. No (Diversional Activity Deficit)
10. Does family need help with home maintenance after patient goes home?
    a. Yes (Impaired Home Maintenance Management)
    b. No

11. Does patient have insurance?
    a. Yes
    b. No (Impaired Home Maintenance Management)
12. Is patient within height and weight norm for age?
    a. Yes
    b. No (Altered Growth and Development)
13. Can patient perform developmental skills appropriate for age level?
    a. Yes (Altered Growth and Development)
    b. No
14. Does patient's cardiogram indicate arrhythmias?
    a. Yes (Decreased Cardiac Output)
    b. No
15. Is patient's jugular vein distended?
    a. Yes (Decreased Cardiac Output)
    b. No
16. Are patient's peripheral pulses within normal limits?
    a. Yes
    b. No (Decreased Cardiac Output or Altered Tissue Perfusion or High Risk
       for Peripheral Neurovascular Dysfunction)
17. Are patient's extremities cold?
    a. Yes (Altered Tissue Perfusion or High Risk for Peripheral Neurovascular
       Dysfunction)
    b. No
18. Does patient have claudication?
    a. Yes (Altered Tissue Perfusion or High Risk for Peripheral Neurovascular
       Dysfunction)
    b. No
19. Does patient have full range of motion?
    a. Yes
    b. No (Impaired Physical Mobility)
20. Does patient have problems moving self in bed or in ambulating?
    a. Yes (Impaired Physical Mobility)
    b. No
21. Is patient paralyzed?
    a. Yes (High Risk for Disuse Syndrome)
    b. No
22. Is patient immobilized by casts or traction?
    a. Yes (High Risk for Disuse Syndrome or High Risk for Peripheral Neuro-
       vascular Dysfunction)
    b. No
23. Does patient have a spinal cord injury at T7 or above and paroxysmal
    hypertension?
    a. Yes (Dysreflexia)
    b. No
24. Does patient have a spinal cord injury at T7 or above and bradycardia or
    tachycardia?
    a. Yes (Dysreflexia)
    b. No
25. Review mental status examination. Is patient exhibiting confusion or
    drowsiness?

    a. Yes (Impaired Gas Exchange)
    b. No
26. Review blood gases. Does patient demonstrate hypercapnia?
    a. Yes (Impaired Gas Exchange or Inability to Sustain Spontaneous Ventilation)
    b. No
27. Were rales (crackles) or rhonchi (wheezes) present on chest auscultation?
    a. Yes (Ineffective Airway Clearance)
    b. No
28. Is respiratory rate increased above normal range?
    a. Yes (Ineffective Airway Clearance or Ineffective Breathing Pattern)
    b. No
29. Is patient on a ventilator? If yes, does the patient have restlessness or an increase from baseline of BP, pulse (P), or respiration (R) when attempts at weaning are tried?
    a. Yes (Dysfunctional Ventilatory Weaning Response)
    b. No
30. Does patient have dyspnea and shortness of breath?
    a. Yes (Ineffective Breathing Pattern or Inability to Sustain Spontaneous Ventilation or Activity Intolerance)
    b. No
31. Is patient exhibiting pursed-lip breathing?
    a. Yes (Ineffective Breathing Pattern)
    b. No

Diagnoses in This Pattern

1. Activity Intolerance, High Risk for or Actual (page 327)
2. Airway Clearance, Ineffective (page 338)
3. Breathing Pattern, Ineffective (page 349)
4. Cardiac Output, Decreased (page 360)
5. Disuse Syndrome, High Risk for (page 374)
6. Diversional Activity Deficit (DVWR) (page 383)
7. Dysfunctional Ventilatory Weaning Response (page 391)
8. Dysreflexia (page 399)
9. Fatigue (page 407)
10. Gas Exchange, Impaired (page 416)
11. Growth and Development, Altered (page 427)
12. Home Maintenance Management, Impaired (page 438)
13. Inability to Sustain Spontaneous Ventilation (page 447)
14. Peripheral Neurovascular Dysfunction: High Risk for (page 454)
15. Physical Mobility, Impaired (page 460)
16. Self-Care Deficit (Feeding, Bathing-Hygiene, Dressing-Grooming, Toileting) (page 472)
17. Tissue Perfusion, Altered (Specify type: Renal, Cerebral, Cardiopulmonary, Gastrointestinal, Peripheral) (page 484)

Conceptual Information

There are several nursing diagnoses included in this pattern that, at first glance, seem to have little relationship with each other. However, closer investigation demonstrates that there is one concept common to all of the diagnoses—immobility.

Immobility or the impulses that control and coordinate mobility can contribute to the development of any of these diagnoses, or any of these diagnoses can ultimately lead to the development of immobility.

Mobility and immobility are end points on a continuum with many degrees of impaired mobility or partial mobility between the two points.[1] Immobility is usually distinguished from impaired mobility by the permanence of the limitation. A person who is quadriplegic has immobility because it is permanent; a person with a long cast on the left leg has impaired mobility because it is temporary.[2]

Mobility is defined as the ability to move freely and is one of the major means by which we define and express ourselves. The central nervous system integrates the stimuli from sensory receptor nerves of the peripheral nervous system and projection tracts of the central nervous system to respond to the internal or external environment of the individual. This integration allows for movement and expressions. A problem with mobility can be a measure of the degree of illness or health problem an individual has.[3]

Patients with self-care deficits are most often those who are experiencing some type of mobility problem.[2] The problem with mobility requires greater energy expenditure, which leads to Activity Intolerance, Diversional Activity Deficit, and Impaired Home Maintenance simply due to the lack of energy or nervous system response to engage in these activities.

Problems with mobility and nervous system response also lead to other physical problems. When a person has impaired mobility or immobility, bed rest is quite often prescribed or is voluntarily sought in an effort to conserve energy. Several authors[3,4,5] describe the physical problems that can occur secondary to prolonged bed rest:

1. *Respiratory*: Decreased chest and lung expansion causes slower and more shallow respiration. Pooling of secretions occurs secondary to decreased respiratory effort and the effects of gravity. The cough reflex is decreased due to decreased respiratory effort, gravity, and decreased muscle strength. Acid-base balance is shifted, causing a retention of carbon dioxide. Respiratory acidosis causes changes in mentation: vasodilation of cerebrovascular blood vessels and increased cerebral blood flow, headache, mental cloudiness, disorientation, dizziness, generalized weakness, convulsions, and unconsciousness. Additionally, because of the buildup of carbon dioxide in the lungs, adequate oxygen cannot be inspired, leading to tissue hypoxia.

2. *Cardiovascular*: Circulatory stasis is caused by vasodilation and impaired venous return. Muscular inactivity leads to vein dilation in dependent parts. Gravity effects also occur. Decreased respiratory effort and gravity lead to decreased changes in thoracic and abdominal pressures, which usually assist in promoting blood return to the heart. Quite often patients have increased use of the Valsalva maneuver, which leads to increases in preload and afterload of cardiac output and ultimately to a decreased cardiac output. Continued limitation of activity leads to decreased cardiac rate, circulatory volume, and arterial pressure due to redistribution of body fluids. Venous stasis contributes to the potential for deep venous thrombosis and pulmonary embolus. After prolonged bed rest, the normal neurovascular mechanism of the cardiovascular system that prevents large shifts in blood volume does not adequately function. When the individual who has experienced extended bed-rest attempts to assume an upright position, gravity pulls an excessive amount of blood volume to the feet and legs, depriving the brain of

adequate oxygen. As a result, the individual experiences orthostatic hypotension.[4]

3. *Musculoskeletal*: Inactivity causes decreased bone stress and decreased muscle tension. Osteoblastic and osteoclastic activities become imbalanced, leading to calcium and phosphorus loss. Decreased muscle use leads to decreased muscle mass and strength due to infrequent muscle contractions and protein loss.

4. *Metabolic: Basal metabolic rate (BMR)* and oxygen consumption decrease, leading to decreased efficiency in using nutrients to build new tissues. Normally, body tissues break down nitrogen, but apparently muscle mass loss with accompanying protein loss leads to nitrogen loss and a negative nitrogen balance. Changes in tissue metabolism lead to increased potassium and calcium excretion. Decreased energy use and decreased BMR lead to appetite loss, which leads to decreased nutrient intake necessary to offset losses.

5. *Skin*: The negative nitrogen balance previously discussed, coupled with continuous pressure on bony prominences, leads to a greatly increased potential for skin breakdown.

Immobility is not the sole causative factor of the nursing diagnoses in this pattern. Many of the diagnoses can be related to specific medical diagnoses such as congestive heart failure or may occur as a result of diagnoses in this pattern, for example, Altered Growth and Development. However, the concept of immobility does serve to point out the interrelatedness of the diagnoses.

Since fatigue plays a major role in determining the quality and amount of musculoskeletal activity undertaken, consideration of the factors that influence fatigue is an essential part of nursing assessment for the activity-exercise pattern. Fatigue might be considered in two general categories — experiential and muscular. The degree to which the individual participates in activity is significant in determining the fatigue experienced. Activities that the person enjoys are less likely to produce fatigue than are those he or she does not enjoy. Preferences should be considered within the framework of capacity and needs. Obviously other factors that must be considered include the physical and medical condition of the person and his or her emotional state, level of growth and development, and state of health in general. Oxygenation needs and extrinsic factors would also need to be addressed. If there is overstimulation, as with noise, extremes of temperature, or interruption of routines, a greater amount of fatigue can be expected. Sensory understimulation with resultant boredom can also contribute to fatigue.

Fatigue can develop as a result of too much waste material accumulating and too little nourishment going to the muscles. Muscle fatigue usually is attributed to the accumulation of too much lactic acid in the muscles. Certain metabolic conditions, such as congestive heart failure, place a person at greater risk for fatigue.

Developmental Considerations

Activity is influenced by diet, musculoskeletal factors, and respiratory and cardiovascular mechanisms. Developmental considerations for diet are addressed in Chapter 3. The developmental considerations discussed below specifically relate to musculoskeletal, respiratory, and cardiovascular factors.

INFANT

Physical and motor abilities are influenced by many things, including genetic, biologic, and cultural factors. Nutrition, maturation of the central nervous system, skeletal formation, overall physical health status, amount of stimulation, environmental conditions, and consistent loving care also play a part in physical and motor abilities.[6] Girls usually develop more rapidly than boys, although the activity level is higher in boys.[6]

All muscular tissue is formed at birth, but growth occurs as the infant uses the various muscle groups. This use stimulates increased strength and function.

The infant engages in various types of play activity at various times in infancy because of developing skills and changing needs. The infant needs the stimulation of parents in this play activity to fully develop. However, parents should be aware of the dangers in overstimulation. Fatigue, inattention, and injury to the infant may result.[6]

Interruptions in the normal developmental sequence of play activities due to illness or hospitalization, for example, can have a detrimental effect on the future development of the infant or child. An understanding of the normal sequence of play development is important to have so that therapeutic interventions can be designed to approximate the developmental needs of the individual.

The structural description of play development focuses on the Piagetian concepts of the increasing cognitive complexity of play activities. Elementary sensorimotor-based games emerge first, with the gradual development of advanced social games in adulthood.[7]

Play activities assist in the child's development of psychomotor skills and cognitive development. Socialization skills are learned and practiced via the interaction with others during play. As the child begins to learn more about his or her body during play, he or she will incorporate more complicated gross and fine motor skills. Play is extremely valuable in the development of language and other communication skills. Play helps the child to establish control over self and the environment and provides a sense of accomplishment. Through play activities, the infant learns to trust the environment. Play also affords the child the opportunity to express emotions that would be unacceptable in other normal social situations.

Practice games begin during the sensorimotor level of cognitive development at 1 to 4 months of age and continue with increasing complexity throughout childhood. These games include skills that are performed for the pleasure of functioning, that is, for the pleasure of practice.

Symbolic games appear later during the sensorimotor period than do practice games—about age 12 to 18 months. Make-believe is now added to the practice game. Elements of absent objects or persons are represented by other objects. As previously stated, activity is influenced by respiratory and cardiovascular mechanisms.

The respiratory mechanisms or air-conducting passages (the nose, pharynx, larynx, trachea, bronchi, bronchioles, and alveoli) and lungs of the infant are small, delicate, and immature. The air that enters the nose is cool, dry, and unfiltered. The nose is unable to filter the air, and the mucous membranes of the upper respiratory tract are unable to produce enough mucus to humidify or warm the inhaled air. Therefore, the infant is more susceptible to respiratory tract infections.[7]

Additionally, the infant is a nose breather. When upper respiratory tract infections do occur, the infant is unable to appropriately clear the airways and may get into some difficulty until he or she learns to breathe through his or her mouth (at about 3 to 4 months of age). The cough of the infant is not very effective, and the infant quickly becomes fatigued with the effort.[7]

In the lungs, the alveoli are functioning, but not all alveoli may be expanded. Therefore, there is a large amount of dead space in the lungs. The infant has to work harder to exchange enough oxygen and carbon dioxide to meet body demands. The elevated respiratory rate of the infant (30 to 60 per minute) reflects this increased work. Additionally, arterial blood gases of the infant may show an acid-base imbalance. The rate and rhythm of respiration in the infant is somewhat irregular, and it is not unusual for the infant to use accessory muscles of respiration. Retractions with respiration are common.

The alveoli of the infant increase in number and complexity very rapidly. By 1 year of age, the alveoli and the lining of the air passages have matured considerably.

Respiratory tract obstructions are common in this age group because of the short trachea and the almost straight-line position of the right main stem bronchus. Additionally, the epiglottis does not effectively close over the trachea during swallowing. Thus, foreign objects are aspirated into the lungs.

In terms of cardiovascular development, the foramen ovale closes during the first 24 hours and the ductus arteriosus closes after several days. The neonate can survive mild oxygen deprivation longer than an adult. The Apgar scoring system is used to measure the physical status of the newborn and includes heart rate, color, and respiration. There is no day-night rhythm to the neonate's heart rate, but from the sixth week on, the rate will be lower at night than during the day. Axillary temperature and age-sized blood pressure cuffs should be used to assess vital signs. The pulse is 120 to 150 beats per minute; respiration ranges from 35 to 50 per minute; and BP ranges from 40 to 90 mm Hg systolic and 6 to 20 mm Hg diastolic. Vital signs become more stable over the first year. Listening for murmurs should be done over the base of the heart rather than at the apex. Breath sounds are bronchovesicular. The neonate has limited ability to respond to environmental temperature changes and will lose heat rapidly. This leads to an increased BMR and an increased work load on the heart. Until age 7, the apex is palpated at the fourth interspace just to the left of the midclavicular line.

TODDLER AND PRESCHOOLER

By this age, the child is walking, running, climbing, and jumping. The toddler is very active and very curious. He or she gets into everything. This helps the toddler organize his or her world and develop spatial and sensory perception.[6] It is during this period that the child begins to see himself or herself as a person separate from his or her parents and the environment. This increasing level of autonomy also presents a challenge for the caregivers. The child alternates between the security of the parents and the exciting exploration of the environment.

The toddler is fairly clumsy, but gross and fine motor coordination is improving. Neuromuscular maturation and repetition of movements help the child further develop skills.[6] Muscles grow faster than bones during these years. Safety is a major concern for children of this age. The toddler, especially, wants to do many things for himself or herself, thus testing control of self and the environment.

Bathing and Hygiene

By the age of 3, the child can wash and dry hands with some wetting of clothes; can brush teeth, but requires assistance to do so adequately. By the fourth birthday the child may bathe himself or herself with assistance. The child will be able to bathe himself or herself without assistance by the age of 5. Both parents and nurses must keep in mind the safety issues involved in bathing; the child requires supervision in selection of water temperature and in the prevention of drowning.

Dressing and Grooming

At age 18 to 20 months the child has the fine motor skills required to unzip a large zipper. By 24 to 48 months the child can unbutton large buttons. The child can put on a coat with assistance by age 2; the child can undress himself or herself in most situations and can put on his or her own coat without assistance by age 3. At $3\frac{1}{2}$ years the child can unbutton small buttons and by 4 years can button small buttons. Dressing without assistance and beginning ability to lace shoes are accomplishments of the 5-year-old. The development of fine motor skills is required for most of the tasks of dressing. It is important that the child's clothing have fasteners that are appropriate for the motor skill development. The child will require assistance with deciding the appropriateness of clothing selected; seasonal variations in weather and culturally accepted norms regarding dressing and grooming are learned by the child with assistance.

Feeding

The child can drink from a cup without much spilling by 18 months. The child will have frequent spills while trying to get the contents of a spoon into his or her mouth at this age. By 2 years of age the child can drink from a cup; use of the spoon has improved at this age, but the child will still spill liquids (soup) from a spoon when eating. The child can eat from a spoon without spilling by $3\frac{1}{2}$ years. Accomplished use of the fork occurs at 5 years.

Toileting

By age 3 the child can go to the toilet without assistance; the child can pull pants up and down for toileting without assistance at this stage as well. The development of food preferences, preferred eating schedules and environment, and toileting behavior are imparted to the child by learning. Toileting, food, and the eating experience may also include pleasures, control issues, and learning tasks in addition to the development of the motor skills required to accomplish the tasks. Delays or regressions in the tasks of self-feeding may reflect issues other than a self-care deficit, for example, discipline, family coping, or role relationships.

During the preschool years, the child seems to have an unlimited supply of energy. However, he or she does not know when to stop and may continue activities past the point of exhaustion. Parents should provide a variety of activities for the age groups, as the attention span is short.

The lung size and volume of the toddler have now increased, and thus the oxygen capacity of the toddler has increased. The toddler is still susceptible to respiratory tract infections but not to the extent of the infant. The rate and rhythm of respiration has decreased, and respirations average 25 to 35 per minute. Accessory muscles of respiration are infrequently used now, and respirations are primarily diaphragmatic.

The respiratory structures (trachea and bronchi) are positioned farther down in the chest now, and the epiglottis is effective in closing off the trachea during swallowing. Thus, aspiration and airway obstruction are reduced in this age group.

The respiratory rate of the preschooler is about 30 per minute. The preschooler is still susceptible to upper respiratory tract infections. The lymphatic tissues of the tonsils and adenoids are involved in these respiratory tract infections. Tonsillectomies and adenoidectomies are not performed routinely any more. These tissues serve to protect the respiratory tract, and valid reasons must be presented to warrant their removal.

The temperature of the toddler ranges around 99° F, ± 1° (orally); pulse ranges around 105 beats per minute ± 35; respirations range from 20 to 35 per minute; and blood pressure ranges from 80 to 100 mm Hg systolic and 60 to 64 mm Hg diastolic. The size of the vascular bed increases in the toddler, thus reducing resistance to flow. The capillary bed has increased ability to respond to environmental temperature changes. Lung volume increases. Breath sounds are more intense and more bronchial, and expiration is more pronounced. The toddler's chest should be examined with the child in an erect position, then recumbent, and then turned to the left side. Arrhythmias and extrasystoles are not uncommon but should be recorded.

The temperature of the preschooler is 98.6° F, ± 1° (orally); pulse ranges from 80 to 100 beats per minute; respiration is 30 per minute, ± 5; and BP is 90/60 mm Hg, ± 15. There is continued increase of the vascular bed, lung volume, and so on, in keeping with physical growth.

SCHOOL-AGE CHILD

Whereas the muscles were growing faster than the bones during the toddler and preschool years, the skeletal system is growing rapidly during these years—faster than the muscles are growing. Children may experience "growing pains" because of the growth of the long bones. There is a gradual increase in muscle mass and strength, and the body takes on a leaner appearance. The child loses his or her baby fat, muscle tone increases, and loose movements disappear. Adequate exercise is needed to maintain strength, flexibility, and balance and to encourage muscular development.[7] Males have a greater number of muscle cells than females. Posture becomes more upright and straighter but is not necessarily influenced by exercise. Posture is a function of the strength of the back muscles and the general state of health of the child. Poor posture may be reflective of fatigue as well as skeletal defects,[7] with fatigue being exhibited by such behaviors as quarrelsomeness, crying, or lack of interest in eating. Skeletal defects such as scoliosis begin to appear during this period.

Neuromuscular coordination is sufficient to permit the school-age child to learn most skills[6]; however, care should be taken to prevent muscle injuries. Hands and fingers manipulate things well. Although children at age 7 have a high energy level, they also have an increased attention span and cognitive skills. Therefore, they tend to engage in quiet games as well as active ones. Seven-year-olds tend to be more directed in their range of activities. Games with rules develop as the child engages in more social contacts. These games characteristically emerge during the operational phase of cognitive development in the school-age child. These rule games may also be practice or symbolic in nature, but now the child attaches social significance and order to the play by imposing the structure of rules.

Eight-year-olds have grace and balance. Nine-year-olds move with less restlessness; strength and endurance increase; and the 9-year-old has good hand-eye coordination.[6] Competition, among peers, is important to test out their strength, agility, and coordination. While 10- to 12-year-old children are better able to control and direct their high energy level, they do have energetic, active, restless movements with tension release through finger drumming, foot tapping, or leg swinging.

The respiratory rate of the school-age child slows to 18 to 22 per minute. The respiratory tissues reach adult maturity, lung volume increases, and the lung capacity is proportionate to body size. The school-age child is still susceptible to respiratory tract infections. The frontal sinuses are fairly well developed by this age, and all the mucous membranes are very vulnerable to congestion and inflammation. The temperature, pulse, and respiration of the school-age child are gradually approaching adult norms, with temperature ranging from 98 to 98.6°F, pulse (resting) 60 to 70 beats per minute, and respiration from 18 to 20 per minute. Systolic BP ranges from 94 to 112 mm Hg and diastolic from 56 to 60 mm Hg. The heart grows more slowly during this period and is smaller in relation to the rest of the body. Since the heart must continue to supply the metabolic needs, the child should be advised against sustained physical activity and be watched for tiring. After age 7 the apex of the heart lies at the interspace of the fifth rib at the midclavicular line. Circulatory functions reach adult capacity. The child will still have some vasomotor instability with rapid vasodilation. A third heart sound and sinus arrhythmias are fairly common but, again, should be recorded.

ADOLESCENT

Growth in skeletal size, muscle mass, adipose tissue, and skin are significant in adolescence. The skeletal system grows faster than the muscles; thus, stress fractures may result. The large muscles grow faster than the smaller muscles, with the occasional result of poor posture and decreased coordination. Males are more clumsy than females. Muscle growth continues in males during late adolescence because of androgen production.[6]

Physical activities provide a way for adolescents to enjoy the stimulation of conflict in a socially acceptable way. Some form of physical activity should be encouraged to promote physical development, prevent overweight, formulate a realistic body image, and promote peer acceptance.

The respiratory rate of the adolescent is 16 to 20 per minute. The body is growing at various rates, but the respiratory system does not grow proportionately. Therefore, the adolescent may have inadequate oxygenation and become more fatigued. The lung capacity correlates with the adolescent's structural form. Males have a larger lung capacity than females due to greater shoulder width and chest size. Males have greater respiratory volume, greater vital capacity, and a slower respiratory rate. The male's lung capacity matures later than the female's. The female's lungs mature at age 17 or 18.

The heart continues to grow during adolescence but more slowly than the rest of the body, so inadequate oxygen and fatigue are common. The heart continues to enlarge until age 17 or 18. Systolic pulse pressure increases, and the temperature is the same as in an adult. The pulse ranges from 50 to 68 beats per minute; respiration ranges from 18 to 20 per minute, and BP is 100 to 120/50 to 70 mm Hg. Females have slightly higher pulse rates and basal body temperature and lower systolic pressures than males. Hypertension incidence increases. Essential hypertension incidence is approximately equal between races for this age group.

Athletes have slower pulse rates than peers. Heart sounds are heard readily at the fifth left intercostal space. Functional murmurs should be outgrown by this time. Chest pain may arise from musculoskeletal changes, but cardiovascular pain should always be investigated. Cardiovascular problems are the fifth leading cause of death in adolescents. Essential hypertension incidence is approximately equal between races for this age group.

More rest and sleep are needed now than earlier. The teenager is expending large amounts of energy and functioning with an inadequate oxygen supply; both of these factors contribute to fatigue, which should be addressed with additional rest. Parents may need to set limits. Rest does not necessarily mean sleep; it can also include quiet activities.[6]

There is a correlation between the maturation of the skeletal system and the reproductive system. Because of the very rapid growth during this period, the adolescent may not have sufficient energy left for strenuous activities. He or she tires easily and may frequently complain of needing to sit down. Gradually the adolescent is able to increase both speed and stamina during exercise. An increase in muscular and skeletal strength, as well as the increased ability of the lungs and heart to provide adequate oxygen to the tissue, facilitates maintenance of hemodynamics and rate of recovery after exercise. The body reaches its peak of physiologic resilience during late adolescence and young adulthood. Both strength and tolerance to strenuous activity can be increased by regular physical training and an individualized conditioning program.

Faulty nutrition is another major cause of fatigue in the adolescent. Poor eating habits established during the school-age years, combined with the typical quick-service, quick-energy food consumption patterns of adolescents, frequently lead to anemia, which in itself can lead to activity intolerance.[7]

The adolescent may be given responsibility for assisting with the maintenance of the family home or may be responsible for his or her own home if living independent from the family of origin. The role exploration characteristic of adolescence may lead to temporary changes in hygiene practices.

Recreational activities in adolescence often take the form of organized sports and other competitive activities. Social relationships are developed and enhanced, specific motor and cognitive skills related to a specific sport are refined, and a sense of mastery can be developed. Group activities and peer approval and acceptance are important. The adolescent responds to peer activities and experiments with different roles and life-styles. The nurse must distinguish self-care practices that are acceptable to the peer group from those that indicate a self-care deficit.

YOUNG ADULT

Growth of the skeletal system is essentially complete by age 25. Muscular efficiency is at its peak between 20 and 30. Energy level and control of energy are high. Thereafter, muscular strength declines, with the rate of muscle aging depending on the specific muscle group and the activity of the person and the adequacy of his or her diet.

Regular exercise is helpful in controlling weight and maintaining a state of high-level wellness. Muscle tone, strength, and circulation are enhanced by exercise. Problems arise especially when sedentary life-styles decrease the amount of exercise available with daily activities. Caloric intake and exercise should be balanced.

Adequate sleep is important for good physical and mental health. Lack of sleep results in progressive sluggishness of both physical and cognitive functions. This age group gets the majority of its activity from work and leisure activities. The young adult should learn to balance his or her work with leisure-time activities. Getting started in a career can be very stressful and can lead to burnout if an appropriate balance is not found. Physical fitness reflects ability to work for a sustained period with vigor and pleasure, without undue fatigue, with energy left over for enjoying hobbies and recreational activities and for meeting emergencies.[6]

Basic to fitness are regular physical exercise, proper nutrition, adequate rest and relaxation, conscientious health practices, and good medical and dental care. Regular physical fitness is a natural tranquilizer, releasing the body's own endorphins that reduce anxiety and muscular tension.

The respiratory system of the young adult has completely matured. Oxygen demand is based on exercise and activity now but gradually decreases between age 20 and 40. The body's ability to use oxygen efficiently is dependent on the cardiovascular system and the needs of the skeletal muscles.

The respiratory and cardiovascular systems change gradually with age, but the rate of change is highly dependent on the individual's diet and exercise pattern. Generally, contraction of the myocardium decreases. The maximum cardiac output is reached between the ages of 20 and 30. The arteries become less elastic. The maximum breathing capacity decreases between ages 20 and 40. Cardiac and respiratory function can be improved with regular exercise. Hypertension (BP 140/90 mm Hg or higher) and mitral valve prolapse syndrome are the most common cardiovascular medical diagnoses of the young adult.

ADULT

Basal metabolism rate gradually decreases. Although there is a general and gradual decline in quickness and level of activity, people who were most active among their age group during adolescence and young adulthood tend to be the most active during middle and old age. In women, there is frequently a menopausal rise in energy and activity.[8] Judicious exercise balanced with rest and sleep modify and retard the aging process. Exercise stimulates circulation to all parts of the body, thereby improving body functions. Exercise can also be an outlet for emotional tension. If the person is beginning exercises after being sedentary, certain precautions should be taken, such as gradually increasing exercise to a moderate level, exercising consistently, and avoiding overexertion. Recent research indicates that cardiovascular risk factors can be reduced in women by low-intensity walking.[9]

The adult is beginning to have a decrease in bone mass and a loss of skeletal height. Muscle strength and mass are directly related to active muscle use. The adult needs to maintain the patterns of activity and exercise of young adulthood and not become sedentary. Otherwise, muscles lose mass structure and strength more rapidly.

Temperature for the adult ranges from 97 to 99.6°F, pulse ranges from 50 to 100 beats per minute, respiration ranges from 16 to 20 per minute, and BP 120/80 mm Hg, ± 15. Cardiac output gradually decreases, and the decreasing elasticity of the blood vessels causes more susceptibility to hypertension and cardiovascular diseases. Females become as prone to coronary disease after menopause as males, so estrogen appears to be a protective agent. BMR generally decreases. Essential and secondary hypertension and angina occur more frequently in this age group.

The lung tissue becomes thicker and less elastic with age. The lungs cannot expand as they once did, and breathing capacity is reduced. The respiratory rate may increase to compensate for the reduced breathing capacity.

The normal adult should be able to perform activities of daily living without assistance. The needs for close relationships and intimacy of adulthood can be initiated by leisure activities with identified partners or a small group of close friends (for example, hiking, tennis, golf, attending concerts or theaters). The middle-aged adult is often interested in the personal satisfaction of diversional activities.

The adult will most likely be responsible for home maintenance as well as outside employment. Role strain or overtaxation of the adult is possible. Illness or injury to the adults in the household will significantly affect the ability of the family unit to maintain the home.

OLDER ADULT

The older adult faces gradual decline in function through the years. A decrease in skeletal mass affects all the bones of the skeleton. Decrease in skeletal mass leads to decreased strength. The tissues of the joints and bones stiffen due to increased collagen; thus, movement and range of motion markedly decrease. The oxygen supply to the muscles may also be decreased as a result of the reduced cardiac output. Mobility is lessened, and the older adult moves more slowly. The older adult should be encouraged to maintain optimum range of motion through planned exercise and activity.

There is a decline in exercise tolerance and work capacity as one ages. Cardiovascular changes, decreased pulmonary function, disuse of muscle groups, poor nutrition, and debilitating diseases may all contribute to less-than-optimum functioning and decreased mobility. With a decreased oxygen supply, the muscles may function, but cardiac output may be so poor that normal activity is impossible. Decreased sensory and motor abilities and muscle weakness may occur more frequently in the older adult.

Lung tissue continues to lose elasticity and becomes thicker. Alveolar sacs collapse, and thus there are fewer functional units exposed to gas exchange. Additionally, the muscles of respiration have become rigid, so lung expansion is not as great. The blood flow through the lungs is decreased because of reduced cardiac output. All these changes result in a reduced breathing capacity, a decreased amount of oxygen in the blood (decreased pO_2), an increase in air trapped in the lungs (increased pCO_2), and changes in respiratory rate, rhythm, and depth. The work of breathing is increased by a decrease in adequate functioning. The ability and effectiveness of the cough is also decreased due to diminished muscle tone and decreased sensitivity to stimuli.[6]

Physiologic cell and tissue changes (increased connective and collagen tissues, disappearance of some cellular elements, reduction in the number of normally functioning cells, increased amount of fat, decreased oxygen utilization, decreased cardiac output, decreased muscle strength) require the heart to work harder to provide adequate oxygenation. Exercise or stress raises heart rate and BP more in the older adult than in the younger adult, and it takes longer for these rates to return to normal. Heart valves become more rigid and thick. This may give rise to the development of murmurs. Inelasticity of vessels, loss of cell integrity, and decrease in cardiac output and stroke volume combine to produce hypoxia. Blood flow through the coronary arteries decreases. Maximum breathing capacity, vital capacity, and inspiratory reserve volume decrease. The area of alveolar contact decreases, as does the diffusing capacity; hence, there is a decrease in the oxygen content of the blood. Congestive heart failure, chronic occlusive arterial disease, and stasis ulcers rise in incidence with this age group. The BP usually measures 140/80 to 150/90 mm Hg, but the rest of the vital signs remain in the same range as for the middle-aged adult. Downward dislocation of the cardiac apex and increased kyphosis may alter isolation of the apical pulse and usual chest landmarks.

Cardiovascular diseases are the highest cause of death in the older adult group, with the most common medical diagnosis being atherosclerosis.

Since there is decreased physical reserve and muscle strength, the older adult should view exercise and activity as a means of promoting and maintaining health and well-being. Activity and exercise can help keep an individual in shape and maintain an optimal functioning level. The older adult should pace exercise and activity and recognize that it will take longer to do things than it once did.[6]

Time available for leisure activities may dramatically increase for the individual at retirement or for the couple who have accomplished child-rearing or career-establishing tasks. Diversional activities provide physical activity as well as reestablish social contacts and form new friendships.

Older adults are more likely to experience the impairments discussed in the physiological section, thereby altering their ability to maintain their own homes. Impaired elderly may live with their adult children, thereby placing additional responsibilities on the adult children for adequate home maintenance.

While changes do occur, the older population is a diverse group, and so individual assessment is of highest priority. The above-cited changes associated with aging may not apply to all older adults. There are many very independent older persons in our society, and the number is increasing.

APPLICABLE NURSING DIAGNOSES
Activity Intolerance, High Risk for or Actual
DEFINITION

High Risk for: A state in which an individual is at risk of experiencing insufficient physiological or psychological energy to endure or complete required or desired daily activities.[10]

Actual: A state in which an individual has insufficient physiological or psychological energy to endure or complete required or desired daily activities.[10]

NANDA TAXONOMY: MOVING 6.1.1.2, 6.1.1.3

DEFINING CHARACTERISTICS[10]

1. High Risk for Activity Intolerance:
   a. Major defining characteristics (risk factors):
      (1) History of previous intolerance
      (2) Deconditioned status

           (3) Presence of circulatory and/or respiratory problems
           (4) Inexperience with the activity
       b. Minor defining characteristics:
          None given
    2. Activity Intolerance:
       a. Major defining characteristics:
           (1) Verbal report of fatigue or weakness (*critical*)
           (2) Abnormal heart rate or blood pressure response to activity
           (3) Exertional discomfort or dyspnea
           (4) Electrocardiographic changes reflecting arrhythmias or ischemia
       b. Minor defining characteristics:
          None given

RELATED FACTORS[10]

    1. High Risk for Activity Intolerance:
       The risk factors also serve as the related factors for this diagnosis.
    2. Activity Intolerance:
       a. Bed rest and/or immobility
       b. Generalized weakness
       c. Sedentary lifestyle
       d. Imbalance between oxygen supply and demand

RELATED CLINICAL CONCERNS

    1. Anemias
    2. Congestive heart failure
    3. Valvular heart disease
    4. Cardiac arrhythmia
    5. Chronic obstructive pulmonary disease
    6. Metabolic disorder
    7. Musculoskeletal disorders

HAVE YOU SELECTED THE CORRECT DIAGNOSIS?

Impaired Physical Mobility   This diagnosis implies that an individual would be able to move independently if something were not limiting the motion. Activity Intolerance implies that the person is freely able to move but cannot endure or adapt to the increased energy or oxygen demands made by the movement or activity. (See page 460.)

Self-Care Deficit   Self-care Deficit indicates that the patient has some dependence on another person. Activity Intolerance implies that the patient is independent but is unable to perform activities because the body is unable to adapt to the increased energy and oxygen demands made. A person may have a Self-Care Deficit due to Activity Intolerance. (See page 472.)

Ineffective Individual Coping   Persons with the diagnosis of Ineffective Individual Coping may be unable to participate in their usual roles or in their usual self-care because they feel they lack control or the motivation to do so. Activity Intolerance, on the other hand, implies that the person is willing and able to participate in activities but is unable to endure or adapt to the increased energy or oxygen demands made by the movement or activity. (See page 892.)

EXPECTED OUTCOME

1. Will verbalize less fatigue and weakness by (date) and/or
2. Will participate in increased self-care activities by (date). Specify which self-care activities, that is, bathing, feeding, dressing, or ambulation, and the frequency, duration, or intensity of the activity.

EX: Will increase walking by at least one block each week for 8 weeks.

TARGET DATE

Appropriate target dates will have to be very individualized according to the degree of activity intolerance. An appropriate range would be 3 to 5 days.

NURSING ACTIONS/INTERVENTIONS WITH RATIONALES

Adult Health

Actions/Interventions	Rationales
• Monitor current potential for desired activities, including: ○ Physical limitations related to illness or surgery ○ Factors that relate to desired activities ○ Realistic expectations for actualizing potential for desired activities ○ Objective criteria by which specific progress may be measured, for example, distance, time, observable signs or symptoms such as apical pulse, or respiration ○ Previous level of activities patient enjoyed	Provides baseline for planning activities and increases in activities.
• Assist patient with self-care activities as needed. Let patient determine how much assistance is needed. • Monitor and record blood pressure, pulse, and respiration before and after activities.	Allows patient to have some control and choice in plan; helps patient to gradually decrease the amount of activity intolerance. Vital signs increase with activity and should return to baseline within 5 to 7 minutes postactivity. Maximal effort should be greater than or equal to 60 to 80 percent over the baseline.
• Encourage progressive activity and increased self-care as tolerated. Schedule moderate increase in activities on a daily basis, for example, will walk 10 feet farther each day.	Gradually increases tolerance for activities.

Continued

Actions/Interventions	Rationales
• Collaborate with physician regarding oxygen therapy.	Promotes teamwork; oxygen may be needed for shortness of breath associated with increased activity.
• Collaborate with a physical therapist in establishing an appropriate exercise plan.	Provides most appropriate activities for patient.
• Collaborate with an occupational therapist for appropriate diversional activity schedule.	
• Teach client appropriate exercise methods to prevent injury, for example, no straight-leg situps; proper muscle stretching and warm-up before aerobic exercise; reaching target heart rate; stopping exercise if experiencing pain, excessive fatigue, nausea, or breathlessness.	Basic safety measures to avoid complicating condition.
• Encourage rest as needed between activities. Assist patient in planning a balanced rest-activity program.	Planned rest assists in maintaining and increasing activity tolerance.
• Provide for a quiet, nonstimulating environment. Limit number of visitors and length of their stay. Teach relaxation and alternate pain relief measures. Assess internal and external motivators for activities, and record here.	Determines various methods to motivate behavior.
• Encourage adequate dietary input by ascertaining patient's food preferences and consulting with dietitian.	Ensures adequate nutrition to meet metabolic demands.
• Assist the patient in weight reduction as required.	Decreased weight requires less energy and oxygen use.
• Teach patient relationship between nutrition and exercise tolerance, and assist in developing a diet that is appropriate for nutritional and metabolic needs. (See Chapter 3 for further information.) Assist patient in acquiring equipment to perform desired exercise. (List needed equipment here; this could include proper shoes, eyeglasses, or weights.)	Assists patient to learn alternate methods to conserve energy in activities of daily living.
• Instruct patient in energy-saving techniques of daily care, for example, prepare meals sitting on a high stool rather than standing.	
• Provide opportunities of 15 to 30 minutes per shift for allowing patient and family to verbalize concerns regarding activity.	
• Introduce necessary teaching according to the readiness of patient and family with appropriate modifications to best meet patient's needs.	Assists in reducing anxiety, promotes long-range planning, and provides a teaching opportunity. Ensures that teaching meets patient's level of understanding and need.

- Provide patient and family opportunities to contribute to plans for activity as appropriate. Allow for individual preference and suggestions on an ongoing basis.
- Provide opportunities for success in meeting expected goals by using subgoals or increments that lead to desired activity.

The more the patient and family participate in planning, the more likely they are to implement the desired regimen.

Achieving success motivates the patient to continue the activity.

Child Health

Actions/Interventions	Rationales
• Provide learning modules and practice sessions with materials suitable for child's age and developmental capacity, for example, dolls, videos, or pictures.	Developmentally appropriate materials will enhance learning; will maintain child's attention.
• Provide for continuity in care by assigning same nurses for care during critical times for teaching and implementation.	Continuity of caregivers fosters trust in the nurse-patient relationship, which enhances learning.
• Modify expected behavior to incorporate appropriate developmental needs, for example, allow for shared cards, messages, or visitors to lobby if possible for adolescent patients.	Valuing of patient's developmental needs fosters self-esteem and serves as a reward for efforts.
• Reinforce adherence to regimen with stickers or other appropriate measures to document progress.	Extrinsic rewards may help to symbolize concrete progress and assist in reinforcing appropriate behaviors for achieving goals.

Women's Health

Actions/Interventions	Rationales

• Provide quiet, supportive atmosphere for interaction with infant:
  ○ Attachment
  ○ Caretaking activities such as breast- or bottle-feeding
	Promotes positive experience for mother and baby.

• Instruct patient in energy-saving activities of daily care:
  ○ Take care of self and baby only.
  ○ Let significant others take care of housework and other children.
  ○ Let significant others take care of baby for a prearranged time during the day, so mother can spend quality time with other children.
	A common problem with a new baby is fatigue on the part of the mother. These measures will assist in decreasing this fatigue.

Continued

Actions/Interventions	Rationales
○ Learn to sleep when baby sleeps. ○ Have specific set times for visiting of friends or relatives. ○ If breast-feeding, significant other can bring infant to mother at night (mother does not always have to get up every time for infant). • Provide patient with factual information about sexual changes during pregnancy and the postpartum period: ○ Answer questions promptly and factually. ○ Introduce patient to people who have had similar experiences. ○ Discuss fears about sexual changes. ○ Discuss aspects of sexuality and intercourse during pregnancy: (1) Positions for intercourse during different stages of pregnancy (2) Frequency of intercourse (3) Effect of intercourse on pregnancy or fetus ○ Describe postpartum healing process and timing of resumption of intercourse.	Provides basic information regarding sexuality before and after pregnancy.

Mental Health

Actions/Interventions	Rationales
• Discuss with client his or her perceptions of activity appropriate to his or her current capabilities.	Provides an understanding of the client's worldview so that care can be individualized and interventions developed that are acceptable to both the nurse and the client.[11]
• If the client estimates a routine that far exceeds current capabilities (as with eating disorder clients or clients experiencing elated mood): ○ Establish appropriate limits on exercise. (The limits and consequences for not maintaining established limits should be listed here.) If the excessive exercise pattern is related to an elated mood, set limits in a manner that allows client some activity while not greatly exceeding metabolic needs until psychologic status is improved.	Negative reinforcement eliminates or decreases behavior.[12] Because of the high energy level, elated clients need some large motor activity that discharges energy but does not present a risk for physical harm.[13]

○ Begin client slowly, that is, with stretching exercise for 15 minutes twice a day.

Goals need to be achievable to promote the sense of accomplishment and positive self-feelings, which will in turn increase motivation.[11]

○ As physical condition improves, gradually increase exercise to 30 minutes of aerobic exercise once per day.

This regimen provides positive cardiovascular fitness without risk of overexertion.[14]

○ Discuss with client appropriate levels of exercise considering his or her age and metabolic pattern.

Overexertion can decrease benefits of exercise by increasing risk for injury.[14]

○ Discuss with client the hazards of overexercise.

○ Establish a reward system for clients who maintain the established exercise schedule. (The schedule for the client should be listed here with those reinforcers that are to be used.)

Positive reinforcement encourages appropriate behavior.[12]

○ Stay with client while he or she is engaged in appropriate exercise.

Interaction with the nurse can provide positive reinforcement.[12]

○ Develop a schedule for the client to be involved in an occupational therapy program to assist client in identifying alternative forms of activity other than aerobic exercise.

Promotes accurate perception of body size, nutrition, and exercise needs.

○ Limit number of walks off the unit to accommodate client's weight, level of exercise on the unit, and physiology (the frequency and length of the walk should be listed here).

• For further information related to eating disorder clients, see Altered Nutrition: Less than Body Requirements.

• If client's expectations are much less than current capabilities (as with depressed or poorly motivated client), implement the following actions:

Goals need to be achievable to promote sense of accomplishment and positive self-feelings that will in turn increase motivation.[11]

○ Establish very limited goals that client can accomplish, for example, a 5-minute walk in a hallway once a day or walking in the client's room for 5 minutes. The goal established should be listed here.

○ Establish a reward system for achievement of goals. (The reward program should be listed here with a list of items the client finds rewarding.)

Positive reinforcement encourages appropriate behavior.[12]

○ Develop a schedule for the client to be involved in an occupational therapy program (note schedule here).

Provides client with opportunity to improve self-help skills while engaged in a variety of activities.

○ Establish limits on the amount of time the client can spend in bed or in his or her

Exercise raises levels of endorphins in the brain, which has a positive effect on

Continued

Actions/Interventions	Rationales
room during waking hours. (Establish limits the client can achieve, and note limits here.)	depression and promotes a general feeling of well-being.[13,15]
○ Stay with client during exercise periods and time out of the room until the client is performing these tasks without prompting.	Interaction with the nurse can provide positive reinforcement.[12]
○ Provide the client with firm support for initiating the activity.	Attention from the nurse can provide positive reinforcement and increase client's motivation to accomplish goal.
○ Place a record of goal achievement where client can see it and mark each step toward the goal with a reward marker.	Provides concrete evidence of goal attainment and motivation to continue these activities that will promote well-being.
○ Provide positive verbal reinforcement for goal achievement and progress.	
• For further information about clients with depressed mood, refer to Ineffective Individual Coping (Chapter 11).	
• Monitor effect that current medications may have on activity tolerance, and teach client necessary adjustments.	Psychotropic medications may cause postural hypotension, and the client should be instructed to change position slowly.
• Schedule time to discuss plans and special concerns with client and client's support system. This could include teaching and answering questions. Schedule daily during initial days of hospitalization and one longer time just before discharge. Note here the scheduled times and the name of the person responsible for the plan.	Recognizes the reciprocity between the client's illness and the family context.[16]

Gerontic Health

NOTE: Research on activity intolerance in older adults is very minimal. Most of the studies that have addressed activity and/or exercise have been conducted on "healthy elders."[17]

Actions/Interventions	Rationales
• Determine, with the assistance of the patient, particular time periods of highest energy, and plan care accordingly.	Maximizes potential to successfully participate in or complete care requirements.
• Teach patient to monitor pulse before, during, and after activity.	Promotes self-monitoring, and provides means of determining progress across care settings.
• Refer to occupational therapy and physical therapy for determination of a progressive activity program.	Collaboration ensures a plan that will result in activity for maximum effect.

• Provide positive feedback for incremental successes. Focus on measurable increases in activity levels.	Provides motivation to continue program.

Home Health

Actions/Interventions	Rationales
• Teach client and family appropriate monitoring of causes, signs, and symptoms of high risk for or actual activity intolerance: 　○ Prolonged bed rest 　○ Circulatory or respiratory problems 　○ New activity 　○ Fatigue 　○ Dyspnea 　○ Pain 　○ Vital signs (before and after activity) 　○ Malnutrition 　○ Previous inactivity 　○ Weakness 　○ Confusion	Provides baseline for prevention and/or early intervention.
• Assist client and family in identifying life-style changes that may be required: 　○ Progressive exercise to increase endurance 　○ Range-of-motion and flexibility exercises 　○ Treatments for underlying conditions (cardiac, respiratory, musculoskeletal, circulatory, and so on) 　○ Motivation 　○ Assistive devices as required (walkers, canes, crutches, wheelchairs, exercise equipment, and so on) 　○ Adequate nutrition 　○ Adequate fluids 　○ Stress management 　○ Pain relief 　○ Prevention of hazards of immobility 　○ Changes in occupations, family, or social roles 　○ Changes in living conditions 　○ Economic concerns	Life-style changes require sufficient support to achieve.
• Teach client and family purposes and side effects of medications and proper administration techniques.	Changes locus of control to client and family and supports self-care.
• Assist client and family in setting criteria to help them determine when physician or other intervention is required.	Provides additional support for client.
• Consult with or refer to appropriate assistive resources as indicated. (See Appendix B.)	

FLOW CHART EVALUATION
Flow Chart Expected Outcome 1

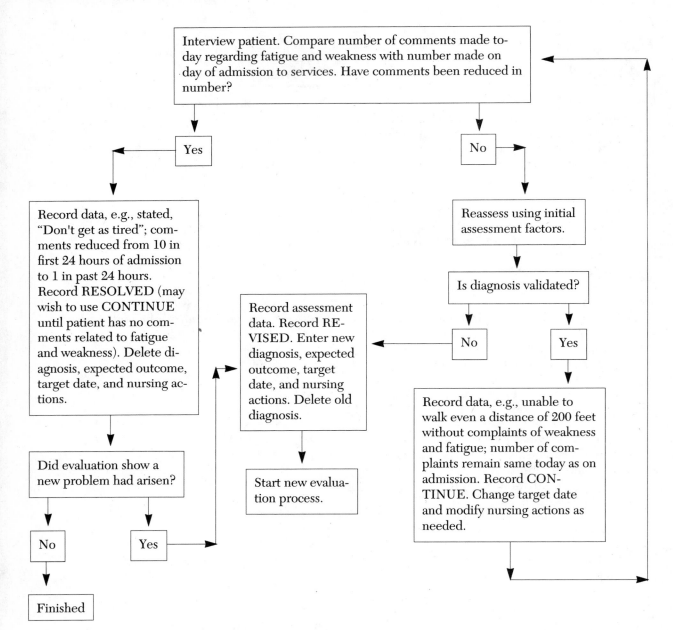

Interview patient. Compare number of comments made to-day regarding fatigue and weakness with number made on day of admission to services. Have comments been reduced in number?

Yes

No

Record data, e.g., stated, "Don't get as tired"; comments reduced from 10 in first 24 hours of admission to 1 in past 24 hours. Record RESOLVED (may wish to use CONTINUE until patient has no comments related to fatigue and weakness). Delete diagnosis, expected outcome, target date, and nursing actions.

Reassess using initial assessment factors.

Is diagnosis validated?

Record assessment data. Record RE-VISED. Enter new diagnosis, expected outcome, target date, and nursing actions. Delete old diagnosis.

No

Yes

Did evaluation show a new problem had arisen?

Start new evalua-tion process.

Record data, e.g., unable to walk even a distance of 200 feet without complaints of weakness and fatigue; number of com-plaints remain same today as on admission. Record CON-TINUE. Change target date and modify nursing actions as needed.

No

Yes

Finished

Flow Chart Expected Outcome 2

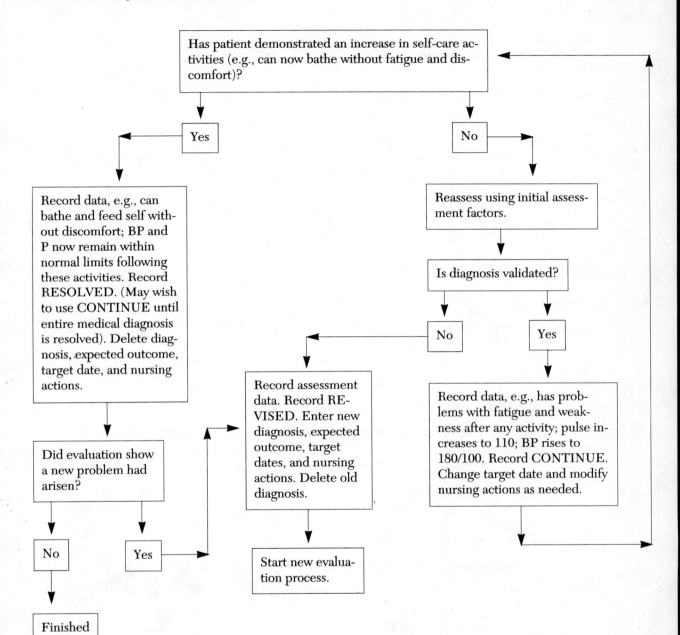

Airway Clearance, Ineffective

DEFINITION

A state in which an individual is unable to clear secretions or obstructions from the respiratory tract to maintain airway patency.[10]

NANDA TAXONOMY: EXCHANGING 1.5.1.2

DEFINING CHARACTERISTICS[10]

1. Major defining characteristics:
   a. Abnormal breath sounds [rales (crackles) and/or rhonchi (wheezes)]
   b. Changes in rate or depth of respiration
   c. Tachypnea
   d. Cough, effective or ineffective, with or without sputum
   e. Cyanosis
   f. Dyspnea
2. Minor defining characteristics:
   None given

RELATED FACTORS[10]

1. Decreased energy or fatigue
2. Tracheobronchial infection, obstruction, secretion
3. Perceptual or cognitive
4. Trauma

RELATED CLINICAL CONCERNS

1. Adult respiratory distress syndrome (ARDS)
2. Pneumonia
3. Cancer of the lung
4. Chronic obstructive pulmonary disease
5. Congestive heart failure
6. Cystic fibrosis
7. Inhalation injuries
8. Neuromuscular diseases

HAVE YOU SELECTED THE CORRECT DIAGNOSIS?

Ineffective Breathing Pattern   This diagnosis implies an alteration in the rate, rhythm, depth, or type of respiration, such as hyperventilation or hypoventilation. These patterns are not effective in supplying oxygen to the cells of the body or in removing the products of respiration. However, air is able to move freely through the air passages. In Ineffective Airway Clearance, the air passages are obstructed in some way. (See page 349.)

Impaired Gas Exchange   This diagnosis means that air has been inhaled through the air passages but that oxygen and carbon dioxide are not appropriately exchanged at the alveolar-capillary level. Air has been able to pass through clear air passages, but a problem arises at the cellular level. (See page 416.)

Fluid Volume Deficit When fluid volume is insufficient to assist in liquifying thick, tenacious respiratory tract secretions, Fluid Volume Deficit then becomes the primary diagnosis. In this instance, the patient would be unable to effectively expectorate the secretions no matter how hard he or she tried, and Ineffective Airway Clearance would result. (See page 155.)

Pain If pain is sufficient to prevent the patient from coughing to clear the airway, then Ineffective Airway Clearance will result secondary to the pain. (See page 546.)

EXPECTED OUTCOME

1. Will have an open, clear airway by (date) and/or
2. Will easily expectorate secretions from airway by (date)

TARGET DATE

Ineffective airway clearance is life-threatening; therefore, progress toward meeting the expected outcome should be evaluated at least on a daily basis.

ADDITIONAL INFORMATION

The various ways of measuring lung volume and capacity are summarized and defined in Table 5.1.

Table 5–1 LUNG CAPACITIES AND VOLUMES

Measurement	Average Value, Adult Male, ml (resting)	Definition
Tidal volume (TV)	500	Amount of air inhaled or exhaled with each breath.
Inspiratory reserve volume (IRV)	3100	Amount of air that can be forcefully inhaled after a normal tidal volume inhalation.
Expiratory reserve volume (ERV)	1200	Amount of air that can be forcefully exhaled after a normal tidal volume exhalation.
Residual volume (RV)	1200	Amount of air left in the lungs after a forced exhalation.
Total lung capacity (TLC)	6000	Maximum amount of air that can be contained in the lungs after a maximum inspiratory effort: TLC = TV + IRV + ERV + RV.
Vital capacity (VC)	4800	Maximum amount of air that can be expired after a maximum inspiration: VC = TV + IRV + ERV. Should be 80% of TLC.
Inspiratory capacity (IC)	3600	Maximum amount of air that can be inspired after a normal expiration: IC = TV + IRV.
Functional residual capacity (FRC)	2400	Volume of air remaining in the lungs after a normal tidal volume expiration: FRC = ERV + RV.

NURSING ACTIONS/INTERVENTIONS WITH RATIONALES

Adult Health

Actions/Interventions	Rationales
• Maintain appropriate emergency equipment as dictated by situation (for example, tracheostomy sterile setup and/or suctioning apparatus).	Basic safety precautions.
• Monitor respiratory rate, depth, and breath sounds at least every 4 hours.	Basic indicators of airway patency.
• Collaborate with physician regarding frequency of blood gas measurements.	Assists in determining changes in ventilatory status. Promotes teamwork.
• Give mucolytic agents via nebulizer or intermittent positive-pressure breathing (IPPB) or continuous positive airway pressure (CPAP) treatments as ordered.	Helps thin and loosen secretion; expands airways.
• Monitor effects and side effects of medications used to open patient's airways (bronchodilators or corticosteroids), for example, aminophylline intravenous (IV) drip: Ensure appropriate dilution, note incompatibility factor, monitor for nausea, increased heart rate, irritability, and so on. Document effect within 30 minutes after administration.	Assists in determining if air flow or lung volume is improved via medication.
• Maintain adequate fluid intake to liquefy secretions. Encourage intake up to 3000 ml per day (unless contraindicated). Measure output each 8 hours.	Assists in liquification of secretions and provides moisture to the pulmonary mucosa.

• Have patient's favorite fluids available:
  ○ Remind patient to drink fluids at least every hour while awake.
  ○ Provide warm or hot drinks instead of cold fluids.	

• Assist patient in coughing, huffing, and breathing efforts to make them more productive:
  ○ Sitting in upright position
  ○ Taking a deep, slow breath while expanding abdomen, allowing diaphragm to expand
  ○ Holding breath for 3 to 5 seconds
  ○ Exhaling the breath slowly through the mouth while abdomen moves inward
  ○ Pausing briefly before next breath
  ○ Coughing with the second breath inward, coughing forcefully from the chest (these should be two short, forceful coughs)
	Deep breathing and diaphragmatic breathing allow for greater lung expansion and ventilation and provide a more effective cough.

- ○ Placing hands on upper abdomen and exerting inward, upward pressure during cough (splint incision or painful areas during procedure)
  - ○ Maintaining adequate humidity in environment (80 percent)
- Observe patient practicing proper breathing techniques 30 minutes twice a day (note time of practice sessions here).
- Assist with cupping and clapping activities every 4 hours while awake at (times). Teach family these procedures.

Cupping and clapping loosen secretions and assist expectoration. Teaching family allows them to participate in care under supervision and promotes continuation of the procedure after discharge.

- Assist patient with clearing secretions from mouth or nose by:
  - ○ Providing tissues
  - ○ Using gentle suctioning if necessary

Removes tenacious secretions from airways.

- Assist patient with oral hygiene at least every 4 hours while awake at (times):
  - ○ Lubricate lips with a moisturizing agent.
  - ○ Do not allow the use of oil-based products around the nose.

Oral hygiene clears away dried secretions and freshens the mouth. Oil-based products may obstruct breathing passages.

- Discuss with the patient importance of maintaining proper position, to include:
  - ○ Side-lying position while in bed
  - ○ Sitting or standing position with shoulders back and back as straight as possible to facilitate expansion of the diaphragm

Facilitates expansion of the diaphragm; decreases probability of aspiration.

- Remind patient of proper positioning as required.
- Promote rest and relaxation by scheduling treatments and activities with appropriate rest periods.

Avoids overexertion and worsening of condition.

- Instruct patient to avoid irritating substances, large crowds, and persons with upper respiratory infections.

Prevents infection or airway spasms.

- Discuss with patient factors contributing to Ineffective Airway Clearance, for example, cigarettes or alcohol. Refer, prior to discharge, to a stop-smoking program at a community agency such as:
  - ○ American Cancer Society
  - ○ American Heart Association
  - ○ American Lung Association

Smoking increases production of mucous and paralyzes or causes loss of cilia.

- Refer for appropriate consultations as needed, for example, respiratory therapy or physical therapy.

Uses resources cost-effectively and promotes follow-up care.

- Provide for appropriate follow-up by scheduling appointments before dismissal.

Child Health

Actions/Interventions	Rationales

• Monitor patient factors that relate to Ineffective Airway Clearance, including:
  ○ Feeding tolerance or intolerance
  ○ Allergens
  ○ Emotional aspects
  ○ Stressors of recent or past activities
  ○ Congenital anomalies
  ○ Parental anxieties
  ○ Infant or child temperament
  ○ Abdominal distention
  ○ Related vital signs, especially heart rate
  ○ Diaphragmatic excursion
  ○ Retraction in respiratory effort
  ○ Choking, coughing
  ○ Flaring of nares
  ○ Appropriate functioning of respiratory equipment
	Provides an individualized data baseline that facilitates individualized care planning.

• Provide appropriate attention to suctioning and related respiratory maintenance:
  ○ Appropriate size for catheter as needed
  ○ Appropriate administration of humidified oxygen as ordered by physician if applicable
  ○ Appropriate follow-up of blood gases
  ○ Documentation of:
    (1) Oxygen administration
    (2) Characteristics of secretions obtained by suctioning
    (3) Vital signs during suctioning
    (4) Reporting apical pulse below 70 or above 149 beats per minute for infant, below 90 or above 120 beats per minute for young child.
	Basic maintenance of airway and respiratory function. Gives priority attention to child's status and developmental level.

• Encourage parent's input in planning care for patient, with attention to individual preferences when possible.	Promotes family empowerment, thus promotes the likelihood of more effective management of therapeutic regimen after discharge.
• Provide health teaching as needed based on assessment and child's situation.	Establishes a basis for home care planning and allows family time to ask questions, practice techniques, and so on before discharge. Assists in reducing anxiety and promotes continuance of therapeutic regimen.
• Plan for appropriate follow-up with health team members. (See Appendix B.)	Provides for long-term support and effective management of therapeutic regimen.
• Reduce apprehension by providing	Sensitivity to individual feelings and needs

comforting behavior and meeting developmental needs of patient and family.
- Allow for diversional activities to approximate tolerance of child.

- Encourage family members to assist in care of patient with use of return-demonstration opportunities for teaching required skills.

- Provide for appropriate safety maintenance, especially with oxygen administration (no smoking) and appropriate precautions for age and developmental level.
- Allow ample time for parental mastery of skills identified in care of child.

builds trust in the nurse-patient-family relationship.
Realistic opportunities for diversion will be measured by what the patient is capable of doing and will leave the patient feeling refreshed and renewed for having participated.
Return-demonstration provides feedback to evaluate skills and serves to provide reinforcement in a supportive environment. Involvement of parents also satisfies emotional needs of both parent and child.
Appropriate safety measures must be taken with the use of combustible potentials whose use out of prescribed parameters may be toxic.

Greater success in compliance and confidence is afforded by providing ample time for mastery-required skills.

Women's Health

NOTE: The following nursing actions pertain to the newborn infant in the delivery room, immediately following delivery. See Adult Health and Home Health for actions related to the mother.

Actions/Interventions	Rationales

• Evaluate and record the respiratory status of the newborn infant.
  ○ Suction mouth and pharynx with bulb syringe.
  ○ Clear mouth and oropharynx with bulb syringe.
  ○ Avoid deep suctioning if possible.
	Basic measures to clear newborn's airway. Deep suctioning would stimulate reflexes, which could result in aspiration.

• Continue to evaluate infant's respiratory status and to act if necessary to resuscitate. Depending on infant's response, the following nursing measures can be taken:
  ○ Administer warm, humid oxygen with face mask.
  ○ If no improvement, administer oxygen with bag and mask.
  ○ If no improvement, be prepared for:
  (1) Endotracheal intubation
  (2) Ventilation with positive pressure
  (3) Cardiac massage
  (4) Transport to neonatal intensive care unit.
	Basic protocol for infant who has difficulty immediately after birth.

Mental Health

Actions/Interventions	Rationales
• Collaborate with physician for possible use of saline gargles or anesthetic lozenge for sore throats. (Report all sore throats to physician, especially if client is receiving antipsychotic drugs and in the absence of other flu or cold symptoms.)	These medications can cause blood dyscrasias which present with the symptoms of sore throat, fever, malaise, unusual bleeding, and easy bruising. Early intervention is important for patient safety.[18]
• Remind client to chew food well, and sit with client during mealtime if cognitive functioning indicates a need for close observation. Note any special adaptations here (for example, soft foods, observation during meals, and so on).	Provides safety for client with alterations of mental status.

Gerontic Health

Actions/Interventions	Rationales
• Encourage coughing and deep-breathing exercises every 2 hours on the (odd/even) hour.	Provides exercise in techniques that assist in clearing the airway.
• Provide small, frequent feedings during periods of dyspnea.	Conserves energy and promotes ventilation efforts.
• Instruct patient regarding early signs of respiratory infections, for example, increased amount or thickness of secretions, increased cough, and/or changes in color of sputum produced.	Early recognition of signs of infection promotes early intervention and avoidance of severe infection.
• Encourage increased mobility, as tolerated, on a daily basis.	Mobility helps to increase rate and depth of respiration as well as decreasing pooling of secretions.
• Teach patient to complete prescribed course of antibiotic therapy.	Due to economic factors, a common problem is stopping therapy before the designated time frame and "saving" of the medication for possible future episodes.
• Monitor for the use of sedative medications that can decrease the level of alertness and respiratory effort.	These medications can decrease the level of alertness and respiratory effort.
• Collaborate with physician regarding the use of cough suppressants.	Decreases episodes of persistent, nonproductive coughing.

Activity-Exercise Pattern

Home Health

Actions/Interventions	Rationales

• Teach client and family appropriate monitoring of signs and symptoms of ineffective airway clearance:
  ○ Cough (effective or ineffective)
  ○ Sputum
  ○ Respiratory status (cyanosis, dyspnea, and rate)
  ○ Abnormal breath sounds (noisy respirations)
  ○ Nasal flaring
  ○ Intercostal, substernal retraction
  ○ Choking or gagging
  ○ Diaphoresis
  ○ Restlessness or anxiety
  ○ Impaired speech
  ○ Collection of mucus in mouth
	Provides for early recognition and intervention for problem.

• Assist client and family in identifying life-style changes that may be required:
  ○ Eliminating smoking
  ○ Treating fear or anxiety
  ○ Treating pain
  ○ Performing pulmonary hygiene
    (1) Clearing the bronchial tree by controlled coughing
    (2) Decreasing viscosity of secretions via humidity and fluid balance
    (3) Postural drainage
  ○ Learning stress management
  ○ Ensuring adequate nutritional intake
  ○ Learning diaphragmatic breathing
  ○ Administering pain relief
  ○ Beginning progressive ambulation (avoid fatigue)
  ○ Maintaining position so that danger of aspiration is decreased
  ○ Maintaining body position to minimize work of breathing and clearing airway
  ○ Ensuring adequate oral hygiene
  ○ Clearing secretions from throat
  ○ Suctioning as needed
  ○ Keeping area free of dust and potential allergens or irritants
  ○ Ensuring adequate hydration (monitor intake and output)
	Provides basic information for client and family that promotes necessary lifestyle changes.

Continued

Actions/Interventions	Rationales
• Teach client and family purposes, side effects, and proper administration techniques of medications.	
• Assist client and family in setting criteria to help them determine when physician or other intervention is required.	Locus of control shifts from nurse to client and family, thus promoting self-care.
• Teach family basic cardiopulmonary resuscitation (CPR).	
• Consult with or refer to appropriate assistive resources as indicated. (See Appendix B.)	Provides additional support for client and family and uses already available resources in a cost-effective manner.

FLOW CHART EVALUATION
Flow Chart Expected Outcome 1

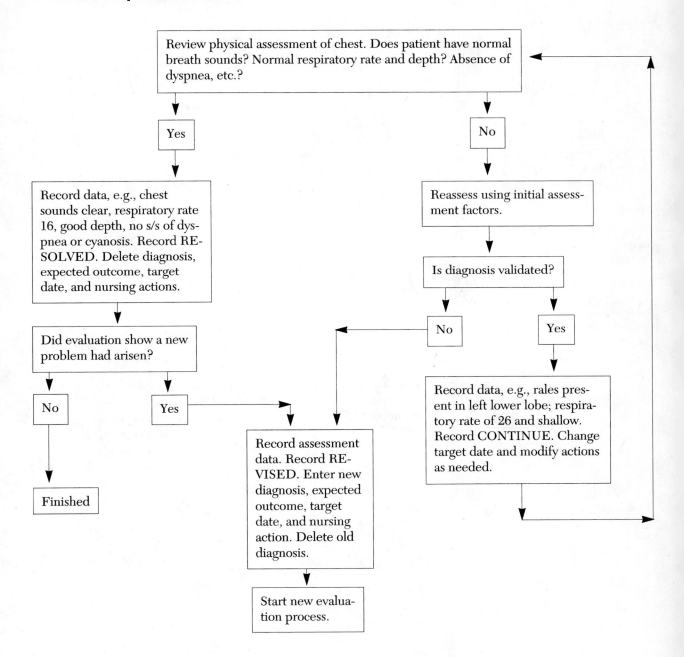

Flow Chart Expected Outcome 2

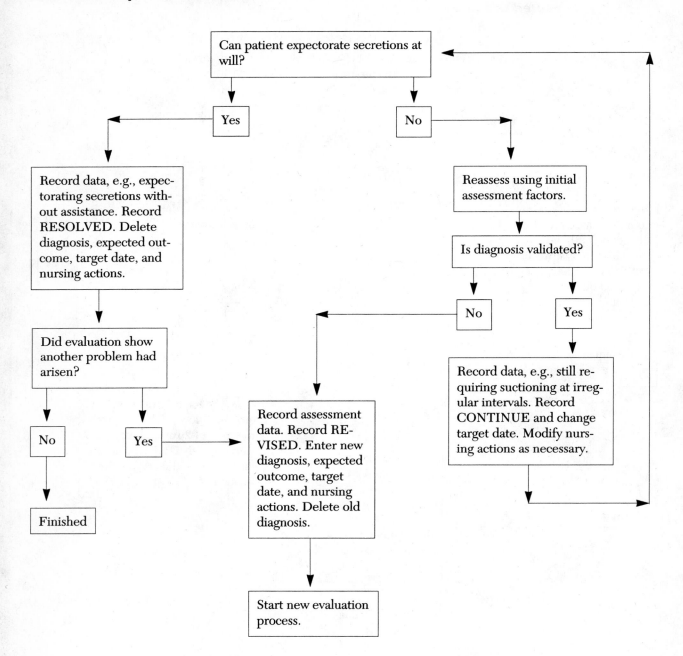

Breathing Pattern, Ineffective

DEFINITION

The state in which an individual's inhalation and/or exhalation pattern does not enable adequate pulmonary inflation or emptying.[10]

NANDA TAXONOMY: EXCHANGING 1.5.1.3

DEFINING CHARACTERISTICS[10]

1. Major defining characteristics:
   a. Dyspnea
   b. Shortness of breath
   c. Tachypnea
   d. Fremitus
   e. Abnormal arterial blood gas
   f. Cyanosis
   g. Cough
   h. Nasal flaring
   i. Respiratory depth changes
   j. Assumption of three-point position
   k. Pursed-lip breathing or prolonged expiratory phase
   l. Increased anteroposterior diameter
   m. Use of accessory muscles
   n. Altered chest excursion
2. Minor defining characteristics:
   None given

RELATED FACTORS[10]

1. Neuromuscular impairment
2. Pain
3. Musculoskeletal impairment
4. Perception or cognition impairment
5. Anxiety
6. Decreased energy or fatigue

RELATED CLINICAL CONCERNS

1. Chronic obstructive or restrictive pulmonary disease
2. Pneumonia
3. Asthma
4. Acute alcoholism (intoxication or overdose)
5. Congestive heart failure
6. Chest trauma
7. Myasthenia gravis

Ineffective Airway Clearance Ineffective Airway Clearance means that something is blocking the air passage, but when air gets to the alveoli, there is adequate gas exchange. In Ineffective Breathing Pattern, the ventilatory effort is insufficient to bring in enough oxygen or to get rid of sufficient amounts of carbon dioxide. However, air is able to freely move through the air passages. (See page 338.)

Impaired Gas Exchange This diagnosis indicates that enough oxygen is brought into the respiratory system and the carbon dioxide that is produced is exhaled, but there is insufficient exchange of oxygen and carbon dioxide at the alveolar-capillary level. There is no problem with either the ventilatory effort or the air passageways. The problem exists at the cellular level. (See page 416.)

EXPECTED OUTCOMES

1. Will demonstrate an effective breathing pattern by (date) as evidence by (specify criteria here, for example, normal breath sounds, arterial blood gases within normal limits, no evidence of cyanosis) and/or
2. Will return-demonstrate methods necessary to improve breathing pattern by (date)

TARGET DATE

Evaluation should be made on an hourly basis since this diagnosis has the potential to be life-threatening. After the patient has stabilized, target dates can be spaced further apart.

NURSING ACTIONS/INTERVENTIONS WITH RATIONALES

Adult Health

Actions/Interventions	Rationales
• Administer oxygen as ordered.	Maintains or improves arterial blood gases (ABGs); reduces anxiety.

• Monitor baseline respiratory data:
  ○ Respiratory rate and pattern
  ○ Use of intercostal and accessory muscles
  ○ Position of comfort
  ○ Nares for flaring
  ○ Grunting or related noises such as stridor
  ○ Coughing, nature of secretions
  ○ Breath sounds
  ○ Related vital signs, especially apical pulse and blood pressure
  ○ Aids required for respiration and airway maintenance
	Basic monitoring of overall condition and its related progress of lack of progress.

○ Skin color, hydration, and elimination
○ Arterial blood gases as ordered
○ Appropriate related equipment such as arterial line or IV
○ Oxygen administration per order
○ Documentation of all the above
- Collaborate with physician on monitoring of blood gases; report abnormal results immediately.
- Perform nursing actions to maintain Airway Clearance. (See Ineffective Airway Clearance—enter those orders here.)
- Reduce chest pain using noninvasive techniques and analgesics.
- Maintain appropriate attention to relief of pain and anxiety via positioning, suctioning, and administration of medications as ordered.
- Maintain appropriate caution for possible side effects of respiratory depression for specific medications such as morphine or Valium.
- Raise head of bed 30 degrees or more if not contraindicated.

- Instruct in diaphragmatic deep breathing and pursed-lip breathing. Have patient return-demonstrate and perform these activities at least every hour.
- Reduce fear and anxiety by spending at least 15 minutes every 2 hours on the (odd/even) hour with patient.
- Administer or assist with IPPB or CPAP as ordered. Remain with patient during treatment.
- Turn every 2 hours on the (odd/even) hour.

- Encourage patient's mobility as tolerated. (See Impaired Physical Mobility.)
- Instruct patient in effects on breathing pattern of smoking, air pollution, and so on prior to discharge.
- Provide teaching based on needs of patient and family regarding:
○ Illness
○ Procedures and related nursing care
○ Implications for rest and relief of anxiety secondary to respiratory failure
○ Advocacy role

ABGs are important indicators of ventilatory effectiveness. Promotes team approach to planning.
Maintains a patent airway for gas exchange.

Promotes chest expansion.

Allows gravity to assist in lowering the diaphragm and provides greater chest expansion.
Promotes lung expansion and slightly increases pressure in the airways, allowing them to remain open longer; increases oxygenation and exhalation of carbon dioxide.
Reduces tension or stress; reduces oxygen demand and work of breathing.

Promotes expansion of airways and exchange of gases; staying with the patient reduces anxiety.
Promotes mobility of any secretions and promotes lung expansion.
Promotes tolerance for activities and helps with lung expansion and ventilation.
Knowledge will assist patient to avoid harmful environments and to protect himself or herself from the effects from such activities.
Reduces anxiety; starts appropriate home care planning; assists family in dealing with health care system.

Child Health

Actions/Interventions	Rationales
• Maintain appropriate emergency equipment in an accessible place. (Specify actual size of endotracheal tube for infant, child, or adolescent, trach set size, and suctioning catheters or chest tube for size of patient.)	Standard accountability for emergency equipment and treatment is basic to patient care and especially so when risk factors are increased.
• Allow at least 5 to 15 minutes per shift for parents and child to verbalize concerns related to illness.	Appropriate time for ventilation may be hard to determine, but effort to do so demonstrates valuing of patient and family needs and serves to reduce anxiety.
• Determine perception of illness by patient and parents.	How the parents and child see (perceive) the patient's problem will provide meaningful data that serves to ensure sensitivity in care and will provide information regarding teaching needs. Provides cues to questions regarding continued implementation of therapeutic regimen.
• Include parents in care of child as appropriate, to include comfort measures, assisting with feeding, and the like.	Parental involvement is critical in maintaining emotional bonds with the child. Also augments sense of contributing to child's care with opportunities for mastering the skills in a supportive environment.
• Collaborate with appropriate related health team members as needed. (See Appendix B.)	Appropriate coordination of services will best meet the patient's needs with attention to the patient's individuality.

Women's Health

Actions/Interventions	Rationales
• Assist patient and significant other in identifying life-style changes that may be required to prevent Ineffective Breathing Pattern during pregnancy, for example, smoking and avoiding crowds during influenza epidemics.	Increased cardiovascular fitness supports increased respiratory effectiveness.
• Develop exercise plan for cardiovascular fitness during pregnancy.	
• Teach patient to avoid wearing constrictive clothing during pregnancy.	Any constriction will contribute to further breathing difficulties, which will become more difficult as the expanding uterus contributes to abdominal contents pressing against the diaphragm.
• Teach and encourage patient to practice correct breathing techniques for labor.	Assists in preventing hyperventilation.

- During the latter stages of pregnancy, encourage patient to:
  - Walk up stairs slowly.
  - Lie on left side, to get more oxygen to fetus.
  - Position herself in bed with pillows for optimum comfort and adequate air exchange.
  - Take frequent rest breaks during the workday.
- Carefully monitor maternal respiration during the laboring process.
- Administer pure oxygen (10 to 12 L per minute) to mother before delivery and until cessation of pulsation in cord.
- Evaluate and record the respiratory status of the newborn infant:
  - Determine the 1-minute Apgar score.
  - Suction mouth and pharynx with bulb syringe.
  - Clear mouth and oropharynx with bulb syringe.
  - Avoid deep suctioning if possible.
- Dry excess moisture off infant with towel or blanket.
- Stimulate (if necessary), using firm but gentle tactile stimulation:
  - Slapping sole of foot
  - Rubbing up and down spine
  - Flicking heel
- Maintain warm environment for infant:
  - Place infant under radiant heat warmer.
  - Place infant next to mother's skin.
  - Cover infant's head with stocking cap.
  - Cover both mother and infant with warm blanket.
- Determine and record the 5-minute Apgar score.
- Continue to evaluate infant's respiratory status and to act if necessary to resuscitate. Depending on infant's response, the following nursing measures can be taken:
  - Administer warm, humid oxygen with face mask.
  - If no improvement, administer oxygen with bag and mask.
  - If no improvement, be prepared for:
    (1) Endotracheal intubation
    (2) Ventilation with positive pressure
    (3) Cardiac massage
    (4) Transport to neonatal intensive care unit

During this stage the chest cavity has less room to expand because of the enlarging uterus.

Analgesics and anesthesia can cause maternal hypoxia and reduce fetal oxygen.

Basic care measures to ensure effective respiration in the newborn infant.

Helps stimulate infant and prevents evaporative heat loss.

Basic protocol to care for the newborn who has respiratory problems.

Mental Health

> NOTE: The following orders are for Ineffective Breathing Pattern related to Anxiety. For those problems related to physiologic problems, refer to Adult Health nursing actions.

Actions/Interventions	Rationales
• Monitor causative factors.	Provides information on client's current status so that interventions can be adapted appropriately.
• Place client in a calm, supportive environment.	Anxiety is contagious, as is calm. A calm, reassuring environment can communicate indirectly to the client that the situation is safe and that the nurse can assist him or her in mobilizing his or her internal resources, thus facilitating client's sense of control.
• Maintain a calm, supportive attitude, reassuring client that you will assist him or her in maintaining control.	
• Give client clear, concise directions.	Anxiety can decrease client's ability to focus on and understand a complex presentation of information.
• Have client maintain direct eye contact with nurse. Modulate based on client's ability to tolerate eye contact. Should not be done in a manner that appears to "stare client down."	Communicates interest in the client and assists client in tuning out extraneous stimuli.
• Instruct client to take slow, deep breaths. Demonstrate breaths to client, and practice with client. Provide client with constant, positive reinforcement for appropriate breathing patterns.	Helps to stimulate relaxation response.
• Remain with client until episode is resolved.	Reassures client of safety and security.
• If client does not respond to the attempts to control breathing, have client breathe into a paper bag.	Rebreathing air with a higher CO_2 content will slow the respiratory rate.
• Distract client from focus on breathing by beginning a deep muscle relaxation exercise that begins at client's feet.	Interrupts pattern of thought that reinforces anxiety and therefore increases breathing difficulties.
• Use successful resolution of a problematic breathing episode as an opportunity to teach client that he or she can gain conscious control over breathing and that these episodes are not out of his or her control.	Promotes client's self-esteem and perceived control. Also provides positive reinforcement for adaptive coping behaviors.
• Teach client and significant others proper breathing techniques to include: ○ Maintaining proper body alignment	Promotes perceived control and adaptive coping behaviors. Provides information that will facilitate positive reinforcement from the

- ○ Using diaphragmatic breathing (see Ineffective Airway Clearance for information on this technique)
- ○ Using deep muscle relaxation before the onset of ineffective breathing pattern begins
- Practice with client diaphragmatic breathing twice a day for 30 minutes. Note practice times here.
- Develop a plan with client for initiating slow, deep breathing when an ineffective breathing pattern begins.
- Identify with client those situations that are most frequently associated with the development of ineffective breathing patterns and assist him or her in practicing relaxation in response to these situations one time a day for 30 minutes. Note time of practice session here.

support system, increasing the probability for the success of the behavior change.[19]

Enhances relaxation response.

Early recognition of problematic situations facilitates client's ability to gain control and utilize adaptive coping behaviors.
Positive imagery promotes positive psychophysiologic responses and enhances self-esteem, promoting possibility for positive outcome.[14]

Gerontic Health

Actions/Interventions	Rationales
• Monitor respiratory rate, depth, effort, and lung sounds every 4 hours around the clock.	Minimum database needed for this diagnosis.
• Due to age-related "air trapping," have patient focus on improving expiratory effort. Instruct patient to inhale to the count of 1 and exhale for 3 counts.[20]	Decreased alveoli and decreased elasticity lead to air trapping, which results in hyperinflation of lungs.
• Collaborate with occupational therapist and respiratory therapist regarding other measures to enhance respiratory function.	Occupational therapist can teach patient less energy-expanding means to complete activities of daily living. Respiratory therapist can assist patient and family in learning how to perform pulmonary toileting at home.
• In the event of a chronic Ineffective Breathing Pattern, refer the patient to a support group such as those sponsored by the American Lung Association.	Provides long-term support for coping with problems; provides updated information; provides role modeling from group's other members.
• Instruct in relaxation techniques, for example, guided imagery or progressive muscle relaxation, to reduce stress.	May assist in decreasing the episodes of acute breathing problems in those with chronic ineffective breathing pattern.
• Where applicable, monitor for knowledge of proper medication use, especially if inhalers are a part of the therapy.	Maximum benefit may be derived from proper drug administration and usage. Inhalers may be difficult to operate due to physical problems and lack of information regarding proper usage.

Home Health

NOTE: If this diagnosis is suspected when caring for a patient in the home, it is imperative that a physician referral be obtained immediately. If the patient has been referred to home health care by a physician, the nurse will collaborate with the physician in the treatment of the patient.

Actions/Interventions	Rationales
• Teach client and family appropriate monitoring of signs and symptoms of Ineffective Breathing Pattern: ○ Cough ○ Sputum production ○ Fatigue ○ Respiratory status: cyanosis, dyspnea, and rate ○ Lack of diaphragmatic breathing ○ Nasal flaring ○ Anxiety or restlessness ○ Impaired speech	Provides for early recognition and intervention for problem.

• Assist client and family in identifying life-style changes that may be required in assisting to prevent ineffective breathing pattern:
○ Stopping smoking
○ Preventing and early treatment of lung infections
○ Avoiding known irritants and allergens
○ Practicing pulmonary hygiene:
  (1) Clearing bronchial tree by controlled coughing
  (2) Decreasing viscosity of secretions via humidity and fluid balance
  (3) Clearing postural drainage
○ Treatment of fear, anxiety, anger, depression, thorax trauma, or narcotic overdoses
○ Adequate nutritional intake
○ Stress management
○ Adequate hydration
○ Breathing techniques (diaphragmatic and/or pursed lips)
○ Progressive ambulation
○ Pain relief
○ Preventing hazards of immobility
○ Appropriate use of oxygen (dosage, route, and safety factors)
	Provides basic information for client and family that promotes necessary life-style changes.

- Teach patient and family purposes, side effects, and proper administration techniques of medication.
- Assist client and family in setting criteria to help them determine when physician or other intervention is required.

    Locus of control shifts from nurse to client and family, thus promoting self-care.

- Teach family basic CPR.

FLOW CHART EVALUATION
Flow Chart Expected Outcome 1

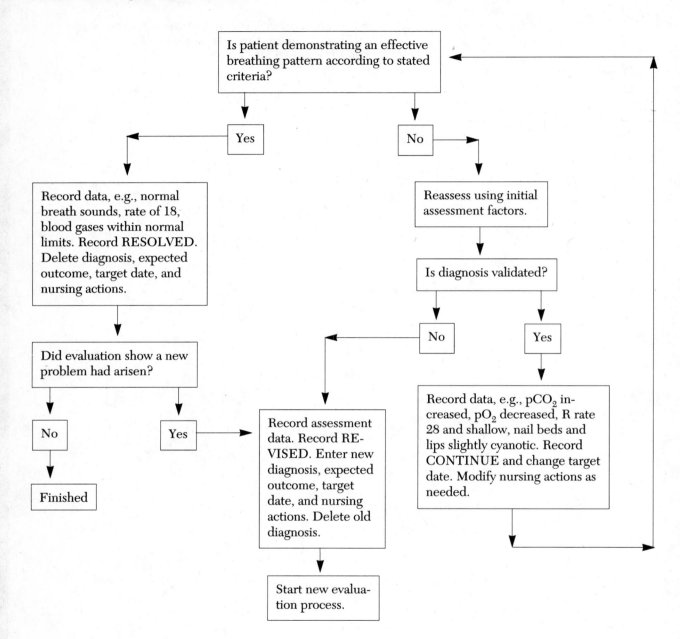

Flow Chart Expected Outcome 2

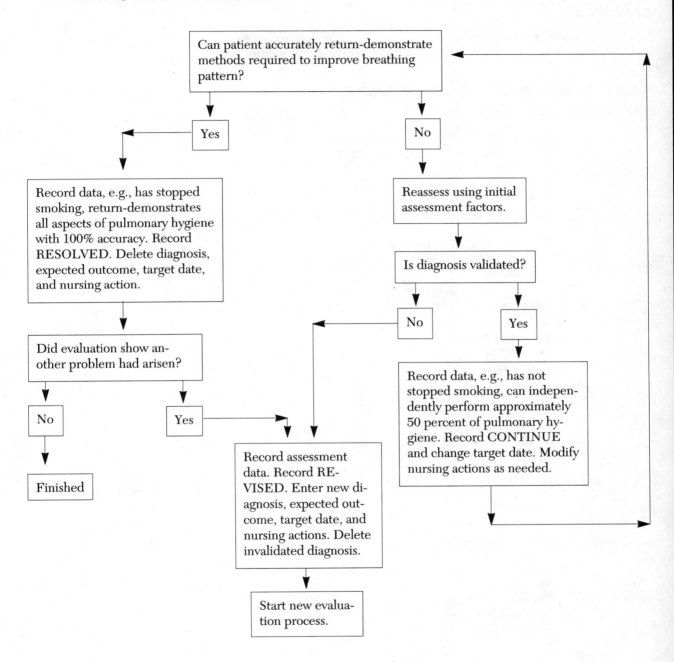

Cardiac Output, Decreased

DEFINITION

A state in which the blood pumped by an individual's heart is sufficiently reduced that it is inadequate to meet the needs of the body's tissues.[10]

NANDA TAXONOMY: EXCHANGING 1.4.2.1

DEFINING CHARACTERISTICS[10]

1. Major defining characteristics:
   a. Variations in blood pressure readings
   b. Arrhythmias
   c. Fatigue
   d. Jugular vein distention
   e. Color changes, skin and mucous membranes
   f. Oliguria
   g. Decreased peripheral pulses
   h. Cold, clammy skin
   i. Rales
   j. Dyspnea, orthopnea
2. Other possible characteristics:
   a. Change in mental status
   b. Shortness of breath
   c. Syncope
   d. Vertigo
   e. Edema
   f. Cough
   g. Frothy sputum
   h. Gallop rhythm
   i. Weakness

RELATED FACTORS

To be developed.

RELATED CLINICAL CONCERNS

1. Congestive heart failure
2. Myocardial infarction
3. Valvular heart disease
4. Inflammatory heart disease, for example, pericarditis
5. Hypertension
6. Shock
7. Chronic obstructive pulmonary disease

HAVE YOU SELECTED THE CORRECT DIAGNOSIS?

Altered Tissue Perfusion   Decreased Cardiac Output relates specifically to a heart malfunction, while Altered Tissue Perfusion relates to deficits in the peripheral circulation which will have cellular-level impact. Tissue perfusion problems may develop secondary to decreased cardiac output but can also exist without cardiac output problems.[21] (See page 484.)

In either diagnosis, close collaboration will be needed with medical practitioners to ensure the best possible interventions for the patient.

EXPECTED OUTCOME

1. Will exhibit no signs or symptoms of decreased cardiac output by (date) and/or
2. Will implement a self-designed plan to decrease the likelihood of future decreased cardiac output episodes by (date)

TARGET DATE

Because the nursing diagnosis Decreased Cardiac Output is life-threatening, progress toward meeting the expected outcomes should be evaluated at least daily for 3 to 5 days. If significant progress is demonstrated, then the target date can be increased to 3-day intervals. Patients who develop this diagnosis should be referred to a medical practitioner immediately and transferred to a critical care unit.

ADDITIONAL INFORMATION

Cardiac output refers to the amount of blood ejected from the left ventricle into the aorta per minute. Cardiac output (CO) is equivalent to the stroke volume (SV), which is the amount of blood ejected from the left ventricle with each contraction times the heart rate (HR), or the number of beats per minute.

$$CO = SV \times HR$$

The average amount of cardiac output is 5.6 L per minute. This amount will vary according to the individual's amount of exercise and body size.

Cardiac output is dependent on the relationship between stroke volume and the heart rate. Cardiac output is maintained by compensatory adjustment of these two variables. If the rate slows, the time for ventricular filling (diastole) increases. This allows for an increase in the preload and a subsequent increase in stroke volume. If the stroke volume falls, the heart rate increases to compensate. Stroke volume is affected by preload, contractility, and afterload.

Preload is related to the amount of stretching of the myocardial fibers. The fibers stretch due to the increase in the volume of blood delivered to the ventricles during diastole. The degree of myocardial stretch before contraction is preload. Preload is determined by the venous return and ejection fraction (amount of blood left in the ventricle at the end of systole). Prolonged excessive stretching will lead to a decrease in cardiac output.

Contractility is a function of the intensity of the actinomycin linkages. Increased contractility increases ventricular emptying and results in increased stroke volume. Contractility can be increased by sympathetic stimulation or by administration of such drugs as calcium and epinephrine. Afterload is the amount of tension developed by the ventricle during contraction. The amount of peripheral resistance will predominantly determine the amount of tension. Excessive increases in the afterload will reduce stroke volume and cardiac output.

The heart rate is predominantly influenced by the autonomic nervous system through both the sympathetic and parasympathetic nervous systems. The sympathetic fibers can increase both rate and force, while the parasympathetic fibers act in an opposite direction. Other factors such as the central nervous system pressoreceptor reflexes, cerebral cortex impulses, body temperature, electrolytes, and hormones also affect the heart rate, but the autonomic nervous system keeps the entire system in balance.[22]

NURSING ACTIONS/INTERVENTIONS WITH RATIONALES

Adult Health

Actions/Interventions	Rationales
• Place on cardiac monitor and continuously monitor cardiac rhythm and rate.	Compromises to cardiac output and myocardial perfusion can be more accurately assessed.
• Monitor, at least every 2 hours on the (odd/even) hour: ○ Vital signs ○ Chest and heart sounds ○ Apical-radial pulse deficit ○ Pedal pulses ○ Pulse pressure ○ Other hemodynamic readings [for example, wedge pressures, PAP, PCWP, central venous pressure (CVP)] ○ Neck vein filling ○ Peripheral edema (extremities, eyelids, or sacral areas) ○ Level of consciousness ○ Activity intolerance ○ Mental status ○ Skin changes ○ Peripheral pulses ○ Liver position	Establishes baseline and allows for accurate monitoring of changes from baselines.
• Collaborate with physician regarding frequency of measurement of the following and closely monitor results: ○ Arterial blood gases ○ Electrolytes ○ Cardiac enzymes	Additional baseline data needed for accurate monitoring of condition.

- ○ Complete blood cell count
- ○ Electrolyte balance
- Explain reasons for tests and monitoring to patient as well as the role he or she plays in ensuring accurate results.
- Administer oxygen and medications as ordered, and monitor effects.
- Monitor flow rate of oxygen.
- Measure urinary output hourly.

- Measure and record intake and total at least every 8 hours. Collaborate with physician regarding limitation of intake.
- Monitor pain, and institute immediate relief measures.
- Keep siderails up and bed in low position particularly during periods of altered mental status.
- Weigh daily at (time) and in same-weight clothing.
- Provide skin care at least every 2 hours on the (odd/even) hour:
  - ○ Change position and support in anatomical alignment.
  - ○ Elevate edematous extremities and use measures such as a bed cradle to keep pressure off edematous parts.
  - ○ Use sheepskin, egg crate mattress, or alternating air mattress under patient.
  - ○ Keep linens free of wrinkles.
  - ○ Keep skin clean and dry. Avoid shearing forces in patient movement.
  - ○ Use cornstarch on bed and skin to facilitate patient's movement.
- Do range-of-motion exercises at least once per shift and position patient carefully.

- Monitor intravenous therapy:
  - ○ Flow rate
  - ○ Insertion site
- Provide adequate rest periods:
  - ○ Schedule at least 5-minute rest after any activity.
  - ○ Schedule 30- to 60- minute rest period after each meal.
- Limit visitors and visiting time. Explain need for restriction to patient and significant others. If presence of significant other promotes rest, allow to stay beyond time limits.

Decreases anxiety and promotes more accurate monitoring results.

Enhances myocardial perfusion and decreases work load.

Fluid overload or underload can compromise cardiac output.

Pain can increase cardiac output; relief measures also decrease anxiety.
Basic patient safety.

Helps to determine changes in fluid volume.

Promotes tissue perfusion; decreases pressure area, thus decreasing the likelihood of impaired tissue integrity.

Promotes circulation; reduces consequences of impaired mobility. Careful positioning assists breathing and avoids pressure.
Prevents fluid overload or underload; monitor for patency of veins and for presence of infection.
Decreases stress on already stressed circulatory system.

Continued

Actions/Interventions	Rationales
• Monitor bowel elimination, abdominal distention, and bowel sounds at least once per shift during waking hours. Collaborate with physician regarding stool softener.	Avoids straining and Valsalva maneuver, which compromise cardiac output.
• Assist patient with stress management and relaxation techniques every 4 hours while awake (state times here). Support patient in usual coping mechanisms.	Decreases anxiety and promotes cardiac output.
• Plan to spend at least 15 minutes every 4 hours providing emotional support to patient and significant others.	Decreases anxiety.
• Collaborate with dietitian regarding dietary restrictions when developing plan of care and reinforce prior to discharge (for example, sodium, fluids, calories, and cholesterol).	These dietary factors can compromise cardiac output.
• Collaborate with occupational therapist and family regarding diversional activities. Refer to: ○ Physical therapist for home exercise program ○ Visiting nurse service	Promotes collaboration and holistic care.

Child Health

Actions/Interventions	Rationales
• Provide in-depth monitoring and documentation related to: ○ Ventilator if applicable: 　(1) If continuous positive airway pressure (CPAP) set according to physician's order 　(2) Peak pressure as ordered 　(3) O_2 percentage desired as ordered ○ Intake and output hourly and as ordered (Notify physician if below 10 ml per hour or as specified for size of infant or child.) ○ Excessive bleeding (If in postop status, notify physician if above 50 ml per hour or as specified.) ○ Tolerance of feedings ○ Notify physician for: 　(1) Premature ventricular contractions (PVCs) or other arrhythmias	These factors constitute the basic measures utilized in monitoring for decompensation of cardiac status. Closely related are respiratory function, hydration status, and hemodynamic status.

(2) Limits of pulse, respiratory rate, output criteria as specified for individual patient

○ Use caution in the administration of medications as ordered, especially digoxin:

(1) Have another RN check dose and medication order.

(2) Validate heart rate to be greater than specified lower-limit parameter (for example, 100 for infant before administering) and documentation of the heart rate.

○ Document if medication withheld because of heart rate.

○ Monitor for signs and symptoms of toxicity, for example, vomiting.

○ Ensure potassium maintenance; collaborate with physician regarding frequency of serum potassium measurement and immediately report results.

○ Maintain digitalizing protocol.

○ Ensure parental understanding of patient's status and treatment.

○ Monitor patient's response to suctioning, x-ray, or other procedures.

- Ensure availability of crash cart and emergency equipment as needed to include:
  ○ Cardiac or emergency drugs
  ○ Defibrillator
  ○ Ambu bag (pedi or infant size)
  ○ Appropriate suctioning equipment

Standard nursing care includes availability and appropriate use of equipment and medications in event of cardiac arrest. Anticipation for need of equipment with a child in high-risk status is required.

- Allow for parents to voice concern on a regular basis; set aside 10 to 15 minutes per shift for this purpose.

Verbalization of concerns helps reduce anxiety. Attempts to set aside time for this verbalization demonstrates the value it holds for the patient's care.

- Encourage parental input in care, such as with feeding, positioning, and monitoring intake and output as appropriate.

Parental input assists in meeting parent's and child's emotional needs for love and augments the care of others. This action also allows for learning essential skills in a supportive environment.

- Encourage patient as applicable to participate in care.

Self-care enhances sense of autonomy and empowerment.

- Allow for sensitivity to time and understanding of diagnosis and seemingly abstract nature of underlying cardiac physiology, especially in noncyanotic heart disease.

Abstract aspects of an illness often prove more difficult to grasp. Congenital cardiac anomalies are often complex in nature, which requires health care personnel to use consistent terms and offer appropriate aids to depict key issues of anatomy.

Continued

Actions/Interventions	Rationales
• Support parents in usual appropriate coping mechanisms.	Emotional security may be afforded by encouragement of usual coping mechanisms for age and developmental status.
• Maintain appropriate technique in dressing change (asepsis and cautious handwashing).	Standard care requires universal precautions to minimize risk factors for infection.
• Limit visitors in immediate postoperative status as applicable.	Visitation may prove overwhelming to all when unlimited in immediate postoperative period. Remember that numerous nursing-medical therapies must be attended to during this time also.
• Help reduce patient and parental anxiety by touching and allowing patient to be held and comforted.	Comforting allows parent and child to feel more secure and will decrease feeling of intimidation parents might perceive from numerous pieces of equipment and activity. Human caring helps offset high tech.
• Provide teaching with sensitivity to patient and parental needs regarding equipment, procedures, or routines, for example, use a doll for demonstration with toddler.	Individualized teaching with appropriate aids will most likely serve to reinforce desired learning and enlist the patient's cooperation.
• Encourage parents to meet parents of similarly involved cardiac patients.	Sharing with similarly involved clientele or families affords a sense of unity, hope, and affirmation of the future far beyond what nurses or others may offer.
• Address need for parents to continue with activities of daily living with confidence regarding knowledge of restrictions in child's status.	Aim should be for normalcy within parameters dictated by the child's condition. Strive to refrain family from labeling child or encouraging child to become a "cardiac cripple."

Women's Health

Actions/Interventions	Rationales
• Assist patient with relaxation techniques.	Assists in stress reduction.

NOTE: Caution the patient never to begin a new vigorous exercise plan while pregnant. Teach the patient to exercise slowly, in moderation, and according to the individual's ability. A good rule of thumb is to use moderation and, with the consent of the physician, continue with the prepregnant established exercise plan. Most professionals discourage aerobics and hot tubs or spas because of the heat. It is not known at this time if overheating by the mother is harmful to the fetus.

• Assist in developing an exercise plan for cardiovascular fitness during pregnancy. Some good exercises are: ○ Swimming ○ Walking	Assists in increasing cardiovascular fitness during pregnancy.

- ○ Bicycling
- ○ Jogging (If patient has done this before and is used to it, she may continue, *but* remember that during pregnancy joints and muscles are more susceptible to strain. If patient feels pain, fatigue, or overheating, she should slow down or stop exercise.)
- Refer patient to support groups that understand the physiology of pregnancy and have developed exercise programs based on this physiology, such as swimming classes for pregnant women at the local YWCA, childbirth education classes, or the exercise videotapes produced by the American College of Obstetricians and Gynecologists (available through ASPO/Lamaze, Post Office Box 952, McLean, VA 22101).
- Teach patient and significant others how to avoid "supine hypotension" during pregnancy (particularly the later stages).

The expanded uterus causes pressure on the large blood vessels.

- Prior to the start of labor, encourage patient to attend childbirth education classes to learn how to work with her body during labor.
- During the second stage of labor:
  - ○ Allow patient to assume whatever position aids her in the second stage of labor (for example, upright, squatting, kneeling position, etc.).
  - ○ Provide patient with proper physical support during the second stage of labor. Such actions might include allowing the partner or support person to sit or stand beside her and support her head or shoulders, or to stand behind her supporting her with his or her body. Other actions might include standing in front of her, allowing her to lean on his or her shoulders with her arms about his or her neck. Supportive equipment can include a birthing bed or chair, pillows, over-the-bed table, or bars.
- *Do not* urge the woman to "push, push" or to hold her breath during the second stage of labor. Allow the woman to bear down with her contractions at her own pace:
  - ○ Keeping pelvic floor muscles relaxed

Avoids straining and the Valsalva maneuver.

Continued

Actions/Interventions	Rationales
○ Keeping shoulders rounded forward ○ Keeping chin tucked against chest ○ Pressing and rounding (rocking pelvis) lower back ○ Encouraging spontaneous, even breathing patterns that flow with the contractions and allow pushing with the diaphragm while relaxing abdominal muscles.[23]	

Mental Health

Actions/Interventions	Rationales
• Monitor risk factors: ○ Medications ○ Past history of cardiac problems ○ Age ○ Current condition of the cardiovascular system ○ Weight ○ Exercise patterns ○ Nutritional patterns ○ Psychosocial stressors	Early identification and intervention help assure better outcome.
• Monitor every (number) hours (depends on level or risk, can be anywhere from 2 to 8 hours) client's cardiac functioning (list times to observe here): ○ Vital signs ○ Chest sounds ○ Apical-radical pulse deficit ○ Mental status	Basic database for further intervention.
• Report alterations to medical practitioner immediately.	
• If acute situation develops, notify medical practitioner and implement adult health nursing actions.	
• If client's condition or other factors necessitate client remaining in the mental health area beyond the acute stage, refer to Adult Health nursing actions for care on an ongoing basis. This is not recommended due to the lack of equipment and properly trained staff to care for this situation on most specialized care units.	
• If client is placed on the psychiatric care unit while in the rehabilitation stage of the	Promotes client's perceived control and supports self-care activities.

decreased cardiac output diagnosis, implement the following nursing actions: Discuss with client current rehabilitation schedule, and record special consideration here.

- Provide appropriate rest periods following activity. This varies according to the client's stage in rehabilitation. Most common times of needed rest are after meals and after any activity. (Note specific limits here.)

- Assist client with implementation of exercise program. List types of activity, time spent in activity, and times of activity here. Also list special motivators the client may need, such as a companion to walk for 30 minutes three times a day at (times).

- Provide meals that adhere to diet restrictions, for example, low sodium, low calorie, low fat, low cholesterol, or fluid restrictions.

- Monitor intake and output each shift.

- Assess for and teach client to assess for:
  ○ Potassium loss (muscle cramps)
  ○ Chest pain
  ○ Dyspnea
  ○ Sudden weight gain
  ○ Decreased urine output
  ○ Increased fatigue

- Assess increased risk factors, and assist client in developing a plan to reduce these, for example, smoking, obesity, and stress— refer to appropriate nursing diagnosis for assistance in developing interventions.

- Spend 30 minutes twice a day teaching client deep muscle relaxation and practicing this process (list times here).

- Discuss with support system the life-style alterations.

- Develop stress reduction program with client, and provide necessary environment for implementation. This could include massage therapy, meditation, aerobic exercise as tolerated, hobbies, music, and so on. (Note specific plan here.)

Prevents excessive stress on the cardiovascular system and prevents fatigue.

Promotes cardiovascular strength and well-being.

Decreases dietary contributions to increased risk factors.

Medications can impact fluid balance, and excessive fluid can increase demands on the cardiovascular system.
Increases client's perceived control and promotes early recognition and treatment of problem.

Increases client's perceived control and decreases risk for further damage to the cardiovascular system.

Relaxation decreases stress on the cardiovascular system.

Enhances possibility for continuation of behavior change.[19]

Gerontic Health

Actions/Interventions	Rationales

• Monitor for possible side effects of diuretic therapy.
• Review the health history for liver or kidney disease in patients on diuretic therapy.
• Whenever possible, give diuretics in the morning.
 	
• Teach proper medication usage, for example, dosage, side effects, dangers related to missed doses, and food-drug interactions.
• Teach patients who are on potassium-wasting diuretics:
  ○ The need for potassium replacement
  ○ Foods that are high in potassium, for example, bananas
  ○ Signs and symptoms of potassium depletion
• Assist patient and/or family to determine environmental conditions that may need to be adapted to promote energy.
	Older adults may have excessive diuresis on normal diuretic dosage.
	Diuretics may need to have adjusted dosages in those with preexisting kidney or hepatic disease to avoid complications.
	Decreases problems with nocturia and consequent distributed sleep-rest pattern or high risk for injury from falls.
	Basic safety for medication administration.
	
	Assists in conservation of energy and balancing oxygen demands with resources.[17]

Home Health

> NOTE: If this diagnosis is suspected when caring for a client in the home, it is imperative that a physician referral be obtained immediately. If the client has been referred to home health care by a physician, the nurse will collaborate with the physician in the treatment of the client.

Actions/Interventions	Rationales

• Teach patient and significant others:
  ○ Risk factors, for example, smoking, hypertension, and obesity
  ○ Medication regimen, for example, toxicity and effects
  ○ Need to balance rest and activity
  ○ Monitoring of:
    (1) Weight (daily)
    (2) Vital signs
    (3) Intake and output
  ○ When to contact health care personnel:
    (1) Chest pain
    (2) Dyspnea
	Provides for early recognition and intervention for problem.

    (3) Sudden weight gain
    (4) Decreased urine output
    (5) Increased fatigue
  ○ Dietary adaptations, as necessary:
    (1) Low sodium
    (2) Low cholesterol
    (3) Caloric restriction
    (4) Soft foods

- Assist patient and family in identifying life-style changes that may be required:
  - Eliminating smoking
  - Cardiac rehabilitation program
  - Stress management
  - Weight control
  - Dietary restrictions
  - Decreased alcohol
  - Relaxation techniques
  - Bowel regimen to avoid straining and constipation
  - Maintenance of fluid and electrolyte balance
  - Changes in role functions in family
  - Concerns regarding sexual activity
  - Monitoring activity and responses to activity. (*Note:* Level of damage to left ventricle should be determined before exercise program is initiated.[24])
  - Providing diversional activities when physical activity is restricted. (See Diversional Activity Deficit.)
  - Pain control.

    Provides basic information for client and family that promotes necessary life-style changes.

- Teach family basic CPR.
- Teach client and family purposes and side effects of medications and proper administration techniques.

    Locus of control shifts from nurse to client and family, thus promoting self-care.

- Teach client and family to refrain from activities that increase the demands on the heart, for example, snow shoveling, lifting, Valsalva maneuver.
- Assist client and family in setting criteria to help them determine when a physician or other intervention is required.

    Provides additional support for client and family and uses already available resources in a cost-effective manner.

- Consult with or refer to appropriate assistive resources as indicated. (See Appendix B.)

FLOW CHART EVALUATION
Flow Chart Expected Outcome 1

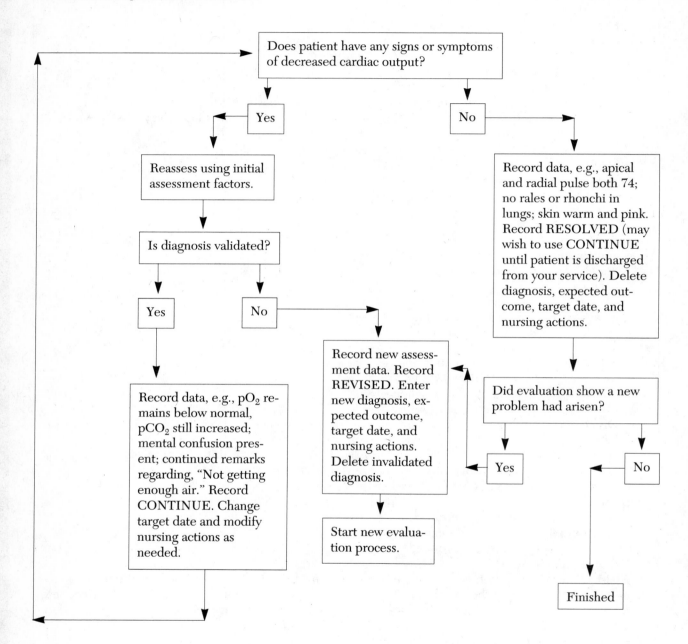

Flow Chart Expected Outcome 2

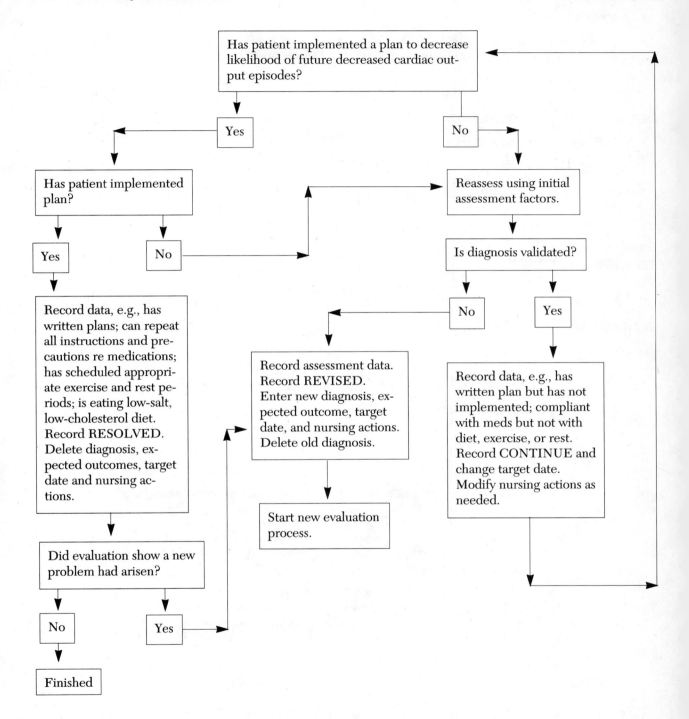

Disuse Syndrome, High Risk for

DEFINITION

A state in which an individual is at risk for deterioration of body systems as the result of prescribed or unavoidable musculoskeletal inactivity.[10]*

NANDA TAXONOMY: EXCHANGING 1.6.1.5

DEFINING CHARACTERISTICS[10]

Presence of risk factors such as:

1. Paralysis
2. Mechanical immobilization
3. Prescribed immobilization
4. Severe pain
5. Altered level of consciousness

RELATED FACTORS[10]

The risk factors also serve as the related factors.

RELATED CLINICAL CONCERNS

1. Cerebrovascular accident
2. Fractures
3. Closed head injury
4. Spinal cord injury or paralysis
5. Rheumatoid arthritis
6. Amputation
7. Cerebral palsy

HAVE YOU SELECTED THE CORRECT DIAGNOSIS?

Activity Intolerance   This diagnosis implies that the individual is freely able to move but cannot endure or adapt to the increased energy or oxygen demands made by the movement or activity. (See page 327.)

Impaired Physical Mobility   With this diagnosis the individual could move independently if something were not limiting the motion. Impaired Physical Mobility could very well be a predisposing factor to High Risk for Disuse Syndrome. (See page 460.)

---

*Complications from immobility can include pressure ulcer, constipation, stasis of pulmonary secretions, thrombosis, urinary tract infection or retention, decreased strength or endurance, orthostatic hypotension, decreased range of joint motion, disorientation, body image disturbance, and powerlessness.

EXPECTED OUTCOME

1. Will exhibit no signs or symptoms of disuse syndrome by (date) and/or
2. Will demonstrate (specify activities) to prevent development of disuse syndrome by (date)

TARGET DATE

Disuse syndrome can develop rapidly after the onset of immobilization. The initial target date, therefore, should be no more than 2 days.

NURSING ACTIONS/INTERVENTIONS WITH RATIONALES

Adult Health

Actions/Interventions	Rationales
• Monitor for contributing factors to pattern of disuse.	Can offset development of Disuse Syndrome or worsening of condition.
• According to patient's status, determine realistic potential and actual levels of functioning with regard to general physical condition: ○ Cognition ○ Mobility, head control, or positioning ○ Communication: receptive and expressive, verbal or nonverbal ○ Augmentive aids for daily living	Improves planning and allows for setting of more realistic goals.
• Turn and anatomically position patient every 2 hours on the (odd/even) hour.	
• Perform active and passive range-of-motion exercises to all joints at least twice a shift while awake. State times here.	Promotes circulation, prevents venous stasis, and helps to prevent thrombosis.
• Teach patient relaxation and pain reduction techniques every shift and have patient return-demonstrate.	Relaxes muscles and promotes circulation.
• Demonstrate and have patient return-demonstrate isotonic exercises.	Helps avoid syndrome; offsets complications of immobility.
• Encourage patient to perform isotonic exercises at least every 4 hours at (state times here).	
• Arrange daily activities with appropriate regard for rest as needed.	
• Maintain adequate nutrition and fluid balance on daily basis.	Provides fluid and nutrients necessary for activity.
• Orient patient to environment as necessary.	Maintains mental activity and reality.
• Monitor patient and family for perceived and actual health teaching needs, including: ○ Patient's status ○ Patient's daily care	Initiates appropriate home care planning.

Continued

Actions/Interventions	Rationales
○ Equipment required for patient's care ○ Signs or symptoms to be reported to physician ○ Medication administration, instructions, and side effects ○ Plans for follow-up • Refer to Impaired Physical Mobility for more detailed nursing actions.	

Child Health

Actions/Interventions	Rationales
• Assist family in development of an individualized plan of care to best meet child's potential. • Assist family in identification of factors that will facilitate progress as well as those factors that may hinder progress in meeting child's potentials. List those factors here, and assist family in planning how to offset factors that hinder progress and encourage factors that facilitate progress. • Encourage patient and family to vent feelings that may relate to disuse problem by scheduling of 15 to 20 minutes each nursing shift for this activity. • Assist family in identification of support system for best possible follow-up care. (See Appendix B.)	Family is the best source for individual preferences and needs as they can related to what daily living for the child involves. Identifies learning needs and reduces anxiety. Fosters a plan that can be adhered to if all involved participate in its development; empowers family. Venting of feelings assists in reducing anxiety and promotes learning about condition. Promotes coordination of care and cost-effective use of already available resources.

Women's Health

This nursing diagnosis will pertain to women the same as to men. Refer to nursing actions for the other sections to meet the needs of women with the diagnosis of High Risk for Disuse Syndrome.

Mental Health

NOTE: The nursing actions in this section reflect the High Risk for Disuse Syndrome related to mental health. This would include use of restraints and seclusion. If the inactivity is related to a physiologic or physical problem, refer to the adult health nursing actions.

Actions/Interventions	Rationales
• Attempt all other interventions before considering immobilizing the client. (See High Risk for Violence, Chapter 9, for appropriate actions).	Promotes client's perceived control and self-esteem.
• Carefully monitor client for appropriate level of restraint necessary. Immobilize the client as little as possible while still protecting the client and others.	Client safety is of primary importance while maintaining, as much as possible, client's perceived control and self-esteem.
• Obtain necessary medical orders to initiate methods that limit the client's physical mobility.	Provides protection of client's rights. This should be done in congruence with the state's legal requirements.
• Carefully explain to client, in brief, concise language, reasons for initiating the intervention and what behavior must be present for the intervention to be terminated.	High levels of anxiety interfere with the client's ability to process complex information. Maintains relationship and promotes client's perceived control.
• Attempt to gain client's voluntary compliance with the intervention by explaining to client what is needed and with a "show of force" (having the necessary number of staff available to force compliance if the client does not respond to the request).	Communicates to client that staff have the ability to maintain control over the situation and provides client with an opportunity to maintain perceived control and self-esteem.
• Initiate forced compliance only if there are an adequate number of staff to complete the action safely. (See High Risk for Violence for a detailed description of intervention with forced compliance.)	Staff and client safety are of primary importance.
• Secure the environment the client will be in by removing harmful objects such as accessible light bulbs, sharp objects, glass objects, tight clothing, metal objects, shower curtain rods, and so on.	Provides safe environment by removing those objects client could use to impulsively harm self.
• If client is placed in four-point restraints, maintain one-to-one supervision.	Promotes client safety and communicates maintenance of relationship while meeting security needs.
• If client is in seclusion or in bilateral restraints, observe client at least every 15 minutes, more frequently if agitated. (List observation schedule here.)	Assures client safety.
• Leave urinal in room with client or offer toileting every hour.	Meets client's physiological needs and communicates respect for the individual.
• Offer client fluids every 15 minutes while awake.	
• Discuss with client his or her feelings about the initiation of immobility, and review at least twice a day the kinds of behavior necessary to have immobility discontinued (note behaviors here).	Promotes client's regaining control and clearly provides the client with alternative behaviors for coping.

Continued

Actions/Interventions	Rationales
• When checking client, let him or her know you are checking by calling him or her by name and orienting him or her to day and time. Inquire about client's feelings, and implement necessary reality orientation.	Promotes sense of security and provides information about client's mental status that will provide information for further interventions.
• Provide meals at regular intervals on paper containers, providing necessary assistance (amount and type of assistance required should be listed here).	Meets physiological needs while maintaining client safety.
• If client is in restraints, remove restraints at least every 2 hours one limb at a time. Have client move limb through a full range of motion and inspect for signs of injury. Apply lubricants such as lotion to area under restraint to protect from injury.	Maintains adequate blood flow to the skin and prevents breakdown. Maintains joint mobility and prevents contractures and muscle atrophy.
• Pad the area of the restraint that is next to the skin with sheepskin or other nonirritating material.	Protects skin from mechanical irritation from the restraint.
• Check circulation in restrained limbs in the area below the restraint by observing skin color, warmth, and swelling. Restraint should not interfere with circulation.	Early assessment and intervention prevents long-term damage.
• Change client's position in bed every 2 hours on the (odd/even) hour. Have client cough and deep-breathe during this time.	Protects skin from ischemic and shearing pressure damage. Promotes normal clearing of airway secretions.
• Place body in proper alignment to prevent complications and injury. Use pillows for support if client's condition allows.	
• If client is in four-point restraints, place on stomach or side or elevate head of bed.	Prevents aspiration or choking.
• Place client on intake and output monitoring to ensure adequate fluid balance is maintained.	Promotes normal hydration, which prevents thickening of airway secretions and thrombus formation.[25]
• Have client in seclusion move around the room at least every 2 hours on the (odd/even) hour. During this time initiate active range of motion and have client cough and take deep breaths.	Assesses client's risk for the development of orthostatic hypotension.
• Administer medications as ordered for agitation.	
• Monitor blood pressure before administering antipsychotic medications.	
• Have client change position slowly, especially from lying to standing.	The combination of immobility and antipsychotic medications can place the client at risk for the development of orthostatic hypotension. Slowing position change allows time for blood pressure to adjust and prevents dizziness and fainting.

- Assist client with daily personal hygiene.
- Have environment cleaned on a daily basis.
- Remove client from seclusion as soon as the contracted behavior is observed for the required amount of time. (Both of these should be very specific and listed here. See High Risk for Violence, Chapter 9, for detailed information on behavior change and contracting specifics.)
- Schedule time to discuss this intervention with client and his or her support system. Inform support system of the need for the intervention and about special considerations related to visiting with the client. This information must be provided with consideration of the support system before and after each visit.

Gives client a sense of control.
Communicates respect for the client.
Promotes client's perception of control and provides positive reinforcement for appropriate behavior.

Promotes family understanding and optimizes potential for positive client response.[19]

Gerontic Health

Actions/Interventions	Rationales
• Monitor for iatrogenesis, especially in the case of institutionalized elderly.	Although OBRA regulations require the least restrictive measures and, ideally, restraint-free care, older adults in long-term care may be placed at risk for Disuse Syndrome secondary to geri-chairs, use of wheelchairs, and lack of properly functioning or fitted adaptive equipment. Additionally there may be reluctance to prescribed occupational therapy or physical therapy based on costs.
• Advocate for older adults to ensure inactivity is not based on ageist perspectives.	Health care providers may be reluctant to ensure early mobilization in older patients, especially the old-old clientele.
• In the event of impaired cognitive function, remind of need for and assist the patient (or caregiver) in mobilizing efforts.	Prompting may encourage increased activity and decreased risk for disuse.

Home Health

Actions/Interventions	Rationales

• Teach client and family appropriate monitoring of causes, signs, and symptoms of High Risk for Disuse Syndrome:
  ○ Prolonged bed rest
  ○ Circulatory or respiratory problems
	Provides for early recognition and intervention for problem.

Continued

Actions/Interventions	Rationales

○ New activity
  ○ Fatigue
  ○ Dyspnea
  ○ Pain
  ○ Vital signs (before and after activity)
  ○ Malnutrition
  ○ Previous inactivity
  ○ Weakness
  ○ Confusion
  ○ Fracture
  ○ Paralysis	

• Assist client and family in identifying life-style changes that may be required:
  ○ Progressive exercise to increase endurance
  ○ Range-of-motion and flexibility exercises
  ○ Treatment for underlying conditions (cardiac, respiratory, musculoskeletal, circulatory, neurologic, and so on)
  ○ Motivation
  ○ Assistive devices as required (walkers, canes, crutches, wheelchairs, ramps, wheelchair access, and so on)
  ○ Adequate nutrition
  ○ Adequate fluids
  ○ Stress management
  ○ Pain relief
  ○ Prevention of hazards of immobility (for example, antiembolism stockings, range-of-motion exercises, or position changes)
  ○ Changes in occupations, family, or social roles
  ○ Changes in living conditions
  ○ Economic concerns
  ○ Proper transfer techniques
  ○ Bowel and bladder regulation
	Provides basic information for client and family that promotes necessary lifestyle changes.

• Teach client and family purposes and side effects of medications and proper administration techniques (for example, anticoagulants or analgesics).	Locus of control shifts from nurse to client and family, thus promoting self-care.
• Assist client and family in setting criteria to help them determine when physician or other intervention is required.	
• Consult with or refer to appropriate resources as indicated. (See Appendix B.)	Provides additional support for client and family and uses already available resources in a cost-effective manner.

FLOW CHART EVALUATION
Flow Chart Expected Outcome 1

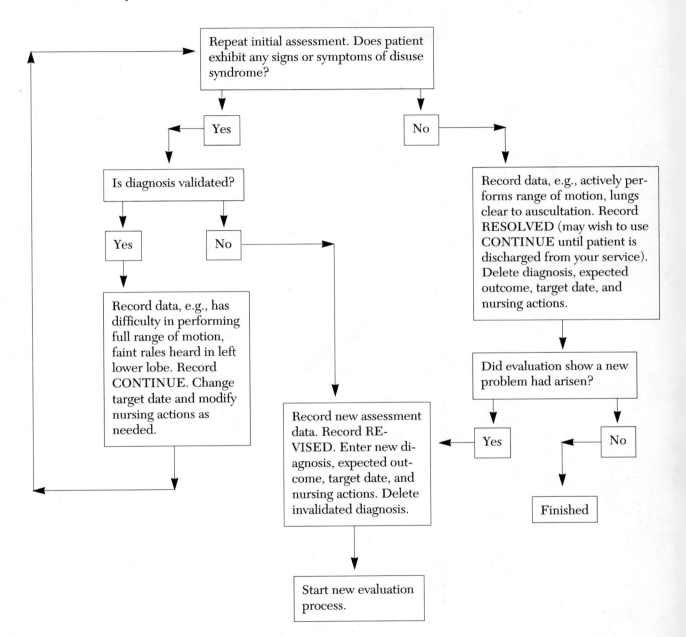

Flow Chart Expected Outcome 2

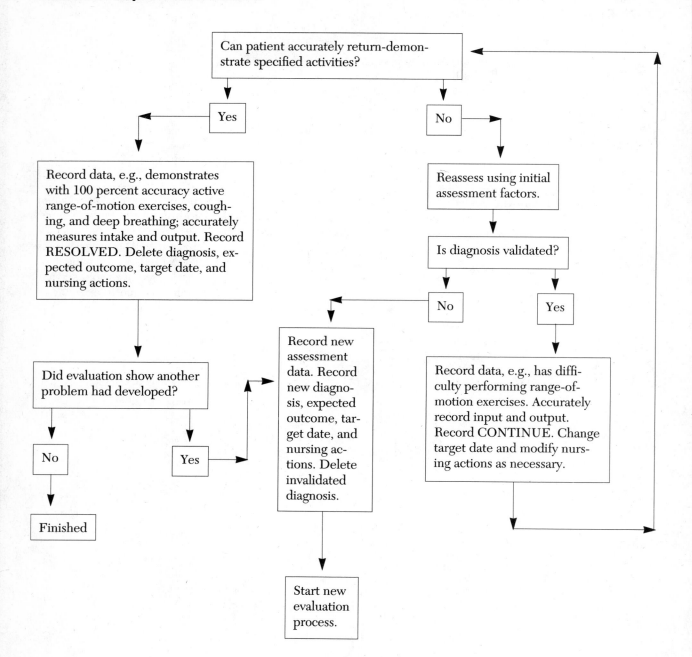

Diversional Activity Deficit

DEFINITION

The state in which an individual experiences a decreased stimulation from or interest or engagement in recreational or leisure activities.[10]

NANDA TAXONOMY: MOVING 6.3.1.1

DEFINING CHARACTERISTICS[10]

1. Major defining characteristics:
   a. Patient expresses feelings of boredom (wishes there were something to do, to read, etc.).
   b. Usual hobbies cannot be undertaken in hospital.
2. Minor defining characteristics:
   None given.

RELATED FACTORS[10]

Environmental lack of diversional activity, as in:

1. Long-term hospitalization
2. Frequent lengthy treatments

RELATED CLINICAL CONCERNS

Any medical diagnosis that could be connected to the related factors.

HAVE YOU SELECTED THE CORRECT DIAGNOSIS?

Activity Intolerance   If the nurse observes or validates reports of the patient's inability to complete required tasks because of insufficient energy, then Activity Intolerance is the appropriate diagnosis, not Diversional Activity Deficit. (See page 327.)

Impaired Physical Mobility   When the patient has difficulty with coordination, range of motion, or muscle strength and control, or he or she has activity restrictions related to treatment, the most appropriate diagnosis is Impaired Physical Mobility. Diversional Activity Deficit is quite likely to be a companion diagnosis to Impaired Physical Mobility. (See page 460.)

Social Isolation   This diagnosis should be considered if the patient demonstrates limited contact with community, peers, and significant others. When patient talks of loneliness rather than boredom, Social Isolation is the most appropriate diagnosis. (See page 781.)

Sensory/Perceptual Alteration   This diagnosis would be the best diagnosis when the patient is unable to engage in his or her usual leisure-time activities due to loss or impairment of one of the senses. (See page 562.)

EXPECTED OUTCOMES

1. Will have decreased number of complaints regarding boredom by (date) and/or
2. Will assist in designing and implementing a plan to overcome diversional activity deficit by (date)

TARGET DATE

Planning and accessing resources will required a moderate amount of time. A reasonable target date would be within 2 to 3 days.

NURSING ACTIONS/INTERVENTIONS WITH RATIONALES

Adult Health

Actions/Interventions	Rationales
• On admission, help patient to review activity likes and dislikes.	Finds the activities the patient would most likely engage in.
• When this diagnosis is made, move patient to semiprivate room if possible and if patient is amenable to move.	Provides companionship, social interaction, and diversion.
• Encourage patient to discuss feelings regarding deficit and causes at least once per day at (time).	Helps patient identify feelings and begin to deal with them.
• Involve patient, to extent possible, in more daily self-care activities.	Increases self-worth and adequacy.
• Alter daily routine (for example, bathe at different times or increase ambulation).	Creates change and provides some diversion.
• Rearrange environment as needed: ○ Provide ample light. ○ Place bed near window. ○ Provide radio as well as television set. ○ Place books, games, and so on within easy reach. ○ Provide clear pathway for wheelchair, ambulation, and so on. ○ Move furniture.	Facilitates activity.
• Provide change of environment at least twice a day at (times), for example, by taking patient out of room to sun deck or outside building or by adding posters to patient's room decor.	Creates change and broadens range of activities.
• Encourage significant others to assist in decreasing deficit: ○ Bringing books, games, hobby materials ○ Visiting more frequently ○ Encouraging other visitors	Reinforces "normal" lifestyle; encourages feelings of self-worth.

- o Bringing a box of wrapped small items, one to be opened each day, for example, paperback book, crossword puzzles, small jigsaw puzzle, or small hand-held games
- Provide for appropriate adaptations in equipment or positioning to facilitate desired diversional activity.
- Provide for scheduling of diversional activity at a time when patient is rested and when there will not be multiple interruptions.
- Refer to individual health care practitioners who can best assist with problem. (See Appendix B.)

Child Health

Actions/Interventions	Rationales
• Monitor patient's potential for activity or diversion according to: o Attention span o Physical limitations and tolerance o Cognitive, sensory, and perceptual deficits o Preferences for gender, age, and interests o Available resources o Safety needs o Pain	Provides essential database for planning desired and achievable diversion.
• Encourage parental input in planning and implementing desired diversional activity plan.	Helps ensure that plan is attentive to child's interests, thus increasing the likelihood of the child's participation.
• Allow for peer interaction when appropriate through diversional activity.	Involvement of peers serves to foster self-esteem and meets developmental socialization needs.

Women's Health

NOTE: The following refers to those women placed on restrictive activities because of threatened abortion, premature labor, multiple pregnancy, or pregnancy-induced hypertension.

Actions/Interventions	Rationales
• Encourage family and significant others to participate in plan of care for patient.	Promotes socialization, empowers family, and provides opportunities for teaching.
• Encourage patient to list life-style adjustments that need to be made as well as ways to accomplish these adjustments.	Basic problem-solving technique that encourages patient to participate in care; will increase understanding of current condition.

Continued

Actions/Interventions	Rationales

• Teach patient relaxation skills and coping mechanisms.
• Maintain proper body alignment with use of positioning and pillows.
• Provide diversional activities:
  ○ Hobbies, for example, needlework, reading, painting, or television
  ○ Job-related activities as tolerated (that can be done in bed), for example, reading, writing, or telephone conferences
  ○ Activities with children, for example, reading to child, painting or coloring with child, allowing child to "help" mother (bringing water to mother, assisting in fixing meals for mother)
  ○ Help and visits from friends and relatives, for example, visits in person, telephone visits, help with child care, or help with housework
	Provides a variety of options to offset deficit.

Mental Health

Actions/Interventions	Rationales
• Assess source of Diversional Activity Deficit. Is the nursing unit appropriately stimulating for the level or type of clients, or is the problem the client's perceptions?	Recognizes the impact of physical space on the client's mood.
Nursing-Unit-Related Problems	
• Develop milieu therapy program: ○ Include seasonal activities for clients such as parties, special meals, outings, or games.	Promotes here-and-now orientation and interpersonal interactions.
○ Alter unit environment by changing pictures, adding appropriate seasonal decorations, updating bulletin boards, or cleaning and updating furniture.	Enhances the aesthetics of the environment and has a positive effect on the client's mood.[13]
○ Alter mood of unit with bright colors, seasonal flowers, and appropriate music.	Colors and sounds impact the client's mood.[13]
○ Develop group activities for clients such as team sports, Ping-Pong, bingo games, activity planning groups, meal planning groups, meal preparation groups, current events discussion groups, book discussion groups, exercise groups, craft groups, and so on.	Provides opportunities to build social skills and alternative methods of coping.

○ Decrease emphasis on television as primary unit activity.

Television does not provide opportunities for learning alternative coping skills and decreases physical activity.

○ Provide books, newspapers, records, tapes, and craft materials.

Resources that assist the clients in meeting belonging needs by facilitating interaction with others on the unit and the world around them.
Provides varied sensory stimulation.

○ Use community service organizations to provide programs for clients.
• Collaborate with occupational therapist for ideas regarding activities and supplies.
• Collaborate with physical therapist regarding physical exercise program.

Client-Perception-Related Problems

• Discuss with client past activities, reviewing those that have been enjoyed and those that have been tried and not enjoyed.

Promotes client's sense of control.

• List those activities that the client has enjoyed in the past with information about what keeps client from doing them at this time.
• Monitor client's energy level and develop activity that corresponds to client's energy level and physiologic needs (for example, manic client may be bored with playing cards and yet physiologic needs require less physical activity than the client may desire, so an appropriate activity would address both these needs.) Note assessment decision here.

Promotes development of alternative coping behaviors by assisting client in choosing appropriate activities.

• Develop with client a plan for reinitiating a previously enjoyed activity. Note that plan here.

Promotes client's sense of control.

• Develop time in the daily schedule for that activity, and note that time here.
• Relate activity to enjoyable time such as a time for interaction with the nurse alone or interaction with other clients in a group area.

Interaction can provide positive reinforcement for engaging in activity.

• Provide positive verbal feedback to client about his or her efforts at the activity.

Positive verbal reinforcement encourages appropriate coping behaviors.

• Assist client in obtaining necessary items to implement activity, and list necessary items here.

Facilitates appropriate coping behaviors.

• Develop plan with client to attempt one new activity—one that has been interesting for him or her but which he or she has not had time or direction to pursue. Note plan and rewards for accomplishing goals here.

Promotes client's perceived control and provides positive reinforcement for the behavior.

Continued

Actions/Interventions	Rationales
• Have client set realistic goals for activity involvement (for example, one cannot paint like a professional in the beginning).	Promotes client's strengths and self-esteem.
• Discuss feelings of frustration, anger, and discomfort that may occur as client attempts a new activity.	Verbalization of feelings and thoughts provides opportunities for developing alternative coping strategies.
• Frame mistakes as positive tools of learning new behavior.	Promotes client's strengths.

Gerontic Health

Actions/Interventions	Rationales
• Discuss with patient whether activities were decreased prior to hospitalization.	If decreased activities were noted prior to admission, there may be ongoing problems that are not related to the acute care setting.
• Provide at least 10 to 15 minutes per shift, while awake, to engage in reminiscing with patient.	Increases self-esteem and focuses on strengths the patient has developed over his or her lifetime.[26]

Home Health

Actions/Interventions	Rationales
• Monitor factors contributing to Diversional Activity Deficit.	Provides database for prevention and/or early intervention.
• Involve client and family in planning, implementing, and promoting reduction in Diversional Activity Deficit: ○ Family conference ○ Mutual goal setting ○ Communication	Involvement improves motivation and improves the outcome.
• Assist client and family in life-style adjustments that may be required: ○ Time management ○ Work, family, social, and personal goals and priorities ○ Rehabilitation ○ Learning new skills or games ○ Development of support systems ○ Stress management techniques ○ Drug and alcohol use	Provides basic information for client and family that promotes necessary life-style changes.
• Refer to appropriate assistive resources as indicated. (See Appendix B.)	Provides additional support for client and family and uses already available resources in a cost-effective manner.

FLOW CHART EVALUATION
Flow Chart Expected Outcome 1

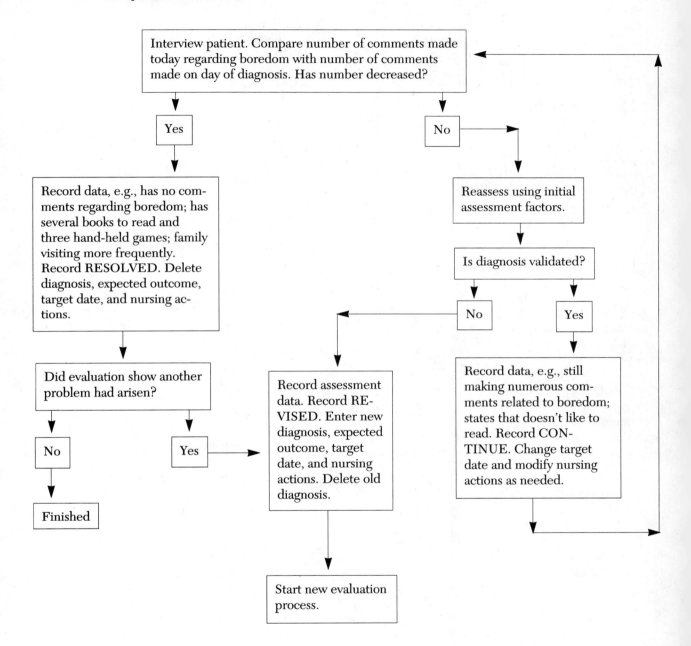

Interview patient. Compare number of comments made today regarding boredom with number of comments made on day of diagnosis. Has number decreased?

Yes

No

Record data, e.g., has no comments regarding boredom; has several books to read and three hand-held games; family visiting more frequently. Record RESOLVED. Delete diagnosis, expected outcome, target date, and nursing actions.

Reassess using initial assessment factors.

Is diagnosis validated?

No

Yes

Did evaluation show another problem had arisen?

Record assessment data. Record REVISED. Enter new diagnosis, expected outcome, target date, and nursing actions. Delete old diagnosis.

Record data, e.g., still making numerous comments related to boredom; states that doesn't like to read. Record CONTINUE. Change target date and modify nursing actions as needed.

No

Yes

Finished

Start new evaluation process.

Flow Chart Expected Outcome 2

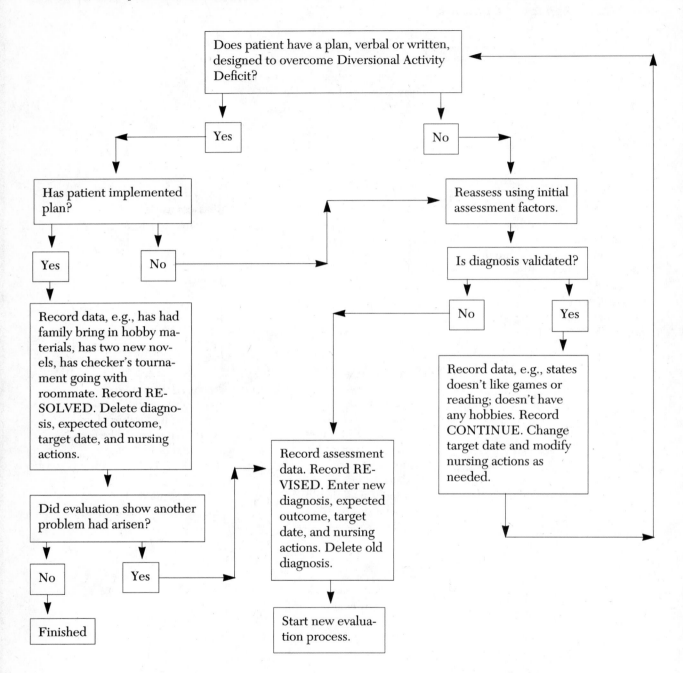

Dysfunctional Ventilatory Weaning Response (DVWR)

DEFINITION

A state in which a patient cannot adjust to lowered levels of mechanical ventilator support, which interrupts and prolongs the weaning response.[27]

NANDA TAXONOMY: EXCHANGING 1.5.1.3.2

DEFINING CHARACTERISTICS[27]

1. Mild DVWR:
   a. Major defining characteristics:
      (1) Restlessness
      (2) Slight increased respiratory rate from baseline
   b. Minor defining characteristic:
      Responds to lowered levels of mechanical ventilator support with:
      (1) Expressed feelings of increased need for oxygen, breathing discomfort, fatigue, or warmth
      (2) Queries about possible machine malfunction
      (3) Increased concentration on breathing
2. Moderate DVWR:
   a. Major defining characteristic:
      Responds to lowered levels of mechanical ventilator support with:
      (1) Slight increase from baseline blood pressure < 20 mm Hg
      (2) Slight increase from baseline heart rate < 20 beats per minute
      (3) Baseline increase in respiratory rate < 5 breaths per minute
   b. Minor defining characteristics:
      (1) Hypervigilence to activities
      (2) Inability to respond to coaching
      (3) Inability to cooperate
      (4) Apprehension
      (5) Diaphoresis
      (6) Eye widening, "wide-eyed look"
      (7) Decreased air entry on auscultation
      (8) Color changes; pale, slight cyanosis
      (9) Slight respiratory accessory muscle use
3. Severe DVWR:
   a. Major defining characteristic:
      Responds to lowered levels of mechanical ventilator support with:
      (1) Agitation
      (2) Deterioration in arterial blood gases from current baseline
      (3) Increase from baseline blood pressure > 20 mm Hg
      (4) Increase from baseline heart rate > 20 beats per minute
      (5) Respiratory rate increase significantly from baseline
   b. Minor defining characteristics:
      None given

RELATED FACTORS[27]

None given.

RELATED CLINICAL CONCERNS

1. Closed head injury
2. Coronary bypass
3. Respiratory arrest
4. Cardiac arrest
5. Cardiac transplant

HAVE YOU SELECTED THE CORRECT DIAGNOSIS?

Ineffective Breathing Pattern In this diagnosis the patient's respiratory effort is insufficient to maintain the cellular oxygen supply. This diagnosis would contribute to the patient's being placed on ventilatory assistance; however, DVWR occurs after the patient has been placed on a ventilator and efforts are being made to reestablish a regular respiratory pattern. The key difference is whether or not a ventilator has been involved in the patient's therapy. (See page 349.)

Impaired Gas Exchange This diagnosis refers to the exchange of oxygen and carbon dioxide in the lungs or at the cellular level. This probably has been a problem for the patient and is one of the reasons the patient was placed on a ventilator. DVWR would develop after the patient has received treatment for the impaired gas exchange via the use of a ventilator. (See page 416.)

EXPECTED OUTCOME

1. Will be able to stay off of the ventilator for at least (number) minutes by (date) and/or
2. Will be weaned from the ventilator by (date)

TARGET DATE

Initial target dates should be in terms of hours as the patient is going through the weaning process. As the patient improves, the target date could be expressed in increasing intervals from 1 to 3 days.

NURSING ACTIONS/INTERVENTIONS WITH RATIONALES

Adult Health

Actions/Interventions	Rationales
• Coach patient to take maximum inspiration and then to exhale all the air that he or she can. Check vital capacity measures (should be at least 10 mg/Kg).	Encourages patient to initiate respiration.
• Measure inspiratory force with pressure manometer (the force needed to optimize successful weaning is -20 to -30).	Measures respiratory muscle strength.

Actions/Interventions	Rationales
• Assess PaO_2 (should be 60 or greater at 40 percent oxygen) and O_2 saturation (with pulse oximeter, should be equal to or more than 94).	Indicates amount of oxygen in alveoli.
• Determine *positive end-expiratory pressure (PEEP)*. Physiologic **PEEP** is generally 5 cm of water.	PEEP should be sufficient to prevent collapse of alveoli.
• Assess tidal volume. Should be at least 3 ml/Kg.	Essential for maintenance of adequate ventilation.
• Assess vital signs and respiratory pattern during weaning.	Essential monitoring of changes in respiratory effort and oxygenation.
• Use weaning technique ordered by physician (T-Piece or IMV technique).	
• Plan goals for weaning and explain weaning procedure. Start weaning process at scheduled time off of ventilator. Stay with patient during weaning process. Stop weaning process before patient becomes exhausted.	Continuously monitors weaning success and ensures that patient can be placed back on ventilator as soon as necessary.
• Reassure patient that you are there in case of problems. Encourage patient that he or she can breathe on his or her own.	Instills trust, decreases anxiety, and increases motivation.
• If unable to wean while patient is still in the hospital, assess resources and support systems at home. Refer to home health or public health department at least 3 days prior to discharge.	Coordinates team efforts and allows sufficient planning time for home care.

Child Health

Actions/Interventions	Rationales
• Monitor for all contributing factors as applicable:[28] ○ Pathophysiologic health concerns, for example, infections, anemia, fever, or pain. ○ Previous respiratory history, especially risk indicators of reactive airway disease and bronchopulmonary dysplasia ○ Previous cardiovascular history, especially risk indicators such as increased or decreased pulmonary blood flow associated with congenital deficits ○ Previous neurologic status ○ Recent surgical procedures ○ Current medication regimen ○ Psychological and emotional stability of parents as well as child	Provides a database that will assist in generating the most individualized plan of care.

Continued

Actions/Interventions	Rationales

• Determine respirator parameters that suggest readiness to begin weaning process.[28] Collaborate with physician, respiratory therapist, and other health care team members:
  ○ Spontaneous respirations for age, for example, rate or depth
  ○ Oxygen saturations in normal range for condition, for example, spontaneous tidal volume of 5 ml/Kg body weight, vital capacity per Wright respirometer of 10 ml/Kg body weight, effective oxygenation with PEEP of 4 to 6 cm water: An exception to the normals would exist if an infant had transposition of the great vessels.
  ○ Blood gases in normal range
  ○ Stable vital signs
  ○ Parental or patient anxiety regarding respirator
  ○ Patient's facial expression and ability to rest
  ○ Resolution of the precipitating cause for intubation and mechanical support
  ○ Tolerance of suctioning and ambuing
  ○ Central nervous system and cardiovascular stability
  ○ Nutritional status, muscle strength, pain, drug-induced respiratory depression, sleep deprivation
	Specific ventilator-related criteria will offer the best decision-making support for determining the best plan of ventilator weaning.

NOTE: Oxygen saturations, blood gases, and vital signs may be abnormal secondary to chronic lung damage with accompanying hypoxemia and hypercapnia but a normal pH with metabolic compensation for chronic respiratory acidosis. In this instance acceptable ranges would be defined.

• Provide constant one-on-one attention to the patient and focus primarily on cardio-respiratory needs. Have CPR backup equipment readily available.
 	
• Monitor the anxiety levels of the patient and family at least once per shift.
• Monitor patient-specific parameters during actual attempts at weaning:
  ○ Arterial blood gases
  ○ Vital signs
  ○ Chest sounds
  ○ Pulse oximetry
	Hierarchy of needs for oxygenation must be met for all vital functions to be effective in homeostasis. Anticipatory safety for a patient on a ventilator demands backup equipment in case of failure of the current equipment. Expression of feelings will assist in monitoring family concerns and help reduce anxiety. Assists in further planning for weaning.

- ○ Chest x-ray
- ○ Hematocrit
- Provide patient teaching as appropriate for patient and family, with emphasis on the often slow pace of weaning.

Assessment of individualized learning needs allows appropriate focus on the patient. Explanation regarding the slow pace encourages a feeling of success rather than failure when each session does not meet the same time limits as the previous session.

- Provide attention to the rising of related emotional problems secondary to the association of ventilators with terminal life-support.

With the need to implement intubation and ventilation, there can arise myriad concerns regarding the patient's prognosis.

- Refer for long-term follow-up as needed. (See Appendix B.)

Fosters long-term support and coping with care at home.

- Administer medications as ordered, with appropriate attention to preparation for weaning, for example, careful use of paralytic agents or narcotics.

The best chance for successful weaning includes appropriate consciousness, no respiratory depression, and adequate neuromuscular strength. Special caution must be taken in positioning the patient receiving neuromuscular blocking agents so that dislocation of joints does not arise.[30]

- Maintain a neutral thermal environment.

Altered oxygenation and metabolic needs occur in instances of hyperthermia and hypothermia.

- Provide parents the option to participate in care as permitted.

Family input offers emotional input and security for the child in times of great stress, thereby allowing for growth in parental-child coping behaviors.

- Communicate with infant or child using age-appropriate methods, for example, infant will enjoy soft music or a familiar voice; older child may be able to use a small magic slate or point to key terms.

Communication effectively allows for expression of or reception of messages of care or concern, thereby acknowledging value of the patient.

Women's Health

The nursing actions for women's health in this diagnosis are the same as those for adult health.

Mental Health

This diagnosis is not appropriate for the mental health care unit.

Gerontic Health

Actions/Interventions	Rationales

• Monitor patient for presence of factors that make weaning difficult, such as:[31]
  ○ Poor nutritional status
  ○ Infection
  ○ Sleep disturbances
  ○ Pain
  ○ Poor positioning
  ○ Large amounts of secretions
  ○ Bowel problems
	These factors can significantly contribute to a delay in the weaning process.

• Ensure that communication efforts are enhanced by the proper use of sensory aids, for example, glasses, hearing aids, adequate lighting, decreased noise level in room, speaking in low-pitched tone of voice, and facing patient when speaking. If written instructions are used, ensure they are brief, jargon-free, printed or written in dark ink, and printed or written in large letters.	Effective communication is critical to success of weaning efforts. Lack of information or misinterpreted information may result in increased anxiety and decreased weaning success.
• Maintain same staff assignments whenever possible.[32] • Contract with patient for short-term and long-term weaning goals, providing reinforcements and rewards for progress. Use wall chart or diary to record progress.	Facilitates communication and decreases anxiety and fear of unfamiliar caregivers.

Home Health

Clients are discharged to the home health setting with ventilators; however, the nursing care required is the same as those actions covered in Adult Health and Gerontic Health.

FLOW CHART EVALUATION
Flow Chart Expected Outcome 1

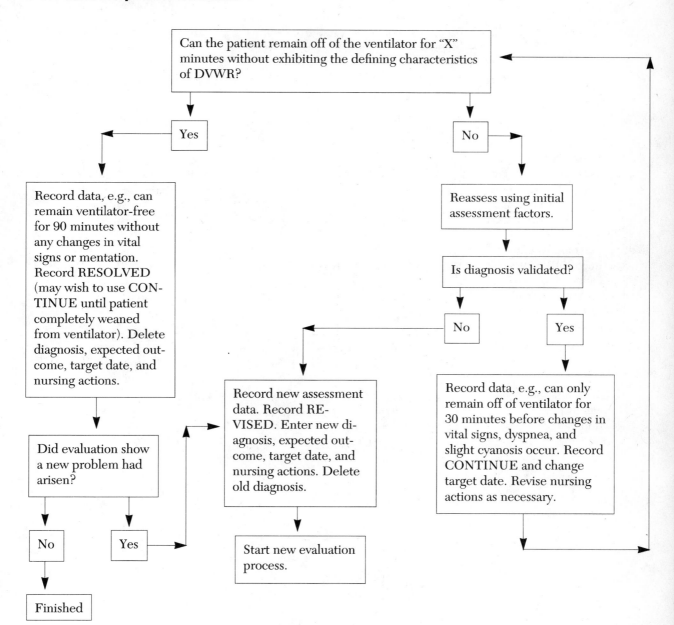

Can the patient remain off of the ventilator for "X" minutes without exhibiting the defining characteristics of DVWR?

Yes

No

Record data, e.g., can remain ventilator-free for 90 minutes without any changes in vital signs or mentation. Record RESOLVED (may wish to use CONTINUE until patient completely weaned from ventilator). Delete diagnosis, expected outcome, target date, and nursing actions.

Reassess using initial assessment factors.

Is diagnosis validated?

No

Yes

Did evaluation show a new problem had arisen?

No

Yes

Record new assessment data. Record REVISED. Enter new diagnosis, expected outcome, target date, and nursing actions. Delete old diagnosis.

Record data, e.g., can only remain off of ventilator for 30 minutes before changes in vital signs, dyspnea, and slight cyanosis occur. Record CONTINUE and change target date. Revise nursing actions as necessary.

Finished

Start new evaluation process.

Flow Chart Expected Outcome 2

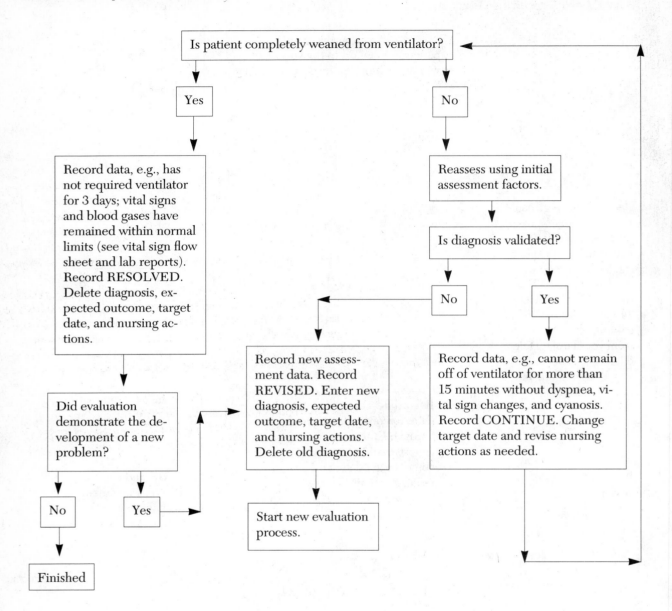

Dysreflexia

DEFINITION

The state in which an individual with a spinal cord injury at T7 or above experiences a life-threatening uninhibited sympathetic response of the nervous system to a noxious stimulus.[10]

NANDA TAXONOMY: EXCHANGING 1.2.3.1

DEFINING CHARACTERISTICS[10]

1. Major defining characteristics:
   a. Paroxysmal hypertension (sudden periodic elevated blood pressure where systolic pressure is over 140 mm Hg and diastolic is above 90 mm Hg)
   b. Bradycardia or tachycardia (pulse rate of less than 60 or over 100 beats per minute)
   c. Diaphoresis (above the injury)
   d. Red splotches on skin (above the injury)
   e. Pallor (below the injury)
   f. Headache (a diffuse pain in different portions of the head and not confined to any nerve distribution area)
2. Minor defining characteristics:
   a. Chilling
   b. Conjunctival congestion
   c. Horner's syndrome (contraction of the pupil, partial ptosis of the eyelid, enophthalmus, and sometimes loss of sweating over the affected side of the face)
   d. Paresthesia
   e. Pilomotor reflex (gooseflesh formation when skin is cooled)
   f. Blurred vision
   g. Chest pain
   h. Metallic taste in mouth
   i. Nasal congestion

RELATED FACTORS

1. Bladder distention
2. Bowel distention
3. Skin irritation
4. Lack of patient and caregiver knowledge

RELATED CLINICAL CONCERN

Spinal cord injury at T7 or above

HAVE YOU SELECTED THE CORRECT DIAGNOSIS?

Decreased Cardiac Output   Dysreflexia occurs only in spinal-cord-injured patients and represents an emergency situation that requires immediate intervention. Decreased Cardiac Output may be suspected because of the changes in blood pressure or arrhythmias;[33,34] but if the patient has a spinal cord injury at T7 or above, Dysreflexia should be considered first. (See page 360.)

Impaired Skin Integrity   Occasionally symptoms of Dysreflexia are precipitated by skin lesions such as pressure sores and ingrown or infected nails.[35] If the patient has a spinal cord injury at T7 or above in combination with impaired skin integrity, the nurse must be extremely alert to the possible development of Dysreflexia. In addition, one of the defining characteristics of Dysreflexia is red splotches, which could lead to a misdiagnosis of High Risk for Impaired Skin Integrity. (See page 239.)

Urinary Retention   Dysreflexia should be suspected in patients with spinal cord injuries at T7 or above who experience bladder spasms, bladder distention, or untoward responses to urinary catheter insertion or irrigation.[35,36] Bowel distention or rectal stimulation may also lead to Dysreflexia. (See page 304.)

EXPECTED OUTCOMES

1. Will have no signs or symptoms of Dysreflexia by (date) and/or
2. Will actively cooperate in care plan to prevent development of Dysreflexia by (date)

TARGET DATE

Dysreflexia is a life-threatening response. For this reason, the target date should be expressed in hours on a daily basis.

NURSING ACTIONS/INTERVENTIONS WITH RATIONALES

Adult Health

Actions/Interventions	Rationales
• Monitor vital signs, especially BP, every 3 to 5 minutes until stable; then every hour for 24 hours; then every 2 hours for 24 hours; then every 4 hours around the clock.	Extreme rises in BP are indicative of sympathetic nervous system stimulation and may lead to cerebrovascular accident and cardiac problems.
• Immediately locate source that may have triggered dysreflexia, for example, bladder distention (76 to 90 percent of all instances); bowel distention (8 percent of all instances);[37,38,39] fractures, acute	Finding precipitating causes prevents worsening of condition and allows further prevention of dysreflexia.

abdomen, narcotic withdrawal, pressure ulcers, childbirth, sunburn, invasive procedures below the level of the spinal cord injury, ingrown toenails, and poor patient positioning.

- Explain to patient reasons for procedures.
- Empty bladder slowly with straight catheter (*do not* use Crede's maneuver or tap bladder[37,39]) or manually remove impacted feces from rectum as soon as possible.
- Elevate head of bed 90 degrees immediately if not contraindicated by spinal injury.
- Send urine specimen to lab for culture and sensitivity.
- Collaborate with physician regarding the administration of emergency antihypertensive therapy.
- Keep patient warm, avoid chilling at all times.
- Monitor intake and output every hour for 48 hours, then every 2 hours for 48 hours, and then every 4 hours. Note time schedule and dates here.
- Collaborate with physician regarding daily monitoring of electrolyte balance.

- Turn, cough, and deep-breathe patient every 2 hours on the (odd/even) hour; keep in anatomic alignment.
- Perform range of motion (active or passive) every 4 hours while awake at (times). Pad bony prominences.
- Instruct patient on isotonic exercises. Encourage patient to perform isotonic exercises at least every 2 hours on (odd/even) hour.
- Instruct on bladder and bowel conditioning. Monitor for bladder and bowel distention every 4 hours at (times).
- Catheterize as necessary; use rectal tube if not contraindicated to assist with flatus reduction.
- Provide appropriate skin care each time patient is turned. Monitor skin integrity at least once per shift at (times).
- Maintain adequate food and fluid balance on a daily basis.
- Involve family in care, such as positioning, feeding, and exercising.

Reduces anxiety.
Alleviates precipitating causes.

Creates orthostatic hypotension.

Assists in determining if infection is a possible cause of episode.
Facilitates lowering of BP; encourages teamwork.

Decreases sensory nervous stimulation.

Monitors adequate functioning of bowel and bladder that are common causative factors for dysreflexia.

Maintains fluid balance and prevents complications that could impact cardiovascular functioning.
Alleviates precipitating causes.

Alleviates precipitating causes; stimulates circulation and muscular activity; decreases incidence of pressure ulcers.
Increases circulation and prevents complications of immobility.

Eliminates the two primary precipitating causes.

Eliminates precipitating causes.

Prevents and monitors for pressure ulcers.

Assists in avoiding constipation.

Assists in teaching and preparing family for home care.

Continued

Actions/Interventions	Rationales
• Be consistent and supportive in approach.	Decreases anxiety and instills confidence in caregivers.
• Use abdominal binders and antiembolic stockings as needed.	Assists in preventing precipitating causes through providing cardiovascular support.
• Administer medications as required.	Medications therapy is generally instituted to help control BP, control heart rate, and block excessive autonomic nerve transmission.
• Encourage family to use community resources. Make referrals as soon as possible after admission.	Cost-effective use of available resources; provides long-range support for patient and family.

Child Health

Actions/Interventions	Rationales
• Administer medications as required to help control the blood pressure at appropriate levels for age and weight.	Assists in preventing seizures and provides appropriate intervention to maintain pressure within desired ranges.
• Monitor the pulse as needed and BP every 5 minutes until stable. Determine parameters for the patient according to the norms for age, site, and condition.	Basic monitoring for initial indications of problem development.
• Monitor family's understanding and perception of the problem. Ensure that proper attention is paid to the family's needs for support during this emergency phase.	Assists in preventing misunderstandings and in identifying learning needs.
• Teach patient, as capable, and family routine for care, including the prevention of infection (particularly urinary and integumentary).	Education enhances care and provides an opportunity for care to be practiced in a supportive environment.

Women's Health

NOTE: This nursing diagnosis will pertain to women the same as to men. The following precautions should be taken when the victim is pregnant.

Actions/Interventions	Rationales

• Position the patient to prevent supine hypotension by:
  ○ Placing the patient on her left side if possible
  ○ Using a pillow or folded towel under the right hip to tip to left
	Keeps the weight of the uterus off the inferior vena cava.

- ○ If neck injury is suspected, placing the patient on a back board and then tipping the board to the left
- Start an IV line for replacement of lost fluid volume.

The pregnant woman has 50 percent more blood volume, and her vital signs may not change until there is a 30 percent reduction in circulating blood volume.

- Monitor fetal status continuously. Monitor for uterine contractions at least once per hour.

Basic data needed to ensure positive outcome.

Mental Health

The expected outcomes and nursing actions for the mental health client are the same as those for adult health.

Gerontic Health

The nursing actions for the gerontic patient are the same as those for adult health.

Home Health

Actions/Interventions	Rationales
• Teach client and family measures to prevent Dysreflexia:[40,41] ○ Bowel and bladder routines ○ Prevention of skin breakdown (for example, turning, transfer, or prevention of incontinence) ○ Use and care of indwelling urinary catheter ○ Prevention of infection	Basic care techniques that can assist in preventing the occurrence of Dysreflexia.

• Assist client and family in identifying signs and symptoms of Dysreflexia:
 ○ Teach family how to monitor vital signs and how to recognize tachycardia, bradycardia, and paroxysmal hypertension.
 ○ Assist client and family in identifying emergency referrals:
   (1) Physician
   (2) Emergency room
   (3) Emergency medical system
	Provides for early recognition and intervention for problem.
	
	Occurrence of this diagnosis is an emergency. This information provides the family with a sense of security by providing routes to and numbers of readily available emergency assistance.

• Teach patient and family appropriate uses and side effects of medications as well as proper administration of the medications.	Locus of control shifts from nurse to client and family, thus promoting self-care.

Continued

Actions/Interventions	Rationales
• Obtain available wallet-sized card which briefly outlines effective treatments in an emergency situation.[41] Have client carry this card with him or her at all times. Family members must be familiar with content and location of card.	
NOTE: Labeled a *Treatment Card*, this card contains information related to Pathophysiology, Common Signs and Symptoms, Stimuli That Trigger AD, Problems, and Recommended Treatment.	

FLOW CHART EVALUATION
Flow Chart Expected Outcome 1

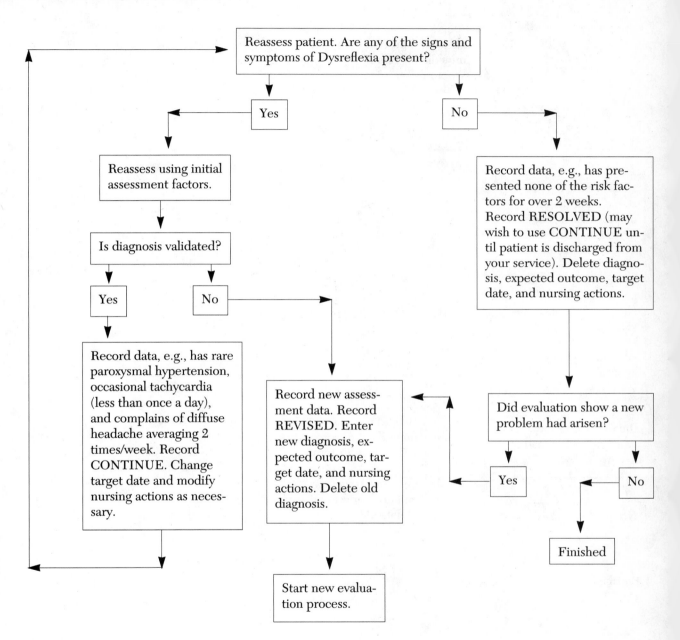

Reassess patient. Are any of the signs and symptoms of Dysreflexia present?

Yes

No

Reassess using initial assessment factors.

Is diagnosis validated?

Yes

No

Record data, e.g., has presented none of the risk factors for over 2 weeks. Record **RESOLVED** (may wish to use **CONTINUE** until patient is discharged from your service). Delete diagnosis, expected outcome, target date, and nursing actions.

Record data, e.g., has rare paroxysmal hypertension, occasional tachycardia (less than once a day), and complains of diffuse headache averaging 2 times/week. Record **CONTINUE**. Change target date and modify nursing actions as necessary.

Record new assessment data. Record **REVISED**. Enter new diagnosis, expected outcome, target date, and nursing actions. Delete old diagnosis.

Did evaluation show a new problem had arisen?

Yes

No

Finished

Start new evaluation process.

Flow Chart Expected Outcome 2

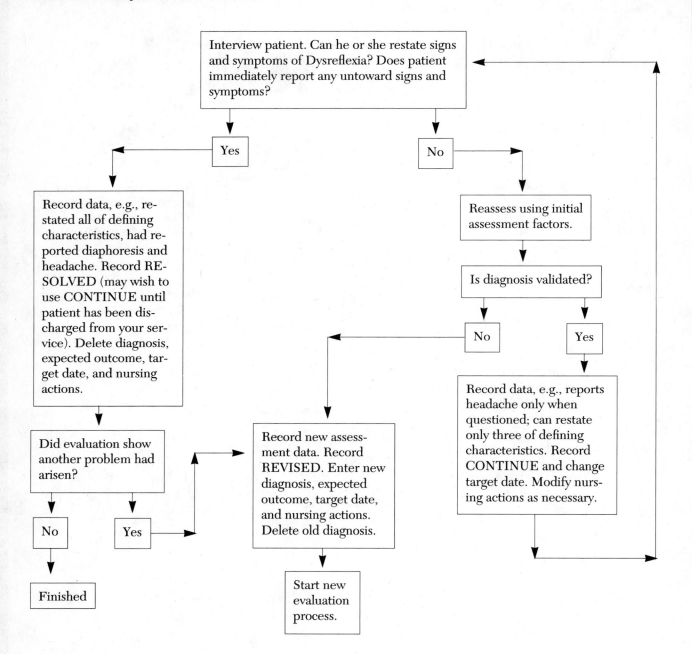

Fatigue

DEFINITION

An overwhelming sustained sense of exhaustion and decreased capacity for physical and mental work.[10]

NANDA TAXONOMY: MOVING 6.1.1.2.1

DEFINING CHARACTERISTICS[10]

1. Major defining characteristics:
   a. Verbalization of an unremitting and overwhelming lack of energy
   b. Inability to maintain usual routines
2. Minor defining characteristics:
   a. Perceived need for additional energy to accomplish routine tasks
   b. Increase in physical complaints
   c. Emotionally labile or irritable
   d. Impaired ability to concentrate
   e. Decreased performance
   f. Lethargic or listless
   g. Disinterest in surroundings or introspection
   h. Decreased libido
   i. Accident prone

RELATED FACTORS[10]

1. Decreased or increased metabolic energy production
2. Overwhelming psychological or emotional demands
3. Increased energy requirements to perform activity of daily living
4. Excessive social and/or role demands
5. States of discomfort
6. Altered body chemistry (for example, medications, drug withdrawal, or chemotherapy)

RELATED CLINICAL CONCERNS

1. Acquired immunodeficiency syndrome
2. Hyper- or hypothyroidism
3. Cancer
4. Menopause
5. Depression
6. Anemia

HAVE YOU SELECTED THE CORRECT DIAGNOSIS?

Sleep Pattern Disturbance   Fatigue is defined as a sense of exhaustion and decreased capacity for mental work regardless of adequate sleep. In this sense Fatigue may be considered an alteration in quality, not quantity, of sleep and is subjective. (See page 507.)

Continued

HAVE YOU SELECTED THE CORRECT DIAGNOSIS?—*Continued*

Decreased Cardiac Output   Decreased oxygenation to the muscles, brain, and so on could result in a sense of fatigue. (See page 360.)

Altered Nutrition: Less than Body Requirements   Decreased nutrition will ultimately lead to decreased muscle mass and decreased energy, which will result in Fatigue. (See page 200.)

EXPECTED OUTCOMES

1. Will have decreased complaints of fatigue by (date) and/or
2. Will have implemented plan to offset fatigue by (date)

TARGET DATE

Fatigue can have far-reaching impact. For this reason the initial target date should be set at no more than 4 days.

NURSING ACTIONS/INTERVENTIONS WITH RATIONALES

Adult Health

Actions/Interventions	Rationales
• Collaborate with diet therapist for in-depth dietary assessment and planning. Monitor patient's food and fluid intake daily.	Adequate, balanced nutrition assists in reducing fatigue.
• Monitor for contributory factors on a daily basis at (time).	Assists in identifying causative factors, which then can be treated.
• Carefully plan activities of daily living and daily exercise schedules with detailed input from patient. Determine how to best foster future patterns that will maintain optimal sleep-rest patterns without fatigue through planning ADL with patient and family.	Realistic schedules based on patient's input promotes participation in activities and a sense of success.
• Assign staff on a consistent basis.	Promotes adherence to planned schedule and facilitates patient's understanding of the need to be consistent in plan.
• Provide frequent rest periods. Schedule at least 30 minutes of rest after any strenuous activity.	Allows patient to gradually increase strength and tolerance for activities.
• Assist patient with self-care as needed. Plan gradual increase in activities over several days.	
• Provide adequate input about usual sleep pattern versus current pattern associated with fatigue.	Increases quantity and quality of rest and sleep.

- Promote rest at night:
  ○ Warm bath at bedtime
  ○ Warm milk at bedtime
  ○ Back massage
- Avoid sensory overload or sensory deprivation. Provide diversional activities.

Sensory aspects can deplete energy stores; diversional activities help prevent overload or deprivation by focusing patient's concentration on an activity he or she personally enjoys.

- Instruct patient in stress reduction techniques. Have patient return-demonstrate at least once a day through day of discharge.

Mental and physical stress greatly contribute to sense of fatigue.

- Assist patient to realistically appraise personal short- and long-term goals.
- Collaborate with physician regarding medical status and condition and its impact on promoting chronic fatigue.
- Assist patient to schedule at least one recreational night per week and one rest evening per week. Have patient sign contract with significant other to promote compliance with this schedule.
- Refer to local exercise center for assistance with regular exercise plan.

Feeling overwhelmed by too many or unrealistic goals can increase fatigue.
Several medical diagnoses include fatigue as a symptom that can be offset by careful planning of care.
Provides distraction from overfocus on work or other such demands. Assists in reducing stress, which contributes to fatigue.

Regular exercise decreases fatigue.

Child Health

Actions/Interventions	Rationales
• Determine a plan to best address contributory factors as determined by verbalized perceptions of fatigue (may be related to parents' perceptions). • Provide daily feedback regarding progress, and reassess child's and family's perception of fatigue. • Ensure safety needs according to child's or infant's age and developmental capacity.	Parents are best able to describe objective behaviors that offer cues to fatigue factors, especially when the patient cannot speak or describe his or her feelings. Due to the ever-changing fatigue factors, close attention to progress will aid in gaining a sense of mastery and will objectify concerns. Standard accountability is to provide for safety needs with special attention to the child's age, developmental capacity, parental education, compliance, and so on.

Women's Health

Actions/Interventions	Rationales
• During pregnancy, schedule rest periods during day.	Realistic planning to offer brief rest periods during the day.
• Find restful area, one time in the morning and one time in the afternoon, to get away from work area and rest 5 to 10 minutes with feet propped above the abdomen.	
• During lunch, leave work area to rest 10 to 15 minutes with feet propped above the abdomen or lying on left side.	
• Have patient research the possibility of split time or job sharing at work during pregnancy.	
• Teach patient relaxation techniques.	Techniques induce a restful state and can be used for short periods of rest as well as more extended periods of rest.
	Assists with relaxation.
• Teach patient to use music of preference during rest periods.	
• Plan for at least 6 to 8 hours of sleep during night. (See Sleep Pattern Disturbance, Chapter 6, for nursing actions to promote sleep.)	
• Involve significant others in discussion and problem-solving activities regarding life-style changes needed to reduce fatigue.	Family can assume more responsibilities to assist in increasing rest time for the patient.
• After delivery, identify a support system that can assist patient with infant care and household duties.	Assists in alleviating fatigue related to trying to manage household as always as well as trying to care for a new baby.
• Learn to rest and sleep when the infant sleeps.	Conserves energy and increases amount of time available for rest.
• Plan daily activities to alleviate unnecessary steps and to allow for frequent rest periods:	
○ If bottle-feeding, prepare formula for 24 hours at a time.	
○ If breast-feeding, let spouse get up at night and bring baby to mother.	
○ Prepare extra when cooking meals for family, and freeze extra for future meals (for example, prepare big batch of stew or spaghetti on one day and freeze portions for future meals).	
• Plan return to work on a gradual basis (for example, work part time for the first 2 weeks, gradually increasing time at work until full time by end of 4 weeks).	Provides gradual return to activities and decreases likelihood of fatigue.

Mental Health

NOTE: All goals established for the nursing actions should be achievable and adjusted as client's condition changes.

Actions/Interventions	Rationales
• Client must be out of bed and dressed by (note time here). Initially this goal may be limited to client's getting out of bed without dressing.	Provides goal client can achieve and enhances self-esteem.
• Assist client with grooming activities (note here the degree of assistance needed as well as any special items needed).	Promotes client's sense of control and enhances self-esteem.
• While assisting client with grooming activities, teach performance of tasks in energy-efficient ways, for example, placing all necessary items in one place before grooming is begun.	Promotes client's control by providing increased opportunity for self-care.
• Provide client with appropriate rewards for accomplishing established goals (note special goals here with the reward for achievement of goal). Establish rewards with client input.	Positive reinforcement encourages appropriate behavior.
• Establish time for client to rest during the day. Initially this will be more frequent and diminish as client's condition changes. Note times and duration of rest periods here.	Meets physiological need for rest. Also provides client with an opportunity for perceived control in determining when these rest periods should be provided.
• Walk with client on unit (number) of minutes (number) times a day.	Promotes cardiorespiratory fitness and promotes self-esteem by providing a goal the client can meet. Interaction with the nurse can provide positive reinforcement for this activity.
• Have client identify pleasurable activities that cannot be performed because of fatigue.	Promotes positive orientation by connecting client with images of past pleasures and provides material for developing positive imaging.
• Identify one pleasurable activity and develop a gradually escalating plan for client involvement in this activity. Provide rewards for accomplishment of each step in this plan.	Promotes positive orientation by providing client with positive goal to work toward. This will increase motivation. Positive reinforcement encourages behavior.
• Provide client with foods that are high in nutritional value and are easy to consume.	Meets physiological needs for nutrition in a manner that conserves energy.
• Talk with client 30 minutes twice a day. Topics for this discussion should include: ○ Client's perception of the problem ○ Identification of thoughts that support the feeling of fatigue ○ Identification of thoughts that decrease feelings of fatigue	Promotes client's sense of control by providing time for his or her input into plan of care on a daily basis; also provides positive reinforcement through social interaction with the nurse and verbal feedback about accomplishments.

Continued

Actions/Interventions	Rationales
○ Identification of unrealistic goals ○ Client's evaluation of and attitudes toward self ○ Identification of circumstances in the client's environment that support continuing feelings of fatigue (for example, family stressors or secondary gain from fatigue) ○ Identification of client's accomplishments	
• After client has verbalized the effects negative thoughts have on feelings and behavior, teach client how to stop negative thoughts and replace them with positive thoughts.	Cognitive maps impact feelings and behavior. When cognitive maps are used inappropriately, they can promote maladaptive thinking, behaving, and feeling. Recognition of dysfunctional maps provides the client with the opportunity for developing positive orientation and adaptive cognitive maps.[13]
• Reward client for positive self-statements.	Positive reinforcement encourages appropriate behavior.
• Assign client tasks on the unit and provide positive reinforcement for task accomplishment. Note task assigned and reward established here.	
• Involve client in group activity with other clients for (number) minutes (number) times a day.	Interaction with peers provides opportunities to increase their social network, share problem-solving strategies, and test perceptions of self and experiences with peers. Family support enhances probability of behavior changes being maintained after discharge.
• Meet with client and client's family to evaluate interaction patterns and provide information that would assist them in assisting the client.	
• Have client identify those factors that will maintain feeling of well-being after discharge, and develop a specific behavioral plan for implementing them. Note plan here.	Reinforces behavior change and new coping skills while providing positive feedback and enhancing self-esteem.[13]

Gerontic Health

Actions/Interventions	Rationales
• Review medications for side effects or possible drug interactions. • Collaborate with physician regarding assessing patient for depression. • Monitor for activities that interrupt the patient's sleep pattern, such as vital signs, daily weights, or treatments. • Plan care activities around periods of least fatigue.	Many medications can contribute to the sensation of fatigue. Depression is often underreported and undertreated in older adults. Environmental noises and inattention to patient's usual sleep pattern may result in sleep fragmentation. Gives attention to patient's circadian rhythm.

Home Health

Actions/Interventions	Rationales
• Assist client and family in identifying risk factors pertinent to the situation: ○ Chronic disease (for example, arthritis, cancer, or heart disease) ○ Medications ○ Pain ○ Role strain • Teach client and family measures to promote capacity for physical and mental work: ○ Use assistive devices as appropriate (wheelchairs, crutches, canes, walkers, adaptive eating utensils, etc.) ○ Maintain sufficient pain control (analgesics, imagery, meditation, etc.) ○ Provide a safe environment to reduce barriers to activity and decrease potential for accidents (throw rugs, stairs, blocked pathways, etc.) ○ Provide balance of work and recreational activities ○ Provide housekeeping assistance as appropriate (for example, homemaker or Meals on Wheels) • Provide diversional activity as appropriate (visiting friends or family, doing hobbies or schoolwork, etc.). • Consult with or refer to appropriate resources as indicated. (See Appendix B.)	Provides additional support for client and family, and uses already available resources in a cost-effective manner.

FLOW CHART EVALUATION
Flow Chart Expected Outcome 1

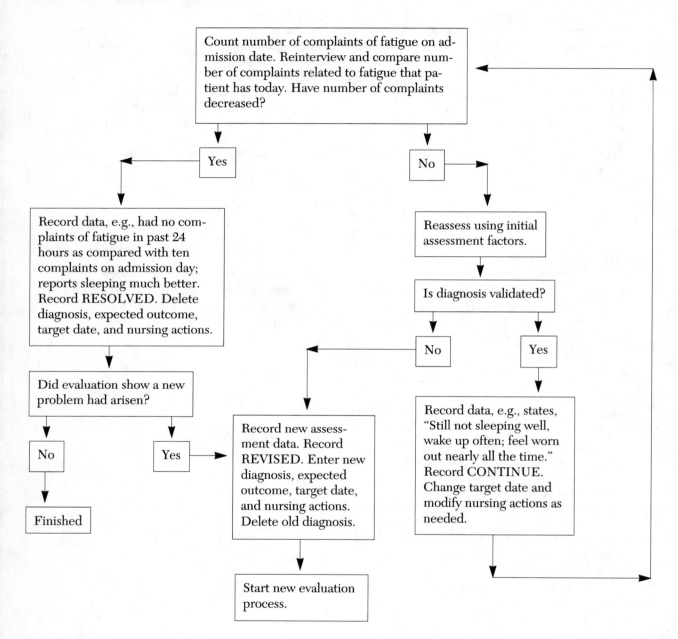

Flow Chart Expected Outcome 2

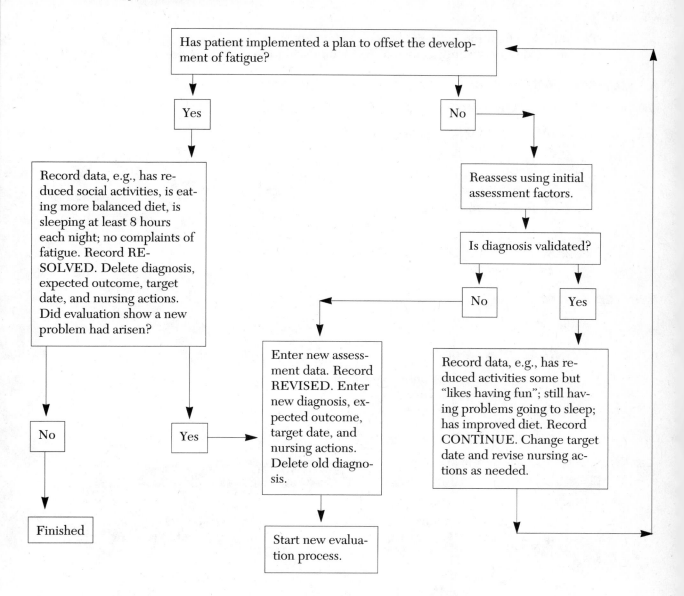

Gas Exchange, Impaired

DEFINITION

The state in which the individual experiences a decreased passage of oxygen and/or carbon dioxide between the alveoli of the lungs and the vascular system.

NANDA TAXONOMY: EXCHANGING 1.5.1.1

DEFINING CHARACTERISTICS[10]

1. Major defining characteristics:
   a. Confusion
   b. Somnolence
   c. Restlessness
   d. Irritability
   e. Inability to move secretions
   f. Hypercapnia
   g. Hypoxia
2. Minor defining characteristics:
   None given

RELATED FACTOR[10]

Ventilation perfusion imbalance.

RELATED CLINICAL CONCERNS

1. Chronic obstructive pulmonary disease
2. Congestive heart failure
3. Asthma
4. Pneumonia
5. Pulmonary tuberculosis

HAVE YOU SELECTED THE CORRECT DIAGNOSIS?

Ineffective Airway Clearance This diagnosis means that something is blocking the air passage but that when and if air gets to the alveoli, there is adequate gas exchange. In Impaired Gas Exchange, the air (oxygen) that reaches the alveoli is not sufficiently diffused across the alveoli-circulatory membrane. (See page 338.)

Ineffective Breathing Pattern This diagnosis suggests that the rate, rhythm depth, and type of ventilatory effort is insufficient to bring in enough oxygen or get rid of sufficient amounts of carbon dioxide. These gases are sufficiently exchanged at the alveoli-circulatory membrane, but the pattern of ventilation makes breathing ineffective. (See page 349.)

Decreased Cardiac Output In this diagnosis, the heart is not pumping a sufficient amount of blood through the lungs to take up enough oxygen or release enough carbon dioxide to meet the body's requirements. There is no impairment in the gas exchange, but there is not enough circulating blood to combine with sufficient amounts of oxygen to supply the body's needs. (See page 360.)

EXPECTED OUTCOMES

1. Will have no signs or symptoms of impaired gas exchange by (date) and/or
2. Will demonstrate improved blood gases and vital signs by (date) (Note initial blood gas measurements and vital signs here.)

TARGET DATE

Because of the extreme danger of Impaired Gas Exchange, progress should be evaluated at least every 8 hours until the client has stabilized. Thereafter, target dates at 3 to 5 days would be acceptable.

NURSING ACTIONS/INTERVENTIONS WITH RATIONALES

Adult Health

Actions/Interventions	Rationales

• Monitor and document:
  ○ Respiratory pattern, rate, and depth at least every 2 hours on (odd/even) hour
  ○ Symptoms noted with respirations, such as pain, difficulty in breathing, retraction of sternum or flaring of nares, or allergies
  ○ Equipment used in ventilation, including ventilator settings for rate, oxygen (FiO_2), peak pressure (PP), and, if needed, CPAP
  ○ Auscultation of breath sounds every 1 hour or as needed, with follow-up chest x-ray as needed
  ○ Tolerance of chest physiotherapy
  ○ Suctioning tolerance, especially pulse rate
  ○ Nature of secretions obtained via suctioning
  ○ Observations of skin and mucous membranes for cyanosis
	Baseline factors that will allow assessment of patient's progress toward improvement or lack of progress.

• Maintain fluid and electrolyte balance:
  ○ Administer appropriate fluids and electrolytes as ordered.
  ○ Monitor hourly intake and output.
  ○ Administer potassium only after voiding is noted.
  ○ Monitor specific gravity four times a day at (times).	

• Administer or assist with IPPB or CPAP as ordered. Stay with patient during treatment. In between treatments, administer oxygen as ordered.	Opens airways and alveoli; improves gas exchange; oxygen reduces the work of breathing and thus enhances gas exchange.
• Perform nursing actions to maintain effective airway clearance. (See Ineffective	Clearing airways of secretions improve ventilation-perfusion relationship.

Continued

Actions/Interventions	Rationales
Airway Clearance for nursing actions and enter those actions here.)	
• Decrease patient's anxiety during periods of increased distress by:	
○ Talking in a calm, slow voice	
○ Reassuring patient that you can provide the necessary assistance	
○ Having patient take slow, deep breaths and follow proper breathing techniques	
○ Staying with client until episode resolves	
• Schedule at least 15 minutes with patient every 2 hours on the (odd/even) hour for discussing concerns, and so on.	Assists in reducing fear and anxiety.
• Raise head of bed to 30 degrees or more if not contraindicated.	Facilitates chest expansion.
• Reduce chest pain by using noninvasive techniques and analgesics.	Relaxes muscles tension; decreases oxygen consumption; decreases carbon dioxide production.
• Encourage drinking 2 to 3 liters of fluid per day unless contraindicated by other medical problems, for example, congestive heart failure.	Assists in liquifying secretions, which makes them easier to expel.
• Maintain adequate nutrition (high protein, low fat, and low carbohydrates) on a daily basis. Collaborate with diet therapist regarding several small meals per day rather than three large meals.	Decreases energy demand for digestion; avoids constriction of chest cavity due to a full stomach.
• Instruct in diaphragmatic deep breathing and pursed-lip breathing: Give patient information in clear, concise manner, providing written notes if necessary. This is especially true for the patient who has altered mental status as a result of hypoxia.	
• Have patient practice proper breathing once every hour while awake. These sessions should be supervised by the nurse until the patient masters the technique. Note schedule for practice sessions here.	Essential knowledge needed for patient to control situation. Will assist in expelling secretions.
• Provide teaching regarding respiratory exercises:	
○ Assume a sitting position with back straight and shoulders relaxed.	
○ Use conscious, controlled deep-breathing techniques that expand diaphragm downward (abdomen should rise).	
○ Breathe in deeply through the nose, hold for 2 to 3 seconds, breathe out slowly	

through pursed lips. Abdomen will sink down with the exhalation.

- Instruct the patient to perform exercises at least twice an hour while awake (practice with and supervise until confident patient can perform exercises accurately).
- Provide teaching regarding bronchial hygiene:
  - Breathe deeply and slowly while sitting up.
  - Use diaphragmatic breathing.
  - Hold the breath for 3 to 5 seconds and then slowly exhale through the mouth as much of the breath as possible.
  - Take another deep breath, hold, and cough forcefully from deep in the chest. Repeat two times.
  - Rest 15 to 20 minutes after coughing session.
- Assist with postural drainage and cupping and clapping exercises. Teach these exercises to significant other.
- Administer bronchodilators and mucolytic agents as ordered.
- Collaborate with physician regarding monitoring of blood gases; report abnormal results immediately.

PCO_2, PO_2, and O_2 saturation are indicators of the efficiency of gas exchange.

- Turn every 2 hours on the (odd/even) hour. Encourage patient's mobility to the extent tolerated without dyspnea.

Position changes modify ventilation-perfusion relationships and enhance gas exchange.

- On day of admission, develop a schedule for activity and rest that provides the patient with the greatest amount of activity with the least amount of fatigue, for example, have chair in bathroom for being seated while doing daily hygiene. Note schedule here.

Conserves energy needed for breathing and gas exchange.

- Discuss with patient the effects smoking has on the respiratory system, and refer him or her to a stop-smoking group if patient is motivated to stop smoking; if not, instruct patient not to smoke 15 minutes before meals and physical activity.

Smoking, or passive smoke for the nonsmoker, greatly increases the risk for development of respiratory and cardiovascular diseases. Smoking immediately before eating or exercise causes vasoconstriction, leading to decreased gas exchange and compounding condition.

- Review the patient's resources and home situation regarding long-term management of Impaired Gas Exchange prior to discharge. Refer to appropriate community resources. (See Appendix B.)

Initiates appropriate home care planning and long-range support for patient and family.

Child Health

Actions/Interventions	Rationales

• Ensure availability of emergency equipment:
  ○ Ambu bag
  ○ Endotracheal tube appropriate for age and size of infant (3.5)
  ○ Suctioning unit and catheters: Infants, 5 or 8 Fr; child, 8 or 10 Fr
  ○ Crash cart with appropriate drugs
  ○ Defibrillation unit with guidelines
  ○ O_2 tank (check amount of oxygen left)
  ○ Tracheostomy sterile set
  ○ Sterile chest tube tray
	Basic emergency preparedness.

• Provide for parental input in planning and implementing care, for example, comfort measures, assisting with feedings, and daily hygienic measures.	Parental involvement provides emotional security for child's parents; offers empowerment and allows practicing of care techniques in a supportive environment.
• Allow at least 10 to 15 minutes per shift to allow family to verbalize concerns regarding child's status and changes. Encourage parents to ask questions as often as needed.	Assists in reducing anxiety; provides teaching opportunity.
• Collaborate with related health care team members as needed. (See Appendix B.)	Promotes coordination of care without undue duplication and fragmentation of care.
• Provide opportunities for parents and child to master essential skills necessary for long-term care, such as suctioning, while in hospital.	Learning of essential skills is enhanced when opportunities for practice are allowed in a safe, secure environment. Compliance is also fostered.
• Ensure that parents and family receive CPR training well before dismissal from hospital.	Anticipatory need for CPR should better prepare parents and other family members in the event of pulmonary arrest. Having this basic knowledge will assist in reducing anxiety regarding home care.
• Encourage parents to use support system to aid in coping with illness and hospitalization.	Reliance on others should afford parents some degree of relief from constant worry based on the likelihood of primary needs with a chronically ill child.
• Allow for sibling visitation as applicable within institution or in specific situation.	Sibling visitation enhances the opportunity for family coping and growth. Provides moral support to both siblings.

Women's Health

NOTE: This nursing diagnosis will pertain to women the same as to men. The following nursing actions will focus only on the fetal-placental unit during pregnancy. Placental function is totally dependent on maternal circulation; therefore, any process that interferes with maternal circulation will affect the oxygen consumption of the placenta and, in turn, the fetus.

Actions/Interventions	Rationales
• Assist patient in developing an exercise plan during pregnancy.	Increases cardiovascular fitness.
• Teach patient and significant others how to avoid "supine hypotension" during pregnancy (particularly during the later stages): ○ Lying on left side to reduce pressure on vena cava ○ Taking frequent rest breaks during the day	
• Assist patient in identifying life-style adjustments that may be needed due to changes in physiologic function or needs during pregnancy: ○ Stop smoking. ○ Avoid lying in supine position. ○ Take no drugs unless so advised by physician.	
• Identify underlying maternal diseases that will affect the fetal-placental unit during pregnancy: ○ Maternal Origin: (1) Maternal hypertension (2) Drug addiction (3) Diabetes mellitus with vascular involvement (4) Sickle cell anemia (5) Maternal infections (6) Maternal smoking (7) Hemorrhage (abruptio placenta or placenta previa) ○ Fetal Origin: (1) Premature or prolonged rupture of membranes (2) Intrauterine infection (3) RH disease (4) Multiple pregnancy	These disorders have direct impact on the gas exchange in the fetal-placental unit.

Actions/Interventions	Rationales
• If client is demonstrating alterations in mental status, assess for increased hypoxia.	The central nervous system is particularly sensitive to impaired gas exchange because of its reliance on simple sugar metabolism for energy production.[25]
• Observe client for signs of respiratory infection.	Infection will increase mucus production, which decreases airway clearance.[25]
• Protect client from respiratory infection by:	Prevents further injury to a system that is stressed and promotes airway patency.
○ Maintaining proper humidity in environment	
○ Placing him or her in private room or monitoring roommate closely for signs and symptoms of respiratory infection and, if present, moving client to another room	
○ Assigning staff members to client who are free of infection	
○ Keeping client away from crowds	
○ Assisting client in obtaining appropriate immunizations against influenza	
○ Having client inform staff of signs or symptoms of respiratory infection when the earliest symptoms appear	
○ Keeping environment as free of respiratory irritants as possible, for example, dust, allergens, or pollution.	
• Discuss with client the effects of alcohol and other depressant drugs on the respiratory system. Refer to a drug-abuse recovery program as necessary.	Sedative effects of drug decrease airway clearance, increasing the risk for the development of infection. Diffusion is also decreased with chronic alcoholism.[42]
• Collaborate with physician regarding supplemental vitamins, especially thiamine, if the impaired gas exchange is secondary to alcohol abuse.	Thiamine is essential for the conversion of glucose to metabolically useful forms. Nerve cell function depends on this glucose. This compensates for the nutritional deficits that result when nutritional calories are replaced by alcohol.[42]
• Spend 30 minutes twice a day with client discussing feelings and reactions to current situation. As feelings are expressed, begin to explore life-style changes with client. Refer to Ineffective Individual Coping (Chapter 11) and Powerlessness (Chapter 8) for specific care plans related to coping styles.	Promotes client's sense of control by facilitating understanding of factors that contribute to maladaptive coping behaviors.
• Develop with client a plan for gradually increasing physical activity. (See Activity Intolerance for specific behavioral interventions.)	Improves cardiorespiratory functioning, thus improving gas exchange.

Gerontic Health

Actions/Interventions	Rationales
• Ensure oxygen delivery system is properly functioning and fits well. Avoid face mask if patient is emaciated. Check proper positioning of nasal cannula (prongs turned inward).	Basic care standards.
• Monitor skin color, mental status, and vital signs every 2 hours on the (odd/even) hour.	
• Check oxygen flow and amount every 4 hours around the clock at (times).	The patient may increase the liter flow during acute episodes of impaired gas exchange and cause respiratory system depression with retention of carbon dioxide.
• Monitor for potential carbon dioxide narcosis, for example, changes in level of consciousness, changes in oxygen and carbon dioxide blood gas levels, flushing, decreased respiratory rate, and headaches. This is especially important for patient on long-term oxygen therapy.[22]	
• Teach patient and family the signs and symptoms of carbon dioxide narcosis, especially patients on long-term oxygen therapy.	Decreases potential for carbon dioxide narcosis.

Home Health

NOTE: If this diagnosis is suspected when caring for a client in the home, it is imperative that a physician referral be obtained immediately. If the client has been referred to home health care by a physician, the nurse will collaborate with the physician in the treatment of the client. Preliminary research[43] indicates that women with chronic bronchitis or chronic obstructive pulmonary disease (COPD) cannot walk as far as men. Activity should be planned according to tolerance, keeping in mind gender differences. There is no doubt that better control of dyspnea is a pressing need with research,[44] indicating that a client's subjective report of health status is a better predictor of level of functioning than is objective measure of the lung function.

Actions/Interventions	Rationales
• Teach client and family appropriate monitoring of signs and symptoms of Impaired Gas Exchange: ○ Pursed-lip breathing ○ Respiratory status: Cyanosis, rate, dyspnea, or orthopnea	Provides for early recognition and intervention for problem.

Continued

Actions/Interventions	Rationales

○ Fatigue
  ○ Use of accessory muscles
  ○ Cough
  ○ Sputum production or change in sputum production
  ○ Edema
  ○ Decreased urinary output
  ○ Gasping
• Assist client and family in identifying life-style changes that may be required:
	Provides basic information for client and family that promotes necessary life-style changes.

○ Prevention of Impaired Gas Exchange: Stopping smoking, prevention or early treatment of lung infections, avoidance of known irritants and allergens, influenza and pneumonia immunizations
  ○ Pulmonary hygiene: Clearing bronchial tree by controlled coughing, decreasing viscosity of secretions via humidity and fluid balance, postural drainage
  ○ Daily activity as tolerated (barriers to activity removed)
  ○ Breathing techniques to decrease work of breathing (diaphragmatic, pursed lips, sitting forward)
  ○ Adequate nutrition intake
  ○ Appropriate use of oxygen (dosage, route of administration, and safety factors)
  ○ Stress management
  ○ Limiting exposure to upper respiratory infections
  ○ Avoiding extreme hot or cold temperatures
  ○ Keeping area free of animal hair and dander or dust
  ○ Assistive devices required (oxygen, nasal cannula, suction, ventilator, etc.)
  ○ Adequate hydration (monitor intake and output)	

• Teach client and family purposes, side effects, and proper administration technique of medications.	
• Assist client and family in setting criteria to help them determine when physician or other intervention is required, for example, change in skin color, increased difficulty with breathing, increase or change in sputum production, or fever.	Locus of control shifts from nurse to client and family, thus promoting self-care.
• Teach family basic CPR.	
• Refer to community resources as needed. (See Appendix B.)	Provides additional support for client and family and uses already available resources in a cost-effective manner.

FLOW CHART EVALUATION
Flow Chart Expected Outcome 1

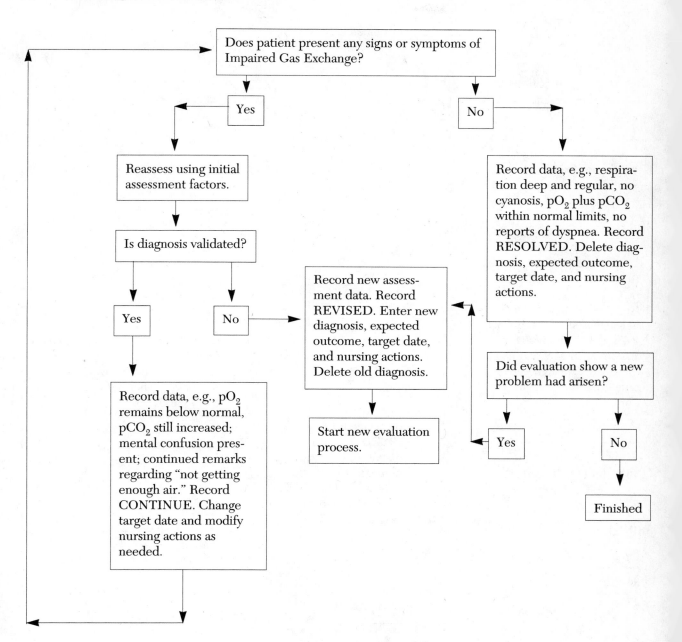

Flow Chart Expected Outcome 2

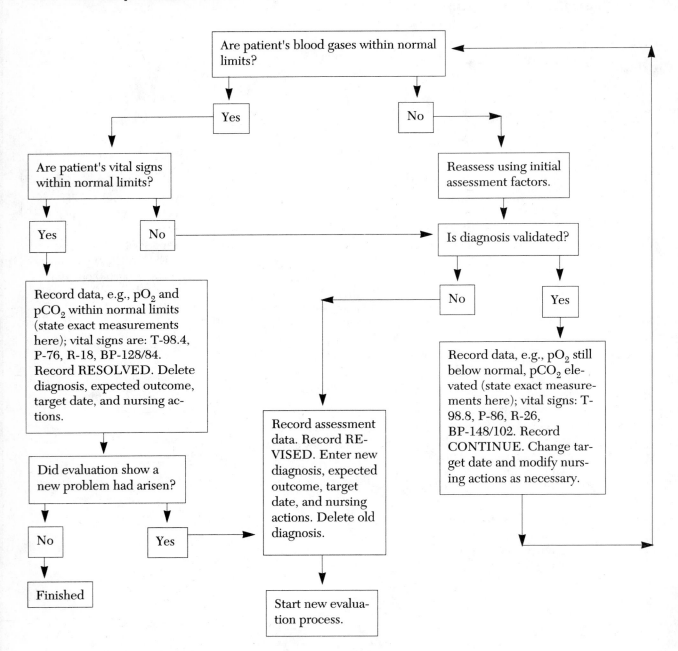

Growth and Development, Altered

DEFINITION

The state in which an individual demonstrates deviations in norms from his or her age group.[10]

NANDA TAXONOMY: MOVING 6.6

DEFINING CHARACTERISTICS[10]

1. Major defining characteristics:
   a. Delay or difficulty in performing skills (motor, social, or expressive) typical of age group
   b. Altered physical growth
   c. Inability to perform self-care or self-control activities appropriate to age
2. Minor defining characteristics:
   a. Flat affect
   b. Listlessness
   c. Decreased responses

RELATED FACTORS[10]

1. Inadequate caretaking
2. Indifference or inconsistent responsiveness
3. Multiple caretakers
4. Separation from significant others
5. Environmental and stimulation deficiencies
6. Effects of physical disability
7. Prescribed dependence

RELATED CLINICAL CONCERNS

1. Hypothyroidism
2. Failure-to-thrive syndrome
3. Leukemia
4. Deficient growth hormone
5. Personality disorders
6. Schizophrenic disorders
7. Substance abuse
8. Dementia
9. Delirium

HAVE YOU SELECTED THE CORRECT DIAGNOSIS?

Sensory/Perceptual Alterations This diagnosis should be considered when blindness, deafness, or neurologic impairment is present. Assisting the patient to adapt to these problems could resolve any developmental problems. (See page 562.)

Continued

HAVE YOU SELECTED THE CORRECT DIAGNOSIS?—*Continued*

Impaired Physical Mobility   When physical disabilities are present, they can definitely impact growth and development. In this example, Impaired Physical Mobility and Altered Growth and Development would be companion diagnoses. (See page 460.)

Altered Nutrition: Less than Body Requirements   Lack of essential vitamins and minerals will also show a direct link to Altered Growth and Development. Assessment should be implemented for both diagnoses. (See page 200.)

   The nursing diagnoses grouped under Self-Perception and Self-Concept Pattern, Role-Relationship Pattern, and Coping-Stress Tolerance Pattern should also be considered when alterations in growth and development are present.

EXPECTED OUTCOMES

1. Will implement plan to offset, as much as possible, altered growth and development factors by (date) and/or
2. Will return, as nearly as possible, to expected growth and development parameter for (specify exact parameter) by (date)

TARGET DATE

Assisting in modifying Altered Growth and Development factors will require a significant time; therefore, an initial target date of 7 to 10 days would be reasonable for evaluating progress.

NURSING ACTIONS/INTERVENTIONS WITH RATIONALES

Adult Health

NOTE: Nursing actions for this diagnosis are varied and complex and incorporate nursing actions associated with other nursing diagnoses. For example, the patient may have either a total self-care deficit or a subdeficit in hygiene, grooming, feeding, or toileting. For an adult, any of these would be an alteration in growth and development. Therefore, it would be appropriate to include the nursing actions associated with these nursing diagnoses in the nursing actions for Altered Growth and Development.

   An adult is generally able to find or initiate diversional and social activities. However, if the adult does not participate in diversional or social activities, it could indicate Altered Growth and Development. Therefore, the nursing actions associated with Diversional Activity Deficit and Social Isolation would be appropriate to be included in the nursing actions for Altered Growth and Development.

Actions/Interventions	Rationales
• Provide adequate opportunities for the patient to be successful in whatever task he or she is attempting.	Success increases motivation.
• Reward and reinforce success, however minor. Downplay relapses. Allow patient to be as independent as possible.	Increases self-esteem and active participation in care.
• Have consistent, nonjudgmental, caring people in the caregiving role.	Caring people instill confidence in patient and a willingness to try new tasks.
• Work collaboratively with other health care professionals and with the patient and family in developing a plan of care.	Facilitates development of a plan that all will use consistently.

Child Health

Actions/Interventions	Rationales
• Monitor and teach parents to monitor child's growth and development status. Determine what alterations there are (that is, delays or precocity).	As a rule, single assessments are not as revealing in growth and development parameters as are serial, longitudinal patterns. Parental involvement offers a more thorough monitoring, fosters their involvement with child, and empowers family.
• Determine what other primary health care needs exist, especially brain damage or residual of same.	In instances of brain damage or retardation, it is often difficult to get an accurate assessment of cognitive capability. The general health of the patient will often influence, to a major degree, what alteration in cognitive functioning exists, for example, sickle cell anemia with resultant infarcts to major organs such as the brain.
• Identify, with child or parents, realistic goals for growth and development.	A plan of care based on individual needs, with parental input, better reflects holistic care and increases probability of effective home management of problem.
• Collaborate with related health care team members as necessary.	Collaboration is required for meeting the special long-term needs for activities of daily living.
• Identify anticipatory safety for child related to Altered Growth and Development, for example, ingestion of objects, falls, or use of wheelchair.	These children may be large physically due to chronological age, and there is a possibility of overlooking the developmental-mental age.
• In case of special diet due to a metabolic component, for example, various enzymes lacking, provide appropriate health teaching for parents.	Appropriate diet can assist in preventing further deterioration or be essential to replace lacking vitamins, enzymes, or other nutrients.

Continued

Actions/Interventions	Rationales
• Refer child and parents to appropriate community resources, such as the early-childhood intervention services, to assist in fostering growth and development.	Offering early intervention assists in fostering development while preventing tertiary delays.
• Help parents to provide for learning needs related to future development, including identification of schools for developmentally delayed children.	Appropriate match of services to needs enhances child's development to the level possible.
• Refer child and parents to state and national support groups, such as National Cerebral Palsy Association.	Support groups assist in empowerment and advocacy at local, state, and national levels.
• Provide with long-term follow-up appointments before discharge.	Promotes implementation of management regimen and provides anticipatory resources and check-point for the patient and family.

Women's Health

NOTE: This nursing diagnosis will pertain to women the same as to men. The following nursing actions pertain only to women with reproductive anatomic abnormalities.

Actions/Interventions	Rationales
• Obtain a thorough sexual and obstetric history, especially noting recurrent miscarriages in the first 3 months of pregnancy.	Provides basic database for determining therapy needs.
• Collaborate with physician regarding assessment for infertility.	
• Refer to gynecologist for further testing if primary amenorrhea is present.	
• Encourage patient to verbalize her concerns and fears.	Decreases anxiety; allows opportunity for teaching and allows correction of any misinformation.
• Encourage communication with significant others to identify concerns and explore options available.	Provides a base to begin teaching and long-range counseling.

Mental Health

Actions/Interventions	Rationales
• Provide a quiet, nonstimulating environment or an environment that does not add additional stress to an already overwhelmed coping ability.	Too little or too much sensory input can result in a sense of disorganization and confusion and result in dysfunctional coping behaviors.[13]
• Sit with client (number) minutes (number) times per day at (list specific times) to discuss current concerns and feelings.	Attention from the nurse can enhance self-esteem. Expression of feelings can facilitate identification and resolution of problematic coping behaviors.
• Provide client with familiar or needed objects. These should be noted here.	Promotes client's sense of control by providing an environment in which client feels safe and secure.
• Discuss with client perceptions of self, others, and the current situation. This should include client's perceptions of harm, loss, or threat. Assist client in altering perception of these situations so they can be seen as challenges or opportunities for growth rather than threats.	Provides positive orientation, which improves self-esteem and provides hope for the future.
• Provide client with an environment that will optimize sensory input. This could include hearing aids, eyeglasses, pencil and paper, decreased noise in conversation areas, appropriate lighting. (These interventions should indicate an awareness of sensory deficit as well as sensory overload, and the specific interventions for this client should be noted here, for example, place hearing aid in when client awakens and remove it before bedtime.)	Appropriate levels of sensory input promotes contact with the reality of the environment, which facilitates appropriate coping.
• Provide client with achievable tasks, activities, and goals (these should be listed here). These activities should be provided with increasing complexity to give client an increasing sense of accomplishment and mastery.	Provides positive reinforcement, which enhances self-esteem and provides motivation for working toward next goal.
• Communicate to client an understanding that all coping behavior to this point has been his or her best effort and that asking for assistance at this time is not failure. A complex problem often requires some outside assistance in resolution. (This will assist client in maintaining self-esteem and diminish feelings of failure.)	Promotes positive orientation, which enhances self-esteem and promotes hope.

Continued

Actions/Interventions	Rationales
• Provide client with opportunities to make appropriate decisions related to care at his or her level of ability. This may begin as a choice between two options and then evolve into more complex decision making. It is important that this be at the client's level of functioning so confidence can be built with successful decision-making experiences.	Promotes client's perception of control, which promotes self-esteem.
• Provide constructive confrontation for client about problematic coping behavior. (See Wilson and Kneisl[12] for guidelines on constructive confrontation.) The kinds of behavior identified by the treatment team as problematic should be listed here.	Provides opportunities for the client to question aspects of behavior, which can promote desire to change.
• Provide client with opportunities to practice new kinds of behavior either with role-play or by applying them to graded real-life experiences.	Provides opportunities to practice new behavior in a safe environment where the nurse can provide positive feedback for gradual improvement of coping strategies. This increases probability for the success of the new behavior in real-life situation, which in turn serves as positive reinforcement for behavior change.
• Provide positive social reinforcement and other behavioral rewards for demonstration of adaptive behavior. (Those things that the client finds rewarding should be listed here with a schedule for use. The kinds of behavior that are to be rewarded should also be listed.)	Positive reinforcement encourages appropriate behavior.
• Assist client in identifying support systems and in developing a plan for their use.	Support systems can provide positive reinforcement for behavior change, increasing the opportunities for client's success, which will enhance self-esteem.
• Assist client with setting appropriate limits on aggressive behavior by (see High Risk for Violence, Chapter 9, for detailed nursing actions if this is an appropriate diagnosis):	Excessive environmental stimuli can increase a sense of disorganization and confusion.
○ Decreasing environmental stimulation as appropriate. (This might include a secluded environment.)	
○ Providing client with appropriate alternative outlets for physical tension. (This should be stated specifically and could include walking, running, talking with a staff member, using a punching bag, listening to music, or doing a deep	Promotes a sense of control and teaches constructive ways to cope with stressors.

muscle relaxation sequence. These outlets should be selected with the client's input.)
- Meet with client and support system to provide information on the client's situation and to develop a plan that will involve the support system in making changes that will facilitate the client's movement to age-appropriate behavior. Note this plan here.
- Refer to appropriate assistive resources as indicated. (See Appendix B.)

Enhances opportunities for success of the treatment plan.

Gerontic Health

The nursing actions for the gerontic patient with this diagnosis are the same as those in Adult Health and Home Health.

Home Health

Actions/Interventions	Rationales
• Monitor for factors contributing to Altered Growth and Development.	Provides database for prevention and/or early intervention.
• Involve client and family in planning, implementing, and promoting reduction or correction of the alteration in growth and development: ○ Family conference ○ Mutual goal setting ○ Communication	Involvement improves motivation and improves the outcome.
• Teach client and family measures to prevent or decrease alterations in growth and development: ○ Expected norms of growth and development with anticipatory guidance. If the caretakers realize, for example, that the newborn begins to roll over by 2 to 4 months or that the 2-year-old can follow simple directions, then appropriate environmental and learning conditions can be provided to protect the child and to promote optimal development. ○ Signs and symptoms of alterations in growth and development that may require professional evaluation, for example, delay in language skills, delay in crawling or walking, below 50 percent on growth chart.	Locus of control shifts from nurse to client and family, thus promoting self-care.

Continued

Actions/Interventions	Rationales
○ Parenting skills, for example, recognition of developmental milestones or nonabusive discipline. ○ Developmentally appropriate nutrition, for example, finger foods for toddlers, appropriate calories for expected developmental stage, or balanced diet. • Assist client and family to identify life-style changes that may be required: ○ Care for handicaps (for example, blindness, deafness, or musculoskeletal or cognitive deficit) ○ Proper use of assistive equipment ○ Adapting to need for assistance or assistive equipment ○ Determining criteria for monitoring client's ability to function unassisted ○ Time management ○ Stress management ○ Development of support systems ○ Learning new skills ○ Work, family, social, and personal goals and priorities ○ Coping with disability or dependency ○ Development of consistent routine ○ Mechanism for alerting to need for assistance ○ Providing appropriate balance of dependence and independence • Assist client and family to obtain assistive equipment as required (depending on alteration present and its severity): ○ Adaptive equipment for eating utensils, combs, brushes, and so on ○ Straw and straw holder ○ Wheelchair, walker, motorized cart, or cane ○ Bedside commode and/or incontinence undergarments ○ Hearing aid ○ Corrective lenses ○ Dressings aids: Dressing stick, zipper pull, button hook, long-handled shoehorn, shoe fasteners, and/or Velcro closures ○ Bars and attachments and benches for shower or tub	Provides basic information for client and family that promotes necessary life-style changes. Assistive equipment improves functioning and increases the possibilities for self-care.

- ○ Hand-held shower device
- ○ Medication organizers or magnifying glass
- ○ Raised toilet seat
- Consult with appropriate assistive resources as indicated. (See Appendix B.)

Provides additional support for client and family and uses already available resources in a cost-effective manner.

FLOW CHART EVALUATION
Flow Chart Expected Outcome 1

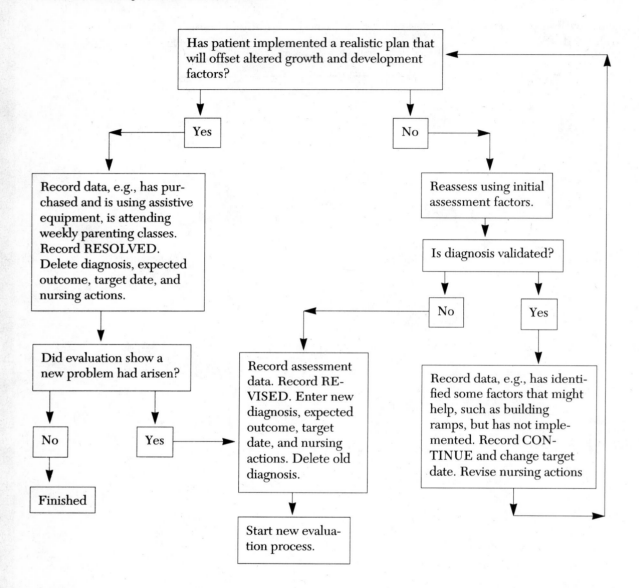

Flow Chart Expected Outcome 2

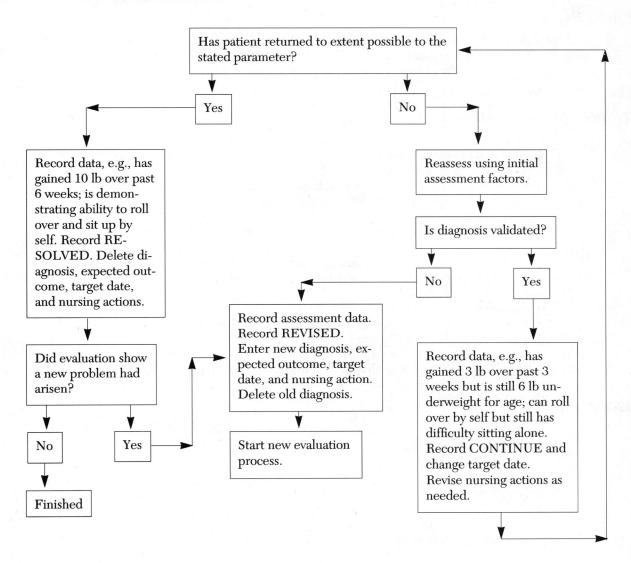

Has patient returned to extent possible to the stated parameter?

Yes

No

Record data, e.g., has gained 10 lb over past 6 weeks; is demonstrating ability to roll over and sit up by self. Record RESOLVED. Delete diagnosis, expected outcome, target date, and nursing actions.

Reassess using initial assessment factors.

Is diagnosis validated?

No

Yes

Did evaluation show a new problem had arisen?

Record assessment data. Record REVISED. Enter new diagnosis, expected outcome, target date, and nursing action. Delete old diagnosis.

No

Yes

Record data, e.g., has gained 3 lb over past 3 weeks but is still 6 lb underweight for age; can roll over by self but still has difficulty sitting alone. Record CONTINUE and change target date. Revise nursing actions as needed.

Finished

Start new evaluation process.

Home Maintenance Management, Impaired

DEFINITION

Inability to independently maintain a safe, growth-promoting immediate environment.[10]

NANDA TAXONOMY: MOVING 6.4.1.1

DEFINING CHARACTERISTICS[10]

1. Subjective:
   a. Household members express difficulty in maintaining their home in a comfortable fashion (*critical*).
   b. Household members request assistance with home maintenance (*critical*).
   c. Household members describe outstanding debts or financial crises (*critical*).
2. Objective:
   a. Disorderly surroundings
   b. Unwashed or unavailable cooking equipment, clothes, or linen (*critical*)
   c. Accumulation of dirt, food wastes, or hygienic wastes (*critical*)
   d. Offensive odors
   e. Inappropriate household temperature
   f. Overtaxed family members, for example, exhausted or anxious (*critical*)
   g. Lack of necessary equipment or aids
   h. Presence of vermin or rodents
   i. Repeated hygienic disorders, infestations, or infections (*critical*)

RELATED FACTORS[10]

1. Individual or family member disease or injury
2. Insufficient family organization or planning
3. Insufficient finances
4. Unfamiliarity with neighborhood resources
5. Impaired cognitive or emotional functioning
6. Lack of knowledge
7. Lack of role modeling
8. Inadequate support systems

RELATED CLINICAL CONCERNS

1. Dementia problems such as Alzheimer's
2. Rheumatoid arthritis
3. Depression
4. Cerebrovascular accident
5. Acquired immunodeficiency syndrome

HAVE YOU SELECTED THE CORRECT DIAGNOSIS?

Activity Intolerance   If the nurse observes or validates reports of the patient's inability to complete required tasks because of insufficient energy, then Activity Intolerance would be the more appropriate diagnosis. (See page 327.)

Knowledge Deficit   The problem with home maintenance may be due to the family's lack of education regarding the care needed and the environment that is essential to promote this care. If the patient or family verbalizes less-than-adequate understanding of home maintenance, then Knowledge Deficit is the more appropriate diagnosis. (See page 536.)

Altered Thought Process   If the patient is exhibiting impaired attention span, impaired ability to recall information, impaired perception, judgment, and decision making, or impaired conceptual and reasoning ability, the most proper diagnosis would be Altered Thought Process. Most likely, Impaired Home Management would be a companion diagnosis. (See page 577.)

Ineffective Individual Coping or Ineffective Family Coping   Suspect one of these diagnoses if there are major differences between reports by the patient and the family of health status, health perception, and health care behavior. Verbalizations by the patient or the family regarding inability to cope also require looking at these diagnoses. (See pages 874 and 892.)

Altered Family Processes   Through observing family interactions and communication, the nurse may assess that Altered Family Processes should be considered. Poorly communicated messages, rigidity of family functions and roles, and failure to accomplish expected family developmental tasks are a few observations to alert the nurse to this possible diagnosis. (See page 710.)

EXPECTED OUTCOMES

1. Will identify factors contributing to impaired home maintenance management by (date) and/or
2. Will demonstrate alterations necessary to reduce impaired home maintenance management by (date)

TARGET DATES

Target dates will depend on the severity of the Impaired Home Maintenance Management. Acceptable target dates for the first evaluation of progress toward meeting this outcome would be 5 to 7 days.

NURSING ACTIONS/INTERVENTIONS WITH RATIONALES

Adult Health

A nurse in an acute care facility might very well receive enough information, while the patient is hospitalized, to make this nursing diagnosis. However, nursing actions specific for this diagnosis will require implementation in the home environment; therefore, the reader is referred to the home health nursing actions for this diagnosis.

Child Health

Actions/Interventions	Rationales

• Monitor risk factors of or contributing factors to Altered Home Maintenance Management, to include:
  ○ Addition of a family member, for example, a birth
  ○ Increased burden of care due to child's illness or hospitalization
  ○ Lack of sufficient finances
  ○ Loss of family member, for example, a death
  ○ Hygienic practices
  ○ History of repeated infections or poor health management
  ○ Offensive odors
	Provides primary database for intervention.

• Identify ways to deal with home maintenance management alterations with assistance of applicable health team members. (See Appendix B.) • Allow for individual patient and parental input in plan for addressing home maintenance management issues. • Monitor educational needs related to illness and the demands of the situation, for example, mother who must attend to a handicapped child and six other children with various school appointments, health care appointments, and so on.	Coordinated activities will be required to meet the entire range of needs related to improving problems with home maintenance management. Parental input offers empowerment and attaches value to family preferences. This in turn increases the likelihood of compliance. Monitoring of educational needs balanced with the home situation will best provide a base for intervention.
• Provide health teaching with sensitivity to patient and family situation, for example, caretaker's seeming inability to manage overwhelming demands of a child's need for care, such as premature infant or child with cerebral palsy who has feeding difficulties.	Teaching to address identified needs will reduce anxiety and promote self-confidence in ability to manage.
• Provide 10 to 15 minutes each 8-hour shift as a time for discussion of patient and family feelings and concerns related to health management.	Setting aside times for discussion shows respect and assigns value to the patient and family.
• Encourage patient and family to identify support groups in the community. • If infant is at risk for sudden infant death syndrome (SIDS) by nature of prematurity or history of previous death in family, assist parents in learning about alarms and	Support groups empower and facilitate family coping. Anticipates appropriate safety and health teaching needs when these risk factors have been identified, for example, with an infant at risk for SIDS, family members will feel more

monitoring respiration, and institute CPR teaching.

able to deal with likelihood of pulmonary arrest if they are taught and receive opportunities to demonstrate techniques for CPR.

- Provide for appropriate follow-up after dismissal from hospital.

Follow-up plans will provide a means of further evaluation for progress in coping with home maintenance management. Ideally, actual home visitation serves to allow the best opportunity for monitoring goal achievement.

Women's Health

Actions/Interventions	Rationales
• Assist the client to describe her perception or understanding of home maintenance as it relates to her life-style and life-style decisions. Include areas related to stress-related problems and effects of environment: ○ Allow patient time to describe work situation. ○ Allow patient time to describe home situation. ○ Encourage patient to describe how she manages her responsibilities as a mother and a working woman. ○ Encourage patient to describe her assets and deficits as she perceives them. ○ Encourage patient to list life-style adjustments that need to be made. ○ Monitor identified possible solutions, modifications, and so on designed to cope with each adjustment. ○ Teach client relaxation skills and coping mechanisms. • Social network and significant others: ○ Identify significant others in patient's social network. ○ Involve significant others if so desired by patient in discussion and problem-solving activities regarding life-style adjustments. • Encourage patient to get adequate rest: ○ Take care of self and baby only. ○ Let significant others take care of the housework and other children. ○ Learn to sleep when the baby sleeps. ○ Have specific, set times for visiting friends or relatives.	Provides database needed to plan changes that will increase ability in home maintenance management. Fatigue can be a major contributor to Impaired Home Maintenance Management.

Continued

Actions/Interventions	Rationales

○ If breast-feeding, significant other can change infant and bring infant to mother at night (mother does not always have to get up every time for infant).
○ Cook several meals at one time for family and freeze them.
○ Prepare baby formula for a 24-hour period and refrigerate until use.
○ Freeze breast milk, emptying breast after baby eats; significant other can then feed infant one time at night so mother can get adequate, uninterrupted sleep.
○ Put breast milk into bottle and directly into freezer:
  (1) Breast milk can be added each time breasts are pumped until needed amount is obtained.
  (2) Breast milk can be frozen for 6 weeks if needed.
  (3) To use, remove breast milk from freezer, and let it thaw to room temperature.
  (4) Once thawed, breast milk must be used within a 12- to 24-hour period. *Do not refreeze.*	

Mental Health

Actions/Interventions	Rationales
• Discuss with client his or her concerns about returning home.	Promotes client's sense of control, which enhances self-esteem.
• Develop with client and significant others a list of potential home maintenance problems.	Promotes client's and support system's sense of control, which increases the willingness of the client to work on goals.
• Teach client and family those tasks that are necessary for home care. Note tasks and teaching plan here.	Provides opportunities for positive reinforcement of approximation of goal achievement.
• Provide time to practice home maintenance skills. This should be a minimum of 30 minutes once a day. Medication administration could be evaluated with each dose by allowing client to administer own medications. The times and types of skills to be practiced should be listed here.	

- If financial difficulties prevent home maintenance, refer to social services or a financial counselor.
- If client has not learned skills necessary to cook or clean home, arrange time with occupational therapist to assess for ability and to teach these skills. Support this learning on unit by (check all that apply):
  - Having client maintain own living area
  - Having client assist with the maintenance of the unit (state specifically those chores client is responsible for)
  - Having client assist with the planning and preparation of unit meals when this is a milieu activity
  - Having client clean and iron own clothing

Provides opportunities to practice new skills in a safe environment and to receive positive reinforcement for approximation of goal achievement.

- If special aids are necessary for client to maintain self successfully, refer to social services for assistance in obtaining these items.
- If client needs periodic assistance in organizing self to maintain home, refer to homemaker service or other community agency.
- If meal preparation is a problem, refer to community agency for Meals on Wheels, or assist family with preparation of several meals ahead of time or exploring nutritious, easy ways to prepare meals.
- Determine with client a list of rewards for meeting the established goals for achievement of home maintenance and then develop a schedule for the rewards. Note the reward schedule here.

Positive reinforcement encourages the maintenance of new behavior.

- Assess environment for impairments to home maintenance, and develop with client and family a plan for resolving these difficulties (for example, recipes that are simplified and written in large print are easier to follow).
- Provide appropriate positive verbal reinforcers for accomplishment of goals or steps toward the goals.

Positive reinforcement encourages maintenance of new behaviors.

- Utilize group therapy once a day to provide:
  - Positive role models
  - Peer support
  - Reality assessment of goals
  - Exposure to a variety of problem solutions
  - Socialization and learning of social skills

Gerontic Health

Actions/Interventions	Rationales
• Refer to local Alzheimer's and related diseases support group if dementia is present.	Alzheimer's support group can provide information on resources and techniques to continue home care.

Home Health

Actions/Interventions	Rationales
• Monitor factors contributing to Impaired Home Maintenance Management (items listed under Related Factors section).	Provides database for prevention and/or early intervention.
• Involve patient and family in planning, implementing, and promoting reduction in the impaired home maintenance management: ○ Family conference ○ Mutual goal setting ○ Communication ○ Family members given specified tasks as appropriate to reduce the impaired home maintenance management (shopping, washing clothes, disposing of garbage and trash, yardwork, washing dishes, meal preparation, and so on.)	Involvement improves motivation and improves the outcome.
• Assist patient and family in life-style adjustments that may be required: ○ Hygiene practices ○ Drug and alcohol use ○ Stress management techniques ○ Family and community support systems ○ Removal of hazardous environmental conditions, such as improper storage of hazardous substances, open heaters and flames, breeding areas for mosquitos or mice, or congested walkways ○ Proper food preparation and storage.	Provides basic information for client and family that promotes necessary life-style changes.
• Refer to appropriate assistive resources as indicated. (See Appendix B.)	Provides additional support for client and family and uses already available resources in a cost-effective manner.

FLOW CHART EVALUATION
Flow Chart Expected Outcome 1

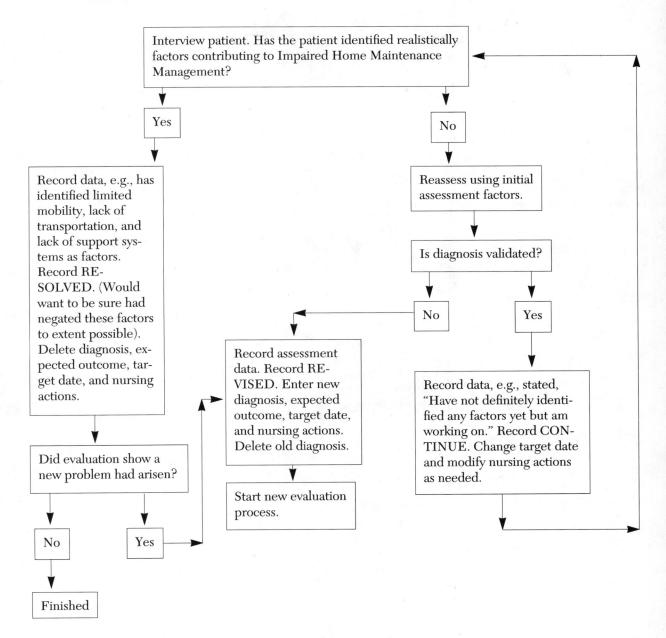

Flow Chart Expected Outcome 2

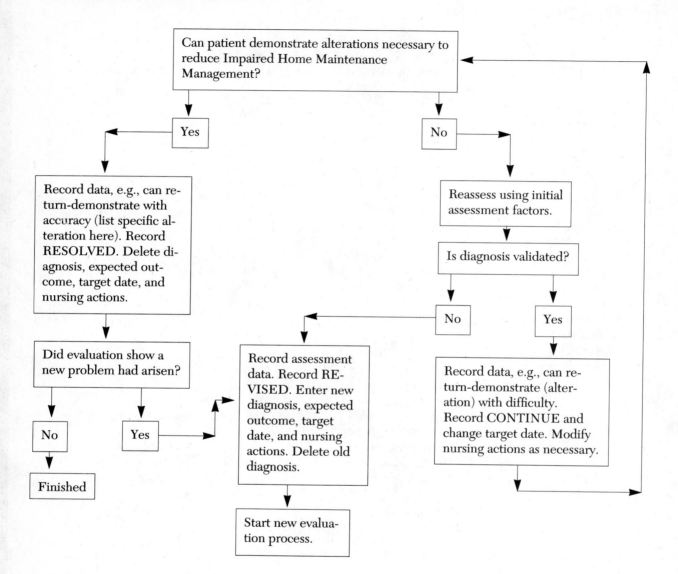

Inability to Sustain Spontaneous Ventilation

DEFINITION

A state in which a patient is unable to maintain adequate breathing to support life. This is measured by deterioration of arterial blood gases, increased work of breathing, and decreasing energy.[27]

NANDA TAXONOMY: EXCHANGING 1.5.1.3.1

DEFINING CHARACTERISTICS[27]

1. Major defining characteristics:
   a. Dyspnea
   b. Increased metabolic rate
2. Minor defining characteristics:
   a. Increased restlessness
   b. Apprehension
   c. Increased use of accessory muscles
   d. Decreased tidal volume
   e. Increased heart rate
   f. Decreased pO_2
   g. Increased pCO_2
   h. Decreased cooperation
   i. Decreased SaO_2

RELATED FACTORS[27]

1. Metabolic factors
2. Respiratory muscle fatigue

RELATED CLINICAL CONCERNS

1. Chronic obstructive pulmonary disease
2. Asthma
3. Closed head injury
4. Respiratory arrest
5. Cardiac surgery
6. Adult respiratory distress syndrome

HAVE YOU SELECTED THE CORRECT DIAGNOSIS?

Ineffective Breathing Pattern In this diagnosis the patient's respiratory effort is insufficient to maintain the cellular oxygen supply. Both diagnoses would contribute to the patient's being placed on ventilatory assistance; however, Inability to Sustain Spontaneous Ventilation would be life-threatening, and a more critical diagnosis than just an Ineffective Breathing Pattern. The major difference would be the criticalness of the patient's condition. (See page 349.)

Impaired Gas Exchange This diagnosis refers to the exchange of oxygen and carbon dioxide in the lungs or at the cellular level. Both this diagnosis and Inability to Sustain Spontaneous Ventilation demonstrate this characteristic, but Inability to Sustain Spontaneous Ventilation is of a more critical nature than an impairment. (See page 416.)

EXPECTED OUTCOME

1. Blood gases will return to normal range by (date) and/or
2. Will not require ventilator support by (date)

TARGET DATE

Due to the life-threatening potential of this diagnosis, initial target dates will need to be stated in terms of hours. After the patient's condition has improved and stabilized, the target date can be increased in increments of 1 to 3 days.

NURSING ACTIONS/INTERVENTIONS WITH RATIONALES

Adult Health

Actions/Interventions	Rationales
• Monitor negative-pressure (pneumobelt or pneumowrap) or positive-pressure (intermittent or continuous) ventilators at least hourly.	Ensures correct functioning of equipment.
• Continuously monitor patient's response to ventilator.	Fear of ventilator malfunction can alter respiratory efforts.
• Provide sedation if needed.	Prevents patient from working against ("bucking") the ventilator.
• Verify ventilator settings every hour.	Ensures adequate functioning of equipment.
• Schedule at least 15 minutes every hour to talk with the patient.	Decreases anxiety; helps prevent patient from working against the ventilator.
• Reassure patient's family while patient is on ventilator.	Essential monitoring of respiratory and ventilator effectiveness.
• Monitor vital signs, especially respiratory status, at least every hour and every time nurse is with patient.	
• Collaborate with physician regarding frequency of ABGs measurements.	Monitors effectiveness of therapy.
• Use pulse oximeter to determine oxygen saturation, and monitor every 15 to 30 minutes.	
• Elevate head of bed 30 degrees if not contraindicated.	Facilitates diaphragmatic excursion.
• Suction as needed.	Removes secretions that may block airways.
• Observe closely for oxygen toxicity.	Inappropriate functioning of ventilator can cause greater oxygen consumption than the body can tolerate.
• Turn every 2 hours on (odd/even) hour.	Facilitates lung expansion; helps to mobilize secretions; improves circulation to extremities; avoids pressure ulcers.
• Explain all procedures and manipulations of ventilator to patient prior to implementing. Keep call light within reach.	Assists in reducing anxiety.

- Provide alternative methods of communication, for example, magic slate, pad and pencil, or flash cards of usual requests (bedpan, urinal, pain, and so on).
- Provide adequate hydration. Monitor and document intake and output at least every shift, total every 24 hours. Weigh patient daily at same time and in same-weight clothing.

Avoids fluid volume deficit, assists in liquifying secretions, and avoids development of pulmonary edema.

- Monitor for respiratory function, for example, temperature, culture, and sensitivity of respiratory sections.

Infection increases the respiratory demand and increases secretions. It will also decrease gas exchange.

- Provide chest physiotherapy and postural drainage if not contraindicated.

Loosens and mobilizes secretions.

- Plan activity-rest schedule on a daily basis. Allow at least 2 hours of uninterrupted rest during the day.

Conserves energy; promotes REM sleep.

- Review patient's resources and support systems for management of ventilator at home.

Initiates timely home care planning.

- Collaborate with respiratory therapist as needed.

Ensures coordination of care.

Child Health

Actions/Interventions	Rationales
<ul><li>Determine parameters for respiratory status:<ul><li>○ Range of acceptable rate, rhythm, and quality of respiration.</li><li>○ Limits for apnea monitor setting.[49] The settings should be set for a range of safety according to age-related norms: (1) *Neonates*: 30 to 60 (2) *Infants*: 25 to 60 (3) *Toddlers*: 24 to 40 (4) *Preschoolers*: 22 to 34 (5) *Adolescents*: 12 to 16</li><li>○ Arterial blood gases</li><li>○ Oxygen saturation levels</li><li>○ Respiratory testing, for example, pneumogram</li><li>○ Other indicators of respiratory function, for example, cyanosis, mottling, diminished pulses, listless behavior, poor feeding, vital signs</li></ul></li></ul>	A specific respiratory assessment will help to individualize the plan of care.

Continued

Actions/Interventions	Rationales
• Provide one-on-one care for infants and children at high risk for apnea or pulmonary arrest.	In high-risk respiratory patients, the possibility of arrest should be planned for. Identification of the actual arrest is a major factor in successful resuscitation.
• Keep emergency medications and equipment (ambu bag, airway, suctioning equipment, crash cart, ventilator, and oxygen) in close proximity.	Success in appropriate treatment of pulmonary arrest requires anticipatory planning with standard treatment modalities according to the American Heart Association guidelines and Pediatric Advanced Life Support guidelines.
• Administer medication as ordered, being especially careful with medications that might affect respirations, for example, narcotics, bronchodilators, or vasoconstrictors. Monitor blood levels for therapeutic parameters of aminophylline-theophylline. Report levels above or below the desired range.	Anticipatory planning for the possibility of respiratory depression or arrest will lessen the likelihood of occurrence in many instances and allow for more success in treatment of these problems. If neuromuscular blocking agents are utilized, exercise caution in positioning due to the possibility of dislocation.[30]
• Encourage family to vent concerns about patient's respiratory status.	Verbalization of concerns helps reduce anxiety and provides subjective data for assessment; provides an opportunity for teaching.
• Allow parental input as an option when it is realistic.	Parental involvement provides emotional security for the child and reinforces parental coping.
• Carry out teaching according to inquiries by patient or family.	Individualized learning is facilitated when it is directed toward stated needs.
• Check level of consciousness (responsiveness) at least every 30 minutes.	Decreased responsiveness is indicative of onset of respiratory failure.
• Monitor and document episodes of crying that result in apnea or loss of usual color for prolonged periods (15 seconds or above).	Breath-holding or crying may seem to cause hypoxia, but often there are underlying causes. Attention to underlying cause can be carried out, but vigilance for possible arrest is necessary.
• Exercise caution in feeding or offering fluids.	Possible aspiration is likely if the infant is apneic, unable to suck well, or has problems swallowing.

• Monitor for contributing factors to problem:
  ○ Central nervous system status
  ○ Airway
  ○ Chest wall
  ○ Respiratory muscles
  ○ Lung tissue
	Alteration in any aspect of respiratory anatomy will affect adequate ventilation.

Additional Information

In the event of a decision to withhold or cease use of the ventilator for the purpose of determining brain death, be aware of the major nursing implications involved in legal acts related to brain death determination in children.

Women's Health

The nursing actions for women's health are the same as those found in Adult Health.

Mental Health

If the client develops this diagnosis while being cared for in a mental health unit, he or she should immediately be transferred to an intensive care unit or adult health unit. A mental health unit is not equipped to handle this type of emergency.

Gerontic Health

Actions/Interventions	Rationales
• Monitor for iatrogenic reactions to medications.	Medication reactions may decrease respiratory drive and effort.
• Observe for signs and symptoms of sleep-pattern disturbance.	Decreased rest secondary to sleep-pattern disturbances further diminishes physiologic reserves in older patients.[45]

Home Health

Should the home health client develop this diagnosis, the nurse should immediately have the client transferred to an acute care setting for the proper care.

FLOW CHART EVALUATION
Flow Chart Expected Outcome 1

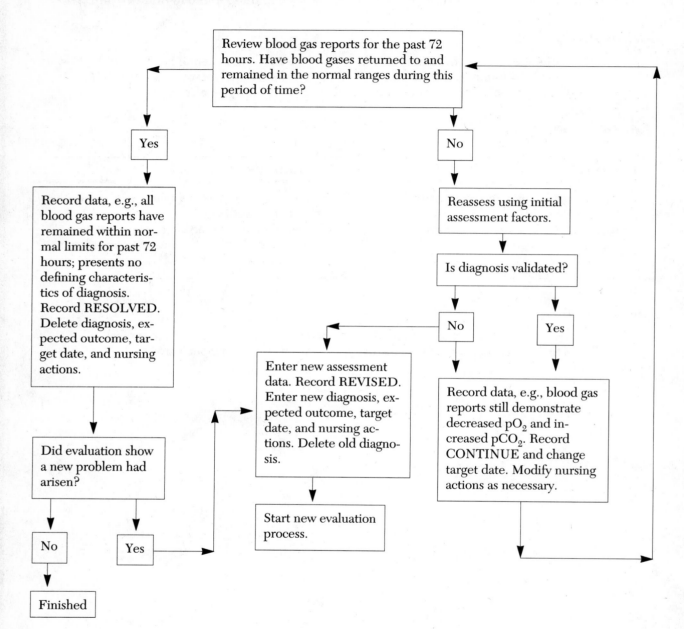

Flow Chart Expected Outcome 2

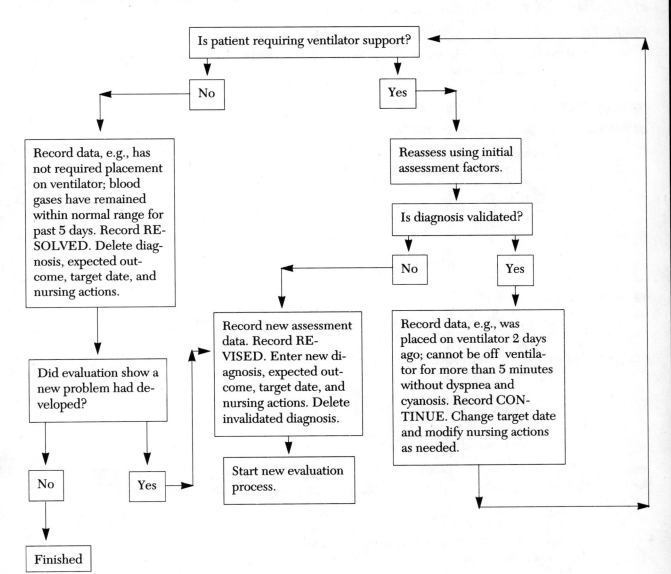

Peripheral Neurovascular Dysfunction, High Risk for

DEFINITION

A state in which an individual is at risk of experiencing a disruption in circulation, sensation, or motion of an extremity.[27]

NANDA TAXONOMY: MOVING 6.1.1.1.1

DEFINING CHARACTERISTICS (RISK FACTORS)[27]

1. Fractures
2. Mechanical compression, for example, tourniquet, cast, brace, dressing, or restraint
3. Orthopedic surgery
4. Trauma
5. Immobilization
6. Burns
7. Vascular obstruction

RELATED FACTORS[27]

The risk factors also serve as the related factors for this high-risk diagnosis.

RELATED CLINICAL CONCERNS

1. Fractures
2. Buerger's disease
3. Thrombophlebitis
4. Burns
5. Cerebrovascular accident

HAVE YOU SELECTED THE CORRECT DIAGNOSIS?

Altered Tissue Perfusion Altered Tissue Perfusion is an actual diagnosis and indicates a definite problem has developed. High Risk for Peripheral Neurovascular Dysfunction indicates that the patient is in danger of developing a problem if appropriate nursing measures are not instituted. (See page 484.)

EXPECTED OUTCOMES

1. Will develop no problems with peripheral neurovascular function by (date) and/or
2. Will be performing at least (number) of activities to offset development of peripheral neurovascular dysfunction by (date)

TARGET DATE

Initial target dates should be stated in hours. After the patient is able to be more involved in self-care and prevention, the target date can be expressed in increments of 3 to 5 days.

NURSING ACTIONS/INTERVENTIONS WITH RATIONALES

Adult Health

Actions/Interventions	Rationales
• Assist patient to do range-of-motion exercises every 2 hours on the (odd/even) hour.	Increases circulation; maintains muscle tone and movement.
• Instruct patient regarding isometric and isotonic exercises. Have patient exercise every 4 hours while awake at (times).	Increases circulation; maintains muscle tone.
• Collaborate with dietitian regarding a low-fat, low-cholesterol diet. Maintain fluid and electrolyte balance.	Maintains hydration; assists in preventing development of atherosclerosis.
• Complete traction checks and peripheral assessments every 2 hours on the (odd/even) hour.	Helps monitor deviations from baseline before problem reaches a serious state.
• Keep extremities warm.	Promotes circulation.
• Turn every 2 hours on the (odd/even) hour.	Prevents sustained pressure on any pressure point.
• Monitor skin integrity every 2 hours on the (odd/even) hour.	Allows intervention before skin breakdown occurs.
• Plan activity-rest schedule on a daily basis.	Increases circulation and maintains muscle tone without fatiguing patient.
• Monitor patient's understanding of effect of smoking, or if nonsmoker, the effects of passive smoke on peripheral circulation.	Smoking constricts peripheral circulation, leading to increased problems with peripheral neurological and vascular functioning.

Child Health

Actions/Interventions	Rationales
• Determine exact parameters to be used in monitoring risk concerns, for example, if the patient is without sensation in specific levels of anatomy, document what the known deficits are: High level of myelomeningocele, Lumbar 4, with apparent sensation in peroneal site.	Specific parameters for assessment of neurodeficits can best guide caregivers in appropriate precautionary treatment.

Continued

Actions/Interventions	Rationales
• Carry out treatments with attention to the neurodeficits, for example, using warm pads for a child unable to perceive heat would require constant attention for signs and/or symptoms of burns.	Common safety measure.
• Provide teaching according to the patient and family's needs, especially with regard to safety.	Appropriate assessment will best foster learning and help prevent injury.
• Include family in care and use of equipment, for example, braces. • Provide dismissal follow-up.	Family involvement meets the child's emotional needs and empowers the parents. Long-term follow-up validates the need for rechecking and offers a time to reassess progress in goal attainment or altered patterns.

Women's Health

> NOTE: Women are at risk for thrombosis in lower extremities during pregnancy and the early postpartum period. Because of decreased venous return from the legs, compression of large vessels supplying legs during pregnancy and during pushing in the second stage of labor, and decreased venous return of blood from the legs during pregnancy, patients need to be continuously assessed for this problem.[50]

Actions/Interventions	Rationales
• Closely monitor patient at each visit and teach patient to self-monitor size, shape, symmetry, color, and edema as well as varicosities in the legs.	Knowledge of the problem and its causative factors can assist in planning and carrying out good health habits during pregnancy. This knowledge can assist in preventing thrombotic complications during pregnancy.
• Encourage the patient to walk daily during the pregnancy and to wear supportive hosiery. • Assist the patient to plan a day's schedule during pregnancy that will allow rest time and time to elevate the legs several times during the day. • Encourage the patient to use a small stool when sitting, for example, at desk, to keep feet elevated and less compression on upper thighs and knees.	
• In the event that thrombophlebitis develops: ◦ Monitor legs for stiffness, pain, paleness, and swelling in the calf or thigh every 4 hours around the clock.	Basic assessment for early detection of complications.
◦ Place patient on strict bed rest with affected leg elevated.	Basic safety measure to avoid dislodging of clots.

- Provide analgesics as ordered for pain relief, and assess for effectiveness within 30 minutes of administration.
- Place a bed cradle on the bed.

Keeps pressure of bed linens off the affected leg.

- Administer and monitor the effects of anticoagulant therapy as ordered. Collaborate with physician regarding the frequency of laboratory exams to monitor clotting factors. *Note*: Breast-feeding mothers on Heparin can continue to breast-feed. *Do not* breast-feed if the mother is on Dicumarol, since it is passed to the infant in breast milk.
- *Do not* rub, massage, or bump affected leg; handle with care when changing linens or giving bath.

Basic safety measures to avoid dislodging clots.

- Assist family to plan for care of infant; include mother in planning process.

Assist patient and family in coping with illness; promotes effective implementation of home care; provides support and teaching opportunity.

- Encourage verbalizations of fears and discouragement of mother and family.

Mental Health

The mental health client with this diagnosis would require the same type of nursing care as in Adult Health. A review of the nursing actions for Activity Intolerance, Impaired Physical Mobility, and Inadequate Tissue Perfusion would also be of assistance.

Gerontic Health

Actions/Interventions	Rationales
- Avoid the use of restraints if at all possible.	Restraint use in older adults can lead to physical and mental deterioration, injury, and death.[46]
- Monitor restraints, if used, at least every 2 hours on the (odd/even) hour. Release restraints and perform range-of-motion exercises before reapplying.	Frequent monitoring decreases the injury risk.

Home Health

Nursing actions for the home health client with this diagnosis would be the same as those for adult health.

FLOW CHART EVALUATION
Flow Chart Expected Outcome 1

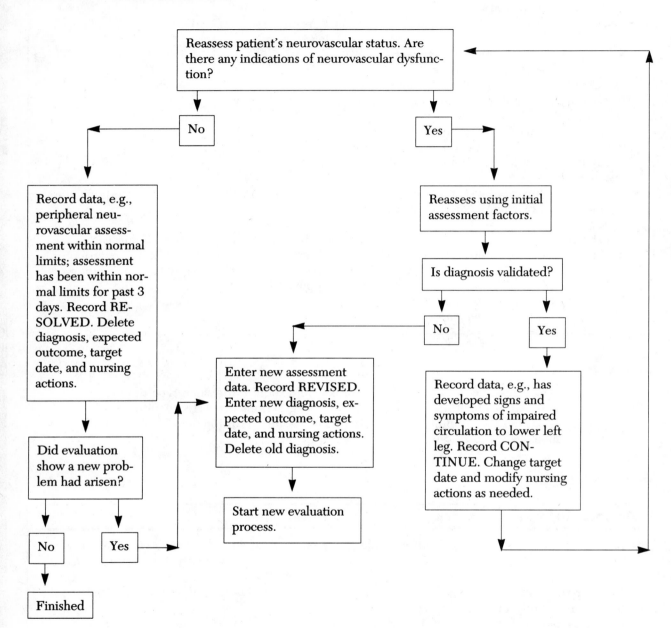

Flow Chart Expected Outcome 2

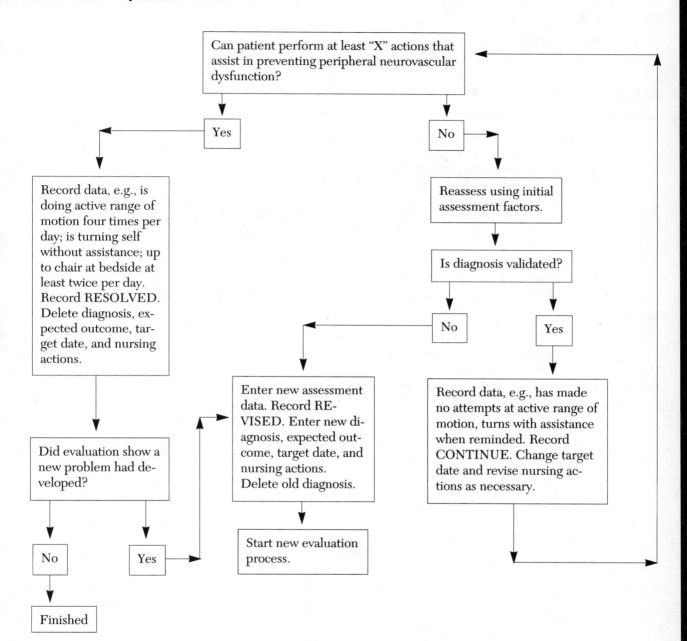

Physical Mobility, Impaired

DEFINITION

A state in which the individual experiences a limitation of ability for independent physical movement.[10]*

NANDA TAXONOMY: MOVING 6.1.1.1

DEFINING CHARACTERISTICS[10]

1. Major defining characteristics:
   a. Inability to purposefully move within the physical environment, including bed mobility, transfer, and ambulation
   b. Reluctance to attempt movement
   c. Limited range of motion
   d. Decreased muscle strength, control, and/or mass
   e. Imposed restrictions of movement, including mechanical or medical protocol
   f. Impaired coordination
2. Minor defining characteristics:
   None given

RELATED FACTORS

1. Intolerance to activity and/or decreased strength and endurance
2. Pain or discomfort
3. Perceptual or cognitive impairment
4. Neuromuscular impairment
5. Depression or severe anxiety

RELATED CLINICAL CONCERNS

1. Fractures that require casting or traction
2. Rheumatoid arthritis
3. Cerebrovascular accident
4. Depression
5. Any neuromuscular disorder

---

*Suggested functional-level classification:

0 = completely independent
1 = requires use of equipment or device
2 = requires help from another person, for assistance, supervision, or teaching
3 = requires help from another person and equipment device
4 = dependent, does not participate in activity

Code adapted by NANDA from E. Jones et al. Patient Classification for Long-Term Care: Users' Manual, HEW, Publication No. HRA-74-3107, November, 1974.

HAVE YOU SELECTED THE CORRECT DIAGNOSIS?

Activity Intolerance This diagnosis implies that the person is freely able to move but cannot endure or adapt to the increased energy or oxygen demands made by the movement or activity. Impaired Physical Mobility indicates that an individual would be able to move independently if something were not limiting the motion.

Impaired Physical Mobility also needs to be differentiated from the respiratory (Impaired Gas Exchange and Ineffective Breathing Pattern) and cardiovascular (Decreased Cardiac Output and Altered Tissue Perfusion) nursing diagnoses. Mobility depends on effective breathing patterns and effective gas exchange between the lungs and the arterial blood supply. Muscles have to receive oxygen and get rid of carbon dioxide for contraction and relaxation. Since oxygen is transported and dispersed to the muscle tissue via the cardiovascular system, it is only logical that the respiratory and cardiovascular diagnoses could impact mobility. (See pages 320, 327, 349, 416, and 484.)

Altered Nutrition: More or Less than Body Requirements Nutritional deficit would indicate that the body is not receiving enough nutrients for its metabolic needs. Without adequate nutrition, the muscles cannot function appropriately. With More than Body Requirements, mobility may be impaired simply because of the excess weight. In someone who is grossly obese, range of motion is limited, gait is altered, and coordination and tone are greatly reduced. (See pages 200 and 215.)

EXPECTED OUTCOMES

1. Will demonstrate measures (identify specifics) to increase mobility by (date) and/or
2. Will demonstrate increased strength and endurance by (date)

TARGET DATE

These dates may be short-term or long-term based on the etiology of the diagnosis. An acceptable first target date would be 5 days.

NURSING ACTIONS/INTERVENTIONS WITH RATIONALES

Adult Health

Actions/Interventions	Rationales
• Maintain proper body alignment at all times; support extremities with pillows, blankets, towel rolls, or sandbags. Use foot boards, firm mattress, and bed boards as necessary to support positioning.	Prevents flexion contractures.

Continued

Actions/Interventions	Rationales
• Implement measures to prevent falls, such as keeping bed in low position, raising siderails, and having items within easy reach.	Basic safety measures.
• Teach patient how to move body in bed.	Prevents shearing forces; participation promotes self-esteem.
• Perform range-of-motion (ROM) exercises (passive, active, and functional) every 2 hours on the (odd/even) hour.	Increases circulation, maintains muscle tone, and prevents joint contractures.
• Turn, cough, and deep-breathe every 2 hours on a schedule opposite from the ROM exercises, for example, if ROM exercises are performed on even hour, then turn, cough, and deep-breathe on odd hour. Massage pressure points after turning.	Increases circulation, promotes maintenance of lung functioning, keeps airways clear, assists in preventing hypostatic pneumonia, and improves tissue oxygenation.
• Monitor skin over pressure areas every 4 hours while awake at (times).	Basic monitoring of skin integrity.
• Implement nursing actions specific to traction, casts, braces, prostheses, slings, and bandages.	Each of these therapies also have complicating side effects.
• Provide progressive mobilization as tolerated. Schedule increased mobilization on a daily basis, for example, increase ambulation length by 25 feet each day.	Maintains muscle tone and prevents complications of immobility.
• Medicate for pain as needed, especially before activity. Document effectiveness of medication within 30 minutes after administering medication.	Pain interferes with ability to ambulate by inhibiting muscle movement.
• Apply heat or cold as ordered.	Aids in muscle healing and promotes relaxation.
• Maintain adequate nutrition on a daily basis.	Provides nutrients for energy and prevents protein loss due to immobility.
• Collaborate with physical therapist regarding exercise program.	Coordinates team approach to care.
• Observe for complications of immobility, for example, negative nitrogen balance or constipation.	Allows early detection and prevention of complications.

• Provide health teaching:
  ○ Transfer methods
  ○ Use of assistive devices
  ○ Safety precautions
  ○ Positioning and body mechanics
  ○ Prescribed exercise
  ○ Self-care activities
	Facilitates understanding of care, encourages participation in care, and promotes effective management of therapeutic regimen.

• Include patient and family or significant other in carrying out plan of care.	Allows time for practice under supervision; increases likelihood of effective management of therapeutic regimen.

Child Health

Actions/Interventions	Rationales

• Monitor alteration in mobility each 8-hour shift according to:
  ○ Actual movement noted and tolerance for the movement
  ○ Factors related to movement, for example, braces used and progress in their use
  ○ Situational factors, for example, previous status, current health needs, or movement permitted
  ○ Pain
  ○ Circulation check to affected limb
  ○ Change in appearance of affected limb or joint
	Provides the primary database for an individualized plan of care.

• Include related health team members in care of patient as needed. (See Appendix B.)	The nurse is in the prime position to coordinate health team members to best match needs and resources.
• Consider patient and family preferences in planning to meet desired mobility goals.	Consideration of preferences increases likelihood of plan's success.
• Encourage family members, especially parents, to participate in care of patient according to needs and situation (feeding and comfort measures).	Involving family in care serves to enhance their skills in care required at home.
• Provide diversional activities appropriate for age and developmental level.	Diversional activity when appropriately planned serves to refresh and relax the patient.
• Maintain appropriate safety guidelines according to age and developmental guidelines.	Basic requirements for maintaining standards of care.
• Devote appropriate attention to traction or related equipment in use, for example, weights hanging free or rope knots tight.	Ensures therapeutic effectiveness of equipment and provides for safety issues related to these interventions.
• Monitor patient and family needs for education regarding patient's situation and any future implications.	Allows timely planning for home care and allows practice of care in a supportive environment.
• Attend to intake and output to ensure adequate fluid balance for each 24-hour period.	Strict intake and output will assist in monitoring hydration status, which is crucial for healing and circulatory adequacy.
• Address related health issues appropriate for patient and family.	Appropriate attention to related health issues fosters holistic care; for example, child may need braces but may also have need for healing, speech follow-up secondary to meningitis, and developmental delays.

Women's Health

NOTE: The following nursing actions apply to those women placed on restrictive activities because of threatened abortion, premature labor, multiple pregnancy, or pregnancy-induced hypertension.

Actions/Interventions	Rationales
• Encourage family and significant others to participate in plan of care for patient.	
• When resting in bed, have patient rest in left lateral position as much as possible.	Will prevent supine hypotension and will allow adequate renal and uterine perfusion.
• Encourage patient to list lifestyle adjustments that will need to be made.	
• Teach patient relaxation skills and coping mechanisms.	Decreases anxiety and muscle tension.
• Encourage adequate protein intake.	Replaces protein lost due to decreasing muscle contraction during immobility.
• Maintain proper body alignment with use of positioning and pillow.	Decreases anxiety and reduces muscle tension. Provides appropriate amounts of activity without danger to pregnancy.
• Provide diversionary activities, for example, hobbies, job-related activities that can be done in bed, or activities with children.	

• Encourage help and visits from friends and relatives:
  ○ Visits in person
  ○ Telephone visits
  ○ Help with child care
  ○ Help with housework	

Mental Health

NOTE: Related to imposed restrictions.

Actions/Interventions	Rationales
• Attempt all other interventions before considering immobilizing client as an intervention. (See High Risk for Violence, Chapter 9, for appropriate nursing actions.)	Promotes client's sense of control and supports self-esteem.
• Carefully monitor client for appropriate level of restraint necessary. Immobilize the client as little as possible while still protecting the client and others.	
• Obtain necessary medical orders to initiate methods that limit the client's physical mobility.	

- Carefully explain to client in brief, concise language reasons for initiating this intervention and what behavior must be present for the intervention to be terminated.

Excessive stimuli can increase confusion; provides client with sense of control.

- Attempt to gain client's voluntary compliance with the intervention by explaining to client what is needed and with a "show of force." (Have the necessary number of staff available to force compliance.)

Promotes client's sense of control and safety. This promotes self-esteem.

- Initiate forced compliance only if there is an adequate number of staff to complete the action safely. (See High Risk for Violence, Chapter 9, for a detailed description of intervention with forced compliance.)

Client and staff safety are of primary concern.

- Secure the environment the client will be in by removing harmful objects such as accessible light bulbs, sharp objects, glass objects, tight clothing, and metal objects such as clothes hangers or shower curtain rods.

Prevents injury by protecting client from impulsive actions of self-harm.

- If client is placed in four-point restraints, maintain one-to-one supervision.

Client safety is of primary concern.

- If client is in seclusion or in bilateral restraints, observe client at least every 15 minutes, more frequently if agitated (list observation schedule here).
- Leave urinal in room with client or offer toileting every hour.
- Offer client fluids every 15 minutes.

Maintains adequate hydration.

- Discuss with client his or her feelings about the initiation of immobility, and review with him or her again, at least twice a day, the behavior necessary to have immobility discontinued.

Exploration of feelings in an accepting environment helps client to identify and explore maladaptive coping behaviors. Promotes client's sense of perceived control.

- When checking client, let him or her know you are checking by calling him or her by name and orienting him or her to day and time. Inquire about client's feelings and implement necessary reality orientation.

Promotes perceived control and promotes an environment of trust.

- Provide meals at regular intervals on paper containers, providing necessary assistance (amount and type of assistance required should be listed here).

Meet biophysical need while providing consistency in a respectful manner that promotes self-esteem and trust.

- If client is in restraints, remove restraints at least every 2 hours, one limb at a time. Have client move limb through a full range of motion and inspect for signs of injury. Apply lubricants such as lotion to area under restraint to protect from injury.

Promotes normal circulation and motion, which prevents injury to the limb.

Continued

Actions/Interventions	Rationales
• Pad the area of the restraint that is next to the skin with sheepskin or other nonirritating material.	Protects skin from mechanical irritation.
• Check circulation in restrained limbs in the area below the restraint by observing skin color, warmth, and swelling. Restraint should not interfere with circulation.	Early assessment and intervention prevent serious injury.
• Change client's position in the bed every 2 hours on the (odd/even) hour.	Prevents disuse syndrome.
• Place body in proper alignment. Use pillows for support if client's condition allows.	Prevents complications and injury.
• If client is in four-point restraints, place him or her on stomach or side.	Prevents aspiration or choking.
• Place client on intake and output monitoring.	Assures that adequate fluid balance is maintained. Prevents complications of immobility.
• Have client in seclusion move around the room at least every 2 hours on the (odd/ even) hour, and during this time initiate active range of motion.	
• Administer medications as ordered for agitation.	Medications reduce anxiety and facilitate interaction with others.
• Monitor blood pressure before administering antipsychotic medications.	Psychotropic medications can cause orthostatic hypotension.
• Assist client with daily personal hygiene. (Record time for this here.)	Communicates positive regard for the client by the nurse, which facilitates the development of positive self-esteem.
• Have environment cleaned on a daily basis.	Promotes sanitary conditions and provides an orderly environment which can decrease the client's disorganization and confusion.
• Review with client the purpose for restraint or seclusion as required and discuss alternative kinds of behavior that will express feelings without threatening self or others.	Promotes client's sense of control by providing him or her with behavioral alternatives and establishing clear limits.
• Remove client from seclusion as soon as the contracted behavior is observed for the required amount of time (both of these should be very specific and listed here). See High Risk for Violence, Chapter 9, for detailed information.	Provides positive reinforcement for appropriate coping behavior and promotes client's sense of control.
◦ If restrictions are due to anxiety, refer to Chapter 8 and the diagnosis of Anxiety.	
◦ If restrictions are due to depressed mood, implement the following interventions: (1) Sit with client for (number) minutes (number) times per shift. Initially	

these times will be brief but frequent, for example, 5 minutes per hour.

(2) Establish clear expectations for these interactions, for example, that client is not expected to talk and that it is okay for these times to be spent in silence.

Communicates respect for the client and facilitates the client's perception of control.

- Explain to client in simple concrete terms the positive effects of physical activity on mood. Note person responsible for this teaching here.

Physical activity can stimulate endorphin production, which has a positive effect on mood.

- Talk with client about activities he or she has enjoyed in the past.

Promotes a positive expectational set based on past positive experiences.

- Develop with client program for increasing physical activity. Note that contact here. Also note rewards for accomplishing goals for activity, and have patient identify ways he or she could assist with this. Note person responsible for assistance here, and note plan when it is developed.

Promotes client's sense of control. Positive reinforcement encourages behavior and enhances self-esteem.

Gerontic Health

Actions/Interventions	Rationales
• Monitor for complications of immobility such as: 　○ Orthostatic hypotension 　○ Thrombosis 　○ Urinary tract infections 　○ Constipation	Normal aging changes in combination with immobility can leave the older adult at increased risks for complications.[47]
• Observe patient, when changing position, pushing a wheelchair, or toileting, for Valsalva maneuver (increased intrathoracic pressure induced by forceful exhalation against a closed glottis).	Valsalva maneuver can produce increased pulse rate and increased BP. This adversely affects patients with cardiovascular disorders, which may lead to their choosing not to engage in physical activity.[47]
• Monitor for behavioral changes that may result from decreased sensory stimulation or decreased socialization, for example, depression, hostility, confusion, or anxiety.	Psychologic changes not addressed may increase problems of physical mobility and lead to prolonged periods of immobility.
• Observe when increasing mobility, transferring, or during early ambulation stage for the high risk for falls.	Older adults may be at risk for falls secondary to orthostatic BP. Changes or problems with balance can occur, especially after prolonged periods of immobility.
• Teach client to perform isometric muscle contraction, namely, tightening of muscle group as hard as possible and then relaxing the muscle.	Isometric contraction helps maintain muscle strength, which can decrease with immobility as much as 5 percent per day.[47]

Home Health

Actions/Interventions	Rationales
• Assist patient and family in identifying risk factors pertinent to the situation: ○ Immobility ○ Malnourishment ○ Confusion or lethargy ○ Physical barriers ○ Neuromuscular deficit ○ Musculoskeletal deficit ○ Trauma ○ Pain ○ Medications that affect coordination and level or arousal ○ Debilitating disease (cancer, stroke, diabetes, muscular dystrophy, multiple sclerosis, arthritis, and so on) ○ Depression ○ Lack of or improper use of assistive devices ○ Casts, slings, traction, IVs, and so on ○ Weather hazards • Teach client and family measures to promote physical activity: ○ Using assistive devices (wheelchairs, crutches, canes, walkers, prostheses, adaptive eating utensils, devices to assist with activities of daily living, and so on) ○ Providing safe environment (reduce barriers to activity such as throw rugs, furniture in pathway, electric cords on floor, doors, steps, and so on) ○ Maintaining skin integrity ○ Using safety devices (ramps, lift bars, tub rails, or tub or shower seat) ○ Using proper transfer techniques	Locus of control shifts from nurse to client and family, thus promoting self-care.
• Assist patient and family in identifying life-style changes that may be required: ○ Alteration in living space (ramps, assistive devices, and so on) ○ Changes in role functions ○ Range-of-motion exercises ○ Positioning and transferring techniques ○ Pain control ○ Progressive activity ○ Use of assistive devices ○ Prevention of injury	Provides basic information for client and family that promotes necessary lifestyle changes.

○ Maintenance of skin integrity
○ Assistance with activities of daily living
○ Special transportation needs
○ Financial concerns

- Consult with or refer to appropriate assistive resources as indicated. (See Appendix B.)

Provides additional support for client and family and uses already available resources in a cost-effective manner.

FLOW CHART EVALUATION
Flow Chart Expected Outcome 1

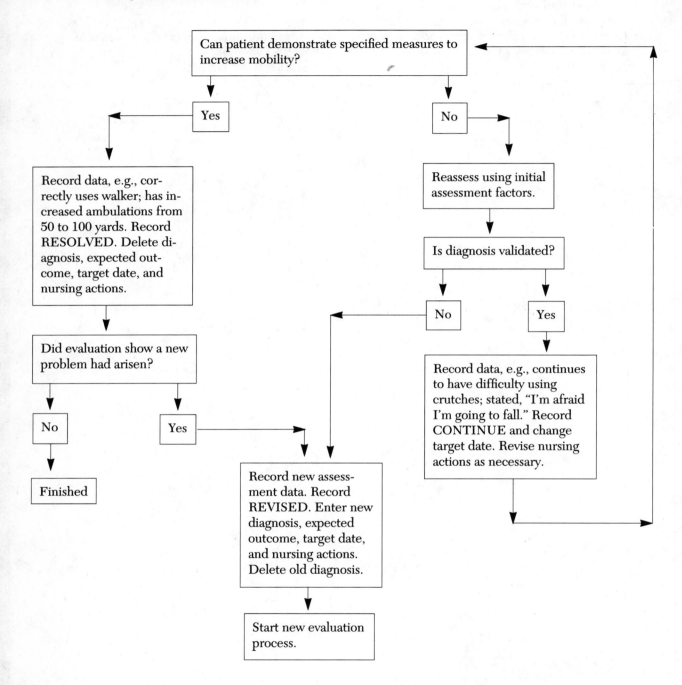

Flow Chart Expected Outcome 2

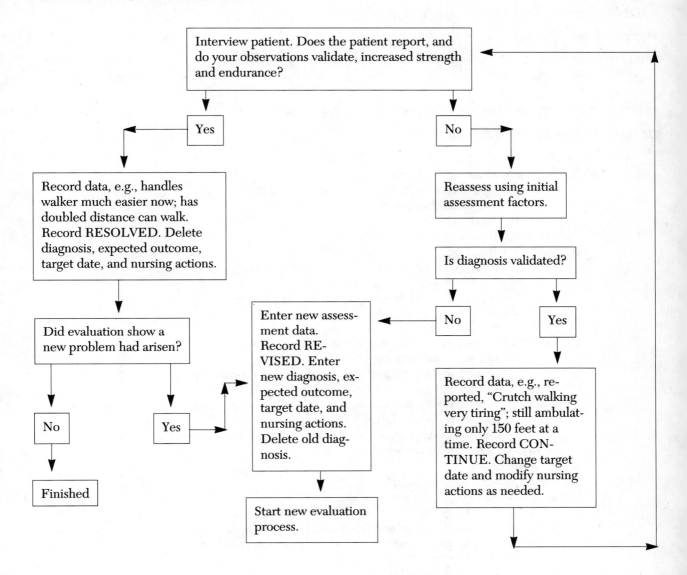

Self-Care Deficit (Feeding, Bathing-Hygiene, Dressing-Grooming, Toileting)

DEFINITION

A state in which the individual experiences an impaired ability to perform or complete feeding, bathing-hygiene, dressing-grooming, or toileting activities for oneself.

NANDA TAXONOMY: MOVING 6.5.1, 6.5.2, 6.5.3, 6.5.4

DEFINING CHARACTERISTICS

1. Feeding Self-Care Deficit:*
   a. Major defining characteristic:
   Inability to bring food from a receptacle to the mouth
   b. Minor defining characteristics:
   None given
2. Bathing-Hygiene Self-Care Deficit:*
   a. Major defining characteristics:
   (1) Inability to wash body or body parts (*critical*)
   (2) Inability to obtain or get to water source
   (3) Inability to regulate temperature or flow of water
   b. Minor defining characteristics:
   None given
3. Dressing-Grooming Self-Care Deficit:*
   a. Major defining characteristics:
   (1) Impaired ability to put on or take off necessary items of clothing (*critical*)
   (2) Impaired ability to obtain or replace articles of clothing
   (3) Impaired ability to fasten clothing
   (4) Inability to maintain appearance at a satisfactory level
   b. Minor defining characteristics:
   None given
4. Toileting Self-Care Deficit:*
   a. Major defining characteristics:
   (1) Unable to get to toilet or commode (*critical*)
   (2) Unable to sit on or rise from toilet or commode (*critical*)
   (3) Unable to manipulate clothing for toileting (*critical*)
   (4) Unable to carry out proper toilet hygiene (*critical*)
   (5) Unable to flush toilet or commode
   b. Minor defining characteristics:
   None given

RELATED FACTORS

1. Feeding, Bathing-Hygiene, Dressing-Grooming Self-Care Deficit
   a. Intolerance to activity and/or decreased strength and endurance
   b. Pain or discomfort

---

*Level 0 to 4; use same code as used in Impaired Physical Mobility.

    c. Perceptual or cognitive impairment
    d. Neuromuscular impairment
    e. Musculoskeletal impairment
    f. Depression or severe anxiety

2. Toileting Self-Care Deficit:
    a. Impaired transfer ability
    b. Impaired mobility status
    c. Intolerance to activity
    d. Decreased strength and endurance
    e. Pain or discomfort
    f. Perceptual or cognitive impairment
    g. Neuromuscular impairment
    h. Musculoskeletal impairment
    i. Depression or severe anxiety

RELATED CLINICAL CONCERNS

1. Cerebrovascular accident
2. Spinal cord injury
3. Dementia
4. Depression
5. Rheumatoid arthritis

HAVE YOU SELECTED THE CORRECT DIAGNOSIS?

Activity Intolerance　　This diagnosis implies that the individual is freely able to move but cannot endure or adapt to the increased energy or oxygen demands made by the movement or activity. Activity Intolerance can be a contributing factor to the development of Self-Care Deficit. (See page 327.)

Impaired Physical Mobility　　This diagnosis is quite often a contributing factor to the development of Self-Care Deficit. It is probable that any time a patient has Impaired Physical Mobility, he or she will also have some degree of Self-Care Deficit. (See page 460.)

Altered Thought Process　　If the patient is exhibiting impaired attention span, impaired ability to recall information, impaired perception, judgment, and decision making, or impaired conceptual and reasoning ability, the most proper diagnosis would be Altered Thought Process. Most likely, Self-Care Deficit would be a companion diagnosis. (See page 577.)

Ineffective Individual Coping or Ineffective Family Coping　　Suspect one of these diagnoses if there are major differences between reports by the patient and the family of health status, health perception, and health care behavior. Verbalizations by the patient or the family regarding inability to cope also require looking at these diagnoses. (See pages 874 and 892.)

Altered Family Processes　　Through observing family interactions and communication, the nurse may assess that Altered Family Processes should be considered. Poorly communicated messages, rigidity of family functions and roles, and failure to accomplish expected family developmental tasks are a few observations to alert the nurse to this possible diagnosis. (See page 710.)

EXPECTED OUTCOMES

1. Will implement a self-care plan by (date) and/or
2. Will return-demonstrate, with 100 percent accuracy, (specify) self-care by (date)

TARGET DATE

Overcoming a self-care deficit will take a significant investment of time; however, 7 days from the date of diagnosis would be an appropriate date to check for progress.

NURSING ACTIONS/INTERVENTIONS WITH RATIONALES

Adult Health

> NOTE: Self-care deficits range from a total self-care deficit to very specific areas of self-care deficits, such as bathing-hygiene or feeding. The nursing actions presented are general in nature and would need to be adapted to fit the exact self-care deficit of the individual. Collaboration with a rehabilitation nurse clinician or review of rehabilitation literature would be excellent sources for current and specific nursing actions related to the specific self-care deficit. Review of the nursing actions for Altered Urinary Elimination Patterns, Activity Intolerance, Impaired Physical Mobility, Impaired Skin Integrity, and Altered Nutrition will also be helpful.

Actions/Interventions	Rationales

• Provide extra time for giving daily care and include:
  ○ Emotional support
  ○ Teaching
  ○ Return-demonstration of self-care activities
	Instills trust, avoids overwhelming patient, facilitates self-motivation, and allows immediate feedback on self-care.

• Provide privacy and safety for patient to practice self-care.	Avoids embarrassment for patient, provides basic safety, and allows practice in closely supervised situation.
• Remind patient to wear corrective appliances, for example, braces, dentures, glasses, or hearing aid.	Promotes self-care by offsetting present limitations.
• Provide positive reinforcement for each self-care accomplishment.	Increases self-esteem and motivation.
• Perform range-of-motion exercises, or assist patient with them, every 4 hours while awake at (times).	Increases circulation and maintains muscle tone and joint mobility.
• Assist patient and significant others in planning measures to overcome or adapt to self-care deficits: ○ Gradual increments in self-care responsibility, for example, getting up in chair independently before ambulating to bathroom by self	Promotes timely home care planning and encourages participation in care.

- ○ Self-care assistive devices, for example, helping hand
- Assist significant others to provide assistive devices, for example, raised toilet seat, buttonhook, or angled extension comb and brush
- Place visual aid in room to help document progress:
  - ○ Chart that allows placement of stars for each day patient accomplishes goal in self-care
  - ○ Calendar on which to document progress
- Monitor:
  - ○ Vital signs every 4 hours while awake at (times)
  - ○ Ambulation: Increase, to extent possible, on a daily basis
- Collaborate with physician regarding pain management.
- Measure intake and output. Total every 8 hours and every 24 hours.
- Monitor bowel elimination at least once daily at (time).
- Establish bowel- and bladder-retraining programs as necessary. See Altered Bowel and Urinary Elimination, Chapter 4.
- Collaborate with dietitian regarding diet, for example, foods to facilitate self-feeding.
- Refer to community support services. (See Appendix B.)
- Have visiting nurse service assist significant others to adapt home environment, at least 3 days prior to discharge:
  - ○ Nonskid rugs
  - ○ Ramps
  - ○ Handrails
  - ○ Safety strips in tub and shower

Visually documents success.

Provides baseline data needed to validate progress and assists in determining physiological impact of progress.

Pain inhibits muscle movement and activity.

Basic monitoring of fluid and electrolyte status that impacts mobility and self-care. Baseline data that assists in determining bowel functioning pattern.
Provides basic education, practice, and reinforcement that facilitates patient's control of these functions.
Promotes self-care and provides motivation to continue striving for improvement.
Provides for long-term support.

Provides time to adapt home for basic safety measures.

Child Health

Actions/Interventions	Rationales
• Monitor patient's and parent's potential for self-care measures appropriate to age and developmental factors.	Provides a database for an individualized plan of care.
• Allow patient and parents to participate in planning for care when possible to help ensure best compliance.	Enhances satisfaction and increases likelihood that care will be continued after discharge from hospital.

Continued

Actions/Interventions	Rationales
• Teach the appropriate skills necessary for self-care in the child's terms, with sensitivity to developmental needs for practice, repetition, or reluctance. • Provide opportunities to enhance the child's confidence in performing self-care.	Individualized teaching best affords reinforcement of learning. Sensitivity to special need attaches value to the patient and family's needs. Confidence in self-care will enhance self-esteem.

Women's Health

Actions/Interventions	Rationales
• Encourage patient to list lifestyle adjustments that need to be made.	Promotes gradual assumption of self-care while avoiding overwhelming patient with activities that must be accomplished.
• Encourage progressive activity and increased self-care as tolerated: ○ Ambulation ○ Bathing ○ Body image and early exercises ○ Bowel care ○ Breast care ○ Perineal care • Encourage patient to get adequate rest: ○ Take care of self and baby only. ○ Let significant other take care of the housework and other children. ○ Learn to sleep when the baby sleeps. ○ Have specific, set times for visiting of friends or relatives. ○ If breast-feeding, significant other can bring infant to mother at night. (Mother doesn't always have to get up every time for infant.)	
• Provide quiet, supportive atmosphere for interaction with infant.	Promotes bonding.
• Instruct patient in infant care and have return-demonstrate: ○ Bathing: (1) *Never* leave infant or small child alone in bath. (2) Bathe in small area (kitchen sink is good) for first weeks. (3) Use warm area in home. (4) Bathing area should be convenient for mother. (5) Avoid drafts.	Basic teaching measures for care of newborn.

      (6) Never run water directly from faucet onto infant, and always test with forearm before placing infant in water (warm, but not too hot).

- Cord care:
  - (1) Clean with alcohol and cotton swabs when changing diapers.
  - (2) Clean around base of cord.
  - (3) Leave alone until it drops off.
  - (4) Alert mother that there will be a small amount of spotting (bleeding) at cord site when it drops off.
- Clothing:
  - (1) How to determine if infant is warm enough: Feel infant's chest or back with hand; never judge infant's body temperature by feeling infant's hands or feet.
  - (2) Discuss the laundering of infant's clothing.
- Diapering:
  - (1) Cloth diapers
  - (2) Disposable diapers
  - (3) Cleaning of infant when changing diapers
- Circumcision care:
  - (1) Explain purpose and care of Yellen clamp (metal clamp).
  - (2) Gently wash penis with water to remove urine and feces.
  - (3) Reapply fresh, sterile Vaseline gauze around glans.
  - (4) It is best to use cloth diapers until circumcision is completely healed (approximately 7 to 10 days).
- Plastic bell:
  - (1) Gently wash penis with water to remove urine and feces.
  - (2) *Do not* apply Vaseline gauze.
  - (3) Leave plastic circle on penis alone until tissue heals and circle falls off.
- Taking baby's temperature and reading a thermometer:
  - (1) Axillary
  - (2) Rectal

- Explain infant alert and rest states and how caretaker can best use these states to interact with infant.

Promotes bonding.

Mental Health

Actions/Interventions	Rationales
• Determine client's optimum level of functioning and note here.	This information assists in establishing realistic goals.
• Develop behavioral short-term goals by:	Goal accomplishment provides positive reinforcement and enhances self-esteem.
○ Listing those activities client can assume	
○ Breaking these activities into their component parts	
○ Determining how much of each activity client could successfully complete and listing achievable activities here with goal achievement dates	
○ Discussing expectations with client	
• Keep instructions simple.	Inappropriate levels of sensory stimuli can contribute to the client's sense of disorganization and confusion.
• Provide support to client during tasks by:	Interaction with the nurse can be a source of positive reinforcement.
○ Spending time with client while he or she is completing the task	
○ Having all items necessary to achieve task readily available	Increases possibility for client's successfully completing the task.
○ Assisting client in focusing on the task at hand	
○ Providing positive verbal feedback as each step of the task is achieved	Positive feedback encourages behavior.
• Keep environment uncluttered, presenting only those items necessary to complete the task in the order needed.	Inappropriate levels of sensory stimuli can contribute to the client's sense of disorganization and confusion.
• Develop a reward schedule for achievement of goals. Discuss with client possible rewards, and list those things client finds rewarding here with the goal to be achieved to gain the reward.	Promotes client's sense of control, and positive feedback encourages behavior.
• Schedule adequate time for client to accomplish task. (Depressed client may need 2 hours to bathe and dress.)	Communicates acceptance of the client, which facilitates the development of trust and self-esteem.
• Decrease environmental stimuli to the degree necessary to assist client in focusing on task.	Promotes client's sense of control.
• Present activities of daily living on a regular schedule, and note that schedule here. This schedule should be developed in consultation with the client.	
• Spend (number) minutes with client twice a day discussing feelings and reactions to current progress and expectations. Times for this and person responsible for this activity should be listed here.	Expression of feelings in a safe environment can facilitate problem identification and the development of coping strategies.

- Allow client to perform activities even though it might be easier at times for staff to complete the task for the client.

Communicates trust and promotes client's sense of control.

- Communicate expectations and goals to all staff members.
- Discuss with family and other support systems and the client the plan and goals. Spend at least 5 minutes with family after each visit to answer questions and explain treatment plan.

Promotes consistency in the treatment and communicates respect for the client. Increases potential for success of treatment plan.

- Have support systems identify how they can assist client in achieving established goals.
- Spend time with client discussing alternative ways of coping with the frustration that may occur while attempting to reach established goals.

Promotes client's sense of control when he or she encounters these difficulties. Successful coping will promote positive self-esteem.

- Collaborate with occupational therapist or physical therapist regarding special adaptations needed to assist client with task accomplishment, for example, exercises to increase muscle strength when the muscles have not been used for a period of time.
- Monitor effects medications might have on goal achievement, and collaborate with physician regarding problematic areas.
- Develop goals and schedules with client, communicating that he or she does have responsibility and control in issues related to care.
- Discuss with client and significant others those things that will facilitate continuance of self-care at home and develop a plan that will assist client in obtaining necessary items.

Facilitates the development of positive coping strategies and increases potential for success when the client returns home. Successful accomplishment of this transition promotes positive self-esteem.

- Refer to community resources as necessary for continued support. (See Appendix B.)

Gerontic Health

Actions/Interventions	Rationales
• Teach self-monitoring skills, such as maintaining a journal or diary to record what factors may increase the self-care deficit.	Encourage patient to identify areas that may need improvement or changes in life-style.[48]
• Contract with the patient for achievement of specific incremental goals and provide rewards or reinforcements when goals are met.	Enhances motivation to increase self-care.

Home Health

Actions/Interventions	Rationales
• Monitor factors contributing to self-care deficit of (specify). This includes items in the Related Factors section.	Provides database for prevention and/or early intervention.
• Involve client and family in planning, implementing, and promoting reduction in the specific self-care deficit: ○ Family conference ○ Mutual goal setting ○ Communication	Involvement improves motivation and improves the outcome.
• Assist client and family to obtain assistive equipment as required: ○ Raised toilet seat ○ Adaptive equipment for eating utensils, combs, brushes, and so on ○ Rocker knife ○ Suction device under plate or bowl ○ Wrist or hand splints ○ Blender, crockpot, or microwave ○ Long-handled reacher (helping hand) ○ Box on seat of chair ○ Raised ledge on utility board ○ Straw and straw holder ○ Washcloth with soap ○ Wheelchair, walker, motorized cart, or cane ○ Bedside commode and/or incontinence undergarments ○ Bars and attachments and benches for shower or tub ○ Hand-held shower device	Assistive equipment improves functioning and increases the possibilities for self-care.

- Long-handled sponge
- Shaver holder
- Medication organizers and/or magnifying glass
- Diet supplements
- Hearing aid
- Corrective lenses
- Dressing aids: Dressing stick, zipper pull, buttonhook, long-handled shoehorn, shoe fasteners, or Velcro closures
- Teach client and family signs and symptoms of overexertion:
  - Pain
  - Fatigue
  - Confusion
  - Decrease or excessive increase in vital signs
  - Injury

Planning activities around physical capabilities prevents further reduction in self-care capacity.

- Assist client and family in life-style adjustments that may be required:
  - Teaching proper use of assistive equipment
  - Adapting to need for assistance or assistive equipment
  - Determining criteria for monitoring client's ability to function unassisted
  - Time management
  - Stress management
  - Development of support systems
  - Learning new skills
  - Setting work, family, social, and personal goals and priorities
  - Coping with disability or dependency
  - Providing environment conducive to self-care privacy, pain relief, social contact, and familiar and favorite surroundings and foods
  - Prevention of injury (falls, aspiration, burns, and so on)
  - Monitoring skin integrity
  - Development of consistent routine
  - Mechanism for alerting to need for assistance

Provides basic information for client and family that promotes necessary life-style changes.

- Refer to appropriate assistive resources as indicated. (See Appendix B.)

Provides additional support for client and family and uses already available resources in a cost-effective manner.

FLOW CHART EVALUATION
Flow Chart Expected Outcome 1

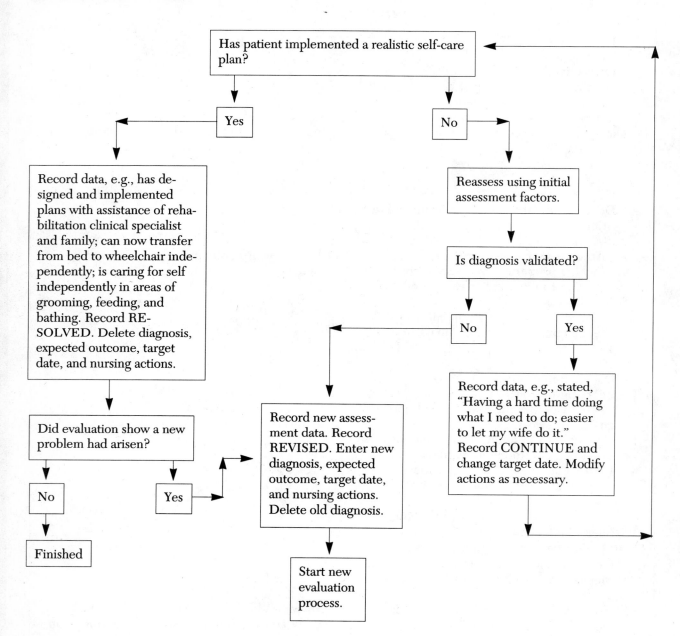

Flow Chart Expected Outcome 2

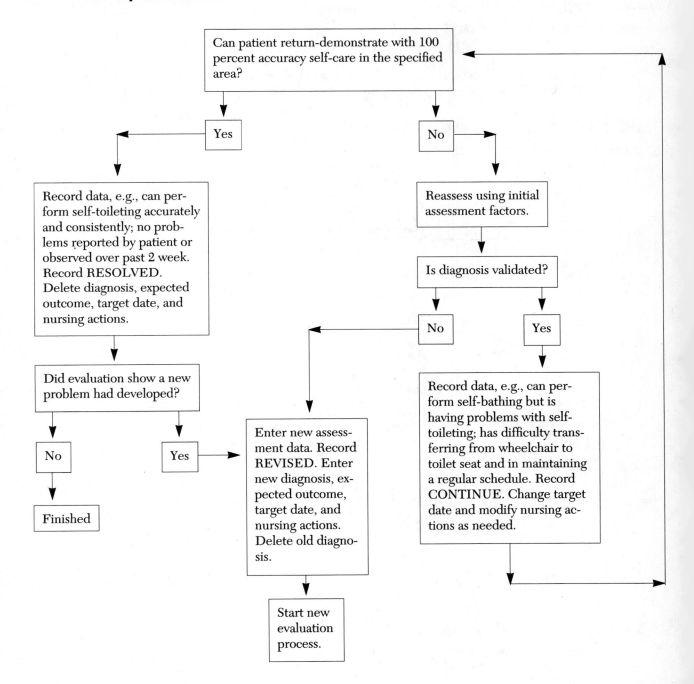

Can patient return-demonstrate with 100 percent accuracy self-care in the specified area?

Yes

No

Record data, e.g., can perform self-toileting accurately and consistently; no problems reported by patient or observed over past 2 week. Record RESOLVED. Delete diagnosis, expected outcome, target date, and nursing actions.

Reassess using initial assessment factors.

Is diagnosis validated?

No

Yes

Did evaluation show a new problem had developed?

No

Yes

Finished

Enter new assessment data. Record REVISED. Enter new diagnosis, expected outcome, target date, and nursing actions. Delete old diagnosis.

Record data, e.g., can perform self-bathing but is having problems with self-toileting; has difficulty transferring from wheelchair to toilet seat and in maintaining a regular schedule. Record CONTINUE. Change target date and modify nursing actions as needed.

Start new evaluation process.

Tissue Perfusion (Specify Type), Altered (Renal, Cerebral, Cardiopulmonary, Gastrointestinal, Peripheral)

DEFINITION

The state in which an individual experiences a decrease in nutrition and oxygenation at the cellular level due to a deficit in capillary blood supply.[10]*

NANDA TAXONOMY: EXCHANGING 1.4.1.1

DEFINING CHARACTERISTICS[10]

	Estimated Sensitivities and Specificities	
Characteristic	Chances That Characteristic Will Be Present in Given Diagnosis	Chances That Characteristic Will Not Be Explained by Any Other Diagnosis
Skin temperature, cold extremities	High	Low
Skin color:		
Dependent blue or purple	Moderate	Low
Pale on elevation; color does not return on lowering of leg (*critical*)	High	High
Diminished arterial pulsations (*critical*)	High	High
Skin quality: Shining	High	Low
Lack of lanugo	High	Moderate
Round scars covered with atrophied skin	High	Moderate
Gangrene	Low	High
Slow-growing, dry, brittle nails	High	Moderate
Claudication	Moderate	High
Blood pressure changes in extremities	Moderate	Moderate
Bruits	Moderate	Moderate
Slow healing of lesions	High	Low

RELATED FACTORS[10]

1. Interruption of arterial flow
2. Interruption of venous flow
3. Exchange problems
4. Hypovolemia
5. Hypervolemia

RELATED CLINICAL CONCERNS

1. Thrombophlebitis
2. Amputation reattachment
3. Varicosities
4. Diabetes mellitus

---

*Further work and development are required for the subcomponents, specifically cerebral, renal, and gastrointestinal.

5. Cardiac infections
6. Anemia

Activity-Exercise Pattern

HAVE YOU SELECTED THE CORRECT DIAGNOSIS?

Decreased Cardiac Output Altered Tissue Perfusion relates to deficits in the peripheral circulation with cellular impact. Altered Cardiac Output relates specifically to a heart malfunction. Tissue perfusion problems may develop secondary to Decreased Cardiac Output but can also exist without cardiac output problems.[21] (See page 360.)

EXPECTED OUTCOMES

1. Will have no signs or symptoms of altered tissue perfusion by (date) and/or
2. Will implement a plan to decrease the likelihood of future alterations in tissue perfusion by (date)

TARGET DATE

A maximum target date would be 2 days from the date of admission because of the dangers involved. A patient who develops this diagnosis should be referred to a medical practitioner immediately.

ADDITIONAL INFORMATION

Perfusion is the movement of blood to and from a body part. Adequate perfusion determines cell survival and depends on an adequate pump and vascular volume as well as adequate functioning of the precapillary sphincters. Factors affecting the adequacy of these structures include vasomotor, metabolic, and neural factors.[22,51]

The basic function of the cardiovascular system is to transport water, oxygen, nutrients, and hormones to the cells and to remove carbon dioxide, waste products, and heat from the cells. The size of the blood vessels decreases along the length of the arterial system, which increases resistance to fluid flow. To perfuse the cells adequately, the mean arterial blood pressure is maintained within a relatively narrow range by such regulatory systems as the baroreceptors, sympathetic nerves, and the cardiac branch of the vagus nerve.[22,51]

NURSING ACTIONS/INTERVENTIONS WITH RATIONALES

Adult Health

Actions/Interventions	Rationales
• Monitor, initially every 2 hours on the (odd/even) hour, then increasing to every 4 hours at (times): ○ Peripheral pulses ○ Capillary refill ○ Skin temperature	Determines changes in physiologic baselines; permits early detection and treatment of complications.

Continued

Actions/Interventions	Rationales
○ Edema: Measure circumference (abdomen and ankles) with tape measure. ○ Motor and sensory status ○ Vital signs ○ Signs and symptoms of pulmonary edema	
• Weigh daily at 7 a.m. • Measure intake and output. Total every 8 and every 24 hours. • Monitor bowel elimination at least daily.	Allows monitoring of fluid balance. Permits assessment of nutritional status and bowel functioning.
• Position patient carefully, and change position at least every hour while awake: ○ Arterial interference: Head and chest elevated, and extremities in dependent position. ○ Venous interference: Extremities elevated. ○ Combined arterial-venous interference: Supine. ○ Apply sheepskin, alternating air mattress, or egg crate mattress to bed. ○ Provide heel and elbow protectors. ○ Provide bed cradle to avoid linen pressure on extremities. ○ Do not use knee gatch or pillows under knees.	Promotes circulation, prevents pressure ulcers, and prevents venous stasis.
• Provide skin and foot care at least once per shift at (times): ○ Cleanse and dry well. ○ Apply lotion. ○ Do not massage if possibility of emboli exists.	Prevents skin integrity problems.
• Collaborate with enterstomal therapist regarding care of open lesions: ○ Cleansing ○ Medicated ointments ○ Dressings	
• Exercise extremities at least every 4 hours while awake at (times): ○ Range of motion ○ Buerger-Allen exercises	Facilitates circulation, assists in preventing complications of immobility.
• Collaborate with physical therapist regarding gradually increasing total exercise program.	
• Apply supportive or antiembolic hose. Remove for at least 30 minutes each shift at (times) and cleanse skin underneath.	Promotes venous return; avoids skin integrity problems.
• Collaborate with physician regarding frequency of each of the following laboratory examinations, and monitor results:	Allows determination of any changes in physiologic indicators of tissue perfusion.

- ○ Electrolytes
- ○ Arterial blood gases
- ○ Blood urea nitrogen
- ○ Cardiac enzymes
- ○ Coagulation time
- Administer, as ordered, and monitor results of medications:
  - ○ Analgesics
  - ○ Anticoagulants
  - ○ Vasodilators
  - ○ Antilipemics

Basic monitoring of the various drugs used in the variety of situations related to altered tissue perfusion.

- Apply, and monitor closely, warm packs for phlebitis.

Promotes venous return; awareness of possibility of burn injury.

- Collaborate with dietitian regarding dietary adaptations:
  - ○ Calorie restrictions
  - ○ Low cholesterol
  - ○ Decreased saturated fats
  - ○ Decreased caffeine and alcohol intake.

Nutritional changes that may assist in avoiding future episodes of tissue perfusion.

- Teach patient, and assist in implementation at least once per shift while awake at (times):
  - ○ Stress management techniques
  - ○ Relaxation techniques

Decreases anxiety; modifies sympathetic nervous system response.

- Teach patient and significant others:
  - ○ Exercise program
  - ○ Dietary adaptations
  - ○ Smoking cessation
  - ○ Avoidance of extremes in temperature
  - ○ Avoidance of prolonged standing, sitting, or crossing of legs
  - ○ Avoiding use of over-the-counter medications
  - ○ Continued use of stress management and relaxation techniques
  - ○ Skin and foot care
  - ○ Prescribed medication regimen: Effects and toxicity

Basic home care planning; promotes participation in care and implementation of prescribed regimen.

- Refer to visiting nurse service.

Provides long-term support.

Child Health

Actions/Interventions	Rationales
• Perform appropriate monitoring and documentation for contributory factors to include:	Provides basic database to ascertain progress and to individualize plan of care.
○ Circulatory monitoring of anatomic site or general signs and symptoms related to peripheral pulses	
○ Apical pulse, blood pressure, temperature, and respiration (monitor at least every hour or as ordered, and check cardiac monitor if applicable)	
○ Intake and output every hour	
○ Nausea or vomiting	
○ Constipation or diarrhea	
○ Tolerance of feeding	
○ Pain or discomfort	
○ Skin color: Temperature or any integrity problems	
○ Circulatory pattern (notify physician of any change in the pattern that suggests lack of oxygenation, for example, cyanosis, arterial blood gas results, or decreased pulses)	
○ Appropriate functioning of equipment such as ventilator, arterial line, or intravenous pump	
○ Maintenance of intravenous line for administration of fluids	
○ Positional demands	
○ Pain or discomfort	
○ Sensory input appropriate for age and developmental status	
○ Fluid and electrolytes	
• Collaborate with other health care providers as needed. (See Appendix B.)	Coordination and implementation of plan of care may involve numerous professionals according to the cause of alteration and the treatment modalities available.
	Basic emergency preparedness.
• Provide for appropriate availability of resuscitative equipment, including:	
○ Ambu bag	
○ Crash cart for pediatrics with drugs and defibrillator	
○ Appropriate respiratory intubation equipment	
• Allow for parental and child health teaching needs by allowing 10 to 15 minutes per 8-hour shift for verbalization of concerns.	Verbalization of health-related concerns may serve as cues for teaching needs and also serve to reduce anxiety.

- Allow for parental participation in care of child at appropriate level, for example, comfort measures and assisting with feeding.
- Encourage rest by scheduling procedures together with devotion to ample time between activities.
- Allow for patient and parental preferences in plan of care.
- Deal with appropriate related factors associated with altered tissue perfusion, for example, minimizing crying by anticipating needs.
- Provide appropriate safety for age, for example, siderails up; positioning as ordered.

- Maintain proper use of equipment, such as Clinitron bed or special K-pads.
- Provide for appropriate follow-up via scheduled appointments after hospitalization.
- Provide patient with teaching appropriate to needs of illness and family, for example, if activities and daily care are to be modified, consider use of pulse oximeter to monitor perfusion; how to do circulatory checks after cast application.
- Ensure that parents have been certified in CPR before child is dismissed from hospital.

Parental involvement in care puts child at ease and provides self-esteem and empowerment for parents.
Appropriate attention to rest needs helps prevent further metabolic demands on already less than ideal homeostasis scenario.
Individualization shows value attached to parents' input.
All efforts to lessen work load on heart and respiratory system will assist in preventing further decompensation.

Safety is a standard part of care and ought to be planned for according to health status, age, and development.
Assists circulation.

Encourages consistency in long-range care.
Demonstrates how to schedule appointments and provides support for parents.
Assists in reducing anxiety; facilitates home management of care.

Basic need for home care when perfusion problem is present.

Women's Health

Actions/Interventions	Rationales

- Assist patient in identifying life-style adjustments that may be needed due to changes in physiological and/or gynecological functions or needs during experiential phases of life (for example, pregnancy, birth, and postpartum period):
  ○ Avoid prolonged sitting, sitting with crossed legs, or standing.
  ○ Develop exercise plan for cardiovascular fitness during pregnancy.
  ○ Avoid wearing constrictive clothing.
  ○ Maintain a balanced diet with adequate hydration.
  ○ Avoid constipation and bearing down to prevent hemorrhoids.
	Decreases factors that could lead to decreased perfusion.

Continued

Actions/Interventions	Rationales

• Monitor patient for signs or pregnancy-induced hypertension (PIH):
  ○ Prenatal weight
  ○ Blood pressure
  ○ Presence of edema
  ○ Proteinuria
  ○ Preeclampsia
  ○ Headaches
  ○ Visual changes such as blurred vision
  ○ Increased edema of face and pitting edema of extremities
  ○ Oliguria
  ○ Hyperreflexia
  ○ Nausea or vomiting
  ○ Epigastric pain
  ○ Eclampsia
  ○ Convulsions
  ○ Coma
	Allows early intervention to avoid perfusion problems.

• Monitor for edema:
  ○ Examine patient for swelling of hands, face, legs, or feet. (*Caution*: Patient may have to remove rings.)
  ○ Patient may need to wear loose shoes or a bigger shoe size.
  ○ Schedule rest breaks during day where patient can elevate legs.
  ○ When lying down, patient should lie on left side to promote placental perfusion and prevent compression of vena cava.
	Provides early warning of perfusion problems and promotes early intervention.

• In collaboration with physician (as appropriate), monitor:[52]
  ○ Intake and output (urinary output not less than 30 ml per hour or 120 ml every four hours)
  ○ Magnesium sulfate ($MgSO_4$) and hydralazine hydrochloride (Apresoline) therapy [Have antidote for $MgSO_4$ (calcium gluconate) available at all times during $MgSO_4$ therapy.]
  ○ Deep tendon reflexes (DTR)
  ○ Respiratory rate, pulse, and BP at least every 2 hours on the (odd/even) hour
  ○ For possibility of seizures
  ○ Amount of noise in patient's environment
  ○ Fetal heart rate and well-being	

• Provide quiet, nonstimulating environment for patient.	Reduces anxiety, promotes rest. Both will assist in maintaining peripheral circulation by avoiding vasoconstriction.

- Provide patient and family factual information and support as needed.

Reduces anxiety and provides teaching opportunity.

- Monitor and teach patient to monitor and report any signs of PIH immediately:

Allows early detection of problem and more rapid intervention.

  - Rapid rise in BP
  - Rapid weight gain
  - Marked hyperreflexia, especially transient or sustained ankle clonus
  - Severe headache
  - Visual disturbances
  - Epigastric pain
  - Increase in proteinuria
  - Oliguria, with urine output of less than 30 ml per hour
  - Drowsiness
- In collaboration with dietitian:

Dietary measures that assist in controlling BP.

  - Obtain nutritional history.
  - Provide high-protein diet (80 to 100 g protein).
  - Provide low-sodium diet (not above 6 g daily or below 2.5 g daily).

Oral Contraceptive Therapy

- Monitor for factors that contraindicate use of oral birth control pills:

These factors will promote side effects and untoward effects from birth control pills.

  - Family history of stroke, diabetes, or reproductive cancer
  - History of thromboembolic disease or vascular problems, hypertension, hepatic disease, and smoking
  - Presence of any breast disease, nodule, or fibrocystic disease

Premenstrual Syndrome

- Assist patient to identify symptoms that occur premenstrually which interfere with normal activities of daily living:

Provides database necessary to plan appropriate intervention.

  - Constipation
  - Bloating (abdominal)
  - Edema in hands and feet
  - Headaches or vertigo
  - Oliguria
  - Irritability
  - Depression
- Provide patient with literature on premenstrual syndrome.
- In collaboration with dietitian:

Dietary measures that assist in reducing the effects of premenstrual syndrome.

  - Obtain nutritional history.
  - Provide diet high in complex carbohydrates and protein.

Continued

Actions/Interventions	Rationales
○ Provide low-sodium diet (not above 6 g daily or below 2.5 g daily). • Teach and encourage patient to: ○ Utilize an exercise program ○ Utilize biofeedback for severe symptoms ○ Stop smoking ○ Utilize relaxation techniques to reduce stress	

Mental Health

NOTE: The nursing actions in this section reflect alteration in tissue perfusion related to the cerebral and peripheral vascular systems since these are the ones most commonly affected in the mental health setting.

Actions/Interventions	Rationales
• Check on orthostatic hypotension by taking blood pressure while client is lying down, then taking blood pressure just after client stands or sits up (provide support for client to prevent injury from a fall).	Psychotropic medications can predispose client to orthostatic hypotension.
• Monitor client's mental status. If compromised, provide information in a clear, concise manner.	
• Discuss with client causes of decreased cerebral blood flow.	Assists in explaining reasons for therapies to client.
• Have client get out of bed slowly by: ○ First, sitting up ○ Second, swinging legs over edge of bed ○ Third, resting in this position for at least 2 minutes ○ Fourth, standing up slowly ○ Fifth, walking slowly	Allows time for cardiovascular system to adapt, thus preventing fainting or dizziness to orthostatic hypotension.
• Teach client to avoid situations in which he or she changes position quickly, for example, bending over to pick something up off the floor or standing quickly from a sitting position.	
• Have client supported while changing positions that cause vertigo until problem is resolved.	
• Assist client in getting in and out of the bathtub.	
• Collaborate with physician regarding alterations in medications.	Promotes changing to a medication that would not interfere with perfusion.

- If situation persists, have client:
  - ○ Sleep sitting up or with head elevated.
  - ○ Use elastic stockings that are waist high.
  - ○ Apply stockings while client is still in bed.
  - ○ Have client raise legs for several minutes.
  - ○ Apply stockings slowly and evenly.
  - ○ Remove stockings after client is lying down at least every 8 hours.
  - ○ When getting out of bed, patient should swing legs over edge of bed. He or she should then rest in this position for at least 2 minutes. Patient should then stand up slowly and walk slowly.
- Develop with client a plan for daily exercise that is very modest, for example, walking the length of the hall for 15 minutes twice a day for 3 days, then increasing distance and time gradually until client is walking for 30 minutes twice a day. Note client's exercise regimen here.
- Develop with the client a reward schedule for implementing exercise plan. List rewards and the reward schedule here.
- Provide the client with positive verbal support for goal accomplishment.
- Do not allow client to participate in unit activities that could produce injury until the condition is resolved, for example, cooking or using sharp objects while standing.
- Discuss with client the effects of alcohol and smoking on blood flow, and help client to develop alternative coping behavior if necessary. Note plan for this here.
- Provide decaffeinated beverages for the client. Consult with dietary department about this adaptation.
- Increase client's fluid intake during times of increased loss, such as exercise or periods of anxiety. Instruct client in the need for this.
- Observe client carefully after injecting medications that have a high potential for producing hypotension. This is especially true for those clients who are very agitated and physically active.
- Inform client of need to change position slowly after injecting medication.
- Teach client and support system about over-the-counter medications that alter blood flow, for example, cold medications, antihistamines, and diet pills.

Provides external support for venous system.

Allows time for cardiovascular system to adapt, thus preventing fainting or dizziness to orthostatic hypotension.

Improves cardiovascular strength; assists in maintaining muscle tone that assists in supporting the venous circulation.

Basic safety measures.

Basic measure to offset the possibility of falling secondary to orthostatic hypotensions.

Continued

Actions/Interventions	Rationales
• Monitor peripheral pulses on affected limbs every 8 hours at (times).	

• Avoid and teach client to avoid pressure in points on affected limbs to include:
  ○ Changing position frequently when sitting or lying down and avoiding pressure in the area behind the knee
  ○ Not crossing legs while sitting
  ○ Making sure shoes fit properly and do not rub feet
  ○ Elevating feet when sitting to reduce pressure on backs of legs
	Avoids compromising circulation by pressure or constriction.

• Keep feet clean and dry and teach client to do same by assessing foot condition once a day at (time). This assessment should include:
  ○ Washing feet
  ○ Checking for sores, reddened areas, and blisters
  ○ Keeping toenails trimmed and caring for ingrown nails
  ○ Applying lotion to feet
  ○ Rubbing reddened areas if client does not have a history of emboli
  ○ Applying clean, dry socks
  ○ Teaching significant others to assist with foot care of elderly client
  ○ Keeping limbs warm (But do not use external heating sources such as heating pads or hot-water bottles.)
	Avoids lower-extremity skin integrity problems and possible infection with the resultant impact on circulation.

• Develop with the client an exercise program and note that program here. Begin slowly, and gradually increase time and distance, for example, walk for 15 minutes two times per day for 1 week. This should be increased until client is walking 1 mile in 30 to 45 minutes 3 times a week.	Promotes normal venous return.

• Instruct client to discontinue exercise if:
  ○ Pulse does not return to resting rate within 3 minutes after exercise.
  ○ Shortness of breath continues for more than 10 minutes after stopping exercise.
  ○ Fatigue is excessive.
  ○ Muscles are painful.
  ○ Client experiences dizziness, pain in the chest, light-headedness, loss of muscle control, or nausea.
	Client safety is of primary importance.

• Encourage client's exercise by:
  ○ Walking with him or her
  ○ Determining things that the client would find rewarding, and supplying these as goals are achieved (note client's specific reward system here)
  ○ Providing positive verbal support as goals are achieved
	Positive reinforcement encourages behavior and enhances self-esteem.

• Monitor client's nutritional status and refer to nutritionist for teaching if necessary.	

• Discuss with client the effects of smoking on peripheral blood flow, and assist him or her in decreasing or eliminating this by:
  ○ Referring to a stop-smoking group
  ○ Encouraging him or her not to smoke before meals or exercise
  ○ Decreasing amount smoked per day
	Nicotine causes vasospasm and vasoconstriction.

• Discuss special needs with client and support system before discharge.	Increases probability of client's behavior change being maintained after discharge.
• Refer to community agencies to provide ongoing care as needed. (See Appendix B.)	

Gerontic Health

The nursing actions for the gerontic patient with this diagnosis are the same as those in Adult Health and Home Health.

Home Health

NOTE: If this diagnosis is suspected when caring for a client in the home, it is imperative that a physician referral be obtained immediately. If the client has been referred to home health care by a physician, the nurse will collaborate with the physician in the treatment of the client.

Actions/Interventions	Rationales

• Teach client and family appropriate monitoring of signs and symptoms of alteration in tissue perfusion:
  ○ Pulse (lying, sitting, or standing)
  ○ Skin temperature and turgor
  ○ Edema
  ○ Motor status
  ○ Sensory status
  ○ Blood pressure (lying, sitting, standing, and pulse pressure)
  ○ Respiratory status (dyspnea, cyanosis, and rate)
	Provides database for prevention and/or early intervention.

Continued

Actions/Interventions	Rationales

○ Weight fluctuations
○ Urinary output
○ Leg pain with walking
• Assist client and family in identifying life-style changes that may be required:
  ○ Eliminating smoking
  ○ Decreasing caffeine
  ○ Decreasing alcohol
  ○ Avoiding over-the-counter medications
  ○ Protecting skin and extremities from injury due to decreased sensation (burns, frostbite, and so on)
  ○ Protecting skin from pressure injury (frequent position changes, sheepskin for pressure areas, and/or foot cradle)
  ○ Improving arterial blood flow (keep extremities warm, elevate head and chest, avoid crossing legs or sitting for long periods of time, wiggle fingers and toes every hour, range-of-motion exercises)
  ○ Performing exercise program as tolerated
  ○ Improving venous blood flow (elevate extremity, use antiembolus stockings, and avoid pressure behind knees)
  ○ Performing skin and foot care
  ○ Decreasing cholesterol and saturated fat
  ○ Performing diversional activities as needed
  ○ Practicing stress management
• Teach family basic CPR.
• Teach client and family purposes, side effects, and proper administration technique of medications.
• Assist client and family in setting criteria to help them determine when a physician or other intervention is required.
• Consult with or refer to appropriate assistive resources as indicated. (See Appendix B.)
	Provides basic information for client and family that promotes necessary life-style changes.
	
	Locus of control shifts from nurse to client and family, thus promoting self-care.
	
	Provides additional support for client and family and uses already available resources in a cost-effective manner.

FLOW CHART EVALUATION
Flow Chart Expected Outcome 1

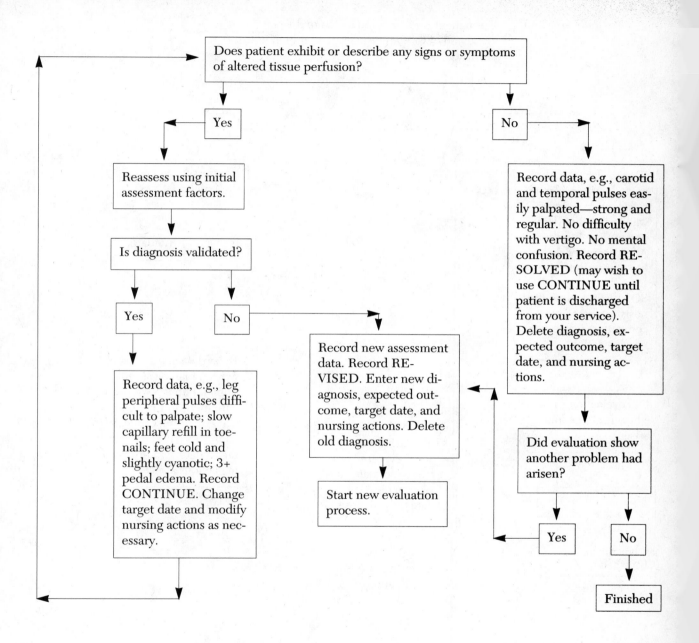

Does patient exhibit or describe any signs or symptoms of altered tissue perfusion?

Yes

No

Reassess using initial assessment factors.

Is diagnosis validated?

Yes

No

Record data, e.g., leg peripheral pulses difficult to palpate; slow capillary refill in toenails; feet cold and slightly cyanotic; 3+ pedal edema. Record CONTINUE. Change target date and modify nursing actions as necessary.

Record new assessment data. Record REVISED. Enter new diagnosis, expected outcome, target date, and nursing actions. Delete old diagnosis.

Start new evaluation process.

Record data, e.g., carotid and temporal pulses easily palpated—strong and regular. No difficulty with vertigo. No mental confusion. Record RESOLVED (may wish to use CONTINUE until patient is discharged from your service). Delete diagnosis, expected outcome, target date, and nursing actions.

Did evaluation show another problem had arisen?

Yes

No

Finished

Flow Chart Expected Outcome 2

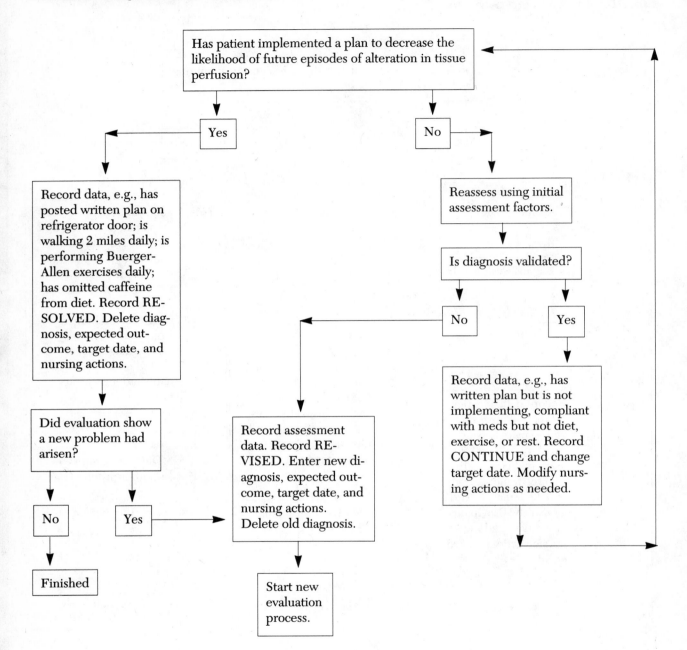

References

1. Potter, PA and Perry, AG: Instructor's Manual for Use with Fundamentals of Nursing: Concepts, Process, and Practice, ed 2. CV Mosby, St. Louis, 1989.
2. Kelly, MA: Nursing Diagnosis Source Book. Appleton-Century-Crofts, East Norwalk, CT, 1985.
3. Mitchell, PH: Motor status. In Mitchell, PH and Loustau, A (eds): Concepts Basic to Nursing. McGraw-Hill, New York, 1981.
4. Lentz, M: Selected aspects of deconditioning secondary to immobilization. Nurs Clin North Am 16:729, 1980.
5. Pardue, N: Immobility. In Flynn, JM and Heffron, PB (eds): Nursing: From Concept to Practice, ed 2. Appleton-Lange, Norwalk, CT, 1988.
6. Murray, RB and Zentner, JP: Nursing Assessment and Health Promotion Strategies through the Life Span, ed 4. Appleton-Lange, Norwalk, CT, 1989.
7. Schuster, CS and Asburn, SS: The Process of Human Development: A Holistic Life-Span Approach, ed 3. JB Lippincott, Philadelphia, 1992.
8. Noble, E: Essential Exercises for the Childbearing Year, ed 3. Houghton Mifflin, Boston, 1988.
9. Duncan, J, Gordon, N, and Scott, C: Women walking for health and fitness: How much is enough? J Am Med Assoc 266:3295, 1991.
10. North American Nursing Diagnosis Association: Taxonomy I, Revised 1990. Author, St. Louis, 1990.
11. Erickson, HC, Tomlin, EM, and Swain, MP: Modeling and Role-Modeling: A Theory and Paradigm for Nursing. Prentice-Hall, Englewood Cliffs, NJ, 1983.
12. Wilson, HS and Kneisl, CR: Psychiatric Nursing, ed 4. Addison-Wesley, Redwood, CA, 1992.
13. Haber, J, et al: Comprehensive Psychiatric Nursing, ed 4. CV Mosby, St. Louis, 1992.
14. Dossey, B, et al: Holistic Nursing. Aspen, Rockville, MD, 1988.
15. Clark, C: Wellness Nursing. Springer, New York, 1986.
16. Leahey, M and Wright, L: Families and Psychosocial Problems. Springhouse Corp., Springhouse, PA, 1987.
17. Maas, M, Buckwalter, K, and Hardy, M: Nursing Diagnosis and Interventions for the Elderly. Addison-Wesley, Fort Collins, CO, 1991.
18. Townsend, M: Drug Guide for Psychiatric Nursing. FA Davis, Philadelphia, 1990.
19. Gilliss, C, et al: Toward a Science of Family Nursing. Addison-Wesley, Menlo Park, CA, 1989.
20. Eliopoulous, C: A Guide to the Nursing of the Aging. Williams & Wilkins, Baltimore, 1987.
21. Doenges, ME and Moorhouse, MF: Nurses' Pocket Guide: Nursing Diagnoses with Interventions. FA Davis, Philadelphia, 1991.
22. Kavanagh, J and Riegger, M: Assessment of the cardiovascular system. In Phipps, WJ, et al (eds): Medical-Surgical Nursing: Concepts and Clinical Practice, ed 4. CV Mosby, St. Louis, 1991.
23. Kitzinger, S: The Experience of Childbirth, ed 5. Cox and Wyman, London, 1984.
24. Folta, A and Metzger, B: Exercise and functional capacity after myocardial infarction. Image 21:215, 1989.
25. Beland, IL and Passos, JY: Clinical Nursing: Pathophysiological and Psychosocial Approaches, ed 4. Macmillan, New York, 1981.
26. Osborn, CL: Reminiscence: When the past erases the present. J of Geronot Nurs 15:6, 1989.
27. North American Nursing Diagnosis Association: Proposed New Nursing Diagnoses: NANDA 10th Conference. St. Louis, Author, 1992.
28. Richless, C: Current trends in mechanical ventilation. Crit Care Nurse 11:41, 1991.
29. Hazinski, MF: Nursing Care of the Critically Ill Child. CV Mosby, St. Louis, 1992.
30. US Department of Health and Human Services: Executive Summary: Guidelines for the Diagnosis and Management of Asthma. Author, Washington, DC, 1991.
31. Norton, LC and Neureuter, A: Weaning the long-term ventilator dependent patient: Common problems and management. Crit Care Nurse 9:42, 1989.
32. Knebel, AR: Weaning from mechanical ventilation: Current controversies. Heart Lung 20:47, 1991.
33. Forrest, G: Atrial fibrillation association with autonomic dysreflexia in patients with tetraplegia. Arch Phys Med Rehabil 72:592, 1991.
34. Pine, A, Miller, S, and Alonso, J: Atrial fibrillation associated with autonomic dysreflexia. Am J Phys Med Rehabil 70:271, 1991.
35. Lindan, R, et al: Incidence and clinical features of autonomic dysreflexia in patients with spinal cord injury. Paraplegia 18:285, 1980.
36. Earnhardt, J and Frye, B: Understanding dysreflexia. Rehabil Nurs 9:28, 1986.
37. Ceron, GE and Rakowski-Reinhardt, AC: Action stat! Autonomic dysreflexia. Nurs 21:33, 1991.
38. Trop, C and Bennett, C: Autonomic dysreflexia and its urological implications. J Urol 146:1461, 1991.
39. Finocchiaro, DN and Herzfeld, ST: Understanding autonomic dysreflexia. Am J Nurs 90:56, 1990.
40. Drayton-Hargrove, S and Reddy, M: Rehabilitation and the long term management of the spinal cord impaired adult. Nurs Clin North Am 21:599, 1986.
41. Braddom, R and Rocco, J: Autonomic dysreflexia. A survey of current treatment. Am J Phys Med Rehabil 70:237, 1991.

42. Luckman, J and Sorensen, KC: Medical-Surgical Nursing: A Psychophysiologic Approach, ed 3. Saunders, Philadelphia, 1987.
43. Thompson, C: Gender differences in walking distances of people with lung disease. Appl Nurs Res 1:141, 1989.
44. Lee, R, Grayder, J, and Ross, E: Effectiveness of psychological well-being, physical status and social support on oxygen dependent COPD patients' level of functioning. Res Nurs Health 14:323, 1991.
45. Fulmer, T and Walker, K: Lessons from the elder boom in ICUs. Geriatr Nur 11:120, 1990.
46. Strumpf, NE and Evans, LK: The ethical problems of prolonged physical restraint. J Gerontol Nurs 17:27, 1991.
47. Mobily, PR and Kelley, LS: Factors of immobility. J Gerontol Nurs 17:5, 1991.
48. Penn, C: Promoting independence. J Gerontol Nurs 14:14, 1988.
49. Whaley, LF and Wong, DL: Nursing Care of Infants and Children, ed 4. CV Mosby, St. Louis, 1991.
50. Reeder, SJ, Martin, LL, and Koniak, D: Maternity Nursing: Family, Newborn and Women's Health Care. JB Lippincott, Philadelphia, 1992.
51. Cunningham, S: Circulatory and fluid-electrolyte status. In Mitchell, PH and Loustau, A (eds): Concepts Basic to Nursing, ed 3. McGraw-Hill, New York, 1981.
52. Bobak, IM and Jensen, MD: Maternity and Gynecologic Care: The Nurse and the Family, ed 4. CV Mosby, St. Louis, 1989.

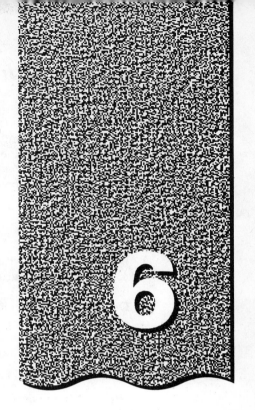

6

Sleep-Rest Pattern

PATTERN INTRODUCTION
Pattern Description

The sleep-rest pattern includes relaxation in addition to sleep and rest. The pattern is based on a 24-hour day and looks specifically at how a person rates or judges the adequacy of his or her sleep, rest, and relaxation in terms of both quantity and quality. The pattern also looks at the patient's energy level in relation to the amount of sleep, rest, and relaxation described by the patient as well as any aids to sleep the patient uses.

Pattern Assessment

1. Does patient report a problem falling asleep?
    a. Yes (Sleep Pattern Disturbance)
    b. No
2. Does patient report interrupted sleep?
    a. Yes (Sleep Pattern Disturbance)
    b. No

Diagnosis in This Chapter

Sleep Pattern Disturbance (page 507)

Conceptual Information

A person at rest feels mentally relaxed, free from anxiety, and physically calm. Rest need not imply inactivity, and inactivity does not necessarily afford rest. Rest is a reduction in bodily work that results in the person's feeling refreshed and having a sense of readiness to perform activities of daily living.

Sleep is a state of rest that occurs for sustained periods. The reduced consciousness during sleep provides time for essential repair and recovery of body systems. A person who sleeps has temporarily reduced interaction with the environment. Sleep restores a person's energy and sense of well-being.

Recent studies confirm that sleep is a cyclical phenomenon. The most common sleep cycle is the 24-hour, diurnal day-night cycle. This 24-hour cycle is also referred to as the *circadian rhythm*. In general, the 24-hour circadian rhythm is governed by light and darkness. Additional factors that influence the sleep-wake cycle of an individual are biological such as the hormonal and thermoregulation cycles. Most people attempt to synchronize activity with the demands of modern society. The two specialized areas of the brain stem that control the cyclical nature of sleep are the reticular activating system in the brain stem, spinal cord, and cerebral cortex, and the bulbar synchronizing portion in the medulla. These two systems function intermittently by activating and suppressing the higher centers of the brain.

After falling asleep, a person passes through a series of stages that afford rest and recuperation physically, mentally, and emotionally. In Stage 1, the individual is in a relaxed, dreamy state, aware of his or her surroundings. In Stages 2 and 3, there is progression to deeper levels of sleep in which the person becomes unaware of his or her surroundings but wakens easily. In Stage 4, there is profound sleep character-ized by little body movement and difficult arousal. Stage 4 restores and allows the body to rest. These stages are known as *non–rapid eye movement (NREM)*. Stage 5 is called *rapid eye movement (REM)*. It is in this stage that everyone dreams. Other characteristics of this stage of sleep are irregular pulse, variable blood pressure, muscular twitching, profound muscular relaxation, and increase in gastric secretions.[1] After REM the individual processes back through Stages, 1, 2, and 3 again.

A person's age, general health status, culture, and emotional well-being will dictate the amount of sleep required. On the whole, older people require the least sleep while young infants require the most sleep. As the nurse assesses the patient's needs for sleep and rest, every effort is made to individualize the care according to this sleep-rest cycle. A major emphasis is to provide patient education regarding the influence of disease process on sleep-rest patterns.

Reports of the occurrence of excessive and pathologic sleep most commonly relate to narcolepsy and hypersomnia. *Narcolepsy* is characterized by attacks of irresistible sleep of brief duration with "auxiliary" symptoms. In sleep paralysis, the narcoleptic patient is unable to speak or move and breathes in a shallow manner. Auditory or visual hypnagogic hallucinations may occur. Cataplexy, a brief form of narcolepsy, is an abrupt and reversible decrease or loss of muscle tone and is most often elicited by emotion. The attacks may last several seconds and almost go undetected or they may last as long as 30 minutes with muscular weakness being evident. In the initial stage of the attack, consciousness remains intact.[2]

Hypersomnia, on the other hand, is characterized by daytime sleepiness and sleep states that are less imperative and of longer duration than those in narcolepsy. Often a deepening and lengthening of night sleep are also noted. Sleep apnea and the Kleine-Levin syndrome are two examples of the hypersomnia disorders.[2]

Sleep apnea may occur in patients with a damaged respiratory center in the brain, brain stem infarction, drug intoxication (barbiturates, tranquilizers, and so on), bilateral cordotomy, and Ondine's Curse syndrome. Patients with the typical "Pickwickian syndrome" show marked obesity and associated alveolar hypoventilation, sleep apnea, and hypersomnia. There are several forms of this condition that may exist without obesity. One such syndrome is that of "Ondine's Curse syndrome," which involves the loss of the automaticity of breathing and manifests during sleep as a recurrent apnea. Another such syndrome is the Kleine-Levin syndrome, which is associated with periods of hypersomnia accompanied by bulimia or polyphagia and mental disturbances. There is also a cyclic hypersomnia reported that is related to the premenstrual period. The typical syndrome, "Pickwickian," is rare, while the atypical variants seem more common.[2]

Various factors influence a person's capability to gain adequate rest and sleep. In the home setting, it is appropriate for the nurse to assist the patient in developing behavior conducive to rest and relaxation. In a health care setting, the nurse must be able to provide ways of promoting rest and relaxation in a stressful environment. Loss of privacy, unfamiliar noises, frequent examinations, tiring procedures, and a general upset in daily routines culminate in a threat to the client's achievement of essential rest and sleep.

Developmental Considerations

In general, as age increases, the amount of sleep per night decreases. The length of each sleep cycle — active REM and quiet NREM — changes with age. For adults, there is no particular change in the actual number of hours slept, but there is a change in the amount of deep sleep and light sleep. As age increases, the amount of deep sleep decreases and the amount of light sleep increases. This helps explain why the older patient wakens more easily and spends time in sleep throughout the day and night. REM sleep decreases in amount from the time of infancy (50 percent) to late adulthood (15 percent). The changes in sleep pattern with age development are:[3]

> *Infant*: Awake 7 hours; NREM sleep, 8.5 hours; REM sleep, 8.5 hours
> *Age 1*: Awake 13 hours; NREM sleep, 7 hours; REM sleep, 4 hours
> *Age 10*: Awake 15 hours; NREM sleep, 6 hours; REM sleep, 3 hours
> *Age 20*: Awake 17 hours; NREM sleep, 5 hours; REM sleep, 2 hours
> *Age 75*: Awake 17 hours; NREM sleep, 6 hours; REM sleep 1 hour

INFANT

The development of sleep and wakefulness can be traced to intrauterine life. A gestational age of 36 weeks seems to be a landmark, for it is at this time that the behavioral states in the fetus and preterm infant begin to take on a more mature character. The joining of physiological variables results in identification of recurrent behavioral states with various parameters. Term birth leads to a number of profound changes, especially in respiratory regulation, but more evidence suggests that continuity of development, rather than discontinuity, prevails.[4]

The newborn begins life with a regular schedule of sleep and activity that is evident during periods of reactivity. For the first hour infants born of unmedicated mothers spend 60 percent of the time in the quiet, alert state and only 10 percent of the time in the irritable, crying state. Five distinct sleep-activity states for the infant have been noted:[5] (1) regular sleep, (2) irregular sleep, (3) drowsiness, (4) alert inactivity, and (5) waking and crying.

After 1 month of age, sleep and wakefulness change dramatically, as do a large number of physiological variables. This period of central nervous system (CNS) reorganization (with a likely increased vulnerability) is immediately followed by a short transient interval at 3 months of age, in which play and wakefulness and, within it, the basic rest-activity cycle, show excessive regularity. This regularity may carry its own risk.

The study of mobility has proven worthwhile in detecting the origin of the basic rest-activity cycle in the fetus. Neonatologists, who deal with the immature infant, often use mobility in prognosis.

Apneas during sleep are common in normal infants and occur most often during the newborn period, with a marked decrease in the first 6 months of life. Long apneas, above 15 seconds, are not usually observed during sleep in laboratory conditions. Obstructive apneas of 6 to 10 seconds are also rarely observed. However, in laboratory studies, paradoxical breathing is observed in neonates, and periodic breathing is associated with REM sleep in normal infants.[4]

When parents find an infant not breathing, the parents usually rush the infant to the hospital. Causes for life-threatening apnea to be investigated include: congenital conditions, especially cardiac disease or arrhythmias; cranial, facial, or other conditions affecting the anatomy of the airway; infections such as sepsis, meningitis, pneumonia, botulism, and pertussis; viral infections such as respiratory syncytial virus; metabolic abnormalities; administration of sedatives; and seizures and chronic hypoxia. If these causes are ruled out, the infant is diagnosed as having "apnea of infancy." Sleep studies, with polygraphic recordings, are required. The term *near miss sudden infant death syndrome (near miss SIDS)* implies that the child is found limp, cyanotic, not breathing, and would have died had caretakers not intervened. Because the relation of the Near Miss SIDS event to SIDS is speculative, *apnea of infancy* is the preferred term.[4]

Obstructive and central apnea identification, hypopnea, prolonged expiration, apnea and reflux, and apnea and cardiac arrhythmia are the current issues being studied in trying to solve this problem. For any infant-related apnea, hospitalization, with special observation for all possible contributing factors and close monitoring of cardiac and respiratory function, is recommended. Attention must be given to parents for the extreme anxiety this problem creates.

The newborn and young infant spend more time in REM sleep than adults. As the infant's nervous system develops, the infant will have longer periods of sleep and wakefulness that become more regular. At approximately 8 months of age, the infant goes through the stage of separation anxiety, with potentially altered sleep patterns. Teething, ear infections, or other disorders affect sleep patterns. Respirations are quiet, with minimal activity noted during deep sleep. The infant sleeps an average of 12 to 16 hours per day.

TODDLER AND PRESCHOOLER

The toddler needs approximately 10 to 12 hours of sleep at night with a nap lasting approximately 2 hours in the afternoon. The percentage of REM sleep is 25 percent. Rituals for preparation for sleep are important, with bedtime associated with separation from family and fun. Quiet time to gradually unwind, a favorite object for security, and a relatively consistent bedtime are suggested. Nightmares may begin to occur due to magical thinking.

The preschooler sleeps approximately 10 to 12 hours per day. Dreams and nightmares may occur at this time, and resistance to bedtime rituals is also common. Unwinding or slowing down from the many activities of the day is recommended to lessen sleep disturbances. Actual attempts to foster relaxation by mental imaging at this age have proven successful. The percentage of REM sleep is 20 percent.

Special needs may be prompted for the toddler during hospitalization. When at all possible, a parent's presence should be encouraged throughout nighttime to lessen fears. Limit setting with safety in mind is also necessary for the toddler due to the surplus of energy and the desire for constant activity. The preschooler may be at risk for fatigue. Sleep may not be necessary at nap time, but rest without disturbance is recommended to supplement night sleep and to prevent fatigue.

SCHOOL-AGE CHILD

The school-age child seems to do well without a nap and requires approximately 10 hours of sleep per day, with REM sleep being approximately 18.5 percent. Individualized rest needs are developed by this age, with a reliable source being the child who can express feelings about rest or sleep. Health status would also determine to a great extent how much sleep the child at this age requires. Permission to stay up late must be considered in view of the potential upset to routine and demands of the next day. When bedtime is assigned a status, peer pressure and power issues may ensue.

When the school-age child alters the usual routines of sleep and rest, fatigue may be a result. Attempts should be made to maintain usual routines even when school is not in session to best maintain the usual sleep-rest pattern.

ADOLESCENT

Irregular sleep patterns seem to be the norm for the adolescent due to high activity levels and usual peer-related activities. There may be a tendency to overexertion that is made more pronounced by the numerous physiologic changes which create increased demands on the body. Fatigue may occur during this time. On the average, the adolescent sleeps approximately 8 to 10 hours per day, with REM sleep being 20 percent.

Rest may be necessary to supplement sleep. Supplementing sleep with rest serves to assist in preventing illness or the risk of illness. Extracurricular activities may also need to be prioritized.

ADULT

The adult sleeps approximately 8 hours per day, with REM sleep being 22 percent. Sleep patterns may be subject to young infants or children in the household or after-hours professional and social demands.

The adult may be at high risk for fatigue due to increasing role expectations, especially in the instance of a new baby being cared for. Sleep deprivation is not a positive means of coping with the many expectations the adult may feel.

Research has shown that women of all ages have higher rates of sleep disturbance than men. Some speculation has occurred that relates this to the reproductive lives of women and hormonal changes. It is well documented that the psychosocial and hormonal changes accompanying pregnancy lead to sleep disturbances.[6] Sleep deprivation during the postpartum period is a well-known fact. A new baby does not allow for uninterrupted sleep for approximately 4 to 6 weeks after birth.[7,8]

The major sleep disturbance in menopause is due to frequent nocturnal hot flashes coupled with early morning awakenings.[6]

OLDER ADULT

The older adult requires less sleep on the average, approximately 5 to 7 hours of sleep per day. The percentage of REM sleep may vary from 20 to 25 percent; however, deep sleep, Stage 4 NREM sleep, is decreased.[9] Older adults report problems in falling asleep and increased periods of waking during the night. Periodic leg movement is also a phenomenon that is reported in sleep disturbances of older adults. The etiology is unknown, and the prevalence is estimated at anywhere from 25 to 37 percent. Those suffering from periodic leg movement have symptoms of leg kicks, insomnia, motor restlessness, and increased daytime sleepiness.[10] Institutionalized older adults may report problems with sleep if their usual sleep pattern does not coincide with the facility schedule. A number of older adults may report taking more naps in the daytime. Safety needs during sleep and rest periods should be kept in mind.

The actual decreased need for sleep may result in fatigue when the older adult is not allowed to divide the sleep time between day and night as he or she might if residing at home. Individualized attention to sleep and potential fatigue is critical to best prevent further loss of activity and self-worth for this client.

Since fatigue plays a major role in determining the quality and amount of musculoskeletal activity undertaken, consideration of the factors that influence fatigue are essential parts of the assessment for the sleep-rest pattern.

APPLICABLE NURSING DIAGNOSIS
Sleep Pattern Disturbance
DEFINITION

Disruption of sleep time causes discomfort or interferes with desired life-style.[11]

NANDA TAXONOMY: MOVING 6.2.1
DEFINING CHARACTERISTICS[11]

1. Major defining characteristics:
   a. Verbal complaints of difficulty falling asleep (*critical*)
   b. Awakening earlier or later than desired (*critical*)
   c. Interrupted sleep (*critical*)
   d. Verbal complaints of not feeling well rested (*critical*)
   e. Changes in behavior and performance (increasing irritability, restlessness, disorientation, lethargy, or listlessness)
   f. Physical signs (mild fleeting nystagmus, slight hand tremor, ptosis of eyelid, expressionless face, dark circles under eyes, frequent yawning, or changes in posture)
   g. Thick speech with mispronunciation and incorrect words
2. Minor defining characteristics:
   None given

RELATED FACTORS[11]

1. Sensory alterations: Internal (illness or psychological stress)
2. Sensory alterations: External (environmental changes or social cues)

RELATED CLINICAL CONCERNS

1. Colic
2. Hyperthyroidism
3. Anxiety
4. Depression
5. Chronic obstructive pulmonary disease
6. Any postoperative state
7. Pregnancy; postpartum

HAVE YOU SELECTED THE CORRECT DIAGNOSIS?

Sleep Pattern Disturbance rarely requires differentiation from any other diagnoses and is quite often a companion diagnosis for any hospitalization.

Ineffective Individual Coping In some instances, patients will use sleep as an avoidance mechanism and might report a sleep pattern disturbance when in reality there is no disturbance. Review of the number of hours of sleep would indicate the patient has a normal sleep pattern but desires to increase

Continued

HAVE YOU SELECTED THE CORRECT DIAGNOSIS?—*Continued*

the amount of sleep to avoid having to deal with stress, anxiety, fear, and so on. These patients will invariably be requesting "a sleeping pill." (See page 892.)

Fatigue   With this diagnosis the patient will talk about lack of energy and difficulty in maintaining his or her usual activities of daily living (ADL). However, when questioned, this fatigue will be seen exist in spite of the amount of sleep. (See page 407.)

Activity Intolerance   Again, a lack of energy will be reported, but there will be no report of inadequate sleep. Indeed, the hours of sleep may have increased. (See page 327.)

EXPECTED OUTCOMES

1. Will demonstrate at least 6 to 8 hours of uninterrupted sleep each night by (date)   (*Note*: Actual hours of uninterrupted sleep will depend on patient's age and developmental level.)   and/or
2. Will verbalize decreased number of complaints regarding loss of sleep by (date)

TARGET DATE

The suggested target date is no less than 2 days after the date of diagnosis and no more than 5 days. This length of time will allow for initial modification of the sleep pattern.

NURSING ACTIONS/INTERVENTIONS WITH RATIONALES

Adult Health

Actions/Interventions	Rationales
• Teach relaxation exercises as needed.	Decreases sympathetic response; decreases stress.
• Suggest sleep preparatory activities such as quiet music, warm fluids, or decreased active exercise at least 1 hour prior to scheduled sleep time. Provide a high-carbohydrate snack.	These winding-down activities promote sleep. Carbohydrates stimulate secretion of insulin. Insulin decreases all amino acids but tryptophan. Tryptophan in larger quantities, in the brain, increases production of serotonin, a neurotransmitter that induces sleep.[12]
• Provide warm, decaffeinated fluids after 6 p.m.; limit fluids after 8 p.m.	Warm drinks are relaxing; limiting fluid reduces the chance of midsleep interruption to go to bathroom.
• Assist patient to bathroom or bedside commode, or offer bedpan at 9 p.m.	The urge to void may interrupt the sleep cycle during the night. Voiding immediately before going to bed lessens the probability of this occurring.

- Schedule all patient therapeutics prior to 9 p.m.
- Maintain room temperature at 68 to 72°F.

- Notify operator to hold telephone calls starting at 9 p.m.
- Ensure adherence, as closely as possible, to patient's usual bedtime routine.

- Close door to room; limit traffic into room beginning at least 1 hour prior to scheduled sleep time.
- Administer required medication, for example, analgesics or sedatives, after all daily activities and therapeutics are completed. Monitor effectiveness of medication 30 minutes after time of administration.
- Give a back massage immediately after administering medication. If no medications are scheduled, give a back massage after toileting.
- Place patient in preferred sleeping position; support position with pillows.
- Ascertain if patient would like a night light.

- Once patient is sleeping, place "do-not-disturb" sign on the door.
- Increase exercise and activity during day as appropriate for patient's condition.
- When appropriate, discuss reasons for Sleep Pattern Disturbance; teach appropriate coping mechanisms.

Promotes uninterrupted sleep.

Environment temperature that is the most conducive to sleep.
Promotes uninterrupted sleep.

Follows patient's established pattern; promotes comfort; allows patient to wind down.
Reduces environmental stimuli.

Promotes action and effect of medication; allows evaluation of medication effectiveness and provides data for suggesting changes in medication if needed.

Relaxes muscles and promotes sleep.

Promotes patient's comfort and follows patient's usual routine.
Promotes sense of orientation in an unfamiliar environment.
Promotes uninterrupted sleep.

Promotes regular diurnal rhythm.

Promotes adaptation that can increase sleep.

Child Health

Actions/Interventions	Rationales
• Give warm bath 30 minutes to 1 hour before scheduled sleep time.	Promotes relaxation and provides quiet time as a part of the sleep routine.
• Feed 15 to 30 minutes before scheduled sleep time—formula and/or snack of protein and simple carbohydrates, no fats.	In young infants and small children, a sense of fullness and satiety, without difficulty in digestion, promotes sleep without the likelihood of upset or disturbances.
• Implement usual bedtime routine—rocking, patting, and favorite stuffed animal or blanket.	A structured approach sets limits yet honors individual preference; provides security and promotes sleep.

Continued

Actions/Interventions	Rationales
• Read a calm, quiet story to child immediately after putting to bed.	Reading allows a passive, meaningful enjoyment that occupies the attention of the young child while creating a bond between parent and child; serendipitous relaxation often follows.
• Provide environment conducive to sleep: room temperature of 74 to 78°F; soft, relaxing music; and/or a night light.	Lack of unpleasant stimuli will provide sensory rest, as well as a chance to tune out need for cognitive-perceptual activity.
• Restrict loud physical activity at least 2 to 3 hours before scheduled sleep time.	Overstimulating physical activity will provide stimulation of the central nervous system along with the resultant activation of bodily function.
• Schedule therapeutics around sleep needs. Complete all therapeutics at least 1 hour before scheduled sleep time.	A valuing of the sleep schedule will show respect and importance to the patient and family and will stress the importance of sleep.
• Assist parents with defining and standardizing general waking and sleeping schedule.	Parents will be able to cope better with developmental issues given the knowledge and opportunity to inquire about sleep-related issues. It is reported that limit setting with confidence by parents helps develop healthy patterns of sleep when no related health problems exist.
• Teach parents and child appropriate age-related relaxation techniques, for example, imagination of the "most-quiet-place" game, or imaging techniques suitable for age.	Improves parent's coping skills in dealing with common developmental issues that affect sleep.

• Discuss with parents difference between inability to sleep and fears related to developmental crises:
  ○ *Infant and toddler*: Separation anxiety
  ○ *Preschooler*: Fantasy versus reality
  ○ *School age*: Ability to perform at expected levels
  ○ *Adolescent*: Role identity versus role diffusion.	

• Ensure child's safety according to developmental and psychomotor abilities, for example, infant placed on abdomen; no plastic, loose-fitting sheets; bedrails up to prevent falling out of bed.	Basic safety standards for infants and children.

Women's Health

Actions/Interventions	Rationales
• Assist patient to schedule rest breaks throughout day.	Knowledge and proper planning can help patient reduce fatigue during pregnancy and the immediate postpartum period.
• Review daily schedule with patient, and assist her to adjust sleep schedule to coincide with infant's sleep pattern.	Knowledge of life changes can help in planning and implementing mechanisms to reduce fatigue and sleep disturbance.
• Identify a support system that can assist patient in alleviating fatigue.	
• Assist patient in identifying life-style adjustments that may be needed due to changes in physiologic function or needs during experiential phases of life, for example, pregnancy, postpartum, or menopause: ○ Possible lowering of room temperature ○ Layering of blankets or covers that can be discarded or added as necessary ○ Practicing relaxation immediately before scheduled sleep time ○ Establishing a bedtime routine, for example, bath, food, fluids, and activity	
• Involve significant others in discussion and problem-solving activities regarding life-cycle changes that are affecting work habits and interpersonal relationships, for example, hot flashes, pregnancy, or postpartum fatigue.	
• Teach patient to experiment with restful activities when she cannot sleep at night rather than lying in bed and thinking about not sleeping.	

Mental Health

Actions/Interventions	Rationales
• Provide only decaffeinated drinks during all 24 hours.	Caffeine stimulates the central nervous system.
• Spend (amount) minutes with client in activity of client's choice at least twice a day.	Increases mental alertness and activity during daytime hours.
• Provide appropriate positive reinforcement for achievement of steps toward reaching a normal sleep pattern.	Positive reinforcement encourages behavior.

Continued

Actions/Interventions	Rationales
• Talk client through deep muscle relaxation exercise for 30 minutes at 9 p.m.	Facilitates relaxation and disengagement from the activities and thoughts of the day to prepare the client both physically and mentally for sleep.
• Sit with client for (amount) minutes three times a day in a quiet environment, and provide positive reinforcement for client's accomplishments. (*Note*: This action is for clients with increased activity.)	Positive reinforcement encourages behavior and enhances self-esteem.
• Go to client's room and walk with him or her to the group area three times a day.	Stimulates wakefulness during daytime hours and facilitates the development of a trusting relationship.
• Spend time out of the room with the client until he or she demonstrates ability to tolerate 30 minutes of interaction with others. (*Note*: This action is for clients with depressed mood.)	Stimulates wakefulness during daytime hours.
• Spend 30 minutes with client discussing concerns 2 hours prior to bedtime.	Facilitates problem solving during daytime hours at a time when normal sleep patterns will not be disturbed.
• If client does not fall asleep within 45 minutes after retiring, have him or her get up and move around unit, sit at nurses' station and read, or engage in some other activity that does not focus on working or going to sleep, but that is not exciting for the client.	Sleep is a spontaneous behavior and cannot be achieved by "working on it." Focuses client's behavior away from "trying to go to sleep."[13]

Gerontic Health

Actions/Interventions	Rationales
• Collaborate with the physician and the pharmacist if a sleeping medication is prescribed to ensure that the drug is one that minimally interferes with the normal sleep cycle.	This assures that the older adult has as natural a sleep pattern as possible.
• Monitor for the presence of pain prior to bedtime. Also monitor to see if the patient is found awake frequently during the night.	Untreated pain may prevent the onset of sleep and interrupt the person's usual sleep pattern.
• Monitor for symptoms of depression,[14] especially if the older adult reports waking very early in the morning with an inability to fall back to sleep and reports feelings of anxiety upon awakening.	Depression is frequently underreported and undertreated in older adults.

Home Health

Actions/Interventions	Rationales
• Involve client and family in planning, implementing, and promoting restful environment and sleep routine: ○ Close door to room. ○ Turn room lights off and provide small night light. ○ Pull blinds to shield from street lights (at night) or sunlight (daytime). ○ Limit activity in room beginning at least 30 minutes before scheduled sleep time. ○ Unplug telephone in room or adjust volume control on bell. ○ Coordinate family activities and client's sleep needs to maximize both schedules. ○ Request that visits and calls be at specified times so that sleep time is not interrupted. ○ Provide favorite music, pillows, bedclothes, teddy bears, and so on. ○ Provide optimal room temperature and ventilation. ○ Support usual bedtime routine as much as possible in relation to medical diagnosis and client's condition. ○ Assist client with bedtime routine as necessary.	Household involvement is important to ensure that the environment is conducive for sleep or rest.
• Maintain pain control via appropriate medications, body positioning, and relaxation.	Pain disturbs or prevents sleep or rest.
• Encourage self-care, exercise, and activity as appropriate and based on medical diagnosis and client's condition.	Sleep-rest patterns are stabilized by a balance of activity and exercise.

FLOW CHART EVALUATION
Flow Chart Expected Outcome 1

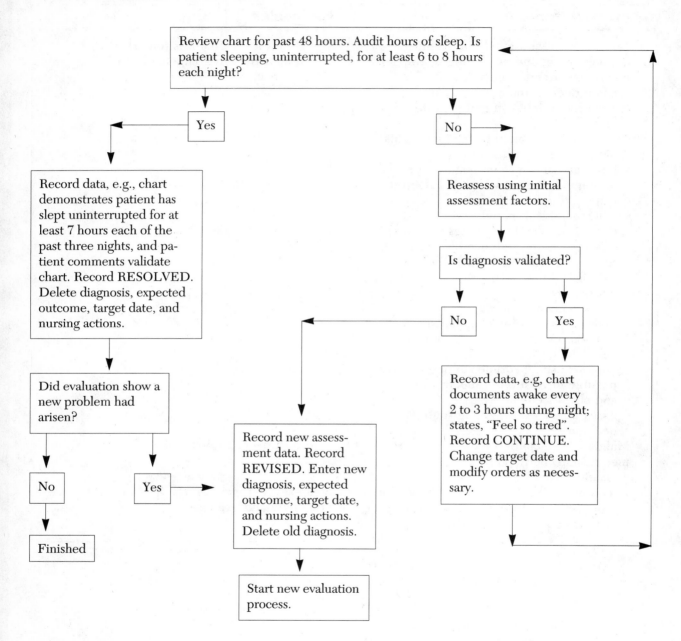

Flow Chart Expected Outcome 2

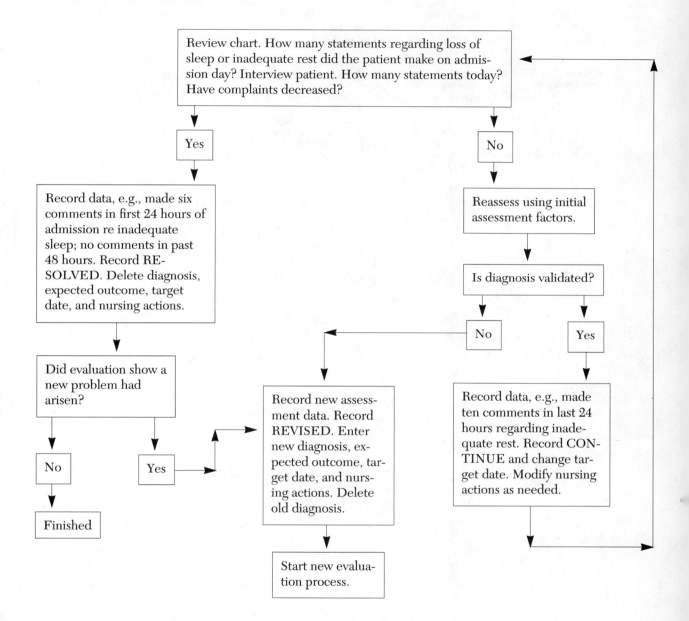

References

1. Hayter, J: The rhythm of sleep. Am J Nurs 80:457, 1980.
2. Roth, B: Narcolepsy and Hypersomnia. Karger, New York, 1980.
3. Lee, K: Rest status. In Mitchell, PH and Loustau, A (eds): Concepts Basic to Nursing, ed 3. McGraw-Hill, New York, 1981.
4. Guilleminault, C: Sleep and Its Disorders in Children. Raven Press, New York, 1988.
5. Whaley, LF and Wong, DL: Nursing Care of Infants and Children, ed 4. CV Mosby, St. Louis, 1991.
6. Mauri, M: Sleep and the reproductive cycle: A review. Health Care Women Int 11:409, 1990.
7. Weiss, ME and Armstrong, M: Postpartum mothers' preferences for nighttime care of the neonate. J Obstet Gynecol Neonatal Nurs 20:290, 1991.
8. Mead-Bennett, E: The relationship of Primigravida sleep experience and select moods on the first postpartum day. J Obstet Gynecol Neonatal Nurs 19:146, 1990.
9. Schirmer, M: When sleep won't come. J Gerontol Nurs 9:16, 1983.
10. Sonia, AI, et al: Periodic leg movements in sleep in community dwelling elderly. Sleep 14:496, 1991.
11. North American Nursing Diagnosis Association: Taxonomy I: Revised 1990. Author, St. Louis, 1990.
12. Wilson, H and Kneisl, C: Psychiatric Nursing, ed 4. Addison-Wesley, Redwood City, CA, 1992.
13. Watzlawicak, P, Weakland, J, and Fisch, R: Change. WW Norton, New York, 1974.
14. Keane, SM and Stella, S: Recognizing depression in the elderly. J Gerontol Nurs 15:21, 1990.

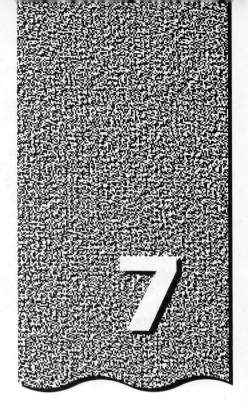

Cognitive-Perceptual Pattern

PATTERN INTRODUCTION
Pattern Description

Rationality, the ability to think, has often been described as the defining attribute of human beings. Thus, the Cognitive-Perceptual Pattern becomes the essential premise for all other patterns used in the practice of nursing. Since this pattern deals with the adequacy of the sensory modes and adaptations necessary to negate inadequacies in the cognitive functional abilities, any failure in recognizing alterations in this pattern will hamper assessment and intervention in all of the other patterns. The nurse must be aware of the Cognitive-Perceptual Pattern as an integral and important part of holistic nursing.

The Cognitive-Perceptual Pattern deals with thought, thought processes, and knowledge as well as the way the patient acquires and applies knowledge. A major component of the process is perceiving. Perceiving incorporates the interpretation of sensory stimuli. Understanding how a patient thinks, perceives, and incorporates these processes to best adapt and function is paramount in helping the patient to return to or maintain the best health state possible. Alterations in the process of cognition and perception is an initial step in any assessment.

Additionally, the nurse-patient relationship identifies human response as a major premise for the nursing process. Ultimately, then, it is this very notion of thought and learning potential that facilitates the self-actualization of human beings.

Pattern Assessment

1. Does patient indicate difficulty in making choices between options for care?
   a. Yes (Decisional Conflict [Specify])
   b. No
2. Is patient delaying decision making regarding care options?
   a. Yes (Decisional Conflict [Specify])
   b. No
3. Does patient indicate lack of information regarding his or her problem?
   a. Yes (Knowledge Deficit [Specify])
   b. No
4. Can patient restate regimen he or she needs to follow for improved health?
   a. Yes
   b. (Knowledge Deficit [Specify])
5. Review mental status exam. Is patient fully alert?
   a. Yes
   b. No (Altered Thought Processes; Sensory-Perceptual Alterations)
6. Does patient or his or her family indicate patient has any memory problems?
   a. Yes (Altered Thought Processes)
   b. No
7. Review sensory exam. Does patient display any sensory problems?
   a. Yes (Sensory-Perceptual Alterations [Specify])
   b. No
8. Does patient use both sides of body?
   a. Yes
   b. No (Unilateral Neglect)

9. Does patient look at and seem aware of affected body side?
   a. Yes
   b. No (Unilateral Neglect)
10. Does patient verbalize that he or she is experiencing pain?
    a. Yes (Pain; Chronic Pain)
    b. No
11. Has pain been experienced for more than 6 months?
    a. Yes (Chronic Pain)
    b. No (Pain)
12. Does patient display any distraction behavior (moaning, crying, pacing restlessness)?
    a. Yes (Pain)
    b. No

Diagnoses in This Pattern

1. Decisional Conflict (Specify) (page 526)
2. Knowledge Deficit (Specify) (page 536)
3. Pain and Chronic Pain (page 546)
4. Sensory-Perceptual Alterations (Specify) (page 562)
5. Thought Process, Altered (page 577)
6. Unilateral Neglect (page 588)

Conceptual Information

A person who is able to carry out the activities of a normal cognitive-perceptual pattern experiences conscious thought, is oriented to reality, solves problems, is able to perceive via sensory input, and responds appropriately in carrying out the usual activities of daily living at the fullest level of functioning. All of these functions rely on a healthy nervous system containing receptors to detect input accurately, a brain that can interpret the information correctly, and transmitters that can transport decoded information. Bodily response is also a basic requisite for responding to the sensory and perceptual demands of the individual.

Cognition is the process of obtaining and using knowledge about one's world through the use of perceptual abilities, symbols, and reasoning. For this reason it includes the use of human sensory capabilities to receive input about the environment. This process usually leads to perception, which is the process of extracting information in such a way that the individual transforms sensory input into meaning. Cognition incorporates knowledge and the process used in its acquisition; therefore, ideas (concepts of mind symbols) and language (verbal symbols) are two tools of cognition. Learning may be considered the dynamic process in which perceptual processing of sensory input leads to concept formation and change in behavior. Cognitive development is highly dependent on adequate, predictable sensory input.

There are two general approaches to contemporary cognitive theory. The information-processing approach attempts to understand human thought and reasoning processes by comparing the mind to a sophisticated computer system that is designed to acquire, process, store, and use information according to various programs or designs.

The second approach is based on the work of the Swiss psychologist Jean Piaget, who considered cognitive adaptation in terms of two basic processes: assimilation and accommodation. Assimilation is the process by which the person integrates new perceptual data or stimulus events into existing schemata or existing patterns of behavior. In other words, in assimilation, a person interprets reality in terms of his or her own model of the world based on previous experience. Accommodation is the process of changing that model by developing the mechanisms to adjust to reality. Piaget believed that representational thought does not originate in a social language but in unique symbols that later provide a foundation for language acquisition.[1]

The American psychologist Jerome Bruner broadened Piaget's concept by suggesting that the cognitive process is affected by three modes: the enactive mode, which involves representation through action; the iconic mode, which uses visual and mental images; and the symbolic mode, which uses language.[1]

Cognitive dissonance is the mental conflict that takes place when beliefs or assumptions are challenged or contradicted by new information. The unease or tension the individual may experience as a result of cognitive dissonance usually results in the person's resorting to defense mechanisms in an attempt to maintain stability in his or her conception of the world and self.

In a broad sense, thinking activities may be considered internally adaptive responses to intrinsic and extrinsic stimuli. The thought processes serve to express inner impulses; but they also serve to generate appropriate goal-seeking behavior by the individual. This behavior is enhanced by perceptual processes as well.

Perception is the process of extracting information in such a way that the individual transforms sensory input into meaning. The senses that serve as the origin of perceptual stimuli are as follows:

1. Exteroceptors (distance sensors)
   a. Visual
   b. Auditory
2. Proprioceptors (near sensors)
   a. Cutaneous or skin senses, which detect and communicate or transduce changes in touch, such as pressure, temperature, and pain
   b. Chemical sense of taste
   c. Chemical sense of smell
3. Interoceptors (deep sensors)
   a. Kinesthetic senses, which detect changes in position of the body and motions of the muscles, tendons, and joints
   b. Static or vestibular senses, which detect changes related to maintaining position in space and the regulation of organic functions such as metabolism, fluid balance, and sensual stimulation.

It is important to note that since perceptual skill processing is an internal event, its presence and development are inferred by changes in overt behavior. For full appreciation of the Cognitive-Perceptual Pattern it is also necessary to understand the normal physiology of the nervous system.

Developmental Considerations

INFANT

The full-term newborn has several sensory capacities. The neonate should have a pupillary reflex in response to light and a corneal reflex in response to touch. The sensory myelinization is best developed at birth for hearing, taste, and smell.

Structurally, the eye is not completely differentiated from the macula. The newborn has the capacity to momentarily fixate on a bright or moving object held within 8 inches and in the midline of the visual field. By approximately 4 months of age, the infant is capable of 20/200 visual acuity. Binocular fixation and convergence to near objects are possible by approximately 4 months of age. In a supine position, the infant follows a dangling toy from the side to past midline. By approximately 15 weeks of age the infant is beginning eye-hand coordination and is capable of accommodation to near objects. Of concern at this age would be any abnormalities noted in any of these tasks plus rubbing of eyes, self-rocking, or other self-stimulating behavior.

At birth all of the structural components of the ear are fully developed. However, the lack of cortical integration and full myelination of the neural pathways prevents specific response to sound. The infant will usually search to locate sounds. The neonate is capable of detecting a loud sound of approximately 90 decibels and reacts with a startle. By approximately 2 months the infant will turn to the appropriate side when a sound is made at ear level. By age of 6 to 8 months the infant will utter sounds and imitate speech. By approximately 20 months the infant will localize sounds made below the ear. A cause for concern might be failure to be awakened by loud noises or abnormalities in any of the above findings.

Smell seems to be a factor in the breast-fed infant's response to the mother's engorgement and leaking. Newborns will turn away from strong odors such as vinegar and alcohol. By approximately 6 to 9 months, infants associate smell with different foods and familiar people of their circle of activity. Avoidance of strong, unpleasant odors occurs also.

The newborn responds to various solutions with the following gustofacial reflexes:

1. A tasteless solution elicits no facial expression.
2. A sweet solution elicits an eager suck and look of satisfaction.
3. A bitter liquid produces an angry, upset expression.

By 1 year of age the infant shows marked taste preference, with similar responses to different flavors as the neonate.

At birth the neonate is capable of touch perception; the mouth, hands, and soles of the feet are very sensitive. There is increasing support for the notion that touch and motion are essential to normal growth and development.

By 1 year of age the infant has a preference for soft textures over rough, grainy textures. The infant relies on the sense of touch for comforting. Overresponse or underresponse to stimuli, for example, pain, is a cause for concern.

At birth, the infant is limited in perceiving itself in space. There is momentary head control. In essence, primitive reflexes, which are protective in nature, enable the neonate to adjust to extrauterine life and can be used to identify congenital anomalies. More complex perception requires deep myelination and total integration of cortical activity. In general, testing more exacting neurologic reflexes of the neonate will provide in-depth supplementary data.

By approximately 3 months of age the infant will reflexively draw up its legs when suspended in a horizontal prone position with the head flexed against the trunk. This is known as the Landau reflex; it remains present until approximately 12 to 24 months of age. Another related reflex is the parachute reflex, in which the infant, on being suspended in a horizontal prone position and suddenly thrust downward, will place hands and fingers forward as an attempt to protect against falling. This reflex appears at approximately 7 months and persists indefinitely.

The neonate responds with total body reaction to a painful stimulus. The primitive reflexes demonstrate this, especially the Moro or startle response to sudden loss of support or loud noises. The neonate is dependent on others for protection from pain. The mother of a newborn is most often the person who assumes this task, along with the father and other primary caregivers. For this reason, management of pain must also include the parents. Distraction, for example, a pacifier, is useful in dealing with painful stimuli.

The infant offers localized reaction to pain at approximately 6 to 9 months of age. Often a physical tugging of the suspected painful body part, as with an earache, will indicate pain in the infant. Crying and irritability may also be manifestations of pain, particularly when the nurse is sure other basic needs have been attended to. The infant is incapable of cooperating in procedures and must be physically restrained.

If chronic pain comes to be a way of life for the infant soon after birth or before much development has occurred, there may be potential alterations in subsequent development. In some instances, infants adapt and develop high tolerances for pain.

The neonate subjected to hypoxia in the perinatal period and the premature infant of less than 38 weeks' gestation are at risk for developmental delays. Apgar scores are typically used as criteria, in addition to neurologic reflexes. Seizures during the neonatal period must also be followed. It is paramount that close examination be performed for basic primitive reflexes and general neonatal status as well as identification of any genetic syndromes or congenital anomalies.

The infant gradually incorporates symbols and interacts with the world through primary caregivers. Any major delays in development should be cause for further close follow-up. Sensory-perceptual deficiencies may indeed bring about impaired thought processes.

TODDLER AND PRESCHOOLER

Binocular vision is well established by 12–15 months. The toddler can distinguish geometric shapes and can demonstrate beginning depth perception. Marked strabismus should be treated at this time to prevent amblyopia. The toddler can begin to name colors.

Smell, taste, and touch all become more related as the toddler initially sees an object and handles it while enjoying, via all the senses, what it is to "know." Regression to previous tactile behavior for comfort is common in this group, as exemplified by a preference for being patted and rocked to sleep during times of stress such as illness. By this time secondary deficits in development may show themselves. There is cause for concern if the toddler shows greater response to movement than to sound or avoids social interaction with other children. By this time speech should be sufficiently developed to validate a basic sense of the toddler's ability to use symbols. Proprioception is not perfected, but "toddling" represents a major milestone. Falls at this age are common.

There is an even greater incorporation of sensory activity in sequencing for the preschooler, in whom major myelination is fully developed. There is refinement of eye-hand coordination, with reading readiness apparent. Visual acuity begins to approach 20/20 and the preschooler will know colors. Before age 5 the child should be screened for amblyopia; amblyopia rarely develops after age 5. Language becomes more sophisticated and is used in social interaction. By this age the child will remember and exercise caution regarding potential dangers, such as hot objects.

Temper tantrums, outbursts, and avoidance of painful stimuli describe the usual response of the toddler to painful stimuli. This will be especially true with invasive procedures. On occasion a toddler may demonstrate tolerance for painful procedures on the basis of understanding the benefits offered; for example, young children with a medical diagnosis of leukemia. This is not the usual case, however. If the toddler must deal with chronic pain, there may be regression to previous behavior as a means of coping.

The preschooler views any invasive procedure as mutilation and attempts to withdraw in response to pain. The preschooler cries out in pain and expresses feelings about pain in his or her own terms. The interpretation of pain is influenced greatly by the parental and familial value systems. Severe pain will probably cause regression to previous behavior levels. The nurse should be aware that pain will bring out fears of abandonment, death, or the unknown in this age group. Also, the effect the pain has on others may serve to further frighten the child.

Play is an ideal noninvasive means of assessment. Difficulties in gait, balance, or the use of upper limbs in symmetry with lower limbs should be noted, as well as related holistic developmental components including speech, motor, cognitive, perceptual, and social components. Allowance should be made for regression to earlier patterns as needed in times of stress such as illness and hospitalization. If a deficit exists, parents should be encouraged to continue appropriate follow-up and intervention.

The preschooler, at ages 4–5, may be aware that he or she is different from peers, although egocentrism continues. Of importance is the mastery of separation from parents for increasing periods of time. The likelihood of sibling integration should be considered also.

The toddler gradually learns to care for himself or herself and is strongly influenced by the family's value system. The child is able to express thoughts.

The preschooler has the capacity for magical thinking and enjoys imitating the parent of the same sex. Resistance to parental authority is common and the child is still egocentric in thought. The child's understanding of abstract concepts and symbols may be rudimentary; for example, death may be perceived as "sleep."

By this age the child explores the world in a meaningful fashion but still relies closely on primary caregivers. Marked delays should be monitored, with a focus on maintaining optimum functioning with developmental sequencing.

The preschooler will enjoy activity and is beginning to enjoy learning colors, using words in sentences, and gradually forming relationships with persons outside the immediate family. If there are delays, they should continue to be monitored. By now major deficits in cognition become more obvious.

SCHOOL-AGE CHILD

The schoolchild has a significant ability to perform logical operations. More complete myelination and maturation enhance the basic physiologic functioning of the central nervous system. Generally, the school-age child is self-motivated and can establish and follow simple rules. Time as an abstract concept is gradually understood. The child understands that death is permanent.

The school-age child begins to interpret the experience of pain with a cognitive component—the cause or source of pain as well as its possible recurrence. By this age the child will attempt to hold still as needed, with an appearance of bravery. The school-age child will give expression to the experience of pain. If the child is particularly shy, the nurse should make special attempts to establish a trusting relationship to best manage pain. A major fear is loss of control. The nurse must consider the need to completely evaluate chronic pain. In some instances, it may signal other altered patterns, especially a distressed family or inability to cope as well. Lower performance in school can be an indicator of chronic pain. Also, the nurse should be aware of the increased complexity required for daily activities of living. The child of this age may have a negative self-image if he or she is unable to perform as peers do. The importance of group activities cannot be overstressed.

With a sense of accomplishment, the school-age child will blossom. When school does not bring success, frustration follows. It is mandatory that caution be exercised in assessing for deficits as distinct from behavioral manifestations of school dislike.

ADOLESCENT

By now, the child has 20/20 vision. Squinting should be investigated, as should any symptoms of prolonged eyestrain.

Hearing should be tested if the adolescent speaks loudly or fails to respond to loud noises.

Overreaction or underreaction to painful stimuli is also cause for further investigation. The adolescent may have food fads, but concern is appropriate if the adolescent overuses spices, especially salt or sugar, or complains of food not "tasting like it used to."

The adolescent should distinguish a full range of odors. The nurse should be concerned if the adolescent is unresponsive to noxious stimuli. Temporary clumsiness may be associated with growth spurts. The nurse should be concerned about patterns of deteriorating gross and fine motor coordination and ataxia.

By now the adolescent is capable of formal operational thought and is able to move beyond the world of concrete reality to abstract possibilities and ideas. Problem solving is evident with inductive and deductive capacity. There is an interest in values, with a tendency toward idealism. Attention must be given to the adolescent's sensitivity to others and potential for rejection if body image is altered. Of particular importance at this time are sports and peer-related activities. As feelings are explored more cautiously there is a tendency to draw into oneself at this stage. There may be major conflicts over independence when self-care is not possible.

The adolescent fears mutilation and attempts to deal with pain as an adult might. The adolescent strives for self-control but may attempt to get secondary gains from pain. Concerns about sexuality may be present in this age group. As with the adult, an attempt to discover the cause and implication of the pain is made. The adolescent experiencing chronic pain will be at risk for abnormal peer interaction and may potentially experience altered self-perception.

The adolescent will most often remain steady in cognitive functioning if there are no major emotional or sensory problems. Of concern at this age would be substance abuse, which could impair thought processes.

ADULT AND OLDER ADULT

The adult is capable of 20/20 vision with a gradual decline in acuity and accommodation. After approximately 40 years of age there is a tendency toward farsightedness. Color discrimination decreases in later ages, with green and blue being the major hues affected. Depending on the cause, corrective aids may be used. However, in degenerative processes, such as macular degeneration, correction may not be possible. Eventually, depth perception and peripheral vision are also affected. There may be sensitivity to light, as with cataract formation. The nurse should be alert for all etiologic components, but especially the retinopathy associated with diabetic alterations.

The adult can accurately discriminate 1600 different frequencies. There should be equal sensation of sounds for the left and right ear. The Rinne test may be done to validate air and bone conduction via a tuning fork. The Weber test may be used to assess lateralization. Equilibrium assessment will provide data regarding the vestibular branch.

With time, hearing acuity gradually diminishes, with detection of high frequencies especially affected. The nurse should be concerned with a lack of response to loud noises and increased volume of speech, and should be alert to clues of decreased hearing such as cupping of the hand on the "better" ear or leaning sideways to catch the conversation on the "better" side.

There may be a gradual deterioration in sensitivity to odors after approximately age 60, although for the most part the sense of smell remains functional in the absence of organic disease. There may be altered gastrointestinal enzyme production, which ultimately interferes with the usual perception of smells.

The ability to taste is well differentiated in adulthood. Sweet and sour can be detected bilaterally. Concern may be raised if the client states the sense of taste has diminished or changed. There is a gradual loss of acuity in taste in later life. This is due in part to decreased enzymatic production and utilization in digestive processes. Oversalting or overspicing of foods may serve as a clue to this loss of taste sensation. The use of dentures may also affect the sensation of taste and enjoyment of food.

The adult is able to discriminate among a wide range of tactile stimuli, including pressure, temperature, texture, and pain or noxious sensation. With aging there is a decrease in subcutaneous fat, loss of skin turgor, increase in capillary fragility, and decrease in conduction of impulses. All of these changes influence the sense of touch, with a loss of acuity in aging.

The adult is well coordinated and has a keen sense of perception of his or her body in space. There are multiple protective mechanisms which aid in maintaining balance. Typically, even with eyes closed, the individual is able to stand and maintain balance.

By now individual tolerance and threshold for pain are well established. The individual has learned various ways to cope with pain and thus may be equipped with a more stable base from which to respond.

The adult is equipped to solve problems and apply principles to everyday living. There is emphasis on seeking a mate for life who is able to satisfy basic companionship needs. There may be difficulties in accepting life's challenges as parents or as adults. In later life, there is a gradual decline in problem-solving capacity which may be exaggerated by illness.

Allowing for potential decrease in bodily perception and functioning with age must be considered. As assessment is carried out, focus should be on risk factors such as chronic illness, financial deficits, resolution of ego integrity versus despair, and obvious etiologic components. The nurse should assist the patient to maintain self-care as the patient desires.

With aging there is a gradual loss of balance, perhaps most related to the concurrent vascular changes. For this reason proprioceptive data may provide an immediate basis for assessing the safety needs of the geriatric client.

In the absence of adversity, the adult enjoys the daily challenges of living. If coping is altered for whatever reason, a risk for impaired thought processes exists. With the process of aging, there are potential risks for impaired thought processes. In addition, there may be potential risks for some regarding degenerative brain and central nervous system (CNS) disorders, which also include impaired thought processes. Two concerns for older adults related to altered thought processes are dementia and delirium or acute confusional states.

APPLICABLE NURSING DIAGNOSES

Decisional Conflict (Specify)

DEFINITION

The state of uncertainty about course of action to be taken when choice among competing actions involves risk, loss, or challenge to personal life values.[2]

NANDA TAXONOMY: CHOOSING 5.3.1.1

DEFINING CHARACTERISTICS[2]

1. Major defining characteristics
   a. Verbalized uncertainty about choices
   b. Verbalization of undesired consequences of alternative actions being considered
   c. Vacillation between alternative choices
   d. Delayed decision making
2. Minor defining characteristics
   a. Verbalized feeling of distress while attempting a decision
   b. Self-focusing
   c. Physical signs of distress or tension (increased heart rate, increased muscle tension, restlessness, and so on)
   d. Questioning personal values and beliefs while attempting a decision

RELATED FACTORS

1. Unclear personal values and beliefs
2. Perceived threat to value system
3. Lack of experience or interference with decision making
4. Lack of relevant information
5. Support system deficit
6. Multiple or divergent sources of information

RELATED CLINICAL CONCERNS

1. Any surgery causing body image change
2. Any illness carrying a potential terminal prognosis
3. Any chronic disease
4. Dementia

HAVE YOU SELECTED THE CORRECT DIAGNOSIS?

Anxiety Anxiety is considered to be a feeling of threat which may not be-known by the person as a specific causative factor. In Decisional Conflict, the patient knows the options but cannot decide between specifics. (See page 605.)

Knowledge Deficit In Knowledge Deficit, the client does not have the information to make a decision. In Decisional Conflict, the information is known. (See page 536.)

Ineffective Individual Coping This diagnosis is closely related in that adaptive behavior and problem-solving abilities are not able to meet the demands of the client's needs. Ineffective Individual Coping and Decisional Conflict may very well be companion diagnoses. (See page 892.)

EXPECTED OUTCOMES

1. Will verbalize at least one concrete personal decision by (date) and/or
2. Will return-demonstrate at least (number) conflict resolution techniques by (date)

TARGET DATE

Value clarification, belief examination, and acquisition of decision-making processes will require a considerable length of time and much support. Therefore, target dates in increments of weeks would be most appropriate.

NURSING ACTIONS/INTERVENTIONS WITH RATIONALES
Adult Health

Actions/Interventions	Rationales
• Instruct patient in stress reduction techniques as needed. Have patient demonstrate specific techniques at least daily.	Reduces anxiety, enabling patient to better process problems.
• Assist patient to focus on problem-solving processes. Help patient to verbalize alternatives and advantages and disadvantages of solutions. Help patient to realistically appraise situations and set realistic short-term objectives daily.	Assists patient in learning to use the problem-solving process.
• Support patient's values as necessary. Do not be judgmental when interacting with patient. Help patient to clarify values and beliefs as needed.	Helps patient focus on what is important to self in decision making rather than being concerned about pleasing others.
• Assist patient to seek, find, and interpret relevant information about problem. Refer to community resources for support.	Helps patient to explore alternatives. Coordinates care of patient.
• Refer to psychiatric nurse clinician as needed.	A nurse specialist may be better able to help the patient focus on the underlying process.

Child Health

Actions/Interventions	Rationales
• Determine who will intervene on behalf of the infant or child: parents or appointed legal guardian.	For legal and ethical reasons, it is essential to determine whether the parents are unable to assume the parental role and obligations and, if not, to make this fact known to all involved in the child's care. It is likewise essential for all caregivers to know who the legal guardian or spokesperson is.
• In instances of conflicting decision makers, ensure that the child's rights are protected according to legal statutes.	Regardless of conflicts in decision making, the infant or child is entitled to appropriate care. In extreme cases of conflict, a state or local judge may appoint guardians or foster parents to assume decision making regarding health matters. In other instances, for example withholding suggested treatment because of religious beliefs, individual states and precedence must be sought by the parties involved.
• Ensure that appropriate documentation is carried out according to situational needs.	Legal documentation according to health care decisions and related matters is to be carried out as standard care, paying attention to the mandates of the institution regarding appropriate forms to be completed.
• Although the child may be ill equipped or unable to participate fully in decision making, encourage developmentally appropriate components for care to assist the child in learning decision making.	Early involvement in decision making fosters safe support for the child, thereby increasing the likelihood of learning effective coping behaviors. This will also empower the child and foster a positive self-image.
• Be certain that choices or options indeed exist when the child is allowed to exercise decision making.	Preferences and individualization will be realistically valued when there are choices or options in the care plan. It is unethical to indicate there are choices when none exist, for example, if medication cannot be given by any other route but intramuscular.
• Provide behavioral reinforcement, which best fosters learning, with appropriate follow-up when the child is involved in decisional conflict.	Appropriate reinforcement will serve to enhance learning and assist the patient in learning decision making.
• Consider potential long-term residual or subsequent effects related to specific decisional conflict for the child or family.	Decision making often has far-reaching effects; for example, in early childhood, values of a lifetime are formulated. Appropriate regard to this fact should guide all involved in this aspect of child rearing and supportive aspects of health care.

Women's Health: Unwanted Pregnancy

Actions/Interventions	Rationales

• Provide an atmosphere that encourages patient to view her options in the event of an unwanted pregnancy. Assure the patient of confidentiality.
• Give clear, concise, complete information to the patient, describing the choices available to her:
  ○ Carrying the pregnancy to term and keeping infant
  ○ Adoption of infant
  ○ Abortion
• Discuss with the patient the advantages and disadvantages of each option.
• Encourage patient to discuss beliefs and practices in a nonthreatening atmosphere and include significant others in conversation and decision as the patient desires.
• Refer patient to proper agency for guidance and treatment.
	Provides information which allows the patient to make an informed choice.

• Discuss and review with patient the different methods of birth control. • Assess the patient's ability to correctly use the different methods of birth control. • Provide factual information, listing the advantages and disadvantages of each method. • Provide patient information on obtaining her method of choice. • Explore with patient and significant other their views on children and family.	Provides information and support to assist patient in planning future pregnancies.

Women's Health: Less-than-Perfect Infant

NOTE: Families faced with the birth of a child with congenital anomalies or developmental defects experience decisional conflict and great confusion about choices that need to be made. Often there is a sense of urgency, as decisions need to be made quickly to save the life of the infant. Many times the infant has been delivered by cesarean section and it is the mother's partner who, alone, must make crucial decisions that could affect the family and the life of the infant. Parents experience confusion, fear, guilt, helplessness, and inadequacy.

Actions/Interventions	Rationales
• Provide accurate information to parents as soon as possible.	Provides information and supportive environment, which helps parents to make decisions.[3,4]
• Let parents see and hold infant if at all possible.	Promotes bonding and provides comfort for both parents and infant.
• Support parents in their grieving process for the loss of the infant and perhaps the death of the infant.[5,6]	
• Keep the parents informed continuously and encourage the health care team to talk to them often.	
• Contact significant persons, of the parents' choice, who can be of support to them.[7]	
• Give parents a private place to be with their support persons.	
• Encourage parents to visit the infant in the neonatal intensive care unit (NICU) as often as possible.	
• Collaborate with NICU staff to plan time for mother-and-infant activities together as much as possible.	
• Refer to support groups and agencies as needed for follow-up care when the infant leaves the hospital.	Support is essential in resolving decisional conflict.

Mental Health

> NOTE: The client who is experiencing a decisional conflict is faced with confusion about alternative solutions. When assisting these clients the nurse should be careful not to connote the client's confusion negatively. Various authors[8-10] have noted the positive role confusion plays in the change process. Erickson[8] frequently encouraged confusion as a way to distract the conscious mind and allow the unconscious to develop solutions. It is from this theoretical base that the following interventions are developed.

Actions/Interventions	Rationales
• Assure the client that the difficulty he or she is experiencing in decision making is positive in that it has placed him or her in a position to look for new, creative solutions. If he or she were not experiencing this difficulty, he or she might be tempted to remain in the same old problem-solution set.	Promotes positive orientation, self-worth, and hope.
• Assist the client in reducing the pressure of time on making a decision.	

- Have the client explain the time he or she has given himself or herself to make a decision. Asking the client, "What is the worst that will happen if a decision is not made right now?" may help this process.

- Assist the client in verbalizing all information that he or she currently has on the choices.

- Have the client explore the feelings and the information related to the choices. This process may extend over several days. The client may be reluctant to verbalize negative feelings related to certain choices if a trusting relationship has not yet been developed with the nurse.

- Have the client discuss how significant others think and feel about the various choices. Have the client evaluate the impact of the feelings of significant others on his or her decision-making process.

- Have the client fantasize an ideal choice.

- Have the client construct a list of solutions (at least 20) that would produce the ideal choice. (These solutions are not to be evaluated at this time.) Encourage client to develop some unrealistic solutions. This may be promoted by asking the client what he or she might tell a friend to do in this situation or by having the client generate three magic-wish solutions; for example, "If you had a magic wand, what would you do to resolve this situation?"

- Sort through the developed list with the client, generating solutions from the ones listed. At this time the client can begin to combine and eliminate ideas after evaluation. Carefully evaluate each solution before it is eliminated. What appears to be a bizarre solution can become useful when altered or combined with another idea.

- As each idea is evaluated, provide all information necessary to evaluate the idea.

- Explore the client's thoughts and feelings about each idea.

- Remind the client that there are no perfect answers and each of us makes the best choice that can be made at the time.

- Remind the client that if a choice that is

Provides time to develop alternative problem solutions and decreases stress on the client.

Aids in understanding client's perception of the situation.

The client's cognitive style and feelings about the situation impact the appraisal of both the situation and possible solutions.[11]

Support system involvement increses the probability of positive outcomes.

Accesses creative problem solutions that bypass the client's self-imposed limits.

Aids in assessing client's commitment to each possible solution.

Promotes positive orientation, self-worth, and hope for the future.

Promotes positive orientation.

Continued

Actions/Interventions	Rationales
made does not resolve the problem, alternative solutions can then be tried. • Remind the client that a solution that does not work provides information about the problem that can be used in developing future solutions. • Meet with the client and support system to allow the support system to be a part of the decision-making process if this is appropriate. • Discuss with the client and the support system any secondary gains from not making a decision. • Once a decision is made, have the client develop a behavioral plan for implementation.	Support system involvement increases the probability of a positive outcome. Assess for positive reinforcement for not resolving the problem. Having a plan to cope with the anticipated situations promotes a perception of greater control over future situations and increases the probability of the client's enacting new coping behaviors

Gerontic Health

Actions/Interventions	Rationales
• Discuss with patient prior examples of decisional conflict and their outcomes.	Emphasizes ability to solve problems and reinforces successes.

Home Health

Actions/Interventions	Rationales

• Teach client and family techniques to decrease decisional conflict:
  ○ Providing appropriate health information
    Joining a support group
    Clarifying values
    Performing stress reduction activities
    Seeking spiritual or legal assistance as needed
    Identifying useful sources of information
	Appropriate knowledge and values clarification between the client and family will reduce conflict.

• Assist client and family in identifying risk factors pertinent to the situation:
  ○ Lack of knowledge
  ○ Developmental or situational crisis
  ○ Role confusion
  ○ Excess stress
  ○ Excess stimuli
	Early identification of risk factors provides opportunity for early intervention.

• Consult with or refer to appropriate resources as indicated. (See Appendix B.)	Use of the network of existing community services provides for effective utilization of resources.

FLOW CHART EVALUATION
Flow Chart Expected Outcome 1

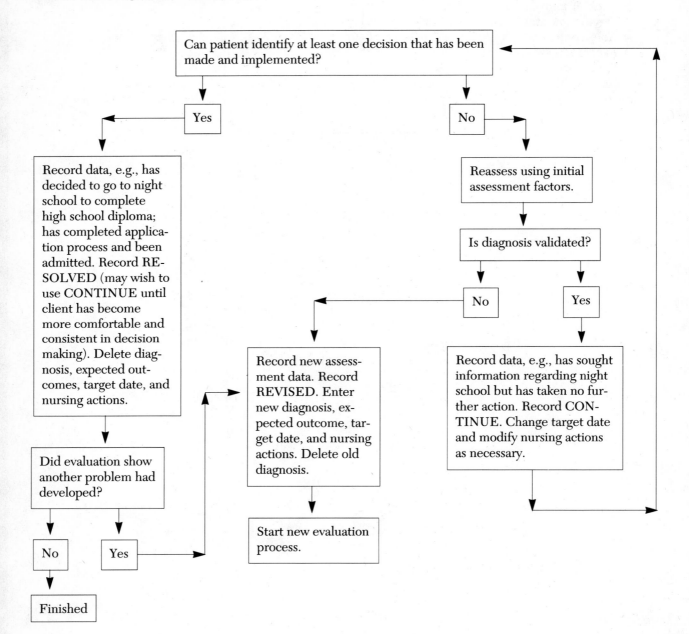

Flow Chart Expected Outcome 2

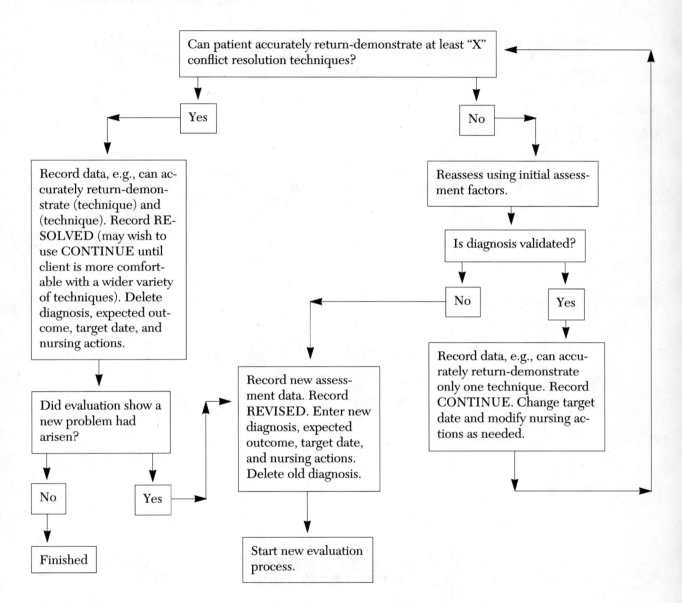

Knowledge Deficit (Specify)

DEFINITION

The situation in which the individual experiences a lack of information or has difficulty in applying information, thus increasing the risk of actual compromise in health care.[12]

NANDA TAXONOMY: KNOWING 8.1.1

DEFINING CHARACTERISTICS[12]

1. Major defining characteristics:
   a. Verbalization of the problem
   b. Inaccurate follow-through of instruction
   c. Inaccurate performance of test
   d. Inappropriate or exaggerated behaviors; for example, hysterical, hostile, agitated, or apathetic
2. Minor defining characteristics:
   None given

RELATED FACTORS[12]

1. Lack of exposure
2. Lack of recall
3. Information misinterpretation
4. Cognitive limitation
5. Lack of interest in learning
6. Unfamiliarity with information resources

RELATED CLINICAL CONCERNS

1. Any diagnosis that is entirely new to the patient
2. Mental retardation
3. Post–head injury
4. Depression
5. Dementia

HAVE YOU SELECTED THE CORRECT DIAGNOSIS?

Noncompliance In Noncompliance the patient can return-demonstrate skills accurately or verbalize the regimen needed but does not follow through on the care. (See page 80.)

Altered Thought Process This diagnosis would be evident by lack of immediate recall on return-demonstration rather than inaccurate or limited demonstration and recall. (See page 577.)

Powerlessness This diagnosis would be reflected by statements such as, "How will this help?" "It's beyond my control" and "Have to rely on others"

> rather than statements related to "Don't really understand" "Not really sure how" or "Is this right?" (See page 657.)
>
> **Altered Health Maintenance** Altered Health Maintenance may include Knowledge Deficit, but it is broader in scope and includes such aspects as limited resources and mobility factors. (See page 38.)

EXPECTED OUTCOMES

1. Will return-demonstrate (specific knowledge deficit activity) by (date) and/or
2. Will restate (specific knowledge deficit material) by (date)

TARGET DATE

Individual learning curves vary significantly. A target date ranging from 3 to 7 days could be appropriate based on the individual's previous experience with this material, education level, potential for learning, and energy level.

NURSING ACTIONS/INTERVENTIONS WITH RATIONALES

Adult Health

Actions/Interventions	Rationales
• Contract with patient regarding what the patient wants and needs to learn. Be sure to include a time frame in the contract. Have patient sign contract to ensure patient consent for teaching. Review the patient's and family's current level of knowledge regarding this illness, hospitalization, and cultural and value beliefs.	Incorporates patient into learning process and provides additional motivation for resolving deficit; allows assessment of patient's readiness to learn; improves learning since it is based on exactly where the patient and family are in their knowledge and avoids needless repetition.
• Design teaching plan specific to patient's deficit area and level of education; for example, self-administration of medication, eighth-grade reading level. Include significant others in teaching sessions. Be sure plan includes content, objectives, methods, and evaluation.	Provides new knowledge based on patient's perceived needs; individuals learn in their own way and in their own time frame; motivates patient to learn; provides support and reinforcement for learning.
• Explain each procedure as it is being done, the rationale for the procedure, and the patient's role.	Incorporates another teaching method; reduces anxiety, thus promoting learning.
• Teach only absolutely relevant information first.	Patient will remember initial information more than subsequent information; avoids overwhelming patient with information. Reinforces learning achieved and promotes positive orientation.
• Provide positive reinforcement as often as possible for patient's progress.	

Continued

Actions/Interventions	Rationales
• Design teaching to stimulate as many of the patient's senses as possible; for example, visual, auditory, touch, smell. Have patient return-demonstrate any psychomotor activities.	Enhances learning, provides mechanism to evaluate learning and teaching effectiveness, and allows clarification of any misunderstandings.
• Have patient restate, in his or her own words, cognitive materials used during teaching session. Have patient repeat them each day until discharge.	Repeated practice of a behavior internalizes and personalizes the behavior.[13]
• Provide quiet, well-lighted, temperature-controlled teaching environment during teaching session.	Avoids distractions.
• Ensure that basic needs are taken care of before and immediately after teaching sessions: ○ Food and fluids ○ Toileting ○ Pain relief	Prevents distractions during teaching session.
• Pace teaching according to patient's rate of learning and preference during teaching session.	Considers patient's learning style and ability to process new information.
• Encourage patient's verbalization of anxiety and concern about self-care. Listen carefully. Redesign plan to incorporate patient's concerns as needed.	Considers patient's input into plan of teaching; increases likelihood of patient's retaining and using information; helps reduce fear and anxiety and provides a means for exploring possible resources.
• In addition to specifics, provide both written and verbal information on: ○ Normal body functioning ○ Signs and symptoms of altered functioning ○ Diet (food and fluid) ○ Exercise and activity ○ Growth and development ○ Self-examination ○ Impact on environment, stress, and change in life-style on health	Provides foundational knowledge on which to build more specific information.
• Start each teaching session with revalidation of the previous session. End each session with a summary.	Reinforces what is known; builds new information on previous knowledge; organizes new knowledge for patient.
• Collaborate with and refer to appropriate assistive resources. (See Appendix B.)	Coordinates team approach to health; provides means to follow-up and reinforce learning.

Child Health

Actions/Interventions	Rationales
• Determine if there are ambiguities in the minds of parents or child.	Clarification and verification will ensure a greater likelihood of understanding and valuing aspects critical to patient teaching.
• Identify the learning capacity of the patient and family.	Realistic capacity for learning should be a primary factor in patient teaching since it serves as one major parameter in expectations of learning.
• Determine the scope and appropriate presentation for patient and family; do not overwhelm the patient.	Developmental needs of all involved will best serve as an essential framework for teaching the patient and family. Potentials and capacity for use of all the sensory-perceptual aspects of cognition should be explored and used to ensure the best opportunity for effective teaching.

• Evaluate appropriately the effectiveness of the teaching-learning experience by:
  ○ Brief verbal discourse to provide concrete data
  ○ Written examination in brief to show progress
  ○ Observation of skills critical for care, such as, change of dressing according to sterile technique
  ○ Allowing child to perform skills in general fashion with use of dolls
	Evaluation is an indicator of both teaching effectiveness and learning. It serves as another essential aspect of patient teaching, with the appropriate focus on individualization by pointing out areas needing reteaching.

Women's Health

Actions/Interventions	Rationales

• Teach normal physiologic changes new mother can expect postpartum:
  ○ Lochia flow
    (1) Normal: rubra, 1–3 days; serosa, 3–10 days; alba, 10–14 days.
    (2) Abnormal: bright red blood and clots with firm uterus, foul odor, pain, fever, persistent lochia serosa or pink to red discharge after 2 weeks.
  ○ Breast changes
    (1) Breast-feeding: engorgement, comfort measures, clothing, positions for mother and infant comfort; hygiene.
	Provides information to assist new mothers in postpartum adaptation.

Continued

Actions/Interventions	Rationales
See also Nutrition diagnoses in Chapter 3. (2) Non-breast-feeding: suppression of lactation (medications, clothing such as tight-fitting bra, comfort measures); importance of holding baby while bottle-feeding (do not prop bottle, burp baby often); formulas (different kinds, preparation). ○ Perineum and rectum: episiotomy, hemorrhoids, hygiene, medications, comfort measures. • Demonstrate infant care to new parents: ○ Bathing ○ Feeding ○ Cord care ○ Holding, carrying, and so on ○ Safety ○ Sleep-wake states of infant • Discuss infant care, taking into consideration age and cultural differences of parents: ○ Teenagers: Involve significant others; have mother return-demonstrate infant care; refer to support systems such as Young Parent Services, church groups, and so on. ○ First-time older mothers: Allow verbalization of fears; involve significant others; provide encouragement. • Adjust teaching to take into consideration different cultural caretaking activities such as preventing the evil eye in Latino culture or mother not holding the baby for several days immediately after birth in some far East Indian cultures. • Demonstrate newborn skills to parents. Use different assessment skills to teach parents about their newborn's capabilities: gestational age assessment, physical examination of newborn, Brazelton Neonatal Assessment Scale, and so on. • Encourage parents to hold and talk to newborn. • Discuss different methods of birth control and the advantages and disadvantages of each method:	Assists new parents in adapting to parenting role; allows parents to practice new skills in a nonthreatening environment and seek clarification from an informed source. Helps parents gain confidence when caring for newborn; provides opportunity for nurse to teach and reinforce teaching. Informs new parents of choices in birth control methods and gives them the opportunity to ask questions.

- ○ Chemical: spermicides, pills
- ○ Mechanical: condom, diaphragm, intrauterine device (IUD)
- ○ Behavioral: abstinence, temperature-ovulation-cervical mucus (Billing's method), coitus interruptus
- ○ Sterilization: vasectomy, tubal ligation, hysterectomy

Mental Health

Actions/Interventions	Rationales
• Ask client about previous learning experiences in general and about those related to the current area of concern. For example, has client learned that he or she is a poor learner or does not have the intellectual ability to learn the type of information that is currently required or that the smallest mistake in the activity to be learned could be fatal?	Helps to determine aspects of the client's cognitive appraisal that could impact learning.
• Monitor client's current level of anxiety. If level of anxiety will inhibit learning, assist client with anxiety reduction. Refer to Anxiety, Chapter 8, for detailed interventions.	Severe anxiety and impaired cognitive functioning can decrease the client's ability to attend to the environment in a manner that facilitates learning.
• Determine what client thinks is most important in the current situation.	Client's cognitive appraisal can impact the client's willingness to attend to the information. This is especially true of adult learners.
• Assist client in meeting the lower-level needs on Maslow's hierarchy so that attention can be focused on the area of learning to be addressed. For example, if client is concerned that children are not being cared for while he or she is hospitalized, he or she may not be able to focus on learning. List the needs to be met here.	Promotes attention to learning; reduces anxiety.
• Include client in group learning experiences.	Provides client with opportunity to learn from others and to discuss new coping behaviors in a safe environment.

Gerontic Health

Actions/Interventions	Rationales
• Determine current knowledge base by interviewing patient, and have patient state current knowledge regarding condition.	Provides a stepping stone to pieces of information that may be incorrect or lacking.
• Ensure that adaptive equipment, if needed, is functioning and used.	Enhances communication process.
• Encourage the patient to set the pace of the teaching sessions.[14]	Assists in keeping sessions focused on patient's ability to acquire new information.
• Monitor for fatigue.	Fatigue interferes with concentration, and thus decreases learning.
• Present small pieces of information in each session.	Avoids overwhelming the patient; promotes learning.
• Use examples that can be related to the individual's life and life-style.	Adds realism to information and makes transferring of information easier.
• Determine if there is increased anxiety during teaching sessions, for example, watch body language. If so, use relaxation techniques prior to session.	Anxiety decreases concentration and ability to learn.
• Use audiovisual aids that are appropriate for the individual in regard to print size, color, volume, and tone pitch.	Promotes visual and sensory input according to individual's needs.
• Use repetition with positive feedback for correct responses.	Reinforces learning and allows evaluation of learning.

Home Health

NOTE: During home health care many of the interactions between clients, families, and the nurse are related to health education. Proper assessment of the potential for or actual knowledge deficit is imperative. The nurse should use techniques based on learning theory to design teaching interventions that will be appropriate to the situation at hand. These techniques include, but are not limited to, readiness of participant, repetition of the material using several senses, reinforcement of learner's progress, positive and enthusiastic approach, and reduction in barriers to learning, for example, language, pain, and physical illness.

Actions/Interventions	Rationales
• Teach client and family measures to reduce knowledge deficit by seeking the following information and learning conditions: ○ Information regarding disease process ○ Rationale for treatment interventions ○ Techniques for improving learning situation (motivation; teaching materials that match cognitive level of participants;	Conditions that support learning will decrease deficit; provides client and family with necessary information.

reduction of discomfort through pain control, familiar surroundings, and so on)
- ○ Enhancement of self-care capabilities
- ○ Written materials to supplement oral teaching (written materials are appropriate to cognitive level and to self-care management)
- ○ Addressing client and family questions
- Coordinate the teaching activities of other health care professionals who may be involved. Reinforce the teaching of range of motion by the physical therapist, for example.

Coordination reduces duplication and enhances planning. This provides an opportunity for health care professionals to clarify any conflicting information before sharing it with the client.

- Involve client and family in planning, implementing, and promoting reduction in knowledge deficit through:
- ○ Family conference
- ○ Mutual goal setting
- ○ Communication
- ○ Making family members responsible for specific tasks or information

Involvement improves motivation and improves the outcome.

- Consult with or refer to assistive resources as indicated. (See Appendix B.)

Use of the network of existing community services provides for effective utilization of resources.

FLOW CHART EVALUATION
Flow Chart Expected Outcome 1

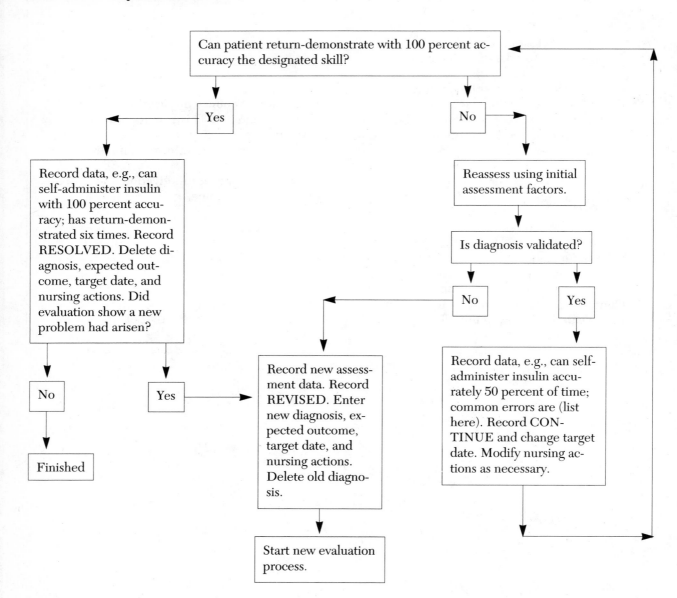

Flow Chart Expected Outcome 2

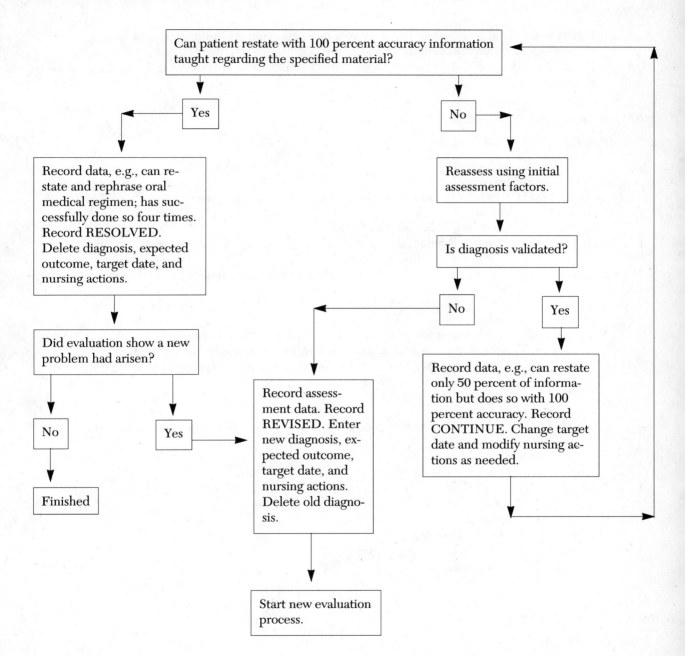

Pain

DEFINITION

Pain is a state in which an individual experiences and reports the presence of severe discomfort or an uncomfortable sensation.

   Chronic Pain is a state in which the individual experiences pain for more than 6 months.[2]

NANDA TAXONOMY: FEELING 9.1.1

DEFINING CHARACTERISTICS[2]

1. Pain:
   a. Subjective:
      (1) Communication (verbal or coded) of pain descriptors
   b. Objective:
      (1) Guarding behavior, protective
      (2) Narrowed focus (altered time perception, withdrawal from social contact, impaired thought process)
      (3) Distraction behavior (moaning, crying, pacing, seeking out other people and/or activities, restlessness)
      (4) Facial mask of pain (eyes lack luster, "beaten look," fixed or scattered movement, grimace)
      (5) Alteration in muscle tone (may span from listless to rigid)
      (6) Autonomic responses not seen in chronic stable pain (diaphoresis, blood pressure and pulse change, pupillary dilation, increased or decreased respiratory rate)
2. Chronic pain:
   a. Major:
      (1) Verbal report or observed evidence of pain experienced for more than 6 months
   b. Minor:
      (1) Fear of reinjury
      (2) Physical and social withdrawal
      (3) Altered ability to continue previous activities
      (4) Anorexia
      (5) Weight changes
      (6) Changes in sleep patterns
      (7) Facial mask
      (8) Guarded movement

RELATED FACTORS

1. Pain:
   a. Injury agents (biological, chemical, physical, psychological)
2. Chronic pain:
   a. Chronic physical and psychosocial disability

RELATED CLINICAL CONCERNS

1. Any surgical diagnosis
2. Any condition labeled chronic; for example, rheumatoid arthritis
3. Any traumatic injury
4. Any infection
5. Anxiety or stress
6. Fatigue

HAVE YOU SELECTED THE CORRECT DIAGNOSIS?

There are no other nursing diagnoses that are easily confused with this diagnosis. Many of the other nursing diagnoses will serve as companion diagnoses and may have pain as a contributing factor to that diagnosis. For example, an individual with chronic pain may be exhausted from trying to deal with the pain and have a companion diagnosis of Fatigue, or may be using alcohol or street drugs to ease the pain and have a companion diagnosis of Ineffective Individual Coping. (See pages 407 and 892.)

EXPECTED OUTCOMES

1. Will verbalize a decreased number of complaints of pain by (date) and/or
2. Will require no more than one medication for pain per 24 hours by (date)

TARGET DATE

For the majority of health disruptions, pain will begin to resolve within 72 hours after the patent has sought health care assistance. Thus, the suggested target date is 3 days after the date of diagnosis.

NURSING ACTIONS/INTERVENTIONS WITH RATIONALES

Adult Health

Actions/Interventions	Rationales
• Monitor for pain at least every 2 hours on the (even/odd) hour. Have patient rank pain on a scale of 0 to 10 at each incidence of pain. Review with patient and document activity engaged in prior to each pain episode. Ask patient to share thoughts and feelings prior to onset of painful episode.	Pain is subjective in nature and only the patient can fully describe it.
• Teach patient to report pain as soon as it starts. Allow patient to talk about pain experience in as much detail as desired.	Initiates a preventive approach before the pain gets too severe.

Continued

Actions/Interventions	Rationales
• Administer pain medication as ordered. Monitor and record amount of pain relief within 30 minutes after administration. Have patient rerank pain (0 to 10). If pain not relieved, collaborate with physician regarding change in medication.	Response to pain and pain medication is unique to each patient.
• Give massage immediately following administration of each pain medication and after each turning.	Assists in muscle relaxation and improves action of pain medication by stimulating peripheral nerve fibers to close the transmission gate.
• Turn at least every 2 hours on (even/odd) hour. Maintain anatomical alignment with pillows or other padded support.	Helps to simulate circulation; alignment helps to prevent pain from malposition; enhances comfort.
• Provide calm, quiet environment. Limit activity for at least 2 hours following pain medication administration.	Promotes action and effect of medication by providing decreased stimuli.
• Monitor vital signs at least every 4 hours while awake at (times).	Detects early changes that might indicate pain.
• Monitor sleep-rest pattern. Promote rest periods during day and at least 8 hours sleep each night. (See nursing actions for Sleep Pattern Disturbance, Chapter 6.)	Fatigue may contribute to an increased pain response or pain can contribute to interrupted sleep.
• Offer 2 to 3 ounces of wine before each meal and at bedtime.	Promotes relaxation and assists in decreasing pain response.
• Promote activity and exercise to extent possible (so long as it does not result in pain). Provide range-of-motion exercises at least every 4 hours while awake at (times).	Promotes natural endorphins and stimulates circulation; prevents complications of immobility secondary to limitation of movement due to pain.
• Apply heat or cold (on 2 hours; off 2 hours). Select heat, cold, dry, moist, according to what patient states provides the best pain relief.	Causes vasoconstriction or vasodilation, either of which, depending on the individual patient's response, will help to decrease swelling, promote healing, and inhibit the transmission of the pain impulse.
• Check bowel elimination at least once per shift.	Immobility caused by pain may decrease the parasympathetic stimulation to the bowel.
• Encourage fluid intake every 2 hours while awake on (even/odd) hour. Encourage up to 3000 ml per day.	Maintains hydration. Patient may limit intake because seeking fluids stimulates pain.
• Provide oral hygiene every 4 hours while awake at (times).	Basic comfort measure.
• Allow time for patient to discuss fears and anxieties related to pain by scheduling at least 15 minutes once per shift to visit with patient on one-to-one basis. Provide accurate information to patient regarding: ○ Pain threshold ○ Pain tolerance ○ Addiction	Just as pain is unique to the individual, so is the pain control intervention. Discussions with the patient provide collaboration and increase patient's compliance, decrease feeling of powerlessness, and initiate basic teaching regarding control of pain.

- ○ Medication effectiveness and ineffectiveness
- ○ Expressing pain
- Apply mentholated or aspirin ointment to affected area every 4 hours while awake at (times) and when needed.

Provides topical relief for pain; dulls peripheral nerve endings that carry pain impulse.

- Use noninvasive pain relief techniques as appropriate:
  - ○ Biofeedback
  - ○ Progressive relaxation
  - ○ Guided imagery
  - ○ Rhythmic breathing
  - ○ Distraction
  - ○ Contralateral stimulation
  - ○ Stress reduction techniques
  - ○ Self-hypnosis

Provides diversion from pain; decreases anxiety and muscle tension; increases comfort and empowers patient.

- Collaborate with physician regarding use of transcutaneous electrical nerve stimulation (TENS).

Collaboration promotes the best approach to pain management.

- Teach patient and significant others:
  - ○ Cause of pain
  - ○ Self-administration of pain medication
  - ○ How to avoid and minimize pain
  - ○ Splinting
  - ○ Gradual increase in activities
  - ○ Use of alternate noninvasive techniques
  - ○ Combining techniques; for example, medication with relaxation technique
  - ○ To alternate various pain relief measures
  - ○ To express anger, frustration, and grief with pain management and change in life-style
  - ○ To be more active in his or her own pain arrangement program: note successes, minimize failure
  - ○ Value of adequate rest and maintaining weight within normal range.

Knowledge assists in the patient in feeling like an active participant on the health team; decreases sense of powerlessness.

- Refer to or collaborate with other health professionals. (See Appendix B.)

Collaboration promotes the best long-range plan for management of pain.

ADDITIONAL INFORMATION Keep current on comparative doses of analgesics, true effect of so-called potentiators, and noninvasive means of pain relief. Do not worry about a patient becoming addicted. With the average length of stay of 3 to 5 days, it is doubtful addiction could occur. Current research in this area shows an extremely low rate of addiction due to medication administration in a health care setting. The same research indicates we undermedicate for pain rather than overmedicate. Undermedication is particularly true in the case of infants, children, and older adults. See the Department of Health and Human Services Guidelines[15] for a discussion of this research as well as further information on pain control.

Child Health

Actions/Interventions	Rationales
• Monitor for contributory factors to pain at least every 8 hours or as required: ○ Physical injury or surgical incision ○ Stressors ○ Fears ○ Knowledge deficit ○ Anxieties ○ Fatigue ○ Description of exact nature of pain, whether per McGill or Elkind tools ○ Vital signs ○ Response to medication ○ Meaning of pain to child and family	Provides the essential database for planning and modification of planning.
• Provide appropriate support in management of pain for the patient and significant others by: ○ Validating the pain. ○ Maintaining self-control to extent feasible. ○ Providing education to deal with applicable specifics. Help patient and family to verbalize the pain experience by allowing at least 30 minutes per shift for such ventilation at (times). ○ Allowing parents to be present and participate in comforting patient. Help child and parents to develop a plan of care that addresses individual needs and is likely to result in a better coping pattern (particularly for chronic pain). ○ Providing appropriate diversional activities for age and developmental level. ○ Paying attention to controlling external stimuli such as noise or light. ○ Using relaxation techniques appropriate for child's capacity. ○ Providing appropriate follow-up of pain tolerance and response to medication as ordered. • Use oral pain medication if possible • If intravenous (IV) route is used, monitor for respiratory and blood pressure depression every 10 minutes for 1 hour following IV administration • Monitor intake and output for decrease due to hypomotility or spasm.	Validation and support of the patient and family will serve to show value and respect for the individual's health need; basic standards of care; ventilation reduces anxiety and parental involvement enhances coping skills.

- Give appropriate emotional support during painful procedures or experiences:
  - Use open and honest explanations at child's level of understanding.
  - Use puppets to demonstrate procedure.
  - Explain to parents that even if child cries excessively, their presence is encouraged.
  - Comfort before, during, and after procedure.
  - Reward the child for positive behavior according to developmental need, for example, with stars on a chart.
  - Discuss and encourage parents and child to share feelings about the painful experience.
- Collaborate with or refer to appropriate health care team members. (See Appendix B.)
- Teach patient and family ways to follow up at home or school with needed pain regimen:
  - Appropriate timing of medication
  - Appropriate administration of medication
  - Need to use aspirin, *not* acetaminophen, for arthritis
- Monitor for stomach alterations or other complications, especially respiratory depression, secondary to administration of pain medication.
- Develop daily plans for pain management to determine those that might be suited for patient on a regular basis.
- Identify need to have several alternate plans to deal with pain.

NOTE: Chronic pain requires long-term follow-up. This follow-up is especially critical since chronic pain places the patient at risk for developmental delays.

Women's Health: Gynecologic Pain

NOTE: A significant amount of the pain experienced by women is associated with the pelvic area and reproductive organs. Determining the origin of the pain is one of the most difficult tasks facing nurses dealing with the gynecologic patient. An organic explanation for pain is never found in approximately 25 percent of women. Because of the close association with the reproductive organs, gynecologic pain can be extremely frightening; it can connote social stigma, affect the perception of the feminine role, cause anger and guilt, and totally dominate the woman's existence. "Pain is culturally more acceptable in certain parts of the body and may elicit more sympathy than pain in other sites."[16]

Actions/Interventions	Rationales
• Identify factors in patient's lifestyle that could be contributing to pain. • Record accurate menstrual cycle and obstetric, gynecologic, and sexual history, being certain to note problems, previous pregnancies, descriptions of previous labors, previous infections or gynecologic problems, and any infections as a result of sexual activities. • Help the client describe her perception of pain as it relates to her. • Include dysmenorrhea pain pattern, being certain to determine if the pain occurs before, during, or after menstruation. • Monitor disturbance of client's daily routine as a result of pain. Have patient describe the location of the pain; for example, lower abdomen, legs, breast, or back. • Have patient describe any edema, especially "bloating," at specific times during the month. • Have the patient describe the onset and character of the pain, for example, mild or severe cramping. • Ascertain whether nausea, vomiting, or diarrhea is associated with the pain. • Identify any precipitating factors associated with pain, for example, emotional upset, exercise, or medication. • Assist patient in identifying various methods of pain relief, including exercise (pelvic rock), biofeedback, relaxation, and medication (analgesics, antiprostaglandins).	Provides the database to adequately assess pain and determine the underlying cause. This information can help to pinpoint source of pain and is useful in devising a plan of care. Individualizes pain control and provides options for patient.

Women's Health: Labor Pain and Nursing

Actions/Interventions	Rationales
• Encourage patient to describe her perception of labor pain, related to her previous labor experiences.[17] • Provide factual information about the labor process. • Refer patient to childbirth preparation group, such as Lamaze.	

- Describe methods of coping with labor pain, for example, relaxation, imaging, breathing, and medication.
- Provide support during labor.
- Encourage involvement of significant others as support during labor process.
- Encourage patient to describe her perception of pain associated with the postpartum period.
- Provide information for pain relief, for example, Kegel exercises, sitz baths, medications.
- Explain etiology of "afterbirth pains" to involution of uterus.
- Explain relationship of breast-feeding to involution and uterine contractions.
- Assist patient in putting on supportive bra.
- Encourage early, frequent breast-feedings to enhance let-down reflex.
- Support patient and provide information on correct breast-feeding techniques, such as changing positions from one feeding to next to distribute sucking pressure and prevent sore nipples.
- Check baby's position on breast; be certain areola, and not just the nipple, is in mouth.
- Provide warm, moist heat for relief of engorged breasts.
- Provide analgesics for discomfort of engorged breasts.
- Pump after infant nurses until breast is relieved. Do not empty breasts, as this will cause more engorgement if infant is not able to empty breasts at each feeding.
- Encourage patient to nurse on least sore side first to encourage let-down reflex.
- Apply ice to nipple just before nursing to decrease pain.

Providing information about the laboring process helps the patient cope with the pain of labor.

Knowing the source of pain increases the patient's sense of control.

Knowledge of how to lessen discomfort during breast-feeding contributes to successful or effective breast-feeding.

Demonstrates to patient various pain relief methods.

Mental Health

Actions/Interventions	Rationales
• Monitor nurse's response to the client's perception of pain. If the nurse has difficulty understanding or coping with the client's expression of pain, this should be	The nurse's response to the client can be communicated and have an effect on the client's level of anxiety; this in turn can then affect the pain response.

Continued

Actions/Interventions	Rationales
discussed with a colleague in an attempt to resolve the nurse's concerns.	
• Note any recurring patterns in the pain experience, such as time of day, recent social interactions, or physical activity. If a pattern is present, begin a discussion of this observation with the client.	Initiates client's awareness of this pattern and allows the nurse to assess the client's perception of this observation.
• Determine effects pain has had on client's life, including role responsibilities, financial impact, cognitive and emotional functioning, and family interactions.	Assesses meaning of pain to the client, amount of anxiety associated with the pain, and possible benefits of pain in the client's life.
• Review client's beliefs and attitudes about the role pain is assuming in client's life. If pain is very important to client's definition of self, assure client that you are not requiring him or her to give up the pain by indicating that you are only interested in that pain that causes undue discomfort or by indicating that you recognize that this client's pain is special and that it would be difficult, if not impossible, for the health care team to get rid of it.	If pain is assuming an important role, it may be difficult for the client to "give up" all of the pain. This should be considered in all further interventions.[8,9]
• Spend brief, goal-directed time with the client when he or she is focusing conversation on pain or pain-related activities.	
• Schedule time with the client when he or she is not complaining about pain. List this schedule here. Focus on special activities in which the client is involved, or follow up on a nonpain-related conversation the client seemed to enjoy.	Provides positive feedback to the client about an aspect of himself or herself that is not pain-related.
• Find at least one nonpain-related activity the client enjoys that can be the source of positive interaction between client and others, and encourage client participation in this activity with positive reinforcement (list client-specific positive reinforcers here along with the activity).	Positive reinforcement encourages a behavior and improves self-esteem.
• Discuss with client alternatives for meeting personal need currently being met by pain. You may need to refer client to another, more specialized care provider if this is a long-standing problem or if client demonstrates difficulty in discussing these concerns. Refer to sections on self-esteem in Chapter 8 for specific interventions.	

- Develop with the client a plan to alter those factors that intensify the pain experience; for example, if the pain increased at 4 p.m. each day and the client associates this with his boss's daily visit at 5 p.m., then the plan might include limiting the visits from the boss or having another person present when the boss visits. List specific interventions here.

  The social milieu can change the basic quality of the pain experience.

- Develop with client a plan for learning relaxation techniques, and have client practice technique for 30 minutes two times a day at (times). Remain with client during practice session to provide verbal cues and encouragement as necessary. These techniques can include:
  - Meditation
  - Progressive deep muscle relaxation
  - Visualization techniques that require the client to visualize scenes that enhance the relaxation response (such as being on the beach or having the sun warm the body, and so on)
  - Biofeedback
  - Prayer
  - Autogenic training

  These techniques decrease anxiety.

- Monitor interaction of analgesic with other medications the client is receiving, especially antianxiety, antipsychotic, and hypnotic drugs.

  These medications may potentiate one another.

- Review client's history for indication of illicit drug use and the effects this may have on client's tolerance to analgesics.

  Client may have developed a cross-tolerance for these drugs.

- If client is to be withdrawn from the analgesic, discuss how alternative coping methods will assist client with the process. Assure client that support will be provided during this process; help client identify those situations that will be most difficult, and schedule one-to-one time with client during these times.

  Promotes perception of control and decreases anxiety.

- If client demonstrates altered mood, refer to Ineffective Individual Coping, Chapter 11, for interventions.

- Consult with occupational therapy unit to assist client in developing diversional activities. Note time for these activities here as well as a list of special equipment that may be necessary for the activity.

  Decreases conscious awareness of pain, thus decreasing the pain experience.

Continued

Actions/Interventions	Rationales
• Involve client in group activities by sitting with him or her during a group activity such as a game, or assign client a responsibility for preparing one part of a unit meal. Begin with activities that require little concentration, and then gradually increase the task complexity.	Alters client's perception of the pain.
• Consult with physician for possible use of hypnosis in pain management.	
• Sit with the client and the family during at least two visits to assess family interactions with the client and the role pain plays in family interaction.	
• Discuss with the client the role of distraction in pain management, and develop a list of those activities the client finds distracting and enjoyable. These could include listening to music, watching TV or special movies, or physical activity. Develop with the client a plan for including these activities in the pain management program, and list that plan here.	Provides other pain relief options for the client.
• Discuss with the client the role that exercise can play in pain management, and develop an exercise program with the client. This should begin at or below the client's capabilities and could include a 15-minute walk twice a day or 10 minutes on a stationary bicycle. Note the plan here with the type of activity, length of time, and time of day it is to be implemented.	Exercise encourages release of natural endorphins.
• Provide positive reinforcement to the client for implementing the exercise program by spending time with the client during the exercise, providing verbal feedback, and allowing client the rewards that have been developed. These rewards are developed with the client.	Positive reinforcement encourages behavior and enhances self-esteem.
• Monitor family's and support system's understanding of the pain and perceptions of the client. If they demonstrate the attitude that the client is closely identified with the pain, then develop a plan to include them in the experiences described above. List that plan here. Consider referral to a clinical specialist in mental health nursing or a family therapist to assist family	Assists family in normalizing and in moving away from a pain-focused identity.

in developing nonpain-related interaction patterns.
- Provide ongoing feedback to client or support system progress.
- Refer to outpatient support systems, and assist with making arrangements for the client to contact these before discharge. (See Appendix B.)

Long-term support enhances the likelihood of effective home management.

Gerontic Health

Actions/Interventions	Rationales
Acute Pain	
• Medicate every 4 to 6 hours rather than prn for the first 48 to 72 hours, especially postoperatively.[18]	Enhances pain control and thus promotes early mobility, which decreases the potential for postoperative complications.
• Encourage physician to prescribe morphine versus Meperidine if a narcotic analgesic is required.	Meperidine is more likely to cause confusion and psychotic behavior when given to the older adult.[19]
• Investigate patient's beliefs regarding pain. Does patient consider pain a punishment for prior misdeeds? That having to take pain medication signals severe illness or a potential for dying?[20]	May be a barrier to seeking pain relief.
• Encourage patient to report pain, especially if medication order is prn.	Patient may not realize that medication will not be given on a scheduled basis.
• Avoid presenting self in a hurried manner.	Older adults are less likely to report pain if caregiver is rushed.[20]
Chronic Pain	
• Explore with patient how he or she has managed chronic pain in the past.	Assists in determining what measures were of significant or of little help.
• Determine use of distraction in helping patient cope with chronic pain.[18]	Music, humor, and relaxation techniques can provide temporary respite from discomfort.
• Monitor skin status when thermal interventions such as ice or heat packs are used.	Changes in sensation may result in thermal injury if not closely monitored.
• In the presence of chronic pain, depression may also exist. Screen for depression.	Chronic pain is exhausting physically and mentally.

Home Health

Actions/Interventions	Rationales
• Teach client and family measures to promote comfort: ○ Proper positioning ○ Appropriate use of medications, for example, narcotics as ordered if pain is severe, nonnarcotic analgesics, and anti-inflammatories ○ Knowledge regarding source of pain or of disease process ○ Self-management of pain and of care as much as is appropriate ○ Relaxation techniques ○ Therapeutic touch ○ Massage (if not contraindicated) ○ Meaningful activities ○ Distraction ○ Breathing techniques ○ Heat or cold (if not contraindicated) ○ Regular activity and exercise ○ Planning and goal setting ○ Biofeedback ○ Yoga or tai chi ○ Imagery or hypnosis ○ Group or family therapy	Involvement of the client and family promotes comfort, decreases self-reported pain and analgesic use.[15]
• Teach client and family factors that decrease tolerance to pain and methods for decreasing these factors: ○ Lack of knowledge regarding disease process or pain control methods ○ Lack of support from significant others regarding the severity of the pain ○ Fear of addiction or loss of control ○ Fatigue ○ Boredom ○ Improper positioning	Reducing these factors can increase the tolerance to pain.[15]
• Involve client and family in planning, implementing, and promoting reduction in pain: ○ Family conference ○ Mutual goal setting ○ Communication ○ Support for caregiver	Involvement improves motivation and improves outcome.
• Assist client and family in life-style adjustments that may be required, such as: ○ Occupational changes	Life-style changes require changes in behavior.

- ○ Family role alterations
- ○ Comfort measures for chronic pain
- ○ Financial situation
- ○ Responses to pain (mood, concentration, ability to complete activities of daily living)
- ○ Coping with disability or dependency
- ○ Altering need for assistance
- ○ Providing appropriate balance of dependence and independence
- ○ Stress management
- ○ Time management
- ○ Use of special equipment, such as cane
- ○ Regular rather than as-needed schedule of pain medication.

- Teach client and family purposes, side effects, and proper administration techniques of medications.

  Provides necessary information for safe self-care.

- Consult with or refer to appropriate community resources as indicated. (See Appendix B.)

  Existing community services network provides effective use of resources.

FLOW CHART EVALUATION
Flow Chart Expected Outcome 1

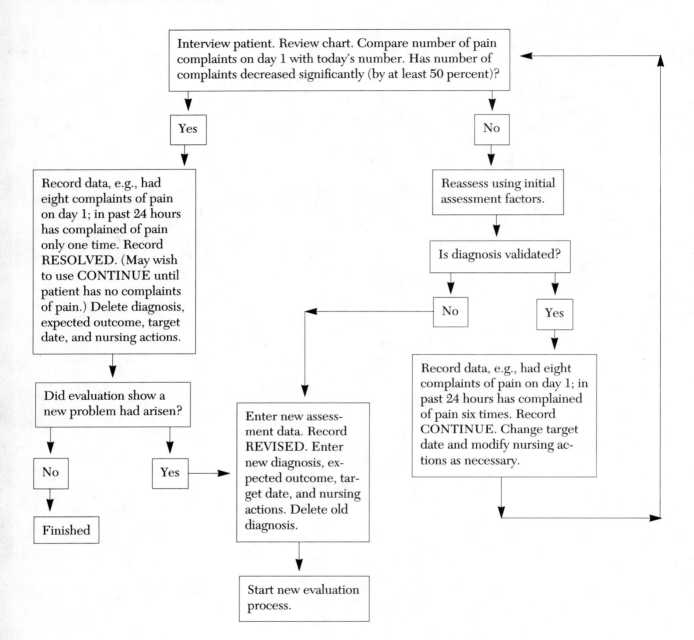

Flow Chart Expected Outcome 2

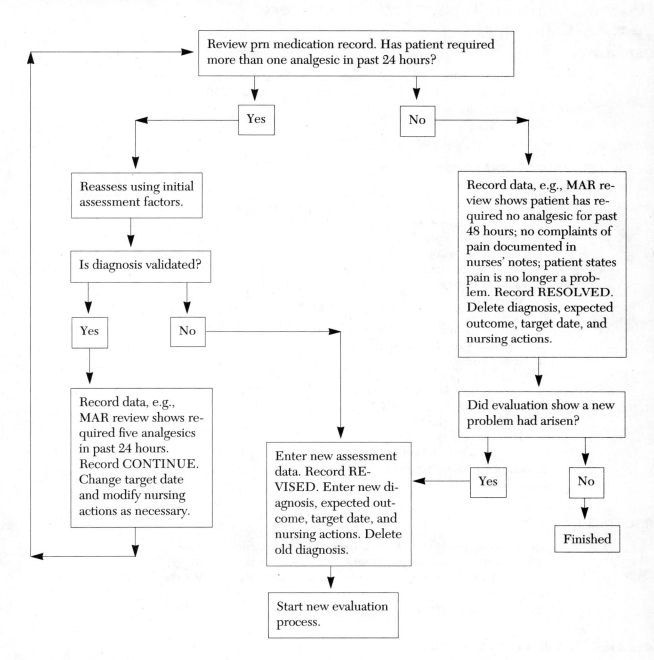

Sensory-Perceptual Alterations (Specify) (Visual, Auditory, Kinesthetic, Gustatory, Tactile, Olfactory)

DEFINITION

A state in which an individual experiences a change in the amount or patterning of oncoming stimuli accompanied by a diminished, exaggerated, distorted, or impaired response to such stimuli.[2]

NANDA TAXONOMY: PERCEIVING 7.2

DEFINING CHARACTERISTICS[2]

1. Major defining characteristics:
   a. Disoriented in time, in place, or with persons
   b. Altered abstraction
   c. Altered conceptualization
   d. Change in problem-solving abilities
   e. Reported or measured change in sensory acuity
   f. Change in behavior pattern
   g. Anxiety
   h. Apathy
   i. Change in usual response to stimuli
   j. Indication of body-image alteration
   k. Restlessness
   l. Irritability
   m. Altered communication patterns
2. Other possible characteristics:
   a. Complaints of fatigue
   b. Alterations in posture
   c. Change in muscular tension
   d. Inappropriate responses
   e. Hallucination

RELATED FACTORS[2]

1. Altered environmental stimuli, excessive or insufficient stimuli
2. Altered sensory reception, transmission, and/or integration
3. Chemical alterations, either endogenous (electrolyte) or exogenous (drugs, and so on)
4. Psychological stress

RELATED CLINICAL CONCERNS

1. Any neurological diagnosis
2. Glaucoma or cataracts
3. Any patient in an intensive care unit
4. Psychosis
5. Substance abuse
6. Toxemia

HAVE YOU SELECTED THE CORRECT DIAGNOSIS?

Impaired Thought Process Impaired Thought Process refers to a patient's cognitive abilities, while Sensory-Perceptual Alterations relate only to sensory input and output. (See page 577.)

Self-Care Deficit Self-Care Deficit deals primarily with ability to care for the self. Sensory-Perceptual Alterations can result in self-care deficits but the focus is on response to sensory input. (See page 472.)

EXPECTED OUTCOME

1. Will identify and initiate at least two adaptive ways to compensate for (specific sensory deficit) by (date) and/or
2. Will verbalize fewer problems with (specific sensory deficit) by (date)

TARGET DATE

Helping the patient to deal with an uncompensated sensory deficit is a long-term process. Also, the patient may never accept the deficit but can be helped to adapt to the deficit. Therefore an appropriate target date would be no sooner than 5 to 7 days from the date of diagnosis.

NURSING ACTIONS/INTERVENTIONS WITH RATIONALES

Adult Health

Actions/Interventions	Rationales
• Provide patient with appropriate prosthesis if the deficit has been previously diagnosed and a prosthesis provided.	Provides immediate assistance with sensory deficit to decrease deficit.
• Maintain prosthesis to ensure optimal functioning.	Prostheses that do not fit or function well tend not to be used.
• Provide calm, nonthreatening environment.	Reinforces reality.
• Orient to room.	
• Check safety factors frequently: ○ Siderails ○ Uncluttered room ○ Lighting: dim at night, increased during day, nonglare ○ Arrange environment to compensate for specific deficit	Basic safety measures.
• Place bedside table, over-the-bed table in same position each time and within easy reach. Ascertain which items patient wants on these tables and where the items are to be placed. Place items in same place each time.	Maintains consistency of environment, which facilitates patient's comfort and decreases anxiety.

Continued

Actions/Interventions	Rationales
• Have significant others bring familiar items from home.	Enhances physical and psychological comfort.
• Promote consistency in care; for example, same nurse and same routine if possible.	Decreases unessential stimuli; inspires trust; reinforces patient's own routine.
• Follow patient's own routine as much as possible; for example, bath, bedtime, meals, grooming. Pace activities to patient's preference.	Promotes comfort; empowers patient.
• Provide reality orientation as necessary: ○ Keep clock and calendar in room ○ Touch patient frequently ○ Check orientation to person, time, and place at least once per shift ○ Listen carefully	Reinforces reality.
• At least once per shift monitor: ○ Intake and output ○ Vital signs ○ Circulatory status ○ Neurologic status ○ Sleep-rest amounts ○ Mental status	Basic monitoring for signs and symptoms of sensory overload or sensory deficit.
• Encourage activity and exercise to extent possible and intersperse with rest periods. Do range of motion at least every 4 hours while awake at (times).	Provides stimulation; avoids complication of immobility.
• Collaborate with occupational therapist regarding appropriate diversionary activity.	Provides stimuli.
• Provide for appropriate follow-up appointments before dismissal.	Providing specific appointments lessens the confusion about the specifics of appointments and increases the likelihood of subsequent follow-through.

Auditory Deficits

• Clean ear with wet washcloth over finger.	Assists in removal of ear wax without damaging inner ear structure.
• If eardrops are ordered, warm to body temperature before applying.	Warm eardrops assist in removal of ear wax and are less likely to cause vertigo problems; increases comfort.
• Speak in low tones when interacting with patient.	Allows for alteration in hearing high-frequency tones, which are lost first.
• Allow patient extended time to respond to verbal messages.	Allows for understanding and interpretation of message.
• Decrease background noise as much as possible when talking with the patient.	Avoids confusion and increases the patient's ability to localize sounds.
• Do not shout when talking with client.	Shouting only accentuates vowel sounds while decreasing consonant sounds.
• Use visual cues as much as possible to enhance verbal messages.	Improves communication.

- Provide message board to use with patient.
- Replace batteries in hearing aids as necessary.

A common problem in hearing deficits.

- Clean ear wax from hearing aid as necessary.

Improves functioning of hearing aid.

- Stand where the patient can watch your lips when you are speaking.
- Make lips visible to the patient by clipping mustache away from lips (males) or wearing lipstick that highlights lips (females).

Provides added cues to what is being said.

- Teach patient and family proper care of ears, for example, using earplugs when in an environment with loud noises, protecting the ears from water while swimming, blowing the nose with both nostrils open.

Protects the eardrum from trauma.

- Teach patient to turn better ear toward speaker. Note here patient's better ear so staff can stand on that side when speaking to patient.

Improves communication.

- Teach patient and family proper maintenance of hearing aid.

Promotes proper functioning of hearing aid.

Visual Deficits

- Provide patient with his or her eyeglasses or contact lenses during waking hours. Note here where they are to be kept when patient is not using them, and place them in that place when patient removes them.

Facilitates patient's use of equipment and assists in avoiding damage to or loss of equipment.

- Provide written information in large print or use audio format.
- Provide telephone dials and other such equipment with large numbers on nonglare surfaces. List here special equipment for this patient and times when the patient may need it.
- Identify patient's room with large numbers or patient's name in large print.
- Provide large-screen TV and pictures with large, colorful images.

Larger images are easier for patient to interpret.

- Place patient in social or group situations so that he or she is not looking directly into an open window.

Glare from window will decrease visual acuity.

- Provide nonglare work surfaces.
- Identify stairs and door frames with contrasting tape or paint.

Increases visual acuity; basic safety measure.

- Verbally address patient as you approach, and approach patient from the front.

Makes patient aware of presence.

- Do not alter the patient's physical environment without telling him or her of the changes.

Promotes consistency in environment and improves safety.

Continued

Actions/Interventions	Rationales
• Address patient by name.	Clearly identifies who you are talking to.
• Ask patient about special environmental adaptations he or she prefers or uses (list those here).	Promotes familiarity of environment while in hospital.
• Provide patient with talking books and large-print periodicals.	Provides diversionary activity.
• Enter patient's environment every hour on the (hour/half hour).	Frequent contact provides assurance that the patient is a matter of concern to the nursing staff.
• Teach patient and family proper maintenance of eyeglasses and other prostheses.	Assures proper functioning; prevents scratching of lenses.
• Teach patient and family methods to improve environmental safety.	
• Assist patient with activities of daily living as necessary. List the activities that require assistance here along with the type of assistance that is needed, for example, assisting patient to eat to extent necessary (feed totally or cut up food and open packages).	Allows patient to be as independent as possible.

Touch and Kinesthesia Deficit

• Remove sharp objects from the patient's environment.	Basic safety measure.
• Protect patient from exposure to excessive heat and cold by:	Basic safety measures to prevent burns.
○ Checking temperature of heat and cold packs carefully before application	
○ Teaching patient to check the temperature of bath and other water with a thermometer	
○ Checking temperature of bath water for patient while he or she is on the nursing unit	
○ Teaching patient to wear protective clothing whenever he or she goes outdoors in the winter	
○ Teaching patient not to use heating pads or hot-water bottles	
• Have patient and family lower the setting on the hot-water heater in the home to 124°F.	
• Instruct patient not to smoke unless someone is with him or her.	
• Have patient change position every 2 hours on the (odd/even) hour.	Promotes circulation; relieves pressure on bony prominences.

- Monitor condition of skin every 4 hours at (times). Note any alteration in integrity. Teach patient to visually inspect skin on a daily basis.

  Guards against skin breakdown.

- Have patient wear well-fitting shoes when walking.

  Prevents blisters and infection.

- Trim toenails and fingernails for patient. Maintain these at a safe length.
- Assist patient in determining if clothing is fitting properly without abrading the skin.
- Perform foot care on a daily basis, including:
  - Bathing feet in warm water
  - Applying moisturizing lotion
  - Trimming nails as needed
  - Checking skin for abrasions or reddened areas
- Note time for foot care here. This process should be taught to the patient and the patient should be assuming primary responsibility for this care before discharge. This should be done with nursing supervision.
- Provide patient with assistance with movement in the environment until he or she is able to make the necessary adaptations to alterations in sensations.
- Consult with physical therapist regarding teaching patient appropriate adaptations for safe and effective movement.

  Demonstrates and promotes self care of extremities for patient.

- Assist patient with care of affected body parts.

  Prevents unilateral neglect; provides cues for patient.

- Assist patient with activities of daily living (ADL). (Note type and amount of assistance needed here.)

  Promotes self-care through demonstrating care to patient.

- Refer to occupational therapy for assisting with learning new self-care behavior.

Smell Deficit

- Assess for extent of neurologic dysfunction on admission.

  Determines what intervention can be planned.

- Determine effect the smell deficit has on patient's appetite, and work with dietitian to make meals visually appealing.

  Assists to compensate for loss of smell.

Child Health

Actions/Interventions	Rationales
• Determine how the parent and child perceive the deficit addressed by setting aside adequate time (30 minutes) each shift for discussion and listening.	Appropriate attention to both subjective and objective data is required to best plan care.
• Stress the importance of follow-up evaluation for any suspected sensory deficits of infants and young children. • Allow for extra safety precautions according to sensory deficit and child's developmental capacity.	Preventing or minimizing secondary and tertiary deficits is enhanced by appropriate attention to sensory-perceptual follow-up. Sensory deficits and developmental capacity increase the risk of accidents.
• Initiate plans for discharge at least 4 days in advance to allow time for confidence in performance of necessary tasks according to deficit.	Adequate practice time in a nonjudgmental situation allows positive feedback and corrective action, lessens anxiety and performance pressures, and increases confidence in giving care at home.

• Provide attention to family coping as it may relate to the deficit:
  ○ Assessment of usual dynamics
  ○ Identification of impact on parents and siblings
  ○ Presence of mental deficits
  ○ Values regarding the deficit
  ○ Support systems
	A child with sensory-perceptual problems and the interventions necessary to deal with this problem place strain on the family; promoting coping will lessen strain for the family while increasing the likelihood that the child's needs will be met.

• Review for appropriate immunization, especially rubella, mumps, and measles.	In the event of early deficits, the likelihood exists for the need to modify the schedule of immunization. This is too often overlooked and will then place the infant or child at unnecessary risk for infectious diseases.
• In presence of ear infections, exercise caution regarding use of ototoxic medications such as gentamicin. • Correlate medical history for potential risk factors such as chronic middle ear infections, upper respiratory infections, or allergies.	Chronic infections, treated with antibiotics by several practitioners, must be carried out with attention to potential side effects. Contributory factors to the pattern of health must be pursued with openness to all possible causes.
• Provide appropriate sensory stimulation for age, beginning slowly so as not to overload child.	Appropriate sensory stimulation will favor gradual progress in development.
• Deal with other contributory factors such as nutrition, illness, and so on.	Related factors must be considered in total health of infant or child with altered sensory-perceptual pattern.

• Include parents in plans for rehabilitation whenever possible by:
  ○ Using basic plan for care
  ○ Adapting intervention as required for child
  ○ Supporting them in their role
	Inclusion of parents provides an opportunity for learning essential skills and enhances security of the infant or child. All efforts contribute to empowerment and potential growth of the family unit.

- ○ Pointing out opportune times for interaction
- ○ Informing them of appropriate safety precautions for age and situation
- ○ Encouraging gentle handling and comforting of infant
- Provide continuity in staffing for nursing care of child and family.
- Introduce new skills sequentially to best actualize potential.

- Especially note, on follow-up, the home environment for nurturing aspects and support systems.

Continuity provides trust and opportunities for reinforcement of learning.
Appropriate introduction of new skills or reinforcement of existing patterns will favor progress.
The home to which the child will go may require reasonable adaptation to foster appropriate resources.

Women's Health

Actions/Interventions	Rationales
Vision	
• Monitor patient for signs of pregnancy-induced hypertension (PIH).	Knowledge of signs of visual disturbances associated with **PIH** can assist the patient in seeking early treatment.
• Monitor for precursor signs and symptoms of eclampsia, for example, headaches, visual changes such as blurred vision, increased edema of face, oliguria, hyperreflexia, nausea or vomiting, and epigastric pain.	
• Teach patient the importance of reporting the above signs and symptoms.	
Smell	
• Be aware of patient's tendency to morning sickness, that is, nausea and vomiting in early pregnancy	
• In collaboration with dietitian: ○ Obtain dietary history ○ Assist patient in planning diet that will provide adequate nutrition for her and the fetus	
• Teach methods for coping with gastric upset, nausea, and vomiting: ○ Eating bland, low-fat foods ○ Increasing carbohydrate intake ○ Eating small, frequent meals ○ Having dry crackers or toast before getting out of bed	Knowledge can help patient to plan actions that decrease incidences of nausea and vomiting and assist in preventing dehydration and possibly hospitalization.

Continued

Actions/Interventions	Rationales
○ Taking vitamins and iron with snack before going to bed ○ Supplementing diet with high-protein liquids, such as soups and eggnog	
Touch during Pregnancy	
• Be aware of expectant mother's sensitivity to extraneous touching: ○ Shyness ○ Protectiveness of unborn child ○ Uterine sensitivity during pregnancy and particularly during labor	Lets pregnant woman know her feelings are normal.
Maternal Touch	
• Encourage visual and tactile contact between mother and infant as soon as possible. • Provide conducive atmosphere for continual mother-infant contact. • Delay newborn eye treatment for 1 hour so that baby can see mother's face.	Provides time for beginning attachment process between mother and infant.
Kinesthesia	
• Be aware of expectant mother's increased physical vulnerability during the third trimester. This is exhibited by: ○ Protectiveness of unborn child ○ Heavy movement ○ Slowed reflexes ○ Fatigue • Assist in and out of difficult furniture that is too low. • Encourage correct body mechanics when lying down or sitting up. • Encourage expectant mother to wear seat belt when traveling in auto (shoulder belt is best).	Reassures mothers that this is a temporary state. Provides for safety measures for mother and fetus.

Mental Health

Actions/Interventions	Rationales
• Monitor client's neurologic status as indicated by current condition and history of deficit; for example, if deficit is recent, assessment would be conducted on a	Client safety is of primary importance. Early recognition and intervention can prevent serious alterations.

schedule that could range from every 15
minutes to every 8 hours. Note frequency
and times of checks here. If checks are to
be very frequent, then keep a record.

- If deficit is determined to result from a
psychologic rather than a physiologic
dysfunction, refer to Ineffective Individual
Coping, Body Image Disturbance, Anxiety,
and Self-Esteem Disturbance for detailed
nursing actions.

Client safety is of primary importance.

NOTE: A comprehensive physical examination and other diagnostic evaluations should be completed before this determination is made. Each of these deficits can be symptoms of severe physiologic or neurologic dysfunction and should be approached with this understanding, especially in a mental health environment where the clients may be assigned without careful assessment. This is a great risk for the client who has a history of mental health problems.

- If deficit is related to a physiologic
dysfunction, attend to needs resulting from
the identified sensory deficit in a matter-of-
fact manner, providing basic care and
having client do the majority of the care.

Provides positive reinforcement for adaptive coping behaviors.

- If deficit is related to a psychologic
dysfunction, spend 15 minutes every hour
with the client in an activity that is not
related to the sensory deficit. If the client
begins to focus on the deficit, terminate the
interaction.

Promotes client's sense of control and increases self-esteem.

- Spend 1 hour twice a day discussing with
the client the effects the deficit will have on
his or her life and developing alternative
coping behavior. Note times for
conversations here. If family is involved in
the client's care, they should be included in
a planned number of these interactions.
- Refer to appropriate mental health
professional if client is going to require
long-term assistance in adapting to the
deficit or if current emotional adaptation
becomes complicated.
- Discuss with client and support system the
alterations that may be necessary in the
home environment to facilitate daily living
activities.

Promotes client's sense of control.

Auditory and Visual Alterations[21–24]

- Observe for signs of hallucinations (intent
listening for no apparent reason, talking to
someone when no one is present, muttering
to self, stopping in mid-sentence, unusual

Interrupts patterns of hallucinations.

Continued

Actions/Interventions	Rationales
posturing). When these symptoms are noted, engage client in here-and-now reality-oriented conversation or involve client in here-and-now activity.	
• Initiate touch only after warning client that you are going to touch him or her.	Client may perceive touch as a threat and respond in an aggressive manner.
• Communicate acceptance to the client to encourage the sharing of the content of the hallucination.	Provides information on the content of the hallucination so that early intervention can be initiated when content suggests harm to client or others.
• If hallucinations place client at risk for self-harm or harm to others, place client on one-on-one observation or in seclusion.	Client and staff safety are of primary importance.
• If client is placed in seclusion, interact with client at least every 15 minutes.	Provides reality orientation and assists client in controlling the hallucinations.
• Have client tell staff when hallucinations are present or when they are interfering with client's ability to interact with others.	Early intervention promotes client's sense of safety and control.
• Maintain environment in a manner that does not enhance hallucinations, for example, television programs that validate client's hallucinations, abstract art on the walls, wallpaper with abstract designs or designs that enhance imagination.	High levels of environmental stimuli can increase the client's disorganization and confusion.
• Teach client to control hallucinations by: ○ Checking ideas out with trusted others. ○ Practicing thought-stopping by singing to self, telling the voices to go away. (This can be done quietly to self, or by asking the voices to come back later but not to talk now.)	Promotes client's sense of control and enhances self-esteem.
• Talk with client about ways to distract himself or herself from the hallucinations, such as physical exercise, playing a game, or using a craft that takes a great deal of concentration. (Note those activities preferred by client here.)	
• When signs of hallucinating are present, assist client in initiating control behaviors.	Reinforces new coping behaviors and increases client's perceived control.
• As client's condition improves, primary nurse will assist client to identify onset of hallucinations and situations that facilitate their onset.	Facilitates the development of alternative coping behaviors.
• As difficult situations are identified, primary nurse can begin working with client on alternative ways of coping with these situations. (Note alternative coping behaviors selected by client here.)	Promotes client's sense of control and self-esteem.

- Refer client and support system to
  appropriate support systems in the
  community, for example, Compeer.
  (Contact local Mental Health Association
  for the program in your community. See
  also Appendix B.)

Gerontic Health

See Adult Health.

Home Health

Actions/Interventions	Rationales

• Teach client and family measures to prevent sensory deficit:
  ○ Use of protective gear, for example, goggles, sunglasses, earplugs, special clothing in hazardous conditions to prevent radiation, sun, or chemical burns
  ○ Avoidance of sharp or projectile toys
  ○ Prevention of injuries to eyes, ears, skin, nose, and tongue
  ○ Prevention of nutritional deficiencies
  ○ Close monitoring of medications that may be toxic to the eighth cranial nerve
  ○ Correct usage of contact lenses
  ○ Prevention of fluid and electrolyte imbalances.
	Family and client involvement in basic safety measures enhances the effectiveness of preventive measures.

• Involve client and family in planning, implementing, and promoting correction or compensation for sensory deficit (specify) by (date):
  ○ Family conference
  ○ Mutual goal setting
  ○ Communication, for example, use of memorabilia and audio- or videotapes provided by family members to stimulate in cases of impaired communication.[25]
	Involvement improves motivation. Communication and mutual goals increase the probability of positive outcomes.

• Assist patient and family in life-style adjustments that may be required:
  ○ Assistance with activities of daily living
  ○ Adjustment to and usage of assistive devices, for example, hearing aid, corrective lenses, magnifying glass
	Life-style changes require change in behavior; self-evaluation and support facilitate these changes.

Continued

Actions/Interventions	Rationales
○ Providing safe environment, for example, protect kinesthetically impaired from burns ○ Stopping substance abuse ○ Changes in family and work role relationships ○ Techniques of communicating with individual with auditory or visual impairment ○ Providing meaningful stimulation ○ Special transportation needs ○ Special education needs • Consult with or refer to appropriate community resources as indicated. (See Appendix B.)	The network of existing community services provides for effective use of resources.

FLOW CHART EVALUATION
Flow Chart Expected Outcome 1

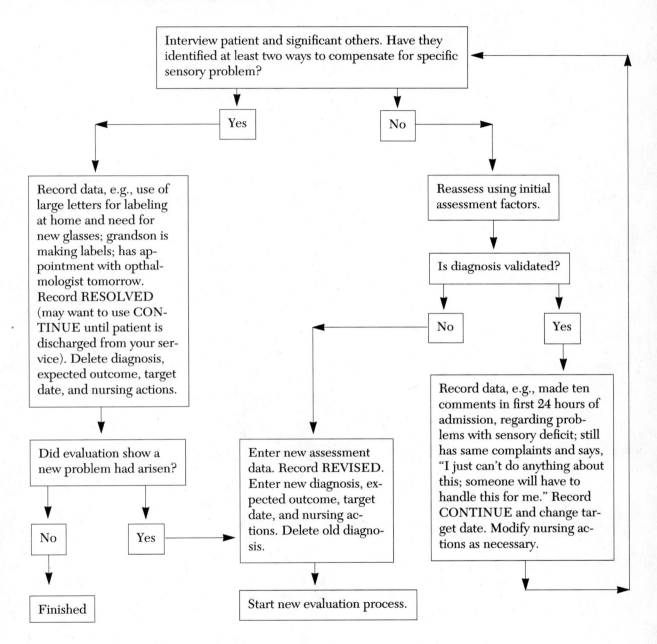

Flow Chart Expected Outcome 2

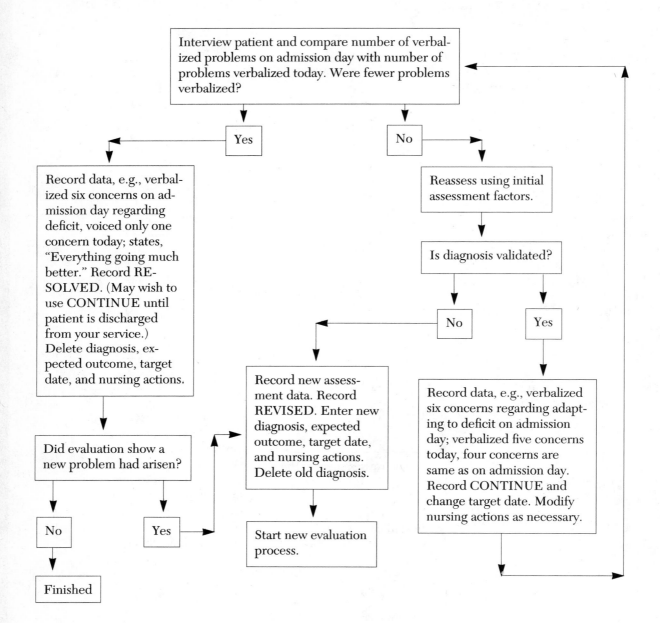

THOUGHT PROCESS, ALTERED

DEFINITION

A state in which an individual experiences a disruption in cognitive operations and activities.[2]

NANDA TAXONOMY: KNOWING 8.3

DEFINING CHARACTERISTICS[2]

1. Major defining characteristics:
   a. Inaccurate interpretation of environment
   b. Cognitive dissonance
   c. Distractibility
   d. Sensory deficit problems
   e. Egocentricity
   f. Hypervigilance or hypovigilance
2. Other possible characteristics:
   a. Inappropriate nonreality-based thinking

RELATED FACTORS[2]

To be developed.

RELATED CLINICAL CONCERNS

1. Dementia
2. Neurologic diseases impacting the brain
3. Head injuries
4. Medication overdose: digitalis, sedatives, narcotics, and so on
5. Major depression
6. Bipolar disorder: manic, depressive, or mixed
7. Schizophrenic disorders
8. Dissociative disorders
9. Obsessive-compulsive disorders
10. Paranoid disorder
11. Delirium
12. Eating disorders

HAVE YOU SELECTED THE CORRECT DIAGNOSIS?

Sensory-Perceptual Alterations This diagnosis refers to deficits or overloads in sensory inputs. If the patient is having difficulty with sight, hearing, or any of the other senses, then a confused patient might well be the result. Double-check the pattern assessment to be sure sensory deficit is not the primary problem. (See page 562.)

Altered Health Maintenance The diagnosis of Altered Thought Process might well contribute to Altered Health Maintenance. In this case, Altered Thought Process and Altered Health Maintenance would be companion diagnoses. (See page 38.)

EXPECTED OUTCOME

1. Will have at least a (number) percent decrease in signs and symptoms of Altered Thought Process by (date) and/or
2. Will be oriented to time, person, and place by (date)

TARGET DATE

A target date of 5 days would be acceptable since this can be a very long-range problem.

NURSING ACTIONS/INTERVENTIONS WITH RATIONALES

Adult Health

Actions/Interventions	Rationales
• Monitor, at least every 4 hours while awake: ○ Vital signs ○ Neurologic status, particularly for signs and symptoms of Increased Intra Cranial Pressure (IICP) ○ Mental status ○ Laboratory values for metabolic alkalosis, hypokalemia, increased ammonia levels, and infection	Assists in determining pathophysiologic causes for altered thought process.
• Collaborate with psychiatric nurse clinician and rehabilitation nurse specialist.	Collaboration provides the best plan of care.
• Consistently provide a safe, calm environment: ○ Provide siderails on bed. ○ Keep room uncluttered. ○ Reorient client at each contact. ○ Reduce extraneous stimuli; for example, limit noise and visitors, reduce bright lighting. ○ Use touch judiciously. Prepare for all procedures by explaining simply and concisely. ○ Provide good, but not intensely bright, lighting. ○ Have family bring clock, calendar, and familiar objects from home.	Basic safety measures; reinforcement of reality.
• Design communications according to patient's best means of communication, for example, writing, visual, sound: ○ Give simple, concise directions. ○ Listen carefully. ○ Present reality consistently. ○ Do not challenge illogical thinking.	Enhances communication and quality of care.

Actions/Interventions	Rationales
• Encourage patient to use prosthetic or assistive devices: glasses, dentures, hearing aid, walker, and so on.	Increases sensory input; reinforces reality.
• Provide frequent rest periods.	Reduces environmental stimuli that could contribute to confusion; helps to avoid sensory overload.
• Provide consistent approach in care: same nurse, same routine.	Inspires trust, reinforces reality, decreases sensory stimuli, and provides memory cues.
• Encourage self-care to the extent possible.	Increases self-esteem, forces reality check, decreases powerlessness, and provides a means of evaluating patient's status.
• Involve significant others in care, and include in teaching sessions.	Provides social support and consistency in management.
• Refer to and collaborate with appropriate community resources. (See Appendix B.)	Provides for long-term support and a more holistic approach to care.

Child Health

Actions/Interventions	Rationales
• Monitor cognitive capacity according to age and developmental capacity.	Basic data needed to plan individualized care.
• Note discrepancies in chronologic age and mastery of developmental milestones.	
• Provide ongoing reality orientation by encouraging family to visit and assessing child's awareness of time, person, and place.	As the patient attempts to reorient, it is helpful to monitor basic orientation as a means for planning gradual increase of activities.
• Anticipate safety issues to reflect greater range of potentials according to psychomotor capacity.	Altered thought process is a high-risk factor for all involved.
• Encourage family members to express concerns about child's condition by allowing 30 minutes each shift for this.	Promotes ventilation, which helps reduce anxiety and offers insight into thoughts about patient's condition.
• Provide for primary health needs, including administration of medications, comfort measures, and control of environment to aid in child's adaptation.	Attention to regular health needs of the whole person must also be considered.
• Structure the room in a manner which suits the child's needs.	Keeping the environment adapted to personal needs will facilitate care, minimize the chance for accidents, and demonstrate the need for structure.
• Allow for ample rest periods according to sleep patterns when healthy and within parameters for age-related sleep needs.	Rest is a key consideration in providing optimal potential for cognitive and perceptual functioning.
• Monitor for existence of other patterns, especially altered coping and role performance.	All contributing factors must be explored to ensure meeting the patient's needs.

Continued

Actions/Interventions	Rationales
• Assist family in discharge plans by referral to appropriate state and community resources.	Improves family adjustment and coping by assisting in preparing for home needs. Empowerment will, hopefully, permit them to develop coping and parenting skills.
• If institutionalization is required, assist family with related issues such as visitation, medical records maintenance, prognosis, and risk factors.	Planning increases the likelihood for coping and adjusting to the move and provides opportunity for clarification. Provides advocacy for patient and family.
• Maintain confidentiality.	Standard practice must include safeguarding patient confidentiality for both ethical and legal reasons.
• Allow for culturally unique aspects in management of care, for example, respect for visitation on religious holidays, family wishes for diet, bathing.	Increases individuation and satisfaction with care; shows respect for family's values; enhances nurse-patient relationship.
• Provide for appropriate follow-up by making appointments for next clinic visits.	Increases likelihood of follow-up and demonstrates the importance of this care.
• Allow family members opportunities for learning necessary care and mastery of content for long-term needs such as resolution of conflicts related to institutionalization or respite care and prognosis.	Anticipatory learning serves to minimize crises related to the child's condition.

Women's Health

See Adult Health.

Mental Health

Actions/Interventions	Rationales
• Monitor client's level of anxiety and refer to Anxiety, Chapter 8, for detailed interventions related to this diagnosis.	Too much information can increase the client's confusion and disorganization. Time of interaction should be guided by the client's attention span.[26]
• Speak to client in brief, clear sentences.	
• Keep initial interactions short but frequent. Interact with client for (number) minutes every 30 minutes. Begin with 5-minute interactions, and gradually increase the length of interactions.	Facilitates the development of a trusting relationship.
• Assign a primary care nurse to the client on each shift to assume responsibility for gaining a relationship of trust with the client.	Facilitates the development of a trusting relationship.

- Be consistent in all interactions with the client.

Facilitates the development of a trusting relationship, and meets the client's safety needs.

- Set limits on inappropriate behavior that may cause harm to the client or others. Note the limits here, as well as any revisions.

Client and staff safety are of primary importance.

- Initially, place client in an area with little stimulation.

Inappropriate levels of sensory stimuli can contribute to client's sense of disorganization and confusion.

- Orient client to the environment, and assign someone to provide one-on-one interaction while client orients to unit.

Promotes client's safety needs while facilitating the development of a trusting relationship.

- Do not make promises that cannot be kept.

Facilitates the development of a trusting relationship.

- Inform client of your availability to talk with him or her; do not pry or ask many questions.

Communicates acceptance of the client and facilitates the development of trust and self-esteem.

- Do not argue with client about delusions. Inform client in a matter-of-fact way that this is not your experience of the situation; for example; "I do not think I am angry with you."

Prevents reinforcement of client's delusional system and promotes the development of a trusting relationship.

- Recognize and support client's feelings; for example, "You sound frightened."

Focuses on client's real feelings and concerns.

- Respond to the feelings being expressed in delusions or hallucinations.

- Initially, have client involved in one-to-one activities; as conditions improve, gradually increase the size of the interaction group. Note current level of functioning here.

High levels of environmental stimuli may increase confusion and disorganization.

- Have client clarify those thoughts you do not understand. Do not pretend to understand that which you do not.

Facilitates the development of a trusting relationship and prevents inadvertent support of delusional thinking.

- Do not attempt to change delusional thinking with rational explanations.

This may encourage client to cling to these thoughts.

- After listening to a delusion once, do not engage in conversations related to this material or focus conversations on this material.

Decreases the possibility of supporting or reinforcing the delusion.

- Focus conversations on here-and-now content related to real things in the environment or to activities on the unit.

Facilitates the client's contact with reality.[22]

- Do not belittle or be judgmental about the client's delusional beliefs.

Protects the client's self-esteem.

- Avoid nonverbal behavior that indicates agreeing with delusional beliefs.

Decreases the possibility of supporting or reinforcing the delusion.

- When client's behavior and anxiety level indicate readiness, place client in small-group situations. Client will spend (number)

Provides feedback about delusional beliefs from peers.

Continued

Actions/Interventions	Rationales
minutes in group activities (number) times a day. (Time and frequency will increase as client's ability to cope with these situations improves.)	
• Develop a daily schedule for the client that encourages focus on the here and now and is adapted to client's level of functioning so that success can be experienced. Note daily schedule here.	Facilitates client's contact with reality. Promotes positive self-image.
• Assign client meaningful roles in unit activities. Provide roles that can be easily accomplished by client to provide successful experiences. Note client responsibilities here.	Facilitates client's contact with reality. Promotes positive self-image.
• Primary nurse will spend (amount) minutes with client twice a day to discuss client's feelings and the effects of the delusions on the client's life. (Number of minutes and the degree of exploration of client's feelings will increase as client develops relationship with nurse.)	Assists in the development of alternative coping behaviors.
• Provide rewards to client for accomplishing task progress on the daily schedule. These rewards should be ones the client finds rewarding.	Positive feedback encourages behavior.
• Spend (number) minutes twice a day walking with client. This should start at 10-minute intervals and gradually increase. This can be replaced by any other physical activity the client finds enjoyable. A staff member should be with the client during this activity to provide social reinforcement to the client for accomplishing the activity.	Facilitates the development of a trusting relationship. Social interaction provides positive reinforcement and helps to increase daytime wakefulness, promoting a normal sleep-wake cycle.
• Arrange a consultation with the occupational therapist to assist client in developing or continuing special interests.	Increases daytime wakefulness, maintaining a normal sleep-rest cycle.
• Monitor delusional beliefs for potential harm to self or others. Note any change in behavior that would indicate a change in the delusional beliefs with a potential for violence.	Patient and staff safety are of primary concern.
• If client is placed in seclusion, interact with client at least every 15 minutes.	Provides reality orientation and assists cilent with controlling hallucinations and delusions. Excessive environmental stimuli can increase confusion and disorganization.
• Maintain environment that does not stimulate client's delusions; for example, if client has delusions related to religion, limit discussions of religion and religious activity	

on unit to very concrete terms. Limit
interaction with people who stimulate
delusional thinking.

• Primary nurse will assist client in identifying signs and symptoms of increasing thought disorganization and in developing a plan to cope with these situations before they get out of control. This will be done in the regular scheduled interaction times between the primary nurse and client.	Promotes client's sense of control and enhances self-esteem.
• As client's condition improves, primary nurse will assist client to identify onset of delusions with periods of increasing anxiety.	Facilitates client's developing alternative coping behaviors.
• As connection is made between thought disorder and anxiety, help client to identify specific anxiety-producing situations and learn alternative coping behaviors. See Anxiety, Chapter 8, for specific interventions.	Promotes client's sense of control and enhances self-esteem.
• Refer client to outpatient support systems and make arrangements for the client to contact these before discharge. (See Appendix B.)	Facilitates client's reintegration into the community.

Gerontic Health

NOTE: Problems related to Altered Thought Process with older adults may present
themselves in various ways. Two conditions, dementia and delirium (acute
confused state), are considered here. Irreversible dementia, such as Alzheimer's
or multi-infarct dementia, is usually progressive, gradual in onset, and of long
duration and has a steady downward course. Delirium, or acute confusional
state, presents with acute onset, is of short duration, has a fluctuating course,
and is often reversible with treatment.[27] Nursing interventions vary depending
on the course of the altered thought process.

Actions/Interventions	Rationales
Dementia	
• Maintain safe environment. Avoid leaving solutions, equipment, or medications near the patient that could result in injury through misuse or ingestion.	Patient is unable to determine the harmful consequences of misuse.
• Monitor environment to prevent overstimulating the patient with light, sounds, and frequent activity.	Patient has a reduced threshold for stress.
• Schedule activities that are of short duration (usually 20-minute sessions).	Prevents stresses on an individual already suffering from attention deficits and anxiety.

Continued

Actions/Interventions	Rationales
• Use short sentences and clear directions when communicating with the patient.	Allows processing of basic information without distraction.
• Determine self-care abilities that are intact, and encourage continued participation in these activities.	Provides stimulation and sense of pride; promotes physical activity.
• Monitor food and fluid intake.	Monitors adequacy of nutritional status.
• Provide consistent staff.	Reduces anxiety.
• Refer family to local support groups for Alzheimer's and related diseases.	Provides long-term support.

Delirium

Actions/Interventions	Rationales
• Monitor for conditions that can induce delirium.	Certain factors such as electrolyte imbalance, preoperative dehydration, unanticipated surgery, intraoperative hypotension, postoperative hypothermia, and a large number of medications have been found to be associated with acute confusional states in older adults.[28,29]
• Provide orienting information to the patient as often as necessary.	Provides information to the patient about the current situation and assists in reducing anxiety and confusion.
• Ensure sensory deficits are corrected to extent possible.	Correcting sensory deficits enhances the patient's ability to use available cues to person, place, and time.
• Provide consistent staff.	Avoids adding to confusion; promotes patient's security.
• Provide sensory stimulation such as bathing, touching, back massages.	Assists in restoring the patient's sense of body image.[30]

Home Health

Actions/Interventions	Rationales

• Teach client and family to monitor for signs and symptoms of impaired thought process:
  ○ Poor hygiene
  ○ Poor decision making or judgment
  ○ Regression in behavior
  ○ Delusions
  ○ Hallucinations
  ○ Changes in interpersonal relationship
  ○ Distractibility
	Basic monitoring allows for earlier intervention.

• Involve client and family in planning, implementing, and promoting appropriate thought processing: ○ Family conference	Involvement improves cooperation and motivation, thereby increasing the probability of an improved outcome.

- ○ Mutual goal setting
- ○ Communication
- Assist client and family in life-style adjustments that may be necessary:
  - ○ Providing safety and prevention of injury
  - ○ Frequent orientation to person, place, and time
  - ○ Reality testing and verification
  - ○ Alterations in role functions in family or at work
  - ○ Stopping substance abuse
  - ○ Alterations in communication
  - ○ Setting limits
  - ○ Learning new skills
  - ○ Decreasing risk for violence
  - ○ Suicide prevention
  - ○ Possible chronicity of disorder
  - ○ Finances
  - ○ Reducing sensory overload
  - ○ Stress management
  - ○ Relaxation techniques
  - ○ Support groups
- Assist client and family in setting criteria to help them determine when professional intervention is required.

  Early identification of issues requiring professional evaluation will increase the probability of successful interventions. Provides necessary information for client and family that promotes safe self-care.

- Teach client and family purposes, side effects, and proper administration of medications.

- Consult with or refer to appropriate resources as required. (See Appendix B.)

  Efficient and cost-effective use of already available resources.

FLOW CHART EVALUATION
Flow Chart Expected Outcome 1

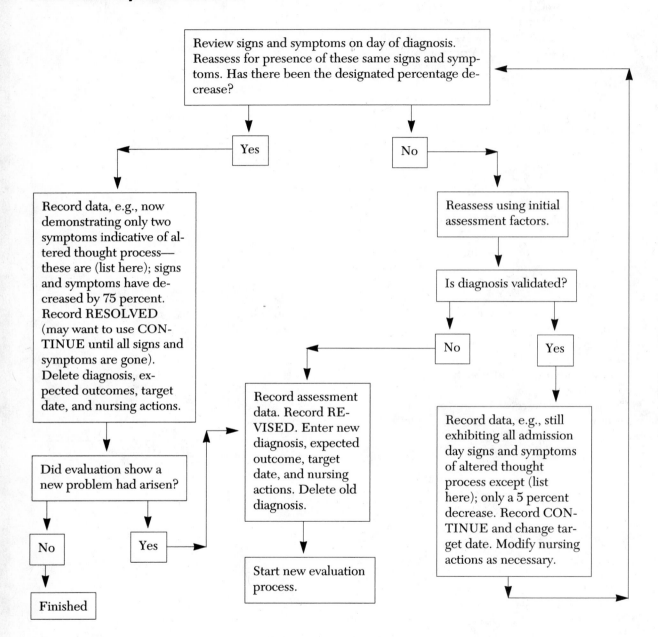

Flow Chart Expected Outcome 2

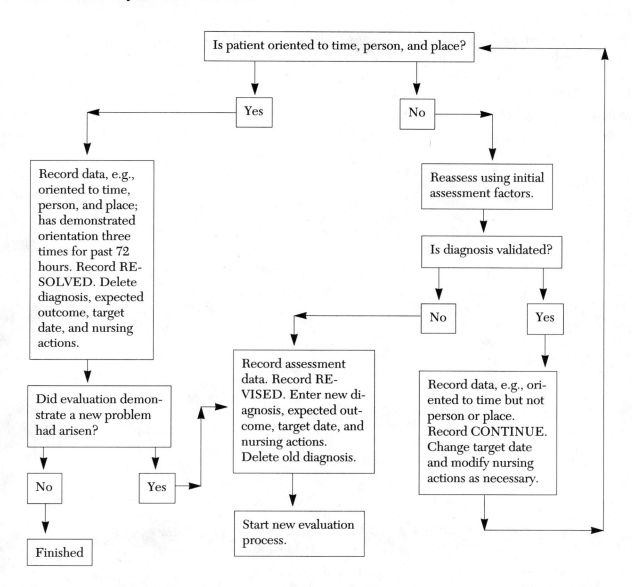

Is patient oriented to time, person, and place?

Yes

No

Record data, e.g., oriented to time, person, and place; has demonstrated orientation three times for past 72 hours. Record RESOLVED. Delete diagnosis, expected outcome, target date, and nursing actions.

Reassess using initial assessment factors.

Is diagnosis validated?

No

Yes

Did evaluation demonstrate a new problem had arisen?

Record assessment data. Record REVISED. Enter new diagnosis, expected outcome, target date, and nursing actions. Delete old diagnosis.

Record data, e.g., oriented to time but not person or place. Record CONTINUE. Change target date and modify nursing actions as necessary.

No

Yes

Finished

Start new evaluation process.

Unilateral Neglect

DEFINITION

A state in which an individual is perceptually unaware of and inattentive to one side of the body.[2]

NANDA TAXONOMY: PERCEIVING 7.2.1.1

DEFINING CHARACTERISTICS[2]

1. Major defining characteristic:
   a. Consistent inattention to stimuli on an affected side
2. Minor defining characteristics:
   a. Inadequate self-care
   b. Positioning and/or safety precautions in regard to the affected side
   c. Does not look toward affected side
   d. Leaves food on plate on the affected side

RELATED FACTORS[2]

1. Disturbed perceptual abilities, for example, hemianopsia
2. One-sided blindness
3. Neurologic illness or trauma

RELATED CLINICAL CONCERNS

1. Cerebrovascular accident
2. Glaucoma
3. Blindness secondary to diabetes mellitus
4. Spinal cord injury
5. Amputation
6. Ruptured cerebral aneurysm
7. Brain trauma

HAVE YOU SELECTED THE CORRECT DIAGNOSIS?

Sensory-Perceptual Alterations   This diagnosis refers to a problem with receiving sensory input and interpretation of this input. Unilateral Neglect could be, as indicated by related factors, an outcome of this disturbance in sensory input and/or perception of this input. (See page 562.)

EXPECTED OUTCOMES

1. Will return-demonstrate at least (number) measures to reduce the effect of unilateral neglect by (date) and/or
2. Will have decreased signs and symptoms of unilateral neglect by (date)

TARGET DATE

A target date between 5 and 7 days would be appropriate to evaluate initial progress.

NURSING ACTIONS/INTERVENTIONS WITH RATIONALES

Adult Health

Actions/Interventions	Rationales
• Frequently remind patient to attend to both sides of his or her body.	Repetition improves brain processing.
• Help patient to touch and feel neglected side of body. Help patient, by providing a variety of sensations (warmth, cool, soft, harsh, and so on), to become more aware of and articulate sensations on neglected side.	Increases brain's awareness of neglected side.
• Help patient with range-of-motion exercises to neglected side of body every 4 hours while awake at (times). Teach extent of movement of each joint on neglected side of body.	Increases brain's awareness of neglected side; maintains muscle tone and joint mobility.
• Help patient to position neglected side of body in a similar way as attended side of body whenever position is changed.	
• Remind patient to turn plate during each meal.	Assists patient to notice all of food and increases cues to brain.
• Turn every 2 hours on the (odd/even) hours. Monitor skin condition on each turning.	Improves circulation, relieves pressure areas, and avoids skin breakdown on affected side.
• Refer to rehabilitation nurse clinician.	Collaboration provides a more holistic plan of care; rehabilitation nurse will have most up-to-date knowledge regarding this diagnsis.

Child Health

NOTE: See nursing actions under Sensory-Perceptual Alterations in addition to those listed here.

Actions/Interventions	Rationales
• Allow 30 minutes every shift for patient and family to express how they perceive the unilateral neglect.	Ventilation of feelings is paramount in understanding the effect the problem has on the patient and the family; it is also critical as a means of evaluating needs.
• Determine how unilateral neglect affects the usual expected behavior or development for the child.	Previous and/or current developmental capacity may be affected by unilateral neglect, depending on the degree of severity.

Continued

Actions/Interventions	Rationales
	To be able to judge the best means of therapy requires this data to be considered; for example, does the child use the affected hand as a helper or not at all?
• Monitor for presence of secondary or tertiary deficits.	Minimizes further sequelae, which can be treated early.
• Establish, with family input, appropriate anticipatory safety guidelines based on the unilateral neglect and the developmental capacity of the child.	Need to structure the environment to allow for appropriate explorative behavior while maintaining safety without overprotection.
• Stress appropriate follow-up prior to discharge with appropriate time frame for family.	Arrangement for follow-up increases the likelihood of compliance and emphasizes its importance.

Women's Health

See Adult Health.

Mental Health

See Adult Health.

Geroritic Health

See Adult Health.

Home Health

Actions/Interventions	Rationales
• Monitor for factors contributing to unilateral neglect, for example, disturbed perceptual abilities, neurologic disease, or trauma.	This action provides the database needed to identify interventions that will prevent or diminish unilateral neglect.

• Involve client and family in planning, implementing, and promoting reduction in effects of unilateral neglect:
  ○ Family conference to discuss concerns family members have.
  ○ Mutual goal setting; for example, establish two measures to offset the effect of unilateral neglect. Be sure roles for the participants are identified.
  ○ Communication.
	Family involvement is important to ensure success. Communication and mutual goals improve the outcome.

- ○ Support for caregiver; for example, plan respite time for primary caregiver. Identify and train alternate caregivers.
- Teach client and family measures to decrease effects of unilateral neglect:
  - ○ Active and passive range-of-motion exercises
  - ○ Ambulation with assistive devices (canes, walkers, crutches)
  - ○ Placement of objects within field of vision and reach
  - ○ Assistive eating utensils
  - ○ Assistive dressing utensils
  - ○ Safe environment; for example, remove objects from area outside field of vision
- Assist family and client to identify life-style changes that may be required:
  - ○ Change in role functions
  - ○ Coping with disability or dependency
  - ○ Obtaining and using assistive equipment
  - ○ Coping with assistive equipment
  - ○ Maintaining safe environment
- Consult with appropriate resources as indicated. (See Appendix B.)

These actions diminish the negative effects of unilateral neglect.

Life-style changes require changes in behavior; self-evaluation and support facilitate these changes.

Existing community services provide effective use of resources.

FLOW CHART EVALUATION
Flow Chart Expected Outcome 1

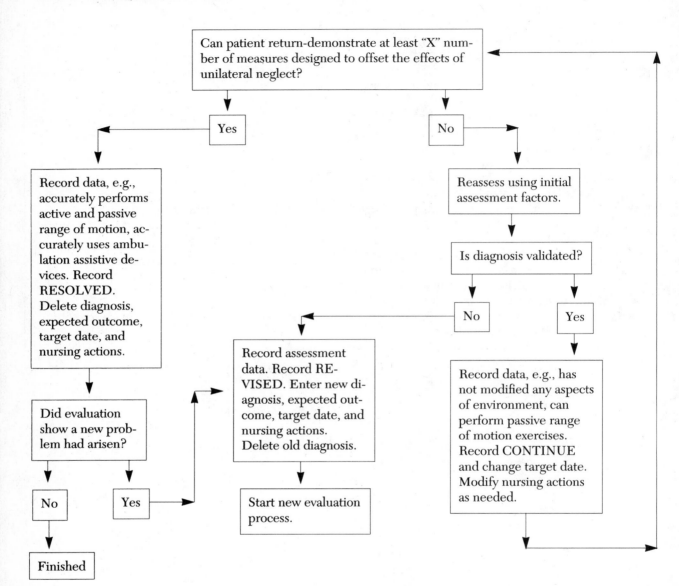

Flow Chart Expected Outcome 2

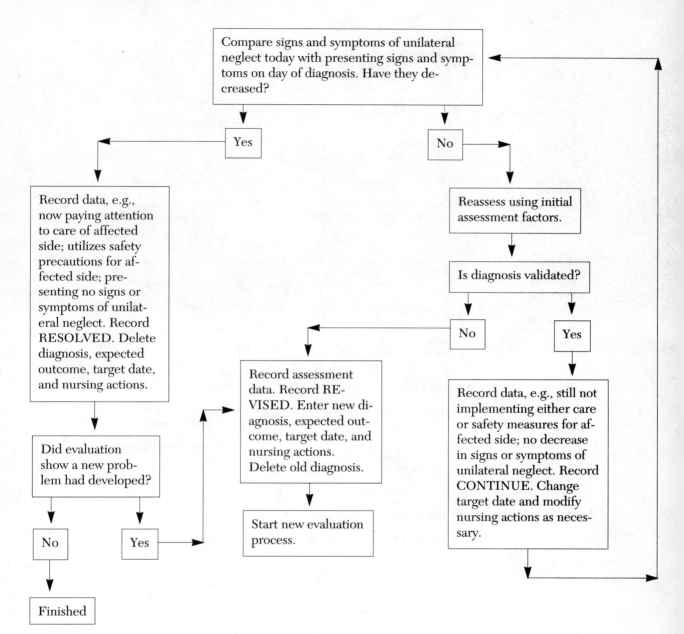

References

1. Murray, RB and Zentner, JP: Nursing Assessment and Health Promotion Strategies through the Lifespan, ed 4. Appleton-Lange, Norwalk, CT, 1989.
2. North American Nursing Diagnosis Association: Taxonomy I: Revised 1990. Author, St. Louis, 1990.
3. Krause, KD and Younger, VJ: Nursing diagnoses as guidelines in the care of the neonatal ECMO patient. J Obstet Gynecol Neonatal Nurs 21:176, 1992.
4. Cox, BE: What if? Coping with unexpected outcomes. Childbirth Instructor 1:24, 1991.
5. Parkman, SE: Helping families to say good-bye. MCH Am J Matern Child Nurs 17:14, 1992.
6. Ryan, PF, Cote-Arsenault, D, and Sugarman, LL: Facilitating care after perinatal loss: A comprehensive checklist. J Obstet Gynecol Neonatal Nurs 20:385, 1991.
7. Ladebauche, P: Unit-based family support groups: A reminder. MCH Am J Matern Child Nurs 17:18, 1992
8. Erickson, M: Healing in Hypnosis. Irvington, New York, 1983.
9. Keeney, BP: Aesthetics of Change. The Guilford Press, New York, 1983.
10. Watzlawick, P, Weakland, J, and Fisch, R: Change. WW Norton, New York, 1974.
11. Aguilera, D and Messick, J: Crisis Intervention: Theory and Methodology. CV Mosby, St. Louis, 1982.
12. North American Nursing Diagnosis Association: Taxonomy I: Revised. Author, St. Louis, 1987.
13. Cresia, J and Parker, B: Conceptual Foundations of Professional Nursing Practice. CV Mosby, St. Louis, 1991.
14. Weinrick, S, Boyd, M, and Nussbaum, J: Continuing education: Adapting strategies to teach the elderly. J Geront Nurs 15:17, 1989.
15. Department of Health and Human Services: Acute Pain Management: Operative on Medical Procedures and Trauma. Clinical Practice Guidelines. Author, Rockville, MD, 1992.
16. Fogel, CI and Woods, NF: Health Care of Women: A Nursing Perspective. CV Mosby, St. Louis, 1981.
17. Gaston-Johansson, F, Fridh, G, and Turner-Norvall, K: Progression of labor pain in primaparas and multiparas. Nurs Res 37:86, 1988.
18. Maas, M, Buckwalter, K, and Hardy, M: Nursing Diagnosis and Interventions for the Elderly. Addison-Wesley, Ft. Collins, CO, 1991.
19. Ferrell, B and Ferrell, B: Easing the pain. Geriatr Nurs 11:175, 1990.
20. Hofland, S: Elder beliefs: Blocks to pain management. J Geront Nurs 18:19, 1992.
21. Haber, J, et al: Comprehensive Psychiatric Nursing, ed 4. CV Mosby, St. Louis, 1992.
22. Puskar, KR, et al: Psychiatric nursing management of medication-free psychotic patients. Arch Psych Nurs 4:78–86, 1990.
23. Townsend, M: Nursing Diagnosis in Psychiatric Nursing, ed 2. FA Davis, Philadelphia, 1991.
24. Schwartz, M and Shockley, E: The Nurse and the Mental Patient. John Wiley & Sons, New York, 1956.
25. Buckwalter, KC, Cusack, D, Kruckeber, T, and Shoemaker, S: Family involvement with communication: Impaired residents in long-term care settings. Appl Nurs Res 4:77, 1991.
26. Friedrick, R and Kus, R: Cognitive impairments in early sobriety: Nursing interventions. Arch Psych Nurs 5:105, 1991.
27. Gomez, G and Gomez, E: Dementia? Or delirium? Geriatr Nurs 11:136, 1989.
28. Foreman, M: Complexities of acute confusion. Geriatr Nurs 11:136, 1990.
29. Bowman, AM: The relationship of anxiety to development of postoperative delirium. J Geront Nurs 18:24, 1992.
30. Faraday, K and Berry, M: The nurse's role in managing reversible confusion. J Geront Nurs 15:17, 1989.

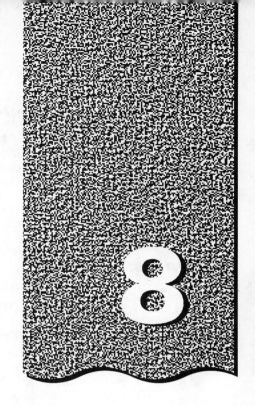

8

Self-Perception and Self-Concept Pattern

PATTERN INTRODUCTION
Pattern Description

As the nurse interacts with the client the most important knowledge the client brings is self-knowledge. It is this knowledge that determines the individual's manner of interaction with others. This knowledge base is most often labeled "self-concept." One's self-concept is composed of beliefs and attitudes about the self, body image, self-esteem, and abilities. The individual's behavior is not only affected by his or her personal history and experiences but also by interactions with the health care system.

Pattern Assessment

1. Does patient express concern regarding current situation?
   a. Yes (Anxiety; Fear)
   b. No
2. Can patient identify source of concern?
   a. Yes (Fear)
   b. No (Anxiety)
3. As a result of this admission, is patient going to have a change in body structure or function?
   a. Yes (Body Image Disturbance)
   b. No
4. Does patient verbalize a change in life-style as a result of this admission?
   a. Yes (Body Image Disturbance)
   b. No
5. Does patient verbalize a negative view of self?
   a. Yes (Self-Esteem Disturbance)
   b. No
6. Does patient believe he or she can deal with the current problem that leads to this admission?
   a. Yes
   b. No (Self-Esteem Disturbance)
7. Does patient or his or her family indicate the self-negating impression is a long-standing (several years) problem?
   a. Yes (Chronic Low Self-Esteem)
   b. No (Situational Low Self-Esteem)
8. Does patient question who he or she is or verbalize lack of understanding regarding his or her role in life?
   a. Yes (Personal Identity Disturbance)
   b. No
9. Does patient appear passive or verbalize passivity?
   a. Yes (Hopelessness)
   b. No
10. Does patient demonstrate decreased verbalization and/or flat affect?
    a. Yes (Hopelessness)
    b. No
11. Does patient verbalize lack of control?
    a. Yes (Powerlessness)
    b. No

12. Is patient participating in care and decision making regarding care?
    a. Yes
    b. No (Powerlessness)

Diagnoses in This Chapter

1. Anxiety (page 605)
2. Body Image Disturbance (page 618)
3. Fear (page 628)
4. Hopelessness (page 640)
5. Personal Identity Disturbance (page 651)
6. Powerlessness (page 657)
7. Self-Esteem Disturbance (page 668)
8. Self-Mutilation, High Risk for (page 680)

Conceptual Information

Definition of the self and of a self-concept has been an issue of debate in philosophy, sociology, and psychology for many years, and many publications are available on this topic.[1] The complexity of the problem of defining self is compounded by the knowledge that external observation provides only a superficial glimpse of the self, and introspection requires that the individual know himself or herself so that information actually gained is self-referential. In spite of these problems, the concept continues to be pervasive in the literature and in the universal experience of "self" or "not-self." Intuitively one would say, of course, "There is a self because I have experiences separate from those around me; I know where I end and they begin." The importance of self is also emphasized by the language in the multitude of self-referential terms such as "self-actualization," "self-affirmation," "ego involvement," and "self-concept."

Turner[2] addresses society's need for the individual to conceptualize the self-as-object. Recognizing the self-as-object allows society to place responsibility, which becomes a very valuable asset in maintaining social control and social order. This returns us to the initial problem of what the self is and how we can understand our own and others' selves.[3]

In this section the assumption is made that self-concept refers to the individual's subjective cognitions and evaluations of self; thus, it is a highly personal experience. This indicates that the self is a personal construct and not a fact or hard reality. It is further assumed that the individual will act, as stated earlier, in congruence with the self-concept. This conceptualization is consistent with the authors who will be discussed and with the assumptions utilized in psychological research.[3] It is also important to recognize that language assists in developing a concept. This becomes crucial when thinking about the concept of self in English because the English language displays a Cartesian dualism which does not express integrated concepts well. Often it will appear that the information presented is separating the individual into various parts when, in fact, an integrated whole is being addressed. For example, James[4] talks about an "I" and a "Me." If these terms were taken at face value, it would appear that the individual is being divided into multiple parts when, in fact, an integrated whole is being discussed and the words describe patterns of the whole person. Unless otherwise stated, it can be assumed that the concepts presented in this book reflect on the individual as an integrated whole.

Symbolic interaction theory provides a basis for understanding the self. The foundation for the self in this theoretical model was developed by James[4] and Mead.[5] James outlines the internal working of the self with his concepts of "I" and "Me." "I" is the thinker or the state of consciousness. "Me" is what the "I" is conscious of and includes all of what people consider theirs. This "Me" contains three aspects: the "material me," the "social me," and the "spiritual me." The self-construction outlined by Mead indicates that there is the "knower" part of the self and that which the knower knows. Mead conceptualizes the thoughts themselves as the "knower" to resolve the metaphysical problem of who the "I" is. In Mead's writings, the consciousness of self is a stream of thought in which the "I" can remember what came before and continues to know what was known. The development of these memories and how they affect one's behavior is expressly addressed by Mead.

Mead describes the self-concept as evolving out of interactions with others in social contexts. This process begins at the moment of birth and continues throughout a lifetime. The definition of self can only occur in social interactions, for one's self only exists in relation to other selves. The individual is continually processing the reactions of others to his or her actions and reactions. This processing is taking place in a highly personalized manner, for the information is experienced through the individual's selective attention, which is guided by the current needs that are struggling to be expressed. This results in an environment that is constructed by one's perceptions. Mead's conceptualization leads to an interesting feedback process in that we can only perceive self as we perceive others perceive us. This continues to reinforce the idea that the self-concept is highly personalized.

Many authors[2-5] have addressed the process of developing a concept of self. The model developed by Harry Stack Sullivan[6] will be presented here because it is consistent with the information presented in the symbolic interaction literature and is used as the theoretical base in much of the nursing literature.

Sullivan describes the self-concept as developing in interactions with significant others. Development of the self-concept is seen by Sullivan as a dynamic process resulting from interpersonal interactions that are directed toward meeting physiologic needs. This process has its most obvious beginnings with the infant and becomes more complex as the individual develops. This increasing complexity results from the layering of experiences that occurs in the developing individual. The biological processes become less and less important in directing the individual the further away from birth one is and as the importance of interpersonal interactions increases. The initial interpersonal interaction is between the infant and the primary caregivers. An infant expresses discomfort with a cry and the "parenting one" responds. This response, whether it be tender or harsh, begins to influence the infant's beliefs about himself or herself and the world in general. If the interaction does not provide the infant with a feeling of security, anxiety results and interferes with the progress toward other life goals. Sullivan makes a distinction between the inner experience and the outer event and describes three modes of understanding experience.

The first developmental experience is the *prototaxic mode*. In this mode the small child experiences self and the universe as an undifferentiated whole. At 3 to 4 months the child moves into the *parataxic mode*. The parataxic mode presents experiences as separated but without recognition of a connectedness or logical sequence. Finally, the individual enters the *syntaxic mode*, in which consensual validation is possible. This allows for events and experiences to be compared with others' experiences and for establishing mutually understandable communication instead of the autistic thinking that has characterized the previous stages.[7,8]

As one experiences the environment through these three modes of thought, the self system or self-concept is developed. Sullivan conceptualized three parts of the self. The part of the self that is associated with security and approval becomes the "good me." That which is within one's awareness but is disapproved of becomes the "bad me." The "bad me" could include those feelings, needs, or desires that stimulate anxiety. Those feelings and understandings that are out of awareness are experienced as "not-me." These not-me experiences are not nonexistent, but are expressed in indirect ways that can interfere with the conduct of the individual's life.[6,7]

As the social sciences adopted a cybernetic worldview, this theoretical perspective has been applied to developing a concept of self. Glasersfeld[9] spoke of the self as a relational entity that is given life through the continuity of relating. This relating provides the intuitive knowledge that our experience is truly ours. This reflects the perspective of knowing presented at the beginning of this section.

Watts[10] describes what many authors feel is the self as it can be understood through a cybernetic worldview. Self is the whole, for it is part of the energy that is the universe and cannot be separated. "At this level of existence 'I' am immeasurably old; my forms are infinite and their comings and goings are simply the pulses or vibrations of a single and eternal flow of energy."[10:12] Within this view, an individual is connected to every other living being in the universe. This places the self in a unique position of responsibility. The self then becomes responsible to everything because it is everything. This conceptual model resolves the issue of responsibility to society without relying on an individual self to which responsibility is assigned.

Although the conceptual model represented here by Watts fits with current theoretical models being utilized in nursing and the social sciences, it is not congruent with the experience of most people in Western society. This limits its usefulness when working with clients in a clinical setting. It is presented here to provide practitioners with an alternative model for themselves.

Sidney Jourard[11] provides direction for interventions related to an individual's self-concept. The healthy self-concept allows individuals to play roles they have satisfactorily played while gaining personal satisfaction from this role enactment. This person also continues to develop and maintain a high level of physical wellness. This high level of wellness is achieved by gaining knowledge of oneself through a process of self-disclosure. Jourard states: "If self-disclosure is one of the means by which healthy personality is both achieved and maintained, we can also note that such activities as loving, psychotherapy, counseling, teaching and nursing, all are impossible—without the disclosure of the client."[11:427] Elaboration of this thought reveals that for the nurse to effectively meet the needs of the client, an understanding of the client's self must be achieved. This understanding must go beyond the interpretation of overt behavior, which is an indirect method of understanding, and access the client's understanding of self through the process of self-disclosure.

Dufault and Martocchio[12] present a conceptual model for hope that also provides a useful perspective for nursing intervention. *Hope* is defined as multidimensional and process-oriented. Hopelessness is not the absence of hope but is the product of an environment that does not activate the process of hoping. Vaillot[13] supports the view presented by Dufault and Martocchio with the existential philosophical perspective that hope arises from relationships and the beliefs about these relationships. One believes that help can come from the outside of oneself when all internal resources are exhausted. Hopelessness arises in an environment where hope is not communicated. This model supports nursing interventions from a systems theory perspective, because it validates the ever-interacting system, the whole. In this perspective the nurse as well as the client contributes to the "hopelessness" and thus the responsibility of nurturing hope is shared.[12-16]

Developmental Considerations

INFANT

In general the sources of anxiety begin in a very narrow scope with the infant and broaden out as the individual matures. Initially the relationship with the primary caregiver is the source of gratification for the infant, and disruptions in this relationship result in anxiety. As the child matures, needs are met from multiple sources and therefore the sources of anxiety expand. Specific developmental considerations are as follows.

The primary source of anxiety for the infant appears to be a sense of "being left." This response begins at about 3 months. Sullivan, as indicated earlier, would contend that the infant could experience anxiety even earlier with any disruption in having needs met by the primary caregiver. At age 8 to 10 months, separation anxiety peaks for the first time. At 5 to 6 months the infant begins to demonstrate stranger anxiety. Primary symptoms of anxiety, across the span from 3 months to 10 months, include disruptions in physiologic functioning and could include colic, sleep disorders, failure-to-thrive syndrome, and constipation with early toilet training. Stranger anxiety and separation anxiety may be demonstrated with screaming, attempting to withdraw, and refusing to cooperate. Both stranger anxiety and separation anxiety are normal developmental responses and should not be considered pathologic as long as they are not severe or prolonged and if the parental response is appropriately supportive of the infant's need.

Erikson[16,17] indicated that he thought hope evolved out of the successful resolution of this first developmental stage, basic trust versus mistrust. Hope was perceived by Erikson to be a basic human virtue. The type of environment that has been identified as promoting the development of this basic trust is warm and loving, one in which there is respect and acceptance for personal interests, ideas, needs, and talents.[14] Several environmental conditions have been associated with early childhood and are seen as increasing the perceptions consistent with hopelessness. These conditions are economic deprivation, poor physical health, being raised in a broken home or a home where parents have a high degree of conflict, having a negative perception of parents, or having parents who are not mentally healthy. From an existential perspective, Lynch[18] identified five areas of human existence that can produce hopelessness. If these areas are not acknowledged in the developmental process, the individual is at greater risk of frustration and hopelessness because hope is being intermingled with a known area of hopelessness. The five areas that Lynch identified are death, personal imperfections, imperfect emotional control, inability to trust all people, and personal areas of incompetence. This supports Erikson's contention that hope evolves out of the first developmental stage, because these basic areas of hopelessness are issues primarily related to the resolution of trust and mistrust. It should be remembered that previously resolved or unresolved developmental issues must be renegotiated throughout life.

Each developmental stage has a set of specific etiologies and symptom clusters related to hopelessness. Since the relationship between self-concept strength and degree of hopefulness is seen as a positive link, many of the etiologies and symptoms of hopelessness at the various developmental stages are similar to those of Self-Esteem Disturbance.[15]

As conceptualized by Erikson, infancy is the primary age for developing a hopeful attitude about life. If the infant does not experience a situation in which trust in another can be developed, then the base of hopelessness has begun. Thus, if the infant experiences frequent changes in caregivers, or if the caregiver does not meet the infant's basic needs in a consistent and warm manner, the infant will become hopeless. Research has indicated that children who have been raised in an environment of despair are at greater risk for experiencing hopelessness.[18] Symptoms of hopelessness in infants resemble infant depression or failure to thrive. Since symptoms in infants are a general response, the diagnosis of Hopelessness must be considered equally with other diagnoses that produce similar symptom clusters, such as Powerlessness and Ineffective Coping.

One's perceptions of place in the larger system and of influence in this system begin at birth. These perceptions are developed through interactions with those in the immediate environment and continue throughout life with each new interaction in each new experience. Thus, the child learns from primary caregivers that his or her expressions of need may or may not have an effect on those around him or her, and also learns what must be done to have an effect. If the caregiver responds to the earliest cries of the infant, a sense of personal influence has begun. The two areas that consistently influence one's perceptions of influence are discipline and communication styles.

Implementation of discipline in a manner that provides the child with a sense of control over the environment while teaching appropriate behavior can produce a perception of mutual system influence. Harsh, overcontrolling methods can produce the perception that the child does not have any influence in the system if acting in a direct manner. This produces an indirect influencing style. An example of indirect influence is the child who always becomes ill just before his or her parents leave for an evening on the town. The parents, out of concern for the child, decide to remain at home and thus never have time together as a couple. Authoritarian styles of interaction can also produce perceptions of powerlessness in adults in unfamiliar environments. If the hospital staff act in an authoritarian manner, the client may develop perceptions of powerlessness.

Double-bind communication can also produce a perception of powerlessness by making the individual feel that "no matter what action I take, it appears to be wrong. I'm damned if I do and damned if I don't." Again, if the individual cannot influence this system in a direct manner, indirect behavior patterns are chosen. Bateson[19] proposes that this is the process behind the symptom cluster identified as schizophrenia. This suggests that if the child is continually placed in the position of being wrong no matter what he or she has done, the child could develop the perception that his or her position is one of powerlessness and carry this attitude with him or her throughout life.

Infants have a need for consistency in having physiologic needs met, and the most important relationship becomes that with the caregiver. If this relationship is disrupted and needs are not met, symptoms related to infant depression or failure to thrive could communicate a perception related to powerlessness.

It is important to remember that self-concept, including body image, is developed throughout life. For the infant, the primary source of developing self-concept and body image is physical interaction with the environment. This includes both the environment's response to physical needs and the body's response to environmental stimuli.

TODDLER AND PRESCHOOLER

The basic sources of anxiety for the toddler and preschooler remain the same as for the infant. Separation anxiety appears to peak again at 18 to 24 months, and stranger anxiety peaks again at 12 to 18 months. Loss of significant others is the primary source of anxiety at this age. In addition to the physiologic responses mentioned above, the child may demonstrate anxiety by motor restlessness and regressive behavior. The preschooler can begin to tolerate longer periods away from the caregiver and enjoys having the opportunity to test new abilities. Lack of opportunity to practice independent skills can increase the discomfort of this age group.

The young child may express or exhibit anxiety about the body and body mutilation, death, or loss of self-control. Increased anxiety can be seen in regressive behavior, motor restlessness, and physiologic response or may be expressed more directly with language and dramatic play as language abilities increase. Anxiety-producing situations may be played out with dolls or other toys; this play can assume a very aggressive nature. The anxieties of the day can also be expressed in dreams and result in nightmares or other sleep disturbances.

Fear is a normal protective response to external threats and will be present at all ages. It becomes dysfunctional at the point that it is attached to situations that do not present a threat or when it prevents the individual from responding appropriately to a situation. Thus, it is important that children have certain fears to protect them from harm. The hot stove, for example, should produce a fear response to the degree that it prevents the child from touching the stove and being injured. Fear is a learned response to situations, and children learn this response from their caregivers. Thus, it becomes the caregivers' responsibility to model and teach appropriate fear. If a mother cannot tolerate being left alone in the house at night with her children, these children will learn to fear being in this situation. When this home is located in a low-crime area with supportive neighbors and appropriate locks, this becomes an inappropriate fear response and the children may be affected by it for a lifetime.

Various developmental stages have characteristic fears associated with them. In the mind of the child these characteristic fears present threats, so the fears can be seen both as a source of "fear" and as a source of anxiety. The characteristic fears result from strong or noxious environmental stimuli such as loud noises, bright lights, or sharp objects against the skin. The response to fears produces physiologic symptoms. The most immediate and obvious response is crying and pulling away from the stressful object or situations.

Fears of this age group evolve from real environmental stimuli and from imagined situations. Typical fears of specific age groups are fear of sudden loud noises (2 years), fear of animals (3 to 4 years), fear of the dark (4 to 6 years), and fear of being lost (6 years). Symptoms of fears include regressive behavior, physical and verbal cruelty, restlessness, irritability, sleep disturbance, dramatic play around issues related to the fear, and increased physical closeness to the caregiver.

Alterations to the body or its functioning place a child at this age at the greatest risk of experiencing hopelessness. If the child experiences a difference between self and other or is ashamed about body functioning, hopelessness can develop in a nonsupportive environment. A specific issue encountered at this stage is toilet training. If the child is required to gain control over bowel and bladder functions before the physical ability to master these functions has developed, the child can experience hopelessness in that he or she truly cannot make his or her body function in the required manner. Peer interactions are also important at this time because they foster the beginnings of trust in someone other than the primary caregivers, thus demonstrating that hope can be gained elsewhere.

Struggle between self-control and control by others becomes the primary psychosocial issue. If appropriate expansion of self-control is encouraged, the child will develop perceptions related to mutual systemic influence. This appropriate support is crucial if the child is to develop a perception of a personal role in the social system. If this struggle for self-control is thwarted, the child can express themes of overcontrol in play or become overly dependent on the primary caregiver and withdraw completely from new situations and learning.

For the preschooler there is a continuation and refinement of a sense of personal influence. Varying approaches are explored and a greater sense of what can be achieved is developed. One of the primary sources of anxiety during this stage is loss of self-control. Symptoms of difficulties in this area include playing out situations with personal influence as a theme and aggressive play.

Sources of the self-concept perceptions are the responses of significant others to exploration of new physical abilities and to the toddler's place in these relationships. The primary concept of self is related to physical qualities, motor skills, sex type, and age. A concept of physical differences and of physical integrity is developed. Thus, situations that threaten the toddler's perception of physical wholeness can pose a threat. This would include physical injury. Toilet training poses a potential threat to the successful development of a positive self-concept or body image. Failure at training could produce feelings of personal incompetence or of bodily shame.

In the preschooler, physical qualities, motor skills, sex type, and age continue to be the primary components of self-concept. Peers begin to assume greater importance in self-perceptions. Physical integrity continues to be important and physical difference can have a profound effect on the preschool child.

SCHOOL-AGE CHILD

Concerns about imagined future events produce the anxieties of the school-age child. The specific concern varies with the developmental age. Typical fears are strange noises, ghosts and imagined phantoms, and natural elements such as fire, drowning, or thunder (6 years); not being liked or being late for school (7 years); and personal failure or inadequacy (8 to 10 years). Symptoms of these fears include physical symptoms of autonomic stimulation, increased verbalization, withdrawal, aggression, sleep disturbance, or obsessive repetition of a specific task.

Peers' perceptions of the individual assume a role in the development of attitudes related to personal hopefulness and influence within the larger social system. This is built on the perceptions achieved during earlier stages of development. The sense of a strong peer group can produce perceptions of help coming from the outside as long as the child thinks and believes along with the group but can produce perceptions of exaggerated personal influence. Problems at this developmental stage can be demonstrated by withdrawal, daydreaming, increased verbalizations of helplessness and hopelessness, angry outbursts, aggressive behavior, irritability, and frustration.

Self-perception expands to include ethnic awareness, ambition, ideal self, ordinal position, and conscience. There is increasing awareness of self as different from peers. Peers become increasingly important in developing a concept of self, and there is increased comparison of real to ideal self.

ADOLESCENT

The developmental theme that elicits anxiety in this age group revolves around the development of a personal identity. This is facilitated by peer relationships, which can also be the source of anxiety. Expression of this anxiety can occur in any of the ways previous discussed and with aggressive behavior. This aggression can take both verbal and physical forms. A certain amount of "normal" anxiety is experienced as the adolescent moves from the family into the adult world. Anxiety would only be considered abnormal if it violates societal norms and is severe or prolonged. Parental education and support during this developmental crisis can be crucial.

Peer relationships, independence, authority figures, and changing roles and relations can contribute to fears for adolescents. Expression of these fears produces cognitive and affective symptoms, including difficulties with attention and concentration, poor judgment, alterations in mood, and alterations in thought content.

The cognitive development of adolescents suggests that their perceptions of situations are guided by hypothetical-deductive thought, which would allow them to develop reasonable models of hopefulness. This cognitive process occurs in conjunction with a lack of life experience and self-discipline and with a heightened state of emotionality, which can result in a situation in which the immediate goal can overshadow future consequences or possibilities. An adolescent who appears very hopeful when cognitive functioning is not overwhelmed by emotions can be filled with despair when involved in a very emotional situation. Consideration of this ability is important when caring for this age group. It is important to distinguish problem behavior from normal behavior and mood swings. Kinds of behavior that could indicate problems in this area include withdrawal and increased or amplified testing of limits. Situations that affect the peer group can place the adolescent at great risk.

Again, issues of dependence-independence assume a primary role. The focus of this struggle is dependence on peers and independence from family. The challenge for the adolescent becomes achieving what Erickson, Tomling, and Swain[20] refer to as affiliated individuation. The adolescent must learn how to be dependent on support systems while maintaining independence from these same support systems and feeling accepted in both positions.

Body image becomes a crucial area of self-evaluation because of changing physical appearance and heightened sexual awareness. This evaluation is based on the cultural ideal as well as that of the peer group. Perceived personal failures are often attributed to physical differences.

ADULT

Changes in role and relationship patterns generate the fears specific to adults. A specific developmental crisis can produce a perception of hopelessness and powerlessness. The situations that place the adult at risk are marriage, pregnancy, parenthood, divorce, retirement, or death of a spouse. Fear expression in these age groups produces cognitive and affective symptoms similar to those described for adolescence.

Concerns about role performance assume an important role in self-perceptions. Perceived failures in meeting role expectations can produce a negative self-evaluation. The number of roles a person has assumed and the personal, cultural, and support system value placed on the identified roles determine the threat that negative evaluation of performance can be to self-perception. Cultural values and personal identity formation determine the degree to which body image remains important in providing a positive evaluation of self. The adult endows unique significance to various body parts. This valuing process is personal, but it is often not in personal awareness until there is a threat to the part.

OLDER ADULT

The older adult faces numerous challenges to self-perception and self-concept. Roles may change secondary to retirement or loss of significant others, such as a spouse or child. Financial resources may become limited or fixed due to illness, retirement, or loss of spouse.[21] Chronic illness that necessitates a decrease in social interactions or increased dependence on others and the resulting loss of control have a negative impact on self-esteem for some elderly.[22]

Negative feedback, such as ageism, sends a message to older adults that they are somehow no longer valuable to the society. In the face of these incremental losses, it is necessary to consider what health care professionals can do to assist the older adult in maintaining a positive regard for self.

APPLICABLE NURSING DIAGNOSES
Anxiety
DEFINITION

A vague uneasy feeling whose source is often nonspecific or unknown to the individual.[23]

NANDA TAXONOMY: FEELING 9.3.1
DEFINING CHARACTERISTICS[23]

1. Subjective
   a. Increased tension
   b. Apprehension
   c. Painful and persistent increased helplessness
   d. Uncertainty
   e. Fearful
   f. Scared
   g. Regretful
   h. Overexcited
   i. Rattled
   j. Distressed
   k. Jittery
   l. Feelings of inadequacy
   m. Shakiness
   n. Fear of nonspecific consequences
   o. Expressed concerns re changes in life events
   p. Worried
   q. Anxious

2. Objective:
   a. Sympathetic stimulation: cardiovascular excitation, superficial vasocon-
      striction, pupil dilation (critical)
   b. Restlessness
   c. Insomnia
   d. Glances about
   e. Poor eye contact
   f. Trembling, hand tremors
   g. Extraneous movement (foot shuffling, hand and arm movements)
   h. Facial tension
   i. Quivering voice
   j. Focus on self
   k. Increased wariness
   l. Increased perspiration

RELATED FACTORS[23]

1. Unconscious conflict about essential values and goals of life
2. Threat to self-concept
3. Threat of death
4. Threat to or change in health status
5. Threat to or change in role functioning
6. Threat to or change in environment
7. Threat to or change in interaction patterns
8. Situational or maturational crises
9. Interpersonal transmission or contagion
10. Unmet needs

RELATED CLINICAL CONCERNS

1. Any hospital admission
2. Failure to thrive
3. Cancer or other terminal illnesses
4. Crohn's disease
5. Impending surgery
6. Hyperthyroidism
7. Substance abuse
8. Phobic disorders
9. Panic disorder
10. Obsessive-compulsive disorder
11. Generalized anxiety disorder
12. Post-traumatic stress disorder
13. Conversion disorder
14. Adjustment disorders
15. Schizophrenic disorders
16. Delusional disorders
17. Psychotic disorders

HAVE YOU SELECTED THE CORRECT DIAGNOSIS?

Fear Fear is the response to an identified threat, while Anxiety is the response to threat that cannot be easily identified. Fear is probably the diagnosis that is most often confused with Anxiety. For example, Fear would be an appropriate diagnosis in the following situation: After being released from jail, the prisoner threatened to kill the judge who placed him in jail. If the judge experiences psychologic stress as a result of this threat, the diagnosis would be Fear. (See page 628.)

Personal Identity Disturbance This diagnosis is the most appropriate if the individual's symptoms are related to a general disturbance in the perception of self. Anxiety would be used when the discomfort is related to other areas. (See page 651.)

Dysfunctional Grieving This would be considered an appropriate diagnosis if the loss is real, whereas the diagnosis of Anxiety would be used when the loss is a threat that is not necessarily real, such as a perceived loss of esteem from others. (See page 732.)

Ineffective Individual Coping This would be the appropriate diagnosis if the individual is not making the necessary adaptations to deal with daily life. This may or may not occur with Anxiety as a companion diagnosis. (See page 892.)

Spiritual Distress This diagnosis occurs if the individual experiences a threat to his or her value or belief system. This threat may or may not produce Anxiety. If the primary expressed concerns are related to the individual's value or belief system, then the appropriate diagnosis would be Spiritual Distress. (See page 923.)

EXPECTED OUTCOMES

1. Will design and implement a plan to reduce anxiety by (date) and/or
2. Will demonstrate, verbally or behaviorally, at least a (number) percent decrease in anxiety by (date)

TARGET DATE

A target date of 3 days would be realistic to start evaluating progress. The sooner anxiety is reduced, the sooner other problems can be dealt with.

NURSING ACTIONS/INTERVENTIONS WITH RATIONALES

Adult Health

Actions/Interventions	Rationales
• Obtain a thorough history upon admission.	Allows identification of all possible contributing factors to anxiety.

Continued

Actions/Interventions	Rationales
• Monitor relationship of anxiety behavior to activity, events, and people every 2 hours on the (odd/even) hour.	When anxiety increases, the ability to follow instruction or cooperate in care plan decreases. Identifying causative factors enhances intervention plans.
• Reassure patient that anxiety is normal. Help patient learn to recognize and identify physical symptoms of anxiety, for example, hyperventilation, rapid heart beat, sweaty palms, inability to concentrate, restlessness.	Helps to identify connection between the precipitating cause and the anxiety experience; reassures the patient that he or she is not "going crazy."
• Provide calm, nonthreatening environment: ○ Explain all procedures and rationale for procedure in clear, concise, simple terms. ○ Decrease sensory input and distraction, for example, lighting, noise. ○ Encourage significant others to stay with patient but not force conversation.	Conveys calm and helps the patient focus on conversation or activity.
• Monitor vital signs at least every 4 hours while awake at (times).	Helps to determine pathological effects of anxiety.
• Attend to primary physical needs promptly.	Conserves patient's energy and allows patient to focus on coping with and reducing anxiety. Failure to attend to physical needs increases anxiety.
• Administer antianxiety medications as ordered. Monitor and document effects of medication within 30 minutes of administration.	Effective medication helps to reduce anxiety to a manageable level.
• Help patient to develop coping skills: ○ Review past coping behaviors and success or lack of success.	Determines what mechanisms have helped and if they are still useful.
○ Help identify and practice new coping strategies, such as progressive relaxation, guided imagery, rhythmic breathing, balancing exercise and rest, appropriate food and fluid intake. Reduce caffeine intake and distraction.	Methods that can be used successfully to decrease anxiety; allows patient to practice and become comfortable with skills in a supporting environment.
○ Challenge unrealistic assumptions or goals.	Helps patient to avoid placing extra stress on himself or herself.
○ Place limits on maladaptive behavior, for example, alcohol abuse, fighting, and so on.	Promotes use of appropriate techniques for reducing anxiety while avoiding harm to self and others.
• Provide at least 20 to 30 minutes every 4 hours while awake for focus on anxiety reduction. List times here. ○ Encourage patient to express feelings verbally and through activity. ○ Answer questions truthfully. ○ Offer realistic reassurance and positive feedback.	Provides opportunity for practice of technique and expression of anxiety-provoking experiences.

- Collaborate with psychiatric nurse clinician regarding care. (See section on Mental Health).

  Collaboration helps to provide holistic care; specialist may discover underlying events for anxiety and assist in designing an alternate plan of care.

- Refer to and collaborate with appropriate community resources. (See Appendix B.)

  Support groups can provide ongoing assistance after discharge.

Child Health

Actions/Interventions	Rationales
• Review with the child and parents coping measures used for daily changes and crises.	The identification of coping strategies will provide essential information to deal with anxiety. Once identified, the nurse can begin to evaluate those strategies that are effective. A major starting point is to describe the feelings and attempt to create a sense of control. In younger infants, rocking is a means of providing soothing repetitive motion when all other measures seem to fail. Allowing the child to plan for meals or snacks with choices when possible or structuring the room to offer a sense of self is conducive to empowerment.
• Identify ways parents can help child to cope with anxiety; for example, setting realistic demands, avoid bribing, telling the truth.	
• Adapt routine, such as meals or putting up posters, to best help child regain control; for example, use a simple but firm speech pattern.	
• Modify procedures, as possible, to help reduce anxiety; for example, do not use intramuscular injections when an oral route is possible.	Unnecessary pain or invasive procedures make overwhelming demands on the already stressed hospitalized child.
• Use child's developmental needs as a basis for care, especially for ventilation of anxiety. Use age-appropriate toys or games.	The developmental level of the patient serves to guide the nurse in care. A holistic approach is more likely to meet health needs. Appropriate time in preparation offers structure and allows focused attention, which empowers and helps reduce anxiety as efforts are directed to what is known.
• Allow child and parents adequate time and opportunities to handle required care issues and thus reduce anxiety; when painful treatments must be done, prepare all involved according to an agreed-upon plan.	
• Encourage family to assist with care as appropriate, including feeding, comfort measures, stories, and so on.	Family involvement provides a sense of empowerment and growth in coping, thereby reducing anxiety and promoting a sense of security in the child.
• Offer sufficient opportunities for rest according to age and sleep requirements.	Proper attention to rest for each individual child will best foster coping capacities by conserving energy for coping.
• Identify knowledge needs and address these by having family explain what they understand about treatments, procedures, needs, and so on.	Allows teaching opportunity that increases patient's and family's knowledge about situation, thus assisting in reducing anxiety.

Continued

Actions/Interventions	Rationales
• Point out and reinforce successes in conquering anxiety.	Positive reinforcement assists in learning.
• Assist patient and family to apply coping to future potential anxiety-producing situations by presenting possible scenarios that would call for new skills: "What if someone pushes ahead of you in line? How should you act if a salesperson is rude?"	Allows practice in a nonanxiety-producing environment; increases skill in using coping strategy; empowers patient and family.

Women's Health

Actions/Interventions	Rationales
Acute Anxiety Attack	
• Provide a realistic, tranquil atmosphere; for example, close door, sit with patient, remind patient you are there to help: ◦ Do not leave the patient alone. ◦ Speak softly using short, simple commands. ◦ Be firm but kind. ◦ Be prepared to make decisions for the patient. ◦ Decrease external stimuli and provide a "safe" atmosphere.	Provides an atmosphere that helps to calm patient and promotes the initiation of coping by the patient.
• Administer antianxiety medication as ordered and monitor effectiveness of medication within 30 minutes of administration.	
Mild or Moderate Anxiety	
• Guide the patient through problem solving related to the anxiety: ◦ Help the patient to verbalize and describe what she thinks is going to happen. ◦ Describe (to the best of your ability) to the patient what will happen and compare with her expectations. ◦ Assist the patient in describing ways she can more clearly express her needs.	
• Help the patient to correct unrealistic expectations by explaining procedures, for example, labor process or sensations during a pelvic exam.	By clarifying misconceptions and providing factual information and support, the nurse enhances the patient's coping abilities.[24]
• Encourage the patient to participate in assertiveness training.	

Pregnancy and Childbirth

- Provide the patient and significant others with factual information about the physical and emotional changes experienced during pregnancy.
- Review daily schedule with the patient and significant other. Assist them to identify life-style adjustments that may be needed for coping with pregnancy.
  - Practicing relaxation techniques when stress begins to build
  - Establishing a routine for relaxing after work
- Refer to a support group, for example, childbirth education classes, MCH nurses in the community.
- Provide the patient and significant other with factual information about sexual changes during pregnancy:
  - Answer questions promptly and factually.
  - Meet people who have had similar experiences.
  - Discuss fears about sexual changes.
  - Discuss aspects of sexuality and intercourse during pregnancy:
    (1) Positions for intercourse during different stages of pregnancy
    (2) Frequency of intercourse
    (3) Effect of intercourse on pregnancy or fetus
  - Describe healing process postpartum and timing of resumption of intercourse.
- Provide patient support during birthing process, for example, Montrice, support person, coach.
- Provide support for significant others during this process:
  - Encourage verbalization of fears.
  - Answer questions factually.
  - Demonstrate equipment.
  - Explain procedures.

Factual information provides the family with the essential knowledge needed in planning for the pregnancy, accomplishing the task of pregnancy, and adapting to a new infant.

Helps to reduce anxiety; increases coping.

Support of significant others leads to more support for patient.

Mental Health

Actions/Interventions	Rationales
• Provide a quiet, nonstimulating environment. For the client experiencing severe or panic anxiety this may be a seclusion setting.	Inappropriate levels of sensory stimuli can contribute to the client's sense of disorganization and confusion.
• Provide frequent, brief interactions that assist the client with orientation. Verbal information should be provided in simple, brief sentences.	Appropriate levels of sensory stimuli promote the client's sense of control.
• If the client is experiencing severe or panic anxiety, provide support in a nondemanding atmosphere.	Communicates acceptance of the client and facilitates the development of trust and self-esteem.
• If the client is experiencing severe or panic anxiety, provide a here-and-now focus.	High levels of anxiety decrease the client's ability to process information.
• Provide the client with a simple repetitive activity until anxiety decreases to the level at which learning can begin.	High levels of anxiety decrease the client's ability to solve problems; promotes client's sense of control.
• If the client is hyperventilating, help him or her to take slow, deep breaths. If necessary, breathe along with the client and provide ongoing, positive reinforcement.	Reestablishes a normal breathing pattern and promotes the client's sense of control.
• Approach the client in a calm, reassuring manner, assessing the caregiver's level of anxiety and keeping this to a minimum.	Anxiety is contagious and can be communicated from the social network to the client.
• Provide a constant, one-on-one interaction for the client experiencing severe or panic anxiety. This should preclude use of physical restraints, which tend to increase the client's anxiety.	Presence of a calm, trusted individual can promote a sense of control in the client.
• Provide the client with alternative outlets for physical tension. This should be stated specifically and could include walking, running, talking with a staff member, using a punching bag, listening to music, doing a deep muscle relaxation sequence (number) times per day at (state specific times). The outlet should be selected with the client's input.	Promotes the client's sense of control and begins the development of alternative, more adaptive coping behaviors.
• Sit with the client (number) times per day at (times) for (number) minutes to discuss feelings and complaints. As the client expresses these openly, the nurse can then explore the onset of the anxiety with the purpose of identifying the sources of the anxiety.	Identification of precipitating factors is the first step in developing alternative coping behaviors and promoting client's sense of control.

- After the source of the anxiety has been identified, the time set aside above can be used to assist the client in developing alternative coping styles.

Promotes the client's sense of control.

- Provide (number) times per day to discuss with the client interests in the external environment (especially with those clients who tend to focus strongly on nonspecific physical complaints).

Provides positive reinforcement through the nurse's attention for improved coping behaviors.

- Talk with the client about the advantages and disadvantages of the current condition. Help the client to identify secondary gain from the symptoms. This would be done in the individual discussion sessions or in group therapy when a trusting relationship has been developed.

Identification of contributing factors is the first step in developing alternative coping behaviors.

- Provide the client with feedback on how his or her behavior affects others. This could be done in an individual or group situation.

Assists client with consensual validation.

- Provide positive feedback as appropriate on changed behavior. The target behavior and goals should be listed here.

Positive feedback encourages behavior and enhances self-esteem.

- Provide appropriate behavioral limits to control the expression of aggression or anger. These limits should be specific to the client and listed here on the care plan; for example, "Client will be asked to go to seclusion room for 15 minutes when he raises his voice to another client." The client should be informed of these limits, which should not exceed the client's capability. The client should be informed of the extent of the limits, for example, "15 minutes." No limit should be set for an indefinite time. All staff should be aware of the limits so that they can be enforced consistently with consistent consequences.

Client safety is of primary importance.

- Provide the client with an opportunity to discuss the situation after the consequences have been met.

Assists client with an opportunity to review behavioral limits and provides the staff with an opportunity to communicate to the client that limit setting is not a punishment. Promotes the development of a trusting relationship.

- Interact with the client in social activities (number) times per day for (number) minutes. This will provide the client with staff time other than that which is used to set limits. The activities selected should be done with the client's input and stated here in the care plan.

Continued

Actions/Interventions	Rationales
• Provide medication as ordered and observe for appropriate side effects (list here).	
• Inform the client of community resources that provide assistance with crisis situations, and provide a phone number before the client leaves the unit.	Promotes the client's sense of control and self-esteem.
• Develop a list of alternative coping strategies that the client can use at home, and have the client practice them before leaving the unit.	Repeated practice of a behavior internalizes and personalizes the behavior.
• Provide the client with a written list of appointments that have been scheduled for outpatient follow-up.	Provides visible documentation of the importance of follow-up; increases likelihood that appointments will be kept.

Gerontic Health

Actions/Interventions	Rationales
• Monitor daily for side effects of antianxiety agents if prescribed.	The potential for side effects and drug interactions is increased with older adults owing to the decreased metabolism of drugs.
• Identify environmental factors that may increase anxiety, such as noise level, harsh lighting, and high traffic flow.	The environmental factors mentioned, if not addressed, induce more stress in the older individual.
• Provide direct, basic information on usual routines and procedures.	May help decrease autonomic nervous system activity and feelings of anxiety.

Home Health

Actions/Interventions	Rationales
• Teach the client and family appropriate monitoring of signs and symptoms of anxiety: ○ Increased pulse ○ Sleep disturbance ○ Fatigue ○ Restlessness ○ Increased respiratory rate ○ Inability to concentrate ○ Short attention span ○ Feeling of dread ○ Faintness ○ Forgetfulness	Provides baseline data for early recognition and intervention.

• Involve the client and family in planning and implementing strategies to reduce and cope with anxiety:	Family and client involvement enhances effectiveness of intervention.
○ *Family conference*: Identify sources of anxiety and interventions designed to decrease anxiety.	
○ *Mutual goal setting*: Identify specific ways to decrease anxiety and specific roles of each family member.	
○ *Communication*: Promote open and honest communication between family members.	
• Assist the client and family in life-style adjustments that may be required:	Lifestyle changes require changes in behavior. Self-evaluation and support facilitate these changes.
○ Relaxation techniques; for example, yoga, biofeedback, hypnosis, breathing techniques, imagery	
○ Problem-solving techniques	
○ Crisis intervention	
○ Maintaining the treatment plan of health care professionals who are guiding the therapy	
○ Redirecting energy to meaningful or productive activities, for example, active games and hobbies, walking, sports	
○ Decreasing sensory stimulation	
• Help the client and family to determine when the intervention of a health care professional is required, for example, when client is unable to perform activities of daily living or is a threat to self or others	Early identification of issues requiring professional evaluation will increase the probability of successful interventions.
• Teach the client and family the purposes, side effects, and proper administration techniques of medications.	Provides necessary information for self-care.
• Consult with or refer to community resources as indicated. (See Appendix B.)	Promotes efficient use of existing community services.

FLOW CHART EVALUATION
Flow Chart Expected Outcome 1

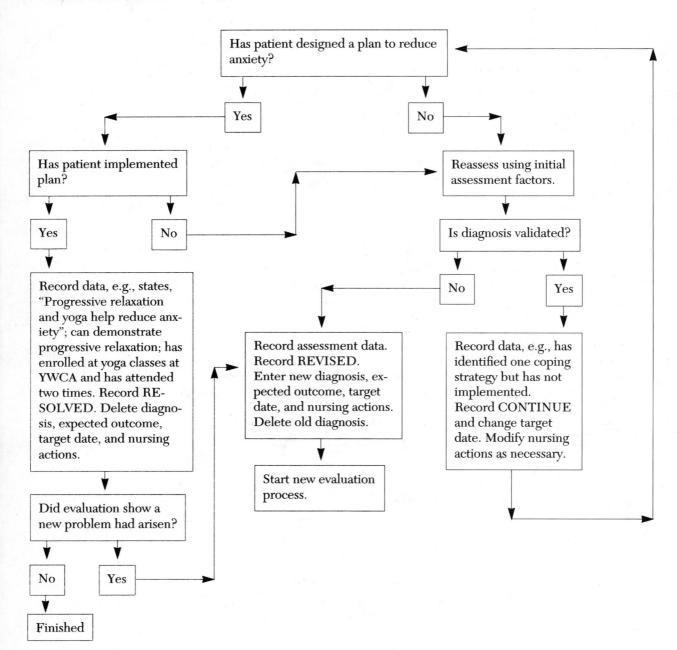

Flow Chart Expected Outcome 2

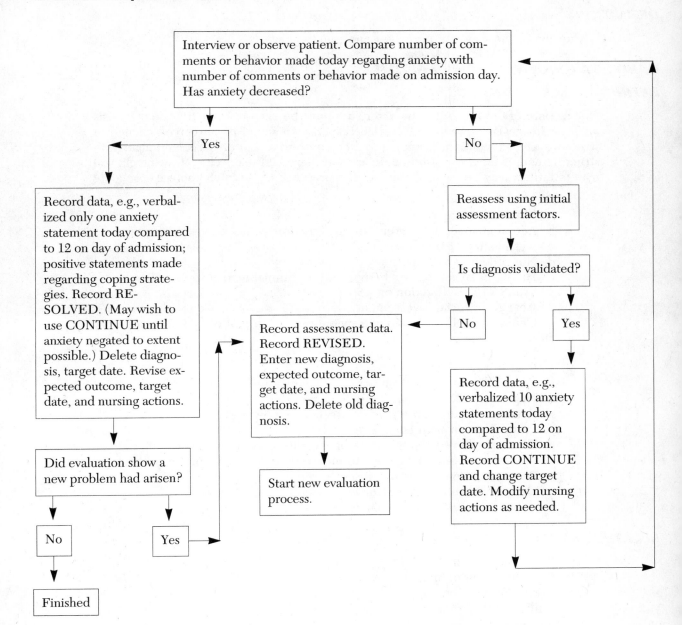

Body Image Disturbance

DEFINITION

Disruption in the way one perceives one's body image.[23]

NANDA TAXONOMY: PERCEIVING 7.1.1

DEFINING CHARACTERISTICS[23]

One or both of the following characteristics must be present to justify the diagnosis of Body Image Disturbance: (1) verbal response to actual or perceived change in structure and/or function; (2) nonverbal response to actual or perceived change in structure and/or function. (*Note*: Both are considered critical.) The following clinical manifestations may be used to validate the presence of these characteristics.

1. Objective:
   a. Missing body part
   b. Actual change in structure and/or function
   c. Not looking at body part
   d. Not touching body part
   e. Hiding or overexposing body part (intentional or unintentional)
   f. Trauma to nonfunctioning part
   g. Change in social involvement
   h. Change in ability to estimate spatial relationship of body to environment
2. Subjective:
   a. Verbalization of change in life-style
   b. Fear of rejection by others
   c. Focus on past strength, function, or appearance
   d. Negative feelings about body
   e. Feelings of helplessness, hopelessness, or powerlessness
   f. Preoccupation with change or loss
   g. Emphasis on remaining strengths, heightened achievement
   h. Extension of body boundary to incorporate environmental objects
   i. Personalization of part or loss by name
   j. Depersonalization of part or loss by impersonal pronouns
   k. Refusal to verify actual change

RELATED FACTORS

1. Biophysical
2. Cognitive, perceptual
3. Psychosocial
4. Cultural
5. Spiritual

RELATED CLINICAL CONCERNS

1. Amputation
2. Mastectomy
3. Acne or other visible skin disorders
4. Visible scarring from surgery or burns
5. Obesity
6. Anorexia nervosa

HAVE YOU SELECTED THE CORRECT DIAGNOSIS?

Self-Esteem Disturbance   This diagnosis addresses the lack of confidence in one's self and is characterized by negative self-statements, lack of concern about personal appearance, and withdrawal from others not related to physical problems or attributes. Body Image Disturbance relates to alterations in the perceptions of self owing to actual or perceived alterations in body structure or function. (See page 668.)

Personal Identity Disturbance   Personal Identity Disturbance is defined as the inability to distinguish between self and nonself. This diagnosis is more involved in the mental health arena. Body Image Disturbance is a reaction to an actual or perceived change in the body structure or function and incorporates the adult health area as well as mental health. (See page 651.)

EXPECTED OUTCOMES

1. Will verbalize at least (number) positive body image statements by (date) and/or
2. Will identify at least (number) measures to overcome body part loss by (date)

TARGET DATES

A target date of 3 to 5 days would be acceptable to use for initial evaluation of progress.

NURSING ACTIONS/INTERVENTIONS WITH RATIONALES

Adult Health

Actions/Interventions	Rationales
• Monitor for pain every 2 hours on the (odd/even) hour. Administer analgesics, monitor effectiveness of analgesic within 30 minutes of administration, and use noninvasive techniques to keep pain under control.	Uncontrolled pain contributes significantly to problems with body functioning, thus promoting the development and continuation of body image disturbance.
• Use anxiety-reducing techniques as often as needed.	Helps the patient to adapt to the changed body image.
• Stay in frequent contact with the patient:	Promotes verbalization of feelings and allows consistent intervention.
○ Be honest with patient.	Any dishonesty in terms of recovery, return of function, or rehabilitation needs causes patient to distrust caregivers and promotes maintenance of body image disturbance.
○ Point out and limit self-negation statements.	Self-negating statements prolong the problem and interfere with rehabilitation potential.

Continued

Actions/Interventions	Rationales
○ Do not support denial. ○ Focus on reality and adaptation (not necessarily acceptance). ○ Set limits on maladaptive behavior. ○ Focus on realistic goals. ○ Be aware of own nonverbal communication and behavior. ○ Avoid moral value judgments. • Assist and encourage patient to look at and use affected body part during activities of daily living. • Promote calm, safe environment throughout hospitalization. • Collaborate with psychiatric nurse clinician regarding care as needed. (See section on Mental Health.) • Teach patient and significant others self-care requirements. • Encourage patient to use available resources: ○ Prosthetic devices ○ Assistive devices ○ Reconstructive and corrective surgery ○ Occupational therapy ○ Physical therapy ○ Rehabilitation services • Refer to and collaborate with community resources. (See Appendix B.)	The patient does not have to accept the problem but he or she does have to, and can, adapt to the problem. Maladaptive behavior supports the continuation of body image disturbance. Supports continued progress, allows positive feedback for achievement, and permits patient to see progress. Any avoidance behavior or nonverbal communication that indicates dismay would support the patient's idea of his or her unacceptability as a damaged person. Helps patient to attend to altered body image constructively and accept self. When using adaptive equipment, the patient's safety must be foremost. A calm environment allows the patient to focus on working with the equipment or techniques without undue pressure. Collaboration promotes a holistic care plan and hastens problem solving. Helps patient to adapt to body change and improves self-care management; provides support for self-care and helps significant others to adapt also. Facilitates adaptation and decreases isolation; provides long-term support. Provides long-term support and cost-effective use of existing support.

Child Health

Actions/Interventions	Rationales
• Monitor for contributory factors for Body Image Disturbance, for example, disfigurement or perceived disfigurement. (Family may perceive such on behalf of the young infant/child.)	Provides database needed to more accurately planned interventions.

Actions/Interventions	Rationales
• Utilize developmentally appropriate communication to assess and determine exact expression of Body Image Disturbance, for example, puppet play or constructive dialogue with the toddler.	Developmental capacity has to guide the interaction to gain accurate information.
• Provide factual information to assist in dealing with Body Image Disturbance, for example, availability of assistive devices, surgery.	Knowledge serves to reduce anxiety and assists patient to cope; provides options to assist in decision making.
• Involve occupational, physical, speech, or other therapists as required.	Promotes a more accurate and holistic plan of care.
• Monitor, on a daily basis, for attitude toward body.	Allows daily evaluation, which promotes changes in plan of care to best meet patient's current status.

NOTE: In some instances, such as an infant or child with an anomaly or a condition offering no hope of resolution, this alteration may accompany other disturbances such as self-esteem, parental coping, and loss.

Women's Health

Actions/Interventions	Rationales
Body Image: Surgery	
• Assist the patient to identify life-style adjustments that may be needed, for example, recuperation time, prosthesis as necessary.	Initiates discharge planning.
• Monitor the patient's anxiety level and discuss, preoperatively:	
○ *Routines related to surgery*: for example, anesthesia, pain, length of surgery, postoperative care	
○ *Physical changes*: for example, cessation of menstruation, menopausal symptoms	
• Allow the patient to grieve for loss and provide an empathetic atmosphere that will allow the patient to ventilate concerns about appearance or reaction of significant others.	
• Dispel "old wives' tales" (usually connected to hysterectomy), such as:	
○ You will no longer feel like a woman (reassure patient that while there will be no more pregnancies or menstruation, hysterectomy does not affect sexual performance, enjoyment, or response).	

Continued

Actions/Interventions	Rationales
○ There will be masculinization (no basis for this belief; does not occur).	
○ There will be weight gain (will not occur if patient follows former life style and participates in an exercise routine and follows proper diet).	
• Involve significant others in discussion and problem-solving activities regarding life-cycle changes that might affect self-esteem and interpersonal relationships, for example, hot flashes, appearance, sexual relationships, ability to have children.	Provides basic information and allows early intervention for anxiety; provides opportunity for teaching and clarification of misinformation.[25]
• In collaboration with physician provide factual information on estrogen replacement therapy.	Assists patient in making decision regarding use or nonuse of estrogen therapy.
Body Image: Pregnancy	
• Assist the patient in identifying life-style adjustments owing to physiologic, physical, and emotional changes that will occur throughout pregnancy and postpartum.	Knowledge that body changes in pregnancy are normal and temporary encourages patient to follow through on care. Helps the patient to cope with the pregnancy and adapt to the changing images.
• Review with patient the body changes that occur during pregnancy and the effect on body image (particularly for teenagers):	
○ Weight gain	
○ Breast tenderness and enlargement	
○ Enlargement of abdomen	
○ Change in gait	
○ Chloasma (mask of pregnancy)	
○ Striations (stretch marks) from pregnancy	
• Consider the patient's age and preparation for pregnancy, including (particularly for teenagers):	Continued home care planning encourages follow-up care.
○ Stress weight loss after delivery usually takes 1 or 2 weeks.	
○ Physical development.	
○ Attitude toward health care providers.	
○ Self-esteem.	
○ Emotional support.	
○ Life-style interruptions.	
○ Encourage the patient to bring an attractive, loose-fitting dress to wear home.	
○ Caution breast-feeding women against purposeful weight loss while lactating.	
○ Encourage nonbreast-feeding mothers to follow low-calorie, high-protein diet for weight loss.	

- ○ Encourage exercise (begin slowly and work up to desired plan).
- ○ Avoid fatigue.

Mental Health

Actions/Interventions	Rationales
• Spend (number) minutes with the client at (times) discussing perception of disruption in life-style necessitated by change.	Promotes client's sense of control and provides information that can be utilized in developing a plan of care that will fit within the client's perception of self.
• Discuss with the client meaning of loss or change from a personal and cultural perspective.	Expression of feelings in an accepting environment can facilitate the client's problem solving.
• Discuss with the client significant others' reaction to loss or change.	Understanding from support system can facilitate the client's adjustment.
• Set an appointment to discuss with the client and significant others effects of the loss or change on their relationships. Time and date of appointment and all follow-up appointments should be listed here.	Expression of feelings and concerns in an accepting environment can facilitate problem solving.
• Spend (number) minutes with the client at (times) to assist with efforts to enhance appearance.	Promotes client's sense of control and enhances self-esteem.
• Provide physical activities two times per day at (times) that provide the client opportunities to define boundaries of body. These activities should be ones the client identifies as enjoyable and that are easily accomplished by the client. Those activities that are selected should be listed here. If this diagnosis is in conjunction with an eating disorder, adjust exercise to appropriate levels for the client.	Assists client in developing a new perception of body.
• Discuss with the client the difference between the cultural ideal of physical appearance and the population norm based on the realities of physiology. This activity should be done by the primary care nurse who has developed a relationship with the client.	Helps to promote reality orientation by contrasting real with ideal and confronts irrational goals.
• Have the client draw a picture of self before and after body change and discuss this with client. This activity can also be done with clay models constructed by the client. This activity should be done by the	Assists client in contrasting and externalizing perceptions of self to facilitate development of congruence between real and ideal.

Continued

Actions/Interventions	Rationales
primary care nurse who has developed a relationship with the client.	
• Have the eating disorder client draw a life-size picture of self on paper hung on the wall; then have the client stand against the picture and trace the real outline and discuss the difference. This activity should be done by the primary care nurse who has developed a relationship with the client.	Assists clients in confronting the difference between their perception of their body and their real body size and shape.
• When the client has begun to discuss issues related to body change with the primary care nurse, the client can then be asked to discuss reactions to image of self in a mirror. One hour should be allowed for this activity. This activity should be done by the primary care nurse who has developed a relationship with the client.	Facilitates the development of a congruence between real and perceived self.
• Discuss with the client the mental images held of what the altered body is like and what life will be like. One hour should be allowed for this activity and it should be implemented by the primary care nurse after a relationship has been established.	Discussion of concerns in a safe environment facilitates the development of strategies of coping.

Gerontic Health

See Adult Health.

Home Health

Actions/Interventions	Rationales
• Involve client and family in planning and implementing strategies to reduce and cope with disturbance in body image: ○ *Family conference*: Discuss meaning of loss or change from family perspective and from perspective of individual members. Discuss the effects of the loss on family relationships and roles. ○ *Mutual goal setting*: Establish realistic goals and identify specific activities for each family member, for example, assistance with activities as required, attendance at support groups as needed.	Family involvement enhances effectiveness of interventions.

○ *Communication*: Clarify responses to Body Image Disturbance.

- Assist the client and family in life-style adjustments that may be required:
  ○ Obtaining and providing accurate information regarding specific Body Image Disturbance and potential for rehabilitation
  ○ Maintaining safe environment
  ○ Encouraging appropriate self-care without encouraging dependence or expecting unrealistic independence
  ○ Maintaining the treatment plan of the health care professionals guiding therapy
  ○ Altering family roles as required

Rehabilitation is a long-term process. Permanent changes in behavior and family roles require evaluation and support.

- Consult with or refer to community resources as indicated. (See Appendix B.)

Use of existing community services is efficient. Rehabilitation therapists and support groups can enhance the treatment plan.

FLOW CHART EVALUATION
Flow Chart Expected Outcome 1

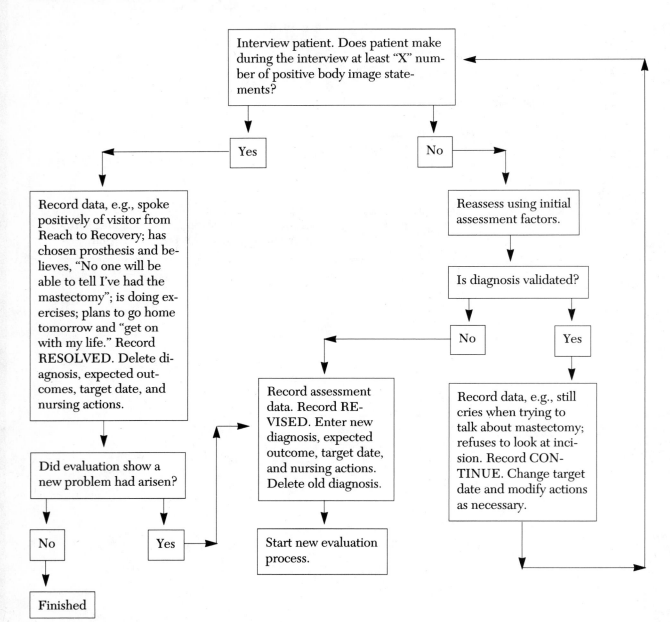

Flow Chart Expected Outcome 2

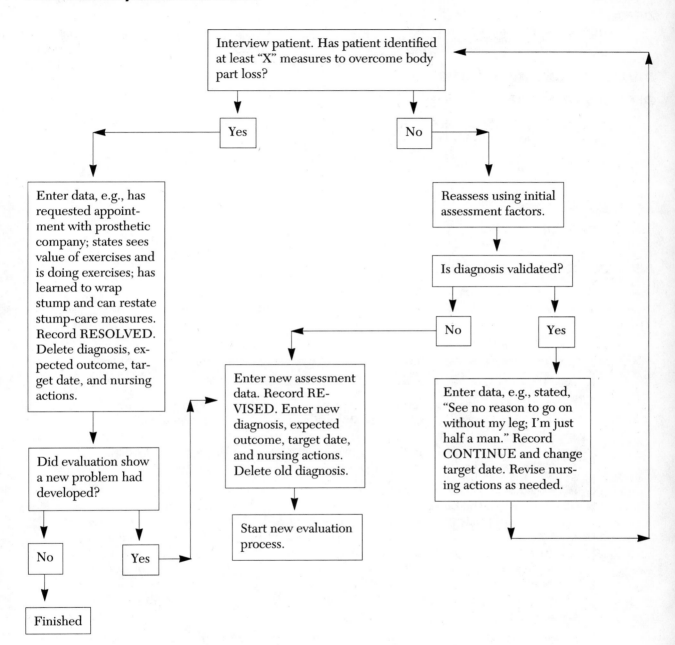

Fear

DEFINITION

Feeling of dread related to an identifiable source that the person validates.[23]

NANDA TAXONOMY: FEELING 9.3.2

DEFINING CHARACTERISTICS[23]

1. Major defining characteristic:
   a. Ability to identify object of fear
2. Minor defining characteristics:
   None given

RELATED FACTORS[23]

To be developed.

RELATED CLINICAL CONCERNS

1. Any hospitalization
2. Any threat of loss of a body part, loss of functioning, or loss of life

HAVE YOU SELECTED THE CORRECT DIAGNOSIS?

Anxiety   Anxiety is the response to a threat that cannot be easily identified, while Fear is the response to an identified threat. Thus, if the individual is responding to the thought of a bear in the woods or actually confronting the bear, the diagnosis is Fear. If the threat cannot be directly identified or attached to a specific situation, the diagnosis is Anxiety. (See page 605.)

Altered Parenting   This diagnosis should be considered as the appropriate diagnosis when the child's fears result from the parent's modeling or reinforcing of a child's fear or when the parent is not providing the appropriate support for the developmental fears. An example might be the child who becomes uncontrollable in the clinic each time an injection is indicated. During the assessment the nurse discovers that the parents tell their children that if they do not behave the nurse or doctor will give them a shot as a reinforcer to discipline at home. In this situation the parent's inappropriate use of the threat of the injection produces fear in the child. (See page 742.)

Knowledge Deficit   If patients indicate that they are afraid they cannot care for themselves, then the most appropriate diagnosis would be Knowledge Deficit. Providing the patient with information and teaching self-care will overcome this diagnosis. (See page 536.)

EXPECTED OUTCOMES

1. Will design and implement a plan to reduce fear by (date) and/or
2. Will be able to identify specific source of fear by (date)

TARGET DATE

A target date of 2 to 3 days would be acceptable, since the sooner the fear can be reduced, the sooner other problems can be resolved.

NURSING ACTIONS/INTERVENTIONS WITH RATIONALES

Adult Health

Actions/Interventions	Rationales
• Assist patient to correct any sensory deficits.	Inability to correctly sense and perceive stimuli may increase fear.

• Maintain calm, safe environment throughout the hospitalization:
  ○ Use frequent reassurance.
  ○ Touch patient frequently.
  ○ Have someone remain with patient.
	A nonthreatening environment decreases fear.

• Administer antianxiety medications as ordered. Observe and record response to medication within 30 minutes after administration.	Determines effectiveness of medication and allows medication to be changed as needed.

• At least every 4 hours while awake, monitor:
  ○ Vital signs
  ○ Degree of confusion
  ○ Degree of reality orientation
	Determines physiologic changes due to fear; assists in determining if physiologic changes are causing pathology.

• Provide information to patient in both written and verbal forms.	Fear interferes with interpretation of verbal input; written forms provide reinforcement and assist patient to focus and attend to activities.

• Sit down and visit with patient at least 15 to 20 minutes every 4 hours while awake:
  ○ Listen carefully.
  ○ Support positive coping.
  ○ Give clear, concise, straightforward information.
	Provides an opportunity for patient to ask questions and verbalize fears.

• Assist patient to increase development of decision-making skills:
  ○ Review decision-making process with patient.
  ○ Provide opportunity for decision making regarding care.
  ○ Assist patient in developing a list of potential solutions to the threatening situation.
	Helps patient to practice, in a nonthreatening environment, the problem-solving process; increases feeling of personal control of situation.

Continued

Actions/Interventions	Rationales
○ Review the developed list of solutions with the patient and assist in evaluating the benefits and costs of each solution. ○ Rehearse with the patient, if necessary, the solution selected, or have patient practice a new response to the threatening situation. ○ Give positive feedback regarding decision making. ○ Involve significant others in promoting patient's decision making. • Collaborate with psychiatric nurse clinician regarding care. (See section on Mental Health.) • Teach patient and significant others: ○ Use of progressive relaxation and guided imagery ○ Use of exercise balanced with rest ○ Proper food and fluid intake • Refer to appropriate community resources for assistance. (See Appendix B.)	 Collaboration promotes a holistic and more total plan of care. Gives additional methods that are successful in dealing with fear. Provides support resources for follow-up on plan after discharge from the hospital.

Child Health

Actions/Interventions	Rationales
• Offer brief interactions that assist the patient and family with orientation, for example, hospital unit, procedures, aspects of care. • In instances of severe fear: ○ Provide support in a nondemanding atmosphere. ○ Provide a here-and-now focus. ○ Provide one-on-one care. ○ Offer simple, direct, repetitive tasks. • Provide patient and family with alternative outlets for physical tension. (This should be stated specifically and could include walking, talking, and so on.) Do this at least (number) times per day at (times). These outlets should be designed with input from patient.	Brief explanations and factual information serve to empower the patient and family as the unknown is made known. The patient and family can then focus on dealing with the identified fear rather than dealing with added fears. Avoids overwhelming patient; promotes a sense of trust. Providing such outlets promotes release of tension.

- Sit with the patient and parents (number) times per day at (times) for (number) minutes to discuss feelings and complaints.

As the patient and parents express these factors openly, the nurse can explore the possible onset of fear with the purpose of individualizing the plan according to patient's needs. The subjective verbalization of fears helps to reduce the preoccupation of the patient with the fear.
Reflection on an ongoing basis demonstrates a sensitivity to need.

- Provide feedback to patient and parents to clarify and reexplore changes regarding feelings about fear.
- Provide appropriate behavioral limits to control the expression of aggression or anger. (These limits should be specific in terms of time, expected behavior, and consequences.)

Structured rules regarding behavioral consequences provide a sense of limit setting that provides security for the child.

- Provide the patient and parents with opportunities to discuss the situation after consequences have been met.
- Provide opportunities for socialization appropriate for patient and family.

Rediscussing and clarification of events serves to update needs and provides feedback for evaluation. Valuing of the patient is also shown.
Socialization is vital as the individual and family assume coping behaviors and learn new coping skills.

- Develop a list of alternative coping strategies to be practiced by patient and family before dismissal, for example, communication, progressive relaxation.
- Ensure follow-up by scheduling appointments for patient before discharge.
- Assist patient and family to view situation represented as something which can be managed. Encourage positive reinforcement of desired behavior patterns.

Allows practice in a nonthreatening environment; increases skills.

Follow-up appointments help ensure follow-up care.
Validation of success in coping will provide a sense of empowerment.

Women's Health

NOTE: Phobias affect approximately 2 to 3 percent of the adult population, and 80 percent of the affected group are female. The most common phobias among women are agoraphobia, fear of animals, and fear of social situations.[26,27]

Actions/Interventions	Rationales

- Obtain a detailed history of patient's fears:
  ○ Encourage patient to discuss signs and symptoms or precipitating event.
  ○ Ascertain how often problem occurs.
  ○ Have patient describe her reaction.
  ○ Identify coping mechanisms that have previously helped.
	Provides essential database for planning appropriate interventions.

Continued

Actions/Interventions	Rationales
○ Identify those factors or coping mechanisms that do not help.	
• Provide a comfortable, nonjudgmental atmosphere to encourage the patient and her significant other to verbalize their fears of: ○ The unknown ○ Safety for herself and her baby ○ Pain during the birthing process ○ Mutilation during the birthing process ○ Loss of control during the birthing process	Assists in decreasing fear through promotion of verbalization.
• Refer patient to appropriate support groups for information: ○ Childbirth education classes in the community ○ Schools of nursing (students in obstetrics who follow up on families of pregnant women) ○ Special national organizations (see Appendix B)	Provides effective use of existing resources and long-range support.
• Monitor patient's level of confidence using prepared childbirth techniques during labor: ○ Encourage use of relaxation and prepared childbirth techniques during labor. ○ Provide ongoing and accurate information, during the labor and birth process, to both the patient and her significant other. ○ Assist patient in using imagery to overcome fears during the birthing process.	Use of relaxation techniques and provision of information regarding progress facilitates the labor process by easing anxiety and promoting comfort.[25]
• Provide continuity of care by remaining with and providing comfort for the laboring woman throughout the birthing process: ○ Provide clear answers to patient's questions. ○ Keep patient informed of her progress in the birthing process.	Encourages involvement in process, which enhances coping.
• Provide the patient and significant other with as many opportunities as possible to make decisions about her care during the birthing process.	

Mental Health

Actions/Interventions	Rationales
• Provide a quiet, nonstimulating environment for the client. This would include removing persons and objects that the person perceives as threatening. If the person is experiencing a thought disorder with delusions and hallucinations, attention should be paid to the details of the environment that could be misinterpreted. At times, a same-sex caregiver can increase fear in the client.	Inappropriate levels of environmental stimuli can increase disorientation and confusion.
• Obtain the clients' understanding of the threat.	Facilitates the development of interventions that directly address the client's concerns.
• Provide a one-on-one relationship for the client with a member of the nursing staff. This should be maintained until the symptoms return to normal levels.	Promotes a trusting relationship and enhances the client's self-esteem.
• Provide clear answers to client's questions.	Inappropriate amounts of sensory stimuli can increase the client's confusion and disorganization.
• Carry on conversations in the client's presence or vision in a voice that the client can hear.	Meets safety needs of client by eliminating stimuli that could be misinterpreted in a personalized manner.
• Inform the client of plans related to care before the plans are implemented. If possible, discuss these with the client; for example, if it is necessary to move the client to another room or institution, the client should be informed of this change before it takes place.	Promotes the client's sense of control and enhances self-esteem.
• Orient the client to the environment.	Promotes safety needs by increasing the client's familiarity with the environment in the accompaniment of a trusted individual.
• Maintain a consistent environment and routine. Record client's daily routine here along with notes about client's special reactions to visitors and staff members.	Promotes the client's sense of safety and trust by maintaining consistency in the environment.
• Provide a primary care nurse for the client on each shift.	Promotes the development of a trusting relationship.
• Sit with the client (number) minutes (number) times per shift. Initially the times should reflect short, frequent contact. This can change with the client's needs.	Promotes the development of a trusting relationship. Interaction with the nurse can provide positive reinforcement and enhance self-esteem.
• Provide the client with objects in the environment that promote security. These may be symbolic items from home or religious objects. List significant ones here.	Meets the need for affiliation by providing meaningful objects to which the client is attached.[20]

Continued

Actions/Interventions	Rationales
• Note the client's desired personal space and respect these limits. The general guidelines should be stated here.	Communicates respect for the client while decreasing the client's anxiety by maintaining a comfortable personal space.
• Assist the client with sorting out the fearful situation by:	Communicates respect for the client while encouraging reality testing.
○ Recognizing that the experience is real for the client even though that is not your experience of the situation ("I can see that you are very upset; I can understand how those thoughts could make you fearful").	
○ Providing feedback about distorted thoughts ("No, I am not going to punish you; I am here to talk with you about your concerns").	
○ Encouraging client to develop an understanding of the threat by talking about it in specific terms and not vague generalizations ("When you say your family is out to get you, who and what do you mean?").	
○ Focusing conversations in the here and now. This would include information about the effects of the client's behavior on those around him or her, your experience of the client, your perceptions of the environment.	
○ Not arguing about client's perceptions; instead, provide feedback in the here and now with your perceptions of the situation. For example, the client tells you that you must have been angry with him or her because of the look you had on your face while reviewing the client's chart. Your response is, "I am not angry with you. When I was looking at your chart, I was thinking about the conversation we had this morning about your job.")	
• Provide the client with as many opportunities as possible to make decisions about his or her care and current situation.	Promotes the client's sense of control and enhances self-esteem.
• Assist the client in developing a list of potential solutions to the threatening situation.	Teaches client problem-solving skills while promoting the client's sense of control and strengths.
• Review developed list of solutions with the client and assist in evaluating the benefits and costs of each solution.	Facilitates the client's decision-making process.

- If necessary, rehearse with the client the solution selected, or have client practice a new response to the threatening situation.
- Provide positive feedback to the client about efforts to resolve the threatening situation.
- Assist the client in developing alternative outlets for the feelings generated by the threatening situation, and provide the opportunity for the use of these outlets. These would be noted in the chart so other staff members would be aware of them and could encourage their use when they notice the client's discomfort increasing.
- Assist the client in identifying early behavioral cues that indicate fear or a fearful situation.
- Encourage the client in alternative coping strategies developed by:
  - Providing the necessary environment
  - Providing the appropriate equipment
  - Spending time with the client doing the activity
  - Providing positive reinforcement for the use of the strategy (this could be verbal as well as with special privileges)
- If fear is related to a specific object or situation, teach the client to use deep muscle relaxation, and then teach this along with progressively real mental images of the threatening situation. This is for those situations that will not cause the client harm if they are approached, such as riding in elevators. Include other methods of relaxation such as music, deep breathing, thought stopping, fantasy, assertiveness training, audiotapes with relaxation images or sequences, yoga, hypnosis, and meditation.
- Explore ways to increase client's feeling of control in threatening situation. For example, a fear of elevators could be lessened by the client's only riding in elevators with emergency phones and only riding when he or she could stand near the phone. The fear may also indicate the client is feeling out of control in an unrelated area of his or her life. This should be explored and ways of increasing control

Rehearsal helps the client learn new skills through the use of feedback and modeling by the nurse.[28]
Positive feedback encourages behavior and enhances self-esteem.

Planned coping strategies facilitate the enactment of new behaviors when the client is experiencing stress.

Early recognition and intervention enhance the opportunities for new coping behaviors to be effective.
Promotes client's perception of control; positive reinforcement encourages behavior.

The relaxation response inhibits the activation of the autonomic nervous system's fight-or-flight response.

Continued

Actions/Interventions	Rationales
should be explored; for example, a woman's fear of driving could indicate that she feels out of control in her marriage, and increased assertive behavior with her husband can remove the fear.	
• If the method to increase control involves interactions with the health care team, these should be noted in specific terms on the client's chart.	Promotes the client's sense of control and enhances self-esteem.
• Assist the client in developing strategies to be used in the community after discharge, and role-play various situations with the client for at least 1 hour for at least 2 days.	Rehearsal provides opportunities for feedback and modeling from the nurse.

Gerontic Health

Actions/Interventions	Rationales
• Assist patient in identifying the source of fear—pain, death, loss of function—by scheduling at least 30 minutes twice a day at (times) to confer with patient about fear.	Identifying the source of fear enables the patient to develop a specific plan of action to reduce the fear.
• Assist the patient in determining what resources are available to enhance his or her coping skills.	Knowledge and use of appropriate resources aid in reducing fear-provoking experiences by increasing the patient's inventory of skills to deal with fear.

Home Health

Actions/Interventions	Rationales
• Teach the client and family appropriate monitoring of signs and symptoms of fear: ○ Increased pulse ○ Flushed face ○ Sweaty palms ○ Shortness of breath ○ Muscle tightness ○ Nausea, vomiting, diarrhea ○ Sleep disturbance ○ Fainting ○ Sweating ○ Urinary frequency, urgency ○ Crying	Provides baseline data for early recognition and intervention.

- Involve the client and family in planning and implementing strategies to reduce and cope with fear.

- Assist the client and family in life-style adjustments that may be required:
  - Relaxation techniques: yoga, biofeedback, hypnosis, breathing techniques, imagery
  - A secure environment: familiar objects and familiar people, predictable events with no surprises
  - Communication techniques: provide responses that reflect reality; orient to person, time, and place; explain activities; provide predictable and consistent situations; and maintain visual, auditory, and tactile contact
  - Problem-solving strategies
- Provide a sense of mastery (that is, accomplishable goals in secure environment).
- Maintain the treatment plan of the health care professional guiding the therapy.
- Help the patient and family to determine when the intervention of a health care professional is required; for example, prolonged nausea, vomiting or diarrhea, uncontrolled crying.
- Consult with or refer to community resources as indicated. (See Appendix B.)

Family involvement is important to insure success. Communication and mutual goal setting will increase the probability of positive outcome.
Life-style changes require changes in behavior. Self-evaluation and support facilitate these changes.

Early identification of situations requiring professional evaluation will increase the probability of successful interventions.

Provides efficient and cost-effective use of already available resources.

FLOW CHART EVALUATION
Flow Chart Expected Outcome 1

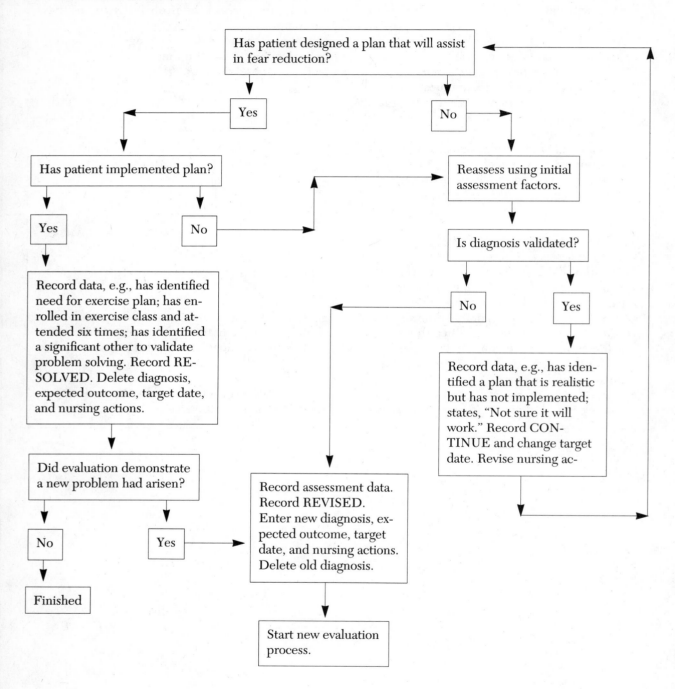

Flow Chart Expected Outcome 2

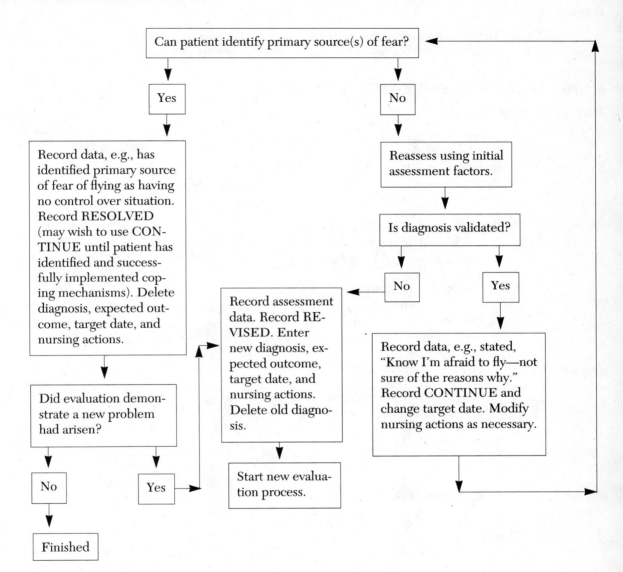

Hopelessness

DEFINITION

A subjective state in which an individual sees limited or no alternatives or personal choices available and is unable to mobilize energy on own behalf.[23]

NANDA TAXONOMY: PERCEIVING 7.3.1

DEFINING CHARACTERISTICS[23]

1. Major defining characteristics:
   a. Passivity, decreased verbalization
   b. Decreased affect
   c. Verbal cues (despondent content, "I can't," sighing)
2. Minor defining characteristics:
   a. Lack of initiative
   b. Decreased response to stimuli
   c. Decreased affect
   d. Turning away from speaker
   e. Closing eyes
   f. Shrugging in response to speaker
   g. Decreased appetite
   h. Increased or decreased sleep
   i. Lack of involvement in care or passivity in allowing care

RELATED FACTORS[23]

1. Prolonged activity restriction creating isolation
2. Failing or deteriorating physiologic condition
3. Long-term stress
4. Abandonment
5. Lost belief in transcendent values or God

RELATED CLINICAL CONCERNS

1. Any disease of a chronic nature
2. Any disease with a terminal diagnosis
3. Any condition where a diagnosis cannot be definitely established

HAVE YOU SELECTED THE CORRECT DIAGNOSIS?

Powerlessness This diagnosis is present when the individual perceives that his or her actions will not change a situation regardless of the options that the person may see in a situation. Hopelessness occurs when the individual perceives that there are few or limited choices in a situation. Powerlessness may evolve out of Hopelessness. Powerlessness is the perception that one's actions will not make a difference, while Hopelessness is the perception that there are no options to act upon. The decision about which is the most appropriate diagnosis is based on the clinical judgment of the nurse about which symptoms predominate. (See page 657.)

Anxiety Anxiety may have as a component a perception of Hopelessness. This could evolve out of the narrowed perception of the anxious client. Hopelessness may have Anxiety as a component. This situation could develop when the client is feeling overwhelmed with the perception that there are no alternatives in a difficult situation. The primary diagnosis evolves from the symptoms sequence. If Anxiety is the predominant symptom cluster, it should be the primary diagnosis because of the strong influence it has on the client's perceptions. (See page 605.)

Altered Thought Process If the individual cannot accurately assess the situation, then a sense of Hopelessness might occur. In this instance Hopelessness would be a companion diagnosis. (See page 577.)

Fear If the client is fearful in a situation, perception can be narrowed and alternative options may be overlooked. When Fear and Hopelessness occur together, Fear should be the primary diagnosis. (See page 628.)

EXPECTED OUTCOMES

1. Will initiate a realistic plan to reduce perception of hopelessness by (date) and/or
2. Will verbalize a decrease in complaints regarding hopelessness by (date)

TARGET DATE

A target date ranging between 3 and 5 days would be appropriate for initial evaluation. A target date over 5 days might lead to increased complications such as potential for self-injury. A target date sooner than 3 days would not provide a sufficient length of time for realizing the effects of intervention.

NURSING ACTIONS/INTERVENTIONS WITH RATIONALES

Adult Health

Actions/Interventions	Rationales
• Establish a therapeutic and trusting relationship with patient and family by actively listening, being nonjudgmental, sitting with patient, touching (as welcomed by patient), and so on.	Promotes a safe, empathetic environment to encourage the patient and/or family to verbalize concerns.
• Identify and deal with other primary nursing needs.	Inattention to basic needs increases feelings of hopelessness and worthlessness.
• Support patent's efforts to objectively describe feelings of hopelessness when interacting with patient.	Assists patient in releasing tension; allows patient to validate reality.
• Help the patient find alternatives to feelings of hopelessness.	Validates reality and encourages use of coping techniques; points out the variety of solutions available.

Continued

Actions/Interventions	Rationales
• Assist the patient to engage in social interaction at least once per shift.	Provides diversion and decreases sense of isolation.
• As health status permits, increase activity level. Have patient participate in self-care management, adding activities such as washing face one day, washing face and arms the next day, and so on; or have patient walk to bathroom first day and ambulate 30 feet down the hall the next day.	Encourages patient to regain control in small increments; decreases the idea that the personal self is responsible for the situation.
• Encourage food and fluid intake to at least 1500 calories per day and at least 2000 cc per day.	Hopelessness may result in unhealthy eating patterns.
• Moderate sleep-wake cycles: ○ Provide diversional activities during the day. ○ *Do not* let patient take naps during the day. ○ Provide massage at bedtime. ○ Darken the room but provide a night light for sleep. ○ Give sleep medication as ordered and monitor effects.	Maintains diurnal rhythm and promotes rest.
• Encourage active participation in activities of daily living. Allow for preferences in day-to-day decisions, for example, bath time. Provide explanations and appropriate teaching for procedures and treatments.	Helps restore sense of being in control.
• Refer to psychiatric nurse clinician as needed. (See section on Mental Health.)	Collaboration promotes a more holistic and complete plan of care.
• Identify religious, cultural, or community support groups prior to discharge. Provide appointments for follow-up.	Support groups can provide advocacy for the patient and continued monitoring and support after discharge from the hospital.

Child Health

Actions/Interventions	Rationales
• Monitor for the etiologic components contributing to hopelessness pattern.	Provides database that results in a more accurate and complete plan of care.
• Encourage patient and family to verbalize feelings about current status. Set aside 30 minutes each shift at (times) for this purpose.	Verbalization helps reduce anxiety and assigns value to the patient's concerns. Allows ongoing assessment.
• Help patient and family to explore growth potential afforded by this specific experience.	Opportunity for growth may be overlooked in times of crisis.
• Allow for opportunities for child to "play	Provides insight into child's coping

out" feelings under appropriate supervision if possible:
- ○ Play with dolls for toddler
- ○ Art and puppets for preschooler
- ○ Peer discussions for adolescents

mechanisms and perceptions in a noninvasive mode; provides valuable data to monitor feelings and concerns.

Women's Health

NOTE: The following nursing actions are for the couple who have been unable to conceive a child.

Actions/Interventions	Rationales
• Provide a nonjudgmental atmosphere to allow the infertile couple to express feelings such as anger, denial, inadequacy, guilt, depression, or grief.	Allows the couple to begin to deal with emotions and lays groundwork for future decision making.[25]
• Support and allow couple to work through grieving process for loss of fertility, loss of children, loss of idealized lifestyle, and loss of female life experiences such as pregnancy, birth, and breast-feeding.	
• Encourage couple to talk honestly with one another about feelings.	
• Encourage couple to seek professional help if necessary to deal with feelings related to sexual relationship, conflicts, anxieties, parenting, coping mechanisms used for dealing with loss of fertility (their own expectations and those of relatives and society).	Allows early intervention and helps avoid complications.
• Be alert for signs of depression, anger, frustration, impending crisis.	
• Provide infertile couples with accurate information on adoption and living without children.	Provides informational support for decision making.

Mental Health

Actions/Interventions	Rationales
• Monitor health care team's interactions with client for verbal and nonverbal behavior that would encourage the client not to be hopeful. If situations are identified, they should be noted here and	Negative attitudes from staff can be communicated to the client.

Continued

Actions/Interventions	Rationales
the team should discuss alternative ways of behaving. The actions needed to support the client's hope should be noted on the client's chart.	
• Sit with client (number) times per day at (times) for 30 minutes to discuss feelings and perceptions the client has about the identified situation. These times should also include discussions about the client's significant others, times the client has enjoyed with these persons, projects or activities the client was planning with or for these persons that have not been accomplished, client's values and beliefs about health and illness, and the attitudes about the current situation.	Promotes positive orientation by assisting the client in remembering past successes and important aspects of life that make it important to succeed this time.[29]
• Identify with client's significant others times that they can talk with the staff about the current situation. Themes to explore during this interaction should be their thoughts and feelings about the current situation, ways in which they can support the client, the importance of their support for the client, questions they may have about the client's situation and possible outcomes. Note the time for this interaction here as well as the name of the person who will be talking with the significant others.	Negative expectations from the support system can be communicated to the client.
• Note times when significant others will be visiting, and schedule this time so there will be a private time for them to interact with the client. Note these times here and designate those times that are scheduled as private visitation times. Inform client and significant others of those places on the unit where they can have privacy to visit.	Assists the client in maintaining connections with the support system and increases awareness of contributions the client has made in the past and can make in the future to this system.
• Identify with client preferences for daily routine, and place this information on the chart to be implemented by the staff. It is vital to the client to have the information shared with all staff so that it will not appear that the time spent in providing information was wasted.	Promotes client's sense of control.
• Provide information to questions in an open, direct manner.	Promotes client's sense of control while building a trusting relationship.
• Provide information on all procedures at a time when the client can ask questions and think about the situation.	

- Allow client to participate in decision making at the level to which he or she is capable. The client who has never made an independent decision would be overwhelmed by the complexity of the decisions made daily by the corporate executive. If necessary, offer decision situations at levels that the client can master successfully. The amount of information that the client can handle should be noted here as well as a list of decisions the client has been presented with.

Promotes the client's sense of control in a manner that increases the opportunities for success. This success serves as positive reinforcement.

- Provide positive reinforcement for behavior changed and decisions made. Those things that are reinforcing for this client should be listed here along with the reward system that has been established with the client; for example, play one game of cards with the client when a decision about ways to cope with a specific problem has been made.

Positive reinforcement encourages behavior while enhancing self-esteem.

- Provide verbal social reinforcements along with behavioral reinforcements.
- Keep promises. Specific promises should be listed on the chart so that all staff will be aware of this information.

Promotes the development of a trusting relationship.

- Accept client's decision if the decision was given to the client to make. These decisions should be noted on the chart.

Promotes the client's sense of control while enhancing self-esteem.

- Provide ongoing feedback to client on progress.

Provides positive reinforcement for accomplishments.

- Spend 30 minutes a day talking with client about current coping strategies and exploring alternative coping methods. Note time for this discussion here as well as the person responsible for this interaction. When alternative coping styles have been identified, this time should be used to assist client with necessary practice. The alternative styles that the client has selected should be noted on the chart and the staff should assist the client in implementing the strategy when appropriate. These could include deep muscle relaxation, visual imagery, prayer, or talking about alternative ways of coping with stressful events.

Interaction with the nurse can provide positive reinforcement. Behavioral rehearsal provides opportunities for feedback and modeling of new behaviors from the nurse.

- Allow client to express anger and assist with discovering constructive ways of expressing this feeling; for example, talking about this feeling, using a punching bag,

Promotes the development of a positive orientation.

Continued

Actions/Interventions	Rationales
playing Ping-Pong, throwing or hitting a pillow. Talk with client about signs of progress and assist him or her in recognizing these as they occur with verbal reminders or by keeping a record of steps taken toward progress.	
• Assist client in establishing realistic goals and expectations for situations. The goals should be short-term and stated in measurable behavioral terms. (Usually dividing the goal set by the client in half provides an achievable goal; this could involve dividing one goal into several smaller goals.) Note goals and evaluation dates here.	Goals that are achieved serve as positive reinforcement for behavior change and enhance self-esteem and a positive expectational set.
• Determine times with the client to evaluate progress toward these goals. These specific times should be listed here, with the name of the person responsible for this activity. Initially, this may need to be done on a daily basis until the client develops competency in making realistic assessments.	Allows nurse to give positive reinforcement for movement toward goal.
• Assist client in developing a list of contingencies for possible blocks to the goals. These would be "what if" and "if then" discussions. This would be done in the goal-setting session, and a record of the alternatives discussed would be made in the chart for future reference.	Provides direction for the client with an opportunity to mentally rehearse situations that could require alteration of goals. This protects the client from all-or-none situations.
• Discuss with client values and beliefs about life and assess importance of formal religion in the client's life. If client requires contact with a person of his or her belief system, arrange this and note necessary information for contacting this person here. Provide client with the time necessary to perform those religious rituals that are personally important. Note the rituals here with the times scheduled and any assistance that is required from the nursing staff.	Spirituality can provide hope-giving experiences.
• Provide the client with opportunities to enjoy aesthetic experiences that have been identified as important, such as listening to favorite music, having favorite pictures placed in the room, enjoying favorite foods, having special flowers in the room. Spend 5 minutes three times a day discussing these	Promotes the client's interest in the positive aspects of life.

experiences and assisting the client in becoming involved in the enjoyment of them. Note here those activities that have been identified by the client as important and times when they will be discussed with the client.

• Help the client develop an awareness of and appreciation for the here and now by focusing attention on the present — pointing out the beauty in the flowers in the room, the warmth of the sunshine as it comes through the window, the calmness or aliveness of a piece of music, the taste and smell of a special food item, the odor of flowers, and so on.	Provides the client with an opportunity to access past positive experiences in the present, thus promoting a positive orientation.
• Establish a time to talk with client about maximizing potential at his or her current level of functioning. Note date and time for this discussion here. This may need to be done in several stages, depending on the client's level of denial. Note person responsible for these discussions here.	Promotes the client's sense of control, thus enhancing self-esteem.

Gerontic Health

See Adult Health and Mental Health.

Home Health

Actions/Interventions	Rationales
• Monitor for factors contributing to the hopelessness: psychologic, social, economic, spiritual, environmental, and so on.	Provides database for earlier recognition and intervention.
• Involve client and family in planning, implementing, and promoting reduction or elimination of hopelessness: ○ Family conference to identify and discuss factors contributing to hopelessness ○ Mutual goal setting, with roles of each family member identified ○ Communication ○ Support for the caregiver	Clarifies roles; personal involvement in planning increases the likelihood of success in resolving problem.
• Assist client and family in life-style adjustments that may be required: ○ Use relaxation techniques: yoga, biofeedback, hypnosis, breathing techniques, imagery.	Life-style changes require significant behavior change. Self-evaluation and support can assist in ensuring changes are not transient.

Continued

Actions/Interventions	Rationales
○ Provide assertiveness training.	
○ Provide opportunities for individual to exert control over situation, give choice when possible, support and encourage self-care efforts.	
○ Provide sense of mastery, accomplishable and meaningful goals in secure environment.	
○ Try to figure out what can be learned from a situation.	
○ Provide treatment for physiologic condition.	
○ Provide grief counseling.	
○ Provide spiritual counseling.	
○ Prevent suicide.	
• Consult with or refer to community resources as indicated. (See Appendix B.)	Effective use of existing community resources helps client.

FLOW CHART EVALUATION
Flow Chart Expected Outcome 1

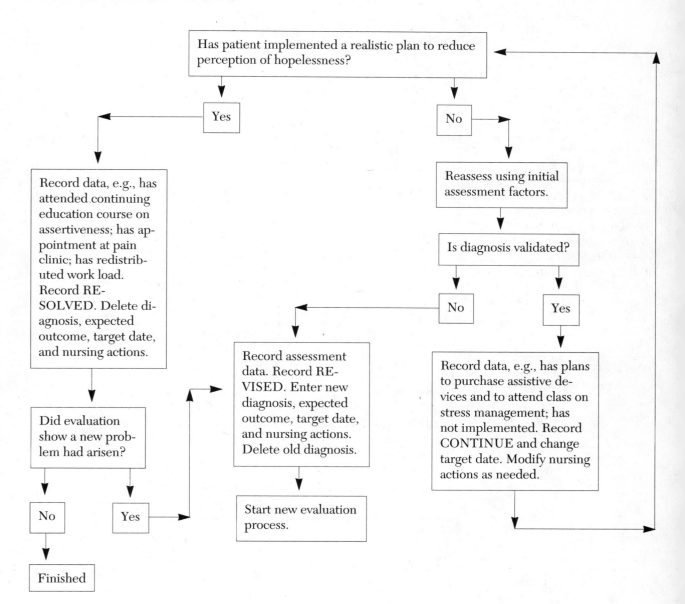

Flow Chart Expected Outcome 2

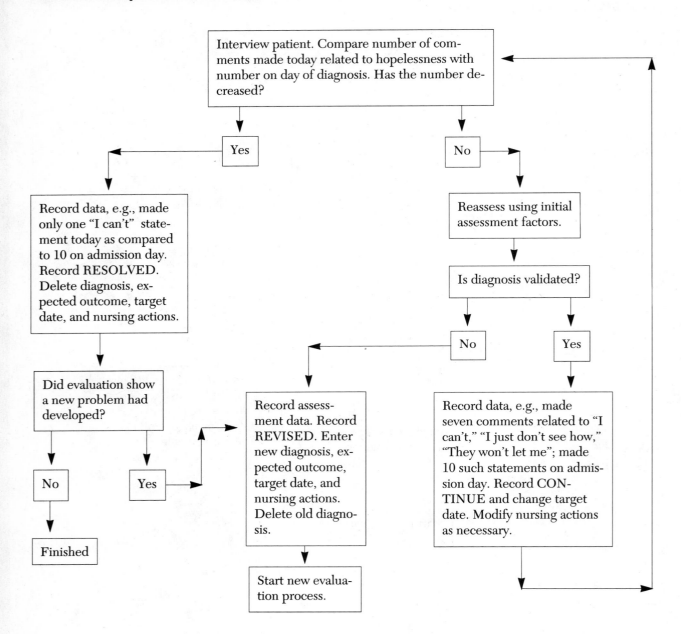

Personal Identity Disturbance

DEFINITION

Inability to distinguish between self and nonself.[23]

NANDA TAXONOMY: PERCEIVING 7.1.3

DEFINING CHARACTERISTICS[23]

To be developed.

RELATED FACTORS[23]

None given.

RELATED CLINICAL CONCERNS

1. Autism
2. Mental retardation
3. Dissociative disorders; for example, psychogenic amnesia, psychogenic fugue, multiple personality, depersonalization disorder
4. Borderline personality disorder

HAVE YOU SELECTED THE CORRECT DIAGNOSIS?

Self-Esteem Disturbance   This diagnosis addresses the lack of confidence in one's self and is characterized by negative self-statements, lack of concern about personal appearance, and withdrawal from others not related to physical problems or attributes. The self is defined. If the client demonstrates an inability to differentiate self from the environment, then the most appropriate diagnosis is Personal Identity Disturbance. An example would be the client who perceives a life-support machine as part of the self. (See page 668.)

Body Image Disturbance   This diagnosis relates to alterations in perceptions of self related to actual or perceived alterations in body structure or function. Again, the self is known with this diagnosis. (See page 618.)

EXPECTED OUTCOME

1. Will verbalize differentiation of self from environment by (date) and/or
2. Will list at least (number) characteristics of self versus nonself by (date)

TARGET DATE

A target date of 5 days would be acceptable for initial evaluation of progress toward expected outcomes.

NURSING ACTIONS/INTERVENTIONS WITH RATIONALES

Adult Health

Should the patient develop this nursing diagnosis on an adult health care unit, referral should be made immediately to a mental health nurse clinician. See Mental Health.

Child Health

Actions/Interventions	Rationales

• Monitor for contributing factors that might predispose the development of Personal Identity Disturbance:
  ○ Risk indicating an altered maternal-infant attachment, for example, overprotecting or ignoring infant
  ○ Altered development norms related to independent functioning, for example, following commands (check for organic or sensory-perceptual deficits)
  ○ Preference for solitary play
  ○ Self-stimulation and/or self-mutilation behaviors
  ○ History of altered identity problems in family
	Provides the database needed to more accurately and completely plan care.

• Provide basic care for other needs with prioritization for safety needs; close observation is mandatory.	In anticipatory safety planning, standards must be in accord with both the known and the unknown self-injury potential of the patient.
• Administer medications as ordered, with attention to hydration and nutritional concerns.	The patient is prone to dehydration and malnutrition owing to inability to rely on usual thirst or appetite regulators.
• Provide appropriate follow-up and collaboration with family.	Appropriate use of specialists will offer a more individualized plan of care with greater likelihood of meeting needs.
• Assist family in decision making regarding long-term care, for example, institutionalization versus day care.	Identification of options helps in decision making, reduces stress, and empowers the family.

Women's Health

See Mental Health.

Mental Health

Actions/Interventions	Rationales
• Provide a quiet, nonstimulating environment.	Inappropriate levels of sensory stimuli can increase confusion and sense of disorganization.
• Provide frequent interactions that assist the client with orientation.	Promotes the development of a trusting relationship within the client's attention span. Interaction with others also helps to reestablish weak ego boundaries.
• Verbal information should be provided in simple, brief sentences.	
• Sit with the client (number) minutes (number) times per day at (times) to provide the client with an opportunity to discuss feelings and thoughts.	Promotes the development of a trusting relationship and provides positive reinforcement for the client, thus meeting needs in a more constructive way.
• Provide the client with honest, direct feedback in all interactions.	Promotes the development of a trusting relationship.
• Utilize constructive confrontation if necessary to include: ○ "I" statements ○ Relationship statements that reflect nurse's reaction to the interaction ○ Responses that will assist the client in understanding, such as paraphrasing and validation of perceptions	Assists client in establishing ego boundaries while supporting self-esteem.
• Discuss with the client the source of the threat.	Assists client in developing more adaptive coping behaviors.
• Develop with the client alternative coping strategies. List here those activities, items, or verbal responses that are rewarding for the client.	Promotes client's sense of control and positive expectational set by providing a concrete plan for responding to stressful situations.
• When the client is presented with a threat, assist with progressing through one of the alternative coping methods, or practice with the client the alternative coping methods (number) minutes twice a day.	Behavioral rehearsal provides opportunities for feedback and modeling from the nurse.
• Develop achievable goals with the client. The goals that are appropriate for this client should be listed here.	Goal achievement enhances self-esteem and promotes a positive expectational set, which encourages client to move on to more complex goals and behavior change.
• As the client masters the first set of goals, develop increasingly complex goals and problems.	Moves client toward health goals in a manner that promotes self-esteem.
• Provide positive reinforcement for accomplishments at any level. Those activities, items, or verbal responses that are rewarding for the client should be listed here.	Positive reinforcement encourages behavior while enhancing self-esteem.

Continued

Actions/Interventions	Rationales
• Do not argue with the client who is experiencing an alteration in thought process. (Refer to Chapter 7 for nursing actions related to Altered Thought Process).	Arguing with the belief interferes with the development of a trusting relationship and does not serve to change the perceptions.
• Monitor the client's mental status before attempting learning or confrontation. If the client is disoriented, orient to reality as needed.	Alterations in mental status can interfere with the client's ability to process information, and teaching at this point could increase stimuli to a level that would only add to the client's confusion and disorganization.
• If disorientation is related to organic brain dysfunction, distract client from those disorientations that are not correct with a brief, simple explanation.	Short-term memory loss will assist with changing the client's orientation without getting into a strong confrontation.

Gerontic Health

If the patient is unable to distinguish between self and nonself, contact a mental health clinician to further assess and devise the plan of care. See Mental Health.

Home Health

Actions/Interventions	Rationales

• Involve client and family in planning and implementing strategies to reduce and cope with disturbance in personal identity:
  ○ *Family conference*: Discuss feelings related to Personal Identity Disturbance of client.
  ○ *Mutual goal setting*: Establish realistic goals and identify roles of each family member. Provide a quiet environment. Provide client with honest and direct feedback.
  ○ *Communication*: Promote clear and honest communication among family members. If organic brain dysfunction is present, use distraction techniques with client.
	Family involvement enhances effectiveness of interventions.

• Assist the client and family in life-style adjustments that may be required:
  ○ Maintaining a safe environment
  ○ Altering roles as necessary
  ○ Maintaining the treatment plan of the health care professionals guiding therapy
	Personal identity disturbance can be a chronic condition that alters family relationships. Permanent changes in behavior and family roles require evaluation and support.

• Consult with or refer to assistive resources as indicated. (See Appendix B.)	Promotes efficient use of existing resources. Psychiatric nurse clinicians and support groups can enhance the treatment plan.

FLOW CHART EVALUATION
Flow Chart Expected Outcome 1

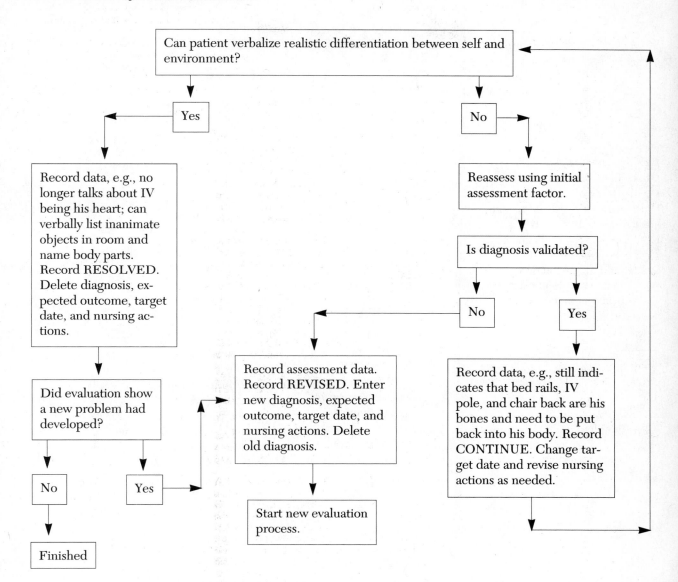

Can patient verbalize realistic differentiation between self and environment?

Yes

No

Record data, e.g., no longer talks about IV being his heart; can verbally list inanimate objects in room and name body parts. Record RESOLVED. Delete diagnosis, expected outcome, target date, and nursing actions.

Reassess using initial assessment factor.

Is diagnosis validated?

No

Yes

Did evaluation show a new problem had developed?

No

Yes

Record assessment data. Record REVISED. Enter new diagnosis, expected outcome, target date, and nursing actions. Delete old diagnosis.

Record data, e.g., still indicates that bed rails, IV pole, and chair back are his bones and need to be put back into his body. Record CONTINUE. Change target date and revise nursing actions as needed.

Finished

Start new evaluation process.

Flow Chart Expected Outcome 2

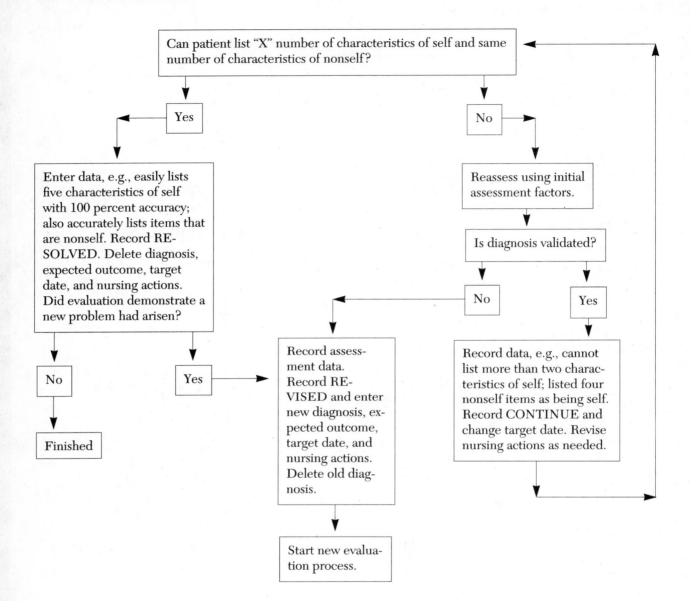

Can patient list "X" number of characteristics of self and same number of characteristics of nonself?

Yes

No

Enter data, e.g., easily lists five characteristics of self with 100 percent accuracy; also accurately lists items that are nonself. Record RE-SOLVED. Delete diagnosis, expected outcome, target date, and nursing actions. Did evaluation demonstrate a new problem had arisen?

Reassess using initial assessment factors.

Is diagnosis validated?

No

Yes

No

Yes

Finished

Record assess-ment data. Record RE-VISED and enter new diagnosis, ex-pected outcome, target date, and nursing actions. Delete old diag-nosis.

Record data, e.g., cannot list more than two charac-teristics of self; listed four nonself items as being self. Record CONTINUE and change target date. Revise nursing actions as needed.

Start new evalua-tion process.

Powerlessness

DEFINITION

Perception that one's own action will not significantly affect an outcome; a perceived lack of control over a current situation or immediate event.[23]

NANDA TAXONOMY: PERCEIVING 7.3.2

DEFINING CHARACTERISTICS[23]

1. Severe:
   a. Verbal expressions of having no control or influence over situation
   b. Verbal expressions of having no control or influence over outcome
   c. Verbal expressions of having no control over self-care
   d. Depression over physical deterioration that occurs despite patient compliance with regimens
   e. Apathy
2. Moderate:
   a. Nonparticipation in care or decision making when opportunities are provided
   b. Expressions of dissatisfaction and frustration over inability to perform previous tasks and/or activities
   c. Does not monitor progress
   d. Expression of doubt regarding role performance
   e. Reluctance to express true feelings
   f. Fearing alienation from caregivers
   g. Passivity
   h. Inability to seek information regarding care
   i. Dependence on others that may result in irritability, resentment, anger, and guilt
   j. Does not defend self-care practices when challenged
3. Low:
   a. Expressions of uncertainty about fluctuation in energy levels
   b. Passivity

RELATED FACTORS[23]

1. Health care environment
2. Interpersonal interaction
3. Illness-related regimen
4. Life-style of helplessness

RELATED CLINICAL CONCERNS

1. Any diagnosis that is unexpected or new to the patient
2. Any diagnosis resulting from a sudden, traumatic event
3. Any diagnosis of a chronic nature
4. Any diagnosis with a terminal prognosis

HAVE YOU SELECTED THE CORRECT DIAGNOSIS?

Anxiety Anxiety may have as a component a perception of Powerlessness. This would evolve into a situation where the anxious client would not attempt to resolve the situation. Powerlessness can also have anxiety as a component. The primary diagnosis is based on the clinical judgment of the nurse about which symptoms predominate. (See page 605.)

Ineffective Individual Coping A perception of Powerlessness can produce Ineffective Individual Coping, because if one perceives that one's own actions cannot influence a situation, appropriate actions may not be taken. If Ineffective Individual Coping is determined to result from a perceived lack of influence, then Powerlessness would be the primary diagnosis. (See page 892.)

Impaired Thought Process This diagnosis can produce a sense of Powerlessness because of the individual's inability to accurately assess the situation. When there is a question of the patients' cognitive ability the most appropriate diagnosis would be Altered Thought Process. (See page 577.)

Fear Fear can produce a sense of Powerlessness, just as Powerlessness can produce Fear. Differentiation is based on the predominant symptom sequence. (See page 628.)

Knowledge Deficit If the client lacks sufficient knowledge about a situation, a perception of Powerlessness may result. Therefore, Knowledge Deficit would be the primary diagnosis. (See page 536.)

EXPECTED OUTCOMES

1. Will describe at least (number) areas of control over self by (date) and/or
2. Will initiate a plan to deal with feelings of powerlessness by (date)

TARGET DATE

A target date of 3 days would be realistic to check for progress toward reduced feeling of powerlessness.

ADDITIONAL INFORMATION

The paradox of the metaphor of power has been presented in the literature. Systems theorists and cyberneticians have presented the most useful information for planning intervention strategies. Keeney[30] presents a summary of the debate over the power metaphor. In sum, most cyberneticians find this to be an invalid metaphor when discussing systems of interaction. The process of a system involves mutual interactions, and within a system each member exerts influence over the other members. Therefore, the individual who acts as if he or she is powerless is exerting "power" over the other parts of the system to act in a manner that would increase this "lost" personal power. The "powerless" one is then actually exercising power to motivate other parts of the system to act in certain ways. Understanding this conceptual model provides the client with an opportunity to know how one's behavior affects the situation and provides nurses with an ópportunity to understand their reactions to and feelings about the client with the diagnosis of Powerlessness. If the power metaphor is not accepted, this affects the concept of internal versus external locus of control. The concepts of internal and external loci of control become metaphors for how a person perceives personal influence within an interactional system. Persons with an external locus of control do not understand their influence on the system, whereas persons with an internal locus of control have an understanding of personal influence.

NURSING ACTIONS/INTERVENTIONS WITH RATIONALES

Adult Health

Actions/Interventions	Rationales
• Plan care with patient on a daily basis: ○ Likes and dislikes ○ Where patient wants personal items placed ○ Routines (to extent possible, according to patient's own pace and schedule) ○ Diet • Encourage patient to provide as much self-care as possible.	Allows patient to have control over environment and care attributes; imparts to patient a sense of power.
• When interacting with the patient, avoid: ○ Reinforcing manipulative behavior ○ Using negative feedback, for example, arguing with patient ○ Overuse of health care terminology • Do not ignore cultural and religious preferences.	Sets limits on behavior; facilitates a nonthreatening environment.
• Provide calm, safe environment throughout hospitalization: ○ Answer question truthfully. ○ Explain all procedures and rationale for procedures. ○ Give positive reinforcement to extent possible. ○ Reduce sensory input; balance high technology with high touch and appropriate attention. ○ Provide diversional activity. ○ Use same staff to degree possible.	Allows for verbalization of feelings and acceptance of those feelings; avoids overwhelming patient and increasing sensation of powerlessness.
• Involve significant others in care.	Promotes their involvement in care and advocacy for patient, thus empowering both patient and significant others.
• Monitor, at least once per shift: ○ Vital signs ○ Exercise	Changes in these signs may signal dysfunctions in other patterns and deterioration of diagnosis to depression.

Continued

Actions/Interventions	Rationales
○ Sleep-rest periods ○ Food and fluid intake • Refer to appropriate community resources prior to discharge. (See Appendix B.)	Support groups can encourage progress in building self-esteem, as well as providing advocacy and long-term support.

Child Health

Actions/Interventions	Rationales
• Perform a thorough assessment appropriate to patient's developmental level to identify specific factors which are causing feelings of powerlessness: ○ Use of art ○ Use of puppetry ○ Use of group therapy	Developmentally appropriate assessment will provide cues and reveal data to generate a more accurate and complete plan of care.
• Allow family to participate in care to the degree that they are able and willing to do so.	Family participation provides security for the child and empowerment for the parents, with increased growth in coping skills.
• Adopt plan of care to best meet child's and family's needs by including them in voicing preferences whenever appropriate.	Valuing individual preferences is demonstrated by frequent encouragement to express choices. Promotes a sense of control.
• Identify and address educational needs that might be contributing to powerlessness.	Misinformation and inadequate knowledge are contributing factors that can be easily overcome by teaching.
• Refer to patient by preferred name or nickname. List that name here.	Promotes personalized communication; points out individuality and serves to empower the patient.
• Allow for privacy and need to withdraw to family as a unit.	Demonstrates appropriate respect for family; attaches value to the family unit.
• Keep patient and family informed as changes occur.	Frequent updates and provision of information helps to clarify actions and reduces anxiety, resulting in a greater sense of control.
• Provide opportunities for parents to demonstrate appropriate care for child so that they will feel in control on discharge from hospital.	Allows practice in a nonthreatening environment, which increases sense of control.

Women's Health

Actions/Interventions	Rationales

• Provide the prospective parents with factual information about the type of choices available for birth, and assist them to identify their preference:
  ○ Traditional obstetric services
  ○ Family-centered maternity care units
  ○ Single-room maternity care
  ○ Mother-baby care
  ○ Birthing center
• Provide answers to questions in an open, direct manner.
• Provide information on all procedures so that the patient can make informed choices:
  ○ Assist the patient and significant others in establishing realistic goals. List goals with evaluation dates here.
  ○ Allow the patient and significant others to participate in decision making.
	Provides basic information that assists family in decision making, thus promoting empowerment of the family unit.[24]

• Allow the patient maximum control over the environment. This could include husband staying in postpartum room to assist with infant care; keeping the newborn with the mother at all times; using different positions for birth, such as squatting or hand-knee position; having grandparents and siblings in the room with mother and newborn; and so on. • Provide positive reinforcement for parenting tasks. • Assist the patient in identifying infant behavior patterns and understanding how they allow her infant to communicate with her. • Support the patient's decisions; for example, to breast-feed or not to breast-feed, which significant others she wants present during the birthing process, and so on. • Reassure the new mother that it takes time to become acquainted with her infant. • Support and reassure the mother in learning infant care—breast-feeding, bathing, changing, holding a newborn, cord care, bottle feeding. • Allow the parents to verbalize fears and	Decreases perception of powerlessness. Promotes decision making and leaves

Continued

Actions/Interventions	Rationales
insecure feelings about their new roles as parents. • Assist the parents in identifying life-style adjustments that may be needed when incorporating a newborn into the family structure. • Involve significant others in discussion and problem-solving activities regarding role changes within the family.	decisions up to the family by providing the guidance and support that is needed. Involvement enhances motivation to stay with plan, thus reinforcing decision-making capacity of new parents.[31]

Mental Health

Actions/Interventions	Rationales
• Sit with the client (number) times per day at (times) for 30 minutes to discuss feelings and perceptions the client has about the identified situation. • Identify client preferences for daily routine and place this information on the chart to be implemented by the staff. • Provide information to questions in an open, direct manner. • Provide information on all procedures at a time when the client can ask questions and think about the situation. • Allow the client to participate in decision making at the level to which he or she is capable. If necessary, offer decision situations in portions that the client can master successfully. The amount of information that the client can handle, as well as a list of decisions the client has been presented with, should be noted here. • Identify the client's needs and how these are currently being met. If these involve indirect methods of influence, discuss alternative direct methods of meeting these needs. The client who requests medication for headache every 15 minutes is requesting attention. The client should be encouraged to approach the nurse and ask to talk when the need for attention arises.	Promotes the development of a trusting relationship and assists client in identifying factors contributing to the feelings of powerlessness. It is vital to this client to have the information shared with all staff so that it will not appear that the time spent in providing information was wasted. Promotes the client's perception of control. Facilitates the development of a trusting relationship. Facilitates the development of a trusting relationship and promotes the client's sense of control. The client who has never made an independent decision would be overwhelmed by the complexity of the decisions made daily by the corporate executive. Promotes the client's sense of control. Assertive direct communication increases the possibility of the client's needs being met. When the client is successful in getting needs met in a direct manner, this will increase the client's sense of control and self-esteem.

- Provide positive reinforcement for behavior changes and decisions made. Those things that are reinforcing for this client should be listed here, along with the reward system that has been established with the client; for example, play one game of cards with the client when a decision about what to eat for dinner is made, or walk with client on hospital grounds when a decision is made about grooming.

Positive reinforcement encourages behavior while enhancing self-esteem.

- Provide verbal and behavioral reinforcements.

Promotes the development of a trusting relationship.

- Keep promises. Specific promises should be listed here so that all staff will be aware of this information.

Promotes positive orientation by assisting client in identifying way in which he or she is already "powerful."

- Assist the client in identifying current methods of influence and in understanding that influence is always there by providing feedback on how influence is being used in the client's interactions with the nurse.

- Accept the client's decisions if the decisions were given to the client to be made. For example, if the decision to take or not take medication was left with the client, the decision not to take the medication should be respected.

Promotes client's sense of control and enhances self-esteem.

- Allow the client maximum control over the environment. This could include where clothes are kept, how room is arranged, times for various activities. Note preferences here.

Promotes client's sense of control.

- Spend 30 minutes twice a day at (times) allowing the client to role-play interactions that are identified as problematic. The specific situations as well as new behavior should be noted here.

Promotes client's sense of control in a manner that increases opportunities for success. This success serves as positive reinforcement.

- Provide opportunities for significant others to be involved in care as appropriate. Careful assessment of the interactions between client and significant others must be made to determine best balance of influencing behavior between client and support system. Specific situation should be listed here.

Provides opportunities for support system and client to practice new ways of interacting while in a situation where they can receive feedback from the health care team.

- Monitor the health care team's interactions with the client for behavior patterns that would encourage the client to choose indirect methods of influence. This could include interactions that encourage the

The role of the nurse in the therapeutic milieu is to promote healthy interpersonal interactions.

Continued

Actions/Interventions	Rationales
adult client to assume a childlike role. If situations are identified they should be noted here.	
• Provide ongoing feedback to the client on progress.	Positive reinforcement encourages behavior.
• Assist the client in establishing realistic goals. List goals with evaluation dates here. (Usually dividing the goal set by the client in half provides an achievable goal; this could also involve dividing one goal into several smaller goals.)	Realistic goals increase the client's opportunities for success, providing positive reinforcement and enhancing self-esteem.
• Refer the client to outpatient support systems, and assist with making arrangements for the client to contact these before discharge. These could be systems that would assist the client in self-assertion and could include assertiveness training groups, battered wives' programs, legal aid, and so on.	Provides the client with support for continuing new behaviors in the community after discharge.

Gerontic Health

Actions/Interventions	Rationales
• Ensure access to call light, telephone, personal care items, and television controls.[22]	Increases patient's ability to take control of some aspects of care.
• Advocate for patient, ensuring that health care professionals are not leaving patient out of the decision loop because of the patient's age.	Stereotyping of older adults is problematic in health care professions.[32]

Home Health

Actions/Interventions	Rationales

• Involve the client and family in planning and implementing strategies to reduce powerlessness:
  ○ *Family conference*: Identify and discuss strategies.
  ○ *Mutual goal setting*: Agree on goals to reduce powerlessness; identify roles of all participants.
	Personal involvement and goal setting according to personal wishes enhances the likelihood of success in resolving problem.

- ○ *Communication*: Promote open communication among family members.
- Assist the client and family in life-style adjustments that may be required:
  - ○ Relaxation techniques, such as yoga, biofeedback, hypnosis, breathing techniques, imagery
  - ○ Providing opportunities for individual to exert control over situation, make choices when possible, and engage in self-care efforts
  - ○ Problem solving and goal setting
  - ○ Providing sense of mastery and achieving accomplishable goals in secure environment
  - ○ Maintaining the treatment plan of the health care professionals guiding therapy
  - ○ Obtaining and providing accurate information regarding condition.
- Consult with or refer to community resources as indicated. (See Appendix B.)
- Help the client and family to determine when the intervention of a health care professional is required; for example, inability to perform activities of daily living, rapid decline in condition.

Lifestyle adjustments require permanent changes in behavior. Self-evaluation and support facilitates the success of these lifestyle changes.

Promotes efficient use of existing resources.

Early identification of issues requiring professional evaluation will increase the probability of successful intervention.

FLOW CHART EVALUATION
Flow Chart Expected Outcome 1

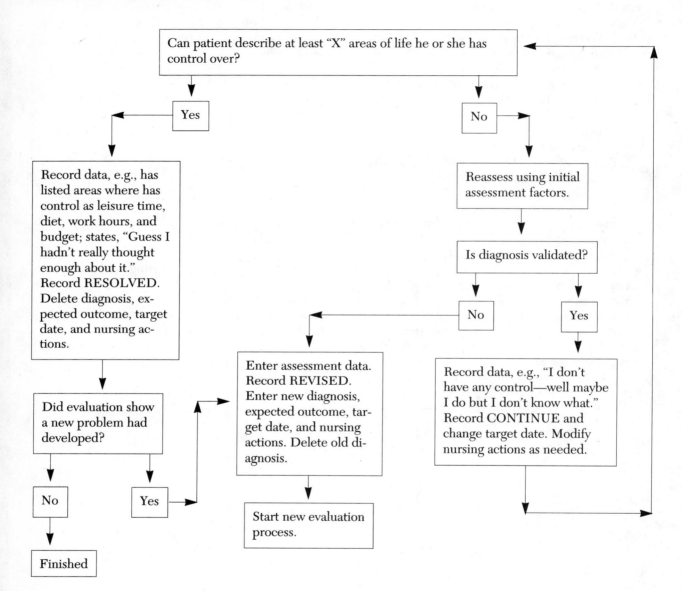

Flow Chart Expected Outcome 2

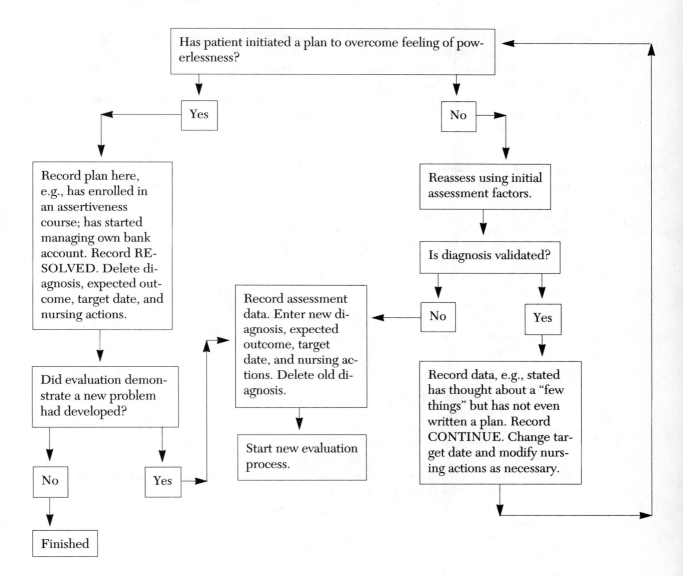

Self-Esteem Disturbance

DEFINITION

Self-Esteem Disturbance: Negative self-evaluation or feelings about self or self capabilities; which may be directly or indirectly expressed.

Chronic Low Self-Esteem: Long-standing negative self-evaluation or feelings about self or self capabilities.

Situational Low Self-Esteem: Negative self-evaluation or feelings about self that develop in response to a loss or change in an individual who previously had a positive self-evaluation.[23]

NANDA TAXONOMY: PERCEIVING 7.1.1., 7.1.2.1., 7.1.2.2

DEFINING CHARACTERISTICS[23]

1. Self-Esteem Disturbance:
   a. Self-negating verbalization
   b. Expressions of shame and guilt
   c. Evaluates self as unable to deal with events
   d. Rationalizes away or rejects positive feedback and exaggerates negative feedback about self
   e. Hesitant to try new things or situations
   f. Denial of problems obvious to others
   g. Projection of blame or responsibility for problems
   h. Rationalizes personal failures
   i. Hypersensitive to slight or criticism
   j. Grandiosity
2. Chronic Low Self-Esteem:
   a. Major defining characteristics:
      (1) Self-negating verbalization
      (2) Expressions of shame and guilt
      (3) Evaluates self as unable to deal with events
      (4) Rationalizes away or rejects positive feedback and exaggerates negative feedback about self
      (5) Hesitant to try new things or situations
   b. Minor defining characteristics:
      (1) Frequent lack of success in work or other life events
      (2) Overly conforming, dependent on others' opinions
      (3) Lack of eye contact
      (4) Nonassertive or passive
      (5) Indecisive
      (6) Excessively seeks reassurance
3. Situational Low Self-Esteem:
   a. Major defining characteristics:
      (1) Episodic occurrence of negative self-appraisal in response to life events in a person with a previous positive self-evaluation
      (2) Verbalization of negative feelings about the self (helplessness, uselessness)
   b. Minor defining characteristics:
      (1) Self-negating verbalizations

(2) Expressions of shame and guilt

(3) Evaluates self as unable to handle situations or events

(4) Has difficulty making decisions

RELATED FACTORS[23]

None given.

RELATED CLINICAL CONCERNS

1. Pervasive developmental disorders
2. Disruptive behavior disorders
3. Eating disorders
4. Organic mental disorders
5. Substance use/dependence/abuse disorders
6. Mood disorders
7. Adjustment disorders
8. Personality disorders
9. Trauma
10. Surgery
11. Medical problems that contribute to the loss of body functions
12. Pregnancy
13. Chronic diseases

HAVE YOU SELECTED THE CORRECT DIAGNOSIS?

Body Image Disturbance This diagnosis relates to alterations in the perception of self when there is an actual or perceived change in body structure or function. If interviewing reveals that the patient perceives a potential change in body structure or function, then Body Image Disturbance is the most appropriate diagnosis. (See page 618.)

Personal Identity Disturbance When the patient cannot differentiate self from nonself, some self-esteem problems may also exist. However, the primary diagnosis would be Personal Identity Disturbance. Working with the Personal Identity Disturbance will take care of the self-esteem problem. (See page 651.)

Ineffective Individual Coping This diagnosis results from the client's inability to appropriately cope with stress. If the client demonstrates a decreased ability to cope appropriately, he or she may also have some defining characteristics related to self-esteem disturbance. Teaching and supporting coping will also assist in correcting the self-esteem problem. (See page 892.)

EXPECTED OUTCOMES

1. Will verbalize an increased number of positive self-statements by (date) and/or
2. Will list at least (number) positive aspects about self by (date)

TARGET DATE

A target date of 3 to 5 days would be acceptable to begin monitoring progress.

NURSING ACTIONS/INTERVENTIONS WITH RATIONALE

NOTE: An attitude of genuine warmth, acceptance of clients, and respect for uniqueness are characteristics required for successful nursing interventions.[31]

Adult Health

Actions/Interventions	Rationales
• Collaborate with psychiatric nurse clinician regarding care. (See section on Mental Health.)	Collaboration promotes a more holistic and total plan of care.
• Teach the patient and significant others patient's self-care requirements as needed. Support patient's self-care management activities.	Self-care increases confidence and self-esteem.
• Control pain with medication, stress management techniques, and diversional activities.	Conserves energy to focus on adaptive coping strategies.
• Encourage patient to use anxiety-reducing techniques such as progressive muscle relaxation, deep breathing, yoga, meditation, assertiveness, and guided imagery.	Helps patient to reduce anxiety and regain self-control, thus increasing self-esteem.
• Encourage assertive behavior in interacting with patient; help patient review passive and aggressive behavior.	Helps patient avoid vacillating from one behavior to another; promotes self-control and a "win-win" situation, which increases self-esteem.
• Promote calm, safe environment by avoiding judgmental attitude, actively listening, using reflection, being consistent in approach, and setting boundaries.	Decreases anxiety and promotes a trusting relationship.
• Allow patient to progress at his or her own rate. Start with simple, concrete tasks. Reward success.	Increases patient's sense of task mastery and promotes self-esteem.
• Use frequent contact with patient, 15 minutes every 2 hours on the (odd/even) hour, to encourage verbalization of feelings: ○ Be honest with patient. ○ Point out and limit self-negation statements. ○ Do not support denial. ○ Focus on reality and adaptation (not necessarily acceptance). ○ Set limits on maladaptive behavior.	Assists in self-understanding and facilitates self-acceptance.

- ○ Focus on realistic goals.
- ○ Be aware of own nonverbal communication and behavior.
- ○ Avoid moral, value judgments.
- ○ Encourage patient to try to note differences in situations and events.
- ○ Help patient to ascertain why he or she can maintain self-esteem in one situation and not in another.
- • Build on coping mechanisms or interpretations that maintain or increase self-esteem. Assist to find alternative coping mechanisms.
- • Encourage patient to use available resources:
  - ○ Prosthetic devices
  - ○ Assistive devices
  - ○ Reconstructive and corrective surgery
- • Refer to and collaborate with community resources. (See Appendix B.)

Supports adaptive coping and helps to broaden inventory or coping strategies.

Decreases feelings of loss and increases self-esteem when patient does not feel "different" from previous self.

Provides ongoing and long-term support.

Child Health

Actions/Interventions	Rationales
• Monitor for contributory factors related to poor self-esteem, including: ○ Family crisis ○ Lack of adequate parenting ○ Lack of sensory stimulation ○ Physical scars, malformation, or disfigurement ○ Altered role performance ○ Social isolation ○ Developmental crisis	Generates the database needed to more accurately and completely plan care.
• Identify ways patient can formulate or reestablish a positive self-esteem according to developmental needs: ○ Coping skills ○ Communication skills ○ Role expectations ○ Self-care ○ Daily activities of living ○ Basic physiologic needs, primary health care ○ Expression of self ○ Peer and social relationships ○ Feelings of self-worth	Developmental norms serve as the conceptual framework for assisting the child to increase self-esteem.

Continued

Actions/Interventions	Rationales
○ Decision making	
○ Validation of self, for example, setting developmentally appropriate expectations	
• Praise and reinforce positive behavior.	Reinforcement of desired behavior serves to enhance permanence of behavior.
• Explore value conflicts and their resolution.	Values must be clarified as patient strives to find his or her identity; a healthy sense of self contributes to positive self-esteem.
• Collaborate with other health care team members as needed. (See Appendix B.)	Collaboration promotes a more holistic plan of care.
• Meet primary health needs in an expedient manner.	Conserves energy, minimizes stress, and enhances trust.
• Provide appropriate attention to other alterations, especially those directly affecting this diagnosis such as High Risk for Violence or Ineffective Parenting.	Related issues must be considered as contributing factors to the diagnosis; inattention to these factors means resolution of problem will not occur.
• Provide for follow-up before child is dismissed from hospital.	Attaches values to follow-up and promotes likelihood of compliance.
• Use developmentally appropriate strategies in care of these children:	Developmentally based strategies are less likely to frighten the child or parent.
○ *Infant and toddlers*: play therapy, puppets	
○ *Preschoolers*: art	
○ *School-age children*: art, role playing	
○ *Adolescents*: discussion, role playing	
• Carry out teaching of appropriate health maintenance. This could be the appropriate way of dealing with crisis related to shyness or poor communication skills.	Personal hygiene and self-care will enhance positive self-esteem as the patient copes with daily living.

Women's Health

Actions/Interventions	Rationales
• Allow the patient to "relive" birthing experience by listening quietly to her perception of the birthing experience.	Promotes ventilation of feelings and provides a database for intervention.
• Encourage the patient to express her concerns about her physical appearance.	Provides a support system that demonstrates adaptive behaviors.
• List activities that will promote positive feelings in the patient:	
○ Join friends or an exercise group with the same goals as the patient.	
○ Encourage activities outside the home as appropriate; for example, parenting support groups or women's groups.	

- ○ Encourage networking with other women with similar interests.
- Encourage the patient to "do something for herself":
  - ○ Buy a new dress.
  - ○ Fix hair differently.
  - ○ Find some time for herself during the day.
  - ○ Take a walk.
  - ○ Take a long bath.
  - ○ Rest quietly.
  - ○ Do a favorite thing—reading, sewing, or some hobby.
  - ○ Spend time with spouse without the children.
- Encourage the patient to engage in positive thinking.
- Encourage the patient to engage in assertiveness training.

Support and positive activities assist in adaptation to new parental role and increase sense of self-worth.

Mental Health

Actions/Interventions	Rationales
• Sit with client (number) minutes (number) times per shift to discuss client's feelings about self.	Expression of feelings and concerns in an accepting environment can facilitate problem solving.
• Answer questions honestly.	Promotes the development of a trusting relationship.
• Provide feedback to client about the nurse's perceptions of the client's abilities and appearance by: ○ Using "I" statements ○ Using references related to the nurse's relationship to the client ○ Describing the client's behavior in situations ○ Describing the nurse's feelings in relationship	Assists client with reality testing in a safe, trusting relationship.
• Provide positive reinforcement. List those things that are reinforcing for the client and when they are to be used. List those things that have been identified as nonreinforcers for this client. Include social rewards.	Positive reinforcement encourages behavior.
• Provide group interaction with (number) persons for (number) minutes three times a day at (times). This activity should be	Disconfirms the client's sense of aloneness and assists client to experience personal importance to others while enhancing

Continued

Actions/Interventions	Rationales
gradual and within the client's ability; for example, on admission the client may tolerate one person for 5 minutes. If the interactions are brief, the frequency should be high; that is, 5-minute interactions should occur at 30-minute intervals.	interpersonal relationship skills. Increasing these competencies can enhance self-esteem and promote positive orientation.
• Protect client from harm by: ○ Removing all sharp objects from environment ○ Removing belts and strings from environment ○ Providing a one-to-one constant interaction if risk for self-harm is high ○ Checking on client's whereabouts every 15 minutes ○ Removing glass objects from environment ○ Removing locks from room and bathroom doors ○ Providing a shower rail that will not support weight ○ Checking to see if client swallows medications	Client safety is of primary concern.
• Reflect back to client negative self-statements made by the client in a supportive manner.	Increases client's awareness of negative evaluations of self.
• Set achievable goals for client.	Goals that can be accomplished increase the client's perception of power and enhance self-esteem.
• Provide activities that the client can accomplish and that the client values.	Activities the client finds demeaning could reinforce the client's negative self-evaluation. Accomplishment of valued tasks provides positive reinforcement and enhances self-esteem.
• Provide verbal reinforcement for achievement of steps toward a goal.	Positive reinforcement encourages behavior while enhancing self-esteem.
• Have the client develop a list of strengths and potentials.	Promotes positive orientation and promotes hope.
• Define the client's lack of goal achievement or failures as simple mistakes that are bound to occur when one attempts something new; for example, learning comes with mistakes, and if one does not make mistakes, one does not learn.	Promotes positive orientation.
• Make necessary items available for the client to groom self.	Physical grooming can facilitate positive self-esteem by encouraging positive feedback from others.
• Spend (number) minutes at (time) assisting the client with grooming, providing	Presence of the nurse can serve as a positive reinforcement. Positive reinforcement

necessary assistance and positive reinforcement for accomplishments.

- Reflect back to the client those statements that discount the positive evaluations of others.
- Focus the client's attention on the here and now.
- Present the client with opportunities to make decisions about care, and record these decisions in the chart.
- Develop with the client alternative coping strategies.

- Practice new coping behavior with client (number) minutes at (times).

- Place the client in a therapy group for (number) minutes once a day where the focus is mutual sharing of feelings and support of each other.
- Identify with the client those situations that are perceived as most threatening to self-esteem.
- Assist the client in identifying alternative methods of coping with the identified situations. These should be developed by the client and listed here.
- Role-play with the client once per day for 45 minutes those high-risk situations that were identified and the alternative coping methods.
- Establish an appointment with the client and significant others to discuss their perceptions of the client's situation. The time of this and follow-up appointments should be listed here.
- Discuss with the client current behavior and reactions of others to this behavior.
- Practice with client (number) minutes twice a day making positive "I" statements.

encourages behavior while enhancing self-esteem.
Raises the client's awareness of this behavior, which facilitates change.

Past happenings are difficult for the nurse to provide feedback on.
Promotes the client's sense of control.

Promotes client's sense of control and enhances opportunities for positive outcome when stressful events are encountered.
Behavioral rehearsal provides opportunities for feedback and modeling of new behaviors from the nurse.
Facilitates awareness of others' perception of client and themselves.

Facilitates developing alternative coping behavior.

Increases the client's opportunities for success, and each success enhances self-esteem.

Behavioral rehearsal provides opportunities for feedback and modeling of new behaviors from the nurse.

Support systems facilitate the maintenance of new behaviors after discharge.[33]

Provides opportunities for feedback on new behaviors in a safe, trusting environment.
Promotes the development of a positive orientation.

Gerontic Health

Actions/Interventions	Rationales
• Assist patient in developing self-care skills needed for managing the current illness.[34]	Enhances perception of control over the situation.
• Assist patient in identifying his or her unique abilities and relate the benefits you as a nurse receive from your interactions with the patient.[34]	Increases recognition of successes that come from the use of personal strengths.
• Review patient's current abilities and how they may require role modification.[34]	Increases perception of functional ability in preferred life roles.
• Assist with personal grooming needs such as removal of excess facial hair and use of cosmetics where applicable.[35]	Attention to personal appearance can have a positive influence on self-esteem, and thus the perception, of the individual.

Home Health

Actions/Interventions	Rationales
• Involve the client and family in planning and implementing strategies to reduce and cope with disturbance in self-esteem: ○ *Family conference*: Discuss perceptions of client's situation and identify realistic strategies. ○ *Mutual goal setting*: Establish goals and identify roles of each family member; for example, provide a safe environment, assist with grooming, focus on the here and now. ○ *Communication*: Promote open and honest communication in the family.	Family involvement improves effectiveness of implementation.
• Assist the client and family in life-style adjustments that may be required:[36] ○ Obtaining and providing accurate information ○ Clarifying misconceptions ○ Maintaining a safe environment ○ Encouraging appropriate self-care without encouraging dependence or expecting unrealistic independence ○ Providing opportunity for expressing feelings ○ Setting realistic goals ○ Providing sense of mastery, accomplishable goals in secure environment	Life-style changes require long-term changes in behavior. Such changes in behavior require support.

- ○ Maintaining the treatment plan of the health care professionals guiding therapy
- ○ Using relaxation techniques: yoga, biofeedback, hypnosis, breathing techniques, imagery
- ○ Altering roles
- Consult with or refer to community resources as indicated. (See Appendix B.)

Promotes efficient use of existing resources. Psychiatric nurse clinician and support groups can enhance the treatment plan.

FLOW CHART EVALUATION
Flow Chart Expected Outcome 1

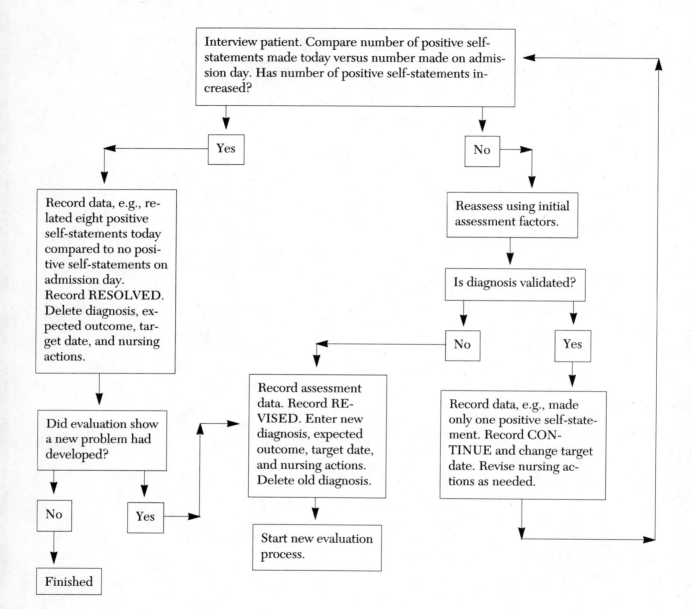

Flow Chart Expected Outcome 2

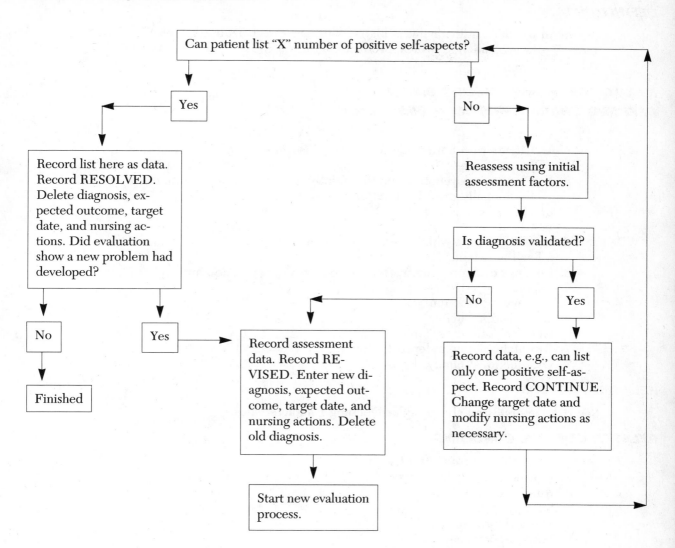

Self-Mutilation, High Risk for

DEFINITION

A state in which an individual is at high risk to perform an act upon the self with the intent to injure, not kill which produces immediate tissue damage and tension relief.[23]

NANDA TAXONOMY: FEELING 9.2.2.1.

DEFINING CHARACTERISTICS[23] (Risk Factors)

1. Groups at risk:
   a. Clients with borderline personality disorder, especially females 16 to 25 years of age
   b. Clients in psychotic state, frequently males in young adulthood
   c. Emotionally disturbed and/or battered children
   d. Mentally retarded and autistic children
   e. Clients with a history of self-injury
2. Inability to cope with increased psychological and/or physiological tension in a healthy manner
3. Feelings of depression, rejection, self-hatred, separation anxiety, guilt, and depersonalization
4. Fluctuating emotions
5. Command hallucinations
6. Need for sensory stimuli
7. Parental emotional deprivation
8. Dysfunctional family

RELATED FACTORS[23]

See risk factors listed above under Defining Characteristics.

RELATED CLINICAL CONCERNS

1. Borderline personality disorder
2. Organic mental disorders
3. Autism
4. Schizophrenia
5. Major depression
6. Multiple personality disorder
7. Sexual masochism
8. Affective disorder, mania

HAVE YOU SELECTED THE CORRECT DIAGNOSIS?

Potential for Violence This diagnosis is very similar to High Risk for Self-Mutilation. However, self-mutilation speaks only to the intent to injure self and specifically exempts suicide. (See page 801.)

Ineffective Individual Coping Certainly self-mutilation would be indicative of ineffective coping. These could be companion diagnoses, but priority should be given to the self-mutilation problem to decrease the life-threatening aspects before working with the client to increase coping abilities. (See page 892.)

EXPECTED OUTCOMES

1. Will demonstrate no self-mutilation attempts by (date) and/or
2. Will verbalize reasons behind self-mutilation threats by (date)

TARGET DATE

Initially, progress should be evaluated on a daily basis owing to the danger involved for the patient. After stabilization has been demonstrated, the target date could be moved to 5 to 7 days.

NURSING ACTIONS/INTERVENTIONS WITH RATIONALES

Adult Health

Should this diagnosis be made for an adult patient, immediately refer to a mental health practitioner. See Mental Health.

Child Health

Refer to Personal Identity Disturbance, above, and High Risk for Violence, Chapter 9, for nursing actions related to this diagnosis.

Women's Health

See Mental Health.

Mental Health

Actions/Interventions	Rationales
• Sit with client (number) minutes (number) times per shift at (times) to assess the client's mood, distress, needs, and feelings.	Promotes the development of a trusting relationship in a nonintrusive manner. Promotes positive orientation.[37]
• If risk for self-injury is high, place the client on a frequent-observation schedule. Note that schedule here. This observation should take place in a nonintrusive manner.	Client safety is of primary importance. Increased attention may inadvertently reinforce injury if it occurs in relation to self-injury episodes.[37]
• Remove objects that could be used to harm self from the environment.	Client safety is of primary importance.
• Use one-to-one observation to protect the client during periods of high risk for self-harming behavior.	Physical and chemical restraints have been demonstrated to escalate behavior. At times clients may escalate their behavior to be placed in restraints.[38]
• Develop a baseline assessment of the self-injury patterns. This should include frequency of behavior, type of behavior, factors related to self-harm, effects of self-harm on client and other clients. Note this information here.	Provides baseline information on which to base criteria for behavioral change and positive reinforcement.

Continued

Actions/Interventions	Rationales
• Answer client's questions honestly.	Promotes the development of a trusting relationship.
• Reframe the client's self-harming behavior as habitual behavior that can be changed. While doing this, do not diminish the client's experience of pain and discomfort.	Promotes a positive orientation and supports the client's strengths.[39]
• Identify, with the client, goals that are reasonable. Note those goals here. For example, "Client will contact staff when feeling need to harm self."	Assists client in gaining internal control of problematic behaviors.[39] Goals that are achieved provide positive reinforcement, which encourages behavior and enhances self-esteem.
• Provide positive verbal reinforcement for positive behavior change.	Positive reinforcement encourages behavior and enhances self-esteem.
• Have client develop a list of "feel-good" reinforcers. Note those reinforcers here.[38]	Promotes the client's sense of control while supporting a positive orientation.
• Provide feel-good reinforcers according to the reinforcement plan developed. Note the plan here.	Provides consistency in behavioral rewards. Positive reinforcement encourages behavior and enhances self-esteem.
• Identify, with the client, those situations and feelings that trigger self-injury.[38]	Promotes client's perception of control by pairing self-injurious behavior to specific situations and decreasing cognitive exaggerations.[40]
• Identify with the client strategies that can be utilized to cope with these situations. Note the identified strategies here.	Promotes the client's sense of control and assists the client with cognitive preparation for coping with these situations.[40]
• Select one identified strategy and spend 30 minutes a day at (times) practicing this with the client. This could be in the form of a role-play. Note the person responsible for this practice here.	Behavioral rehearsal provides opportunities for feedback and modeling from the nurse.
• Meet with the client just prior to and after trigger situations to assist with planning coping strategies and processing outcome to revise plans for future situations.[38]	Promotes the client's sense of control and provides an opportunity for the nurse to provide positive reinforcement for adaptive coping mechanisms.
• Initiate the client's coping strategy or provide distraction, such as physical activity, when the client identifies the urge to self-harm as strong. Acknowledge that the distraction will not increase comfort as much as self-harm would at the present time, but that the feelings of mastery will be satisfying.[39]	Provides opportunity for the client to practice new behaviors in a supportive environment where positive feedback can be provided. Promotes the client's sense of control and enhances self-esteem. Promotes positive orientation.
• Identify, with the client, areas of social skill deficits and develop a plan for improving these areas. This could include assertiveness training, communication skills training, and/or relaxation training to reduce anxiety	Enhances interpersonal skills by providing the client with more adaptive ways of achieving interpersonal goals.

in trigger situations. Note plan and schedule for implementation here. This should be a progressive plan with rewards for accomplishment of each step.[38–40]

- Develop a schedule for the client to attend group therapy. Note this schedule here.

Provides an opportunity for the client to practice interpersonal skills in a supportive environment and to observe peers modeling interpersonal skills.

- Meet with the client and the client's support system to plan coping strategies that can be used at home. Assist system in obtaining resources necessary to implement this plan.

Gerontic Health

See Mental Health.

Home Health

NOTE: See Mental Health nursing actions for additional interventions.

Actions/Interventions	Rationales

• Monitor for factors contributing to risk for self-mutilation.
• Involve client and family in planning, implementing, and promoting reduction or elimination of risk for self-mutilation:
  ○ *Family conference*: Discuss perspective of each family member.
  ○ *Mutual goal setting*: Develop short-term and long-term goals with evaluative criteria. Tasks and roles of each family member should be specified.
  ○ *Communication*: Promote open, direct, reality-oriented communication.
• Assist client and family in life-style adjustments that may be required:
  ○ Development and use of support networks
  ○ Provision of safe environment
  ○ Protection of client from harm
  ○ Long-term care, if required
• Consult with or refer to community resources as indicated. (Appendix B.)
	Provides database for early recognition and intervention.
	Family involvement enhances effectiveness of interventions.
	
	Adjustments in life-style require long-term behavioral changes. Such changes are enhanced by education and support.
	
	Promotes efficient use of existing resources. A psychiatric nurse clinician, support groups, and mental health or mental retardation experts can enhance the treatment plan.

FLOW CHART EVALUATION
Flow Chart Expected Outcome 1

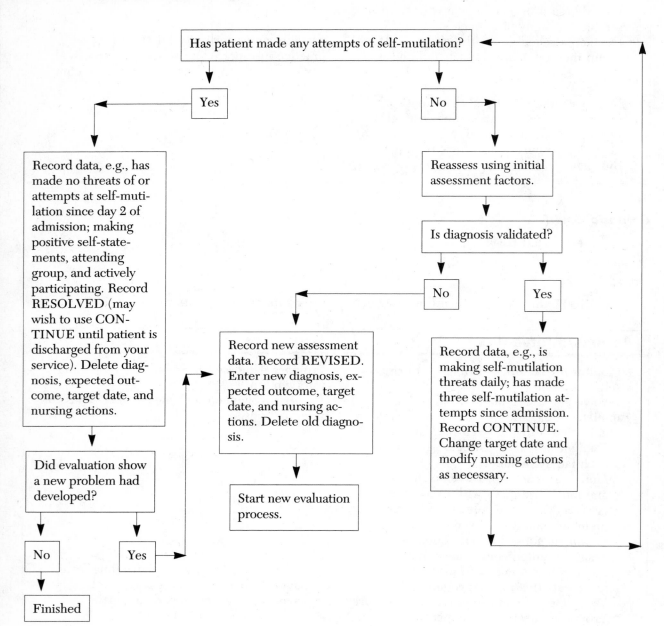

Flow Chart Expected Outcome 2

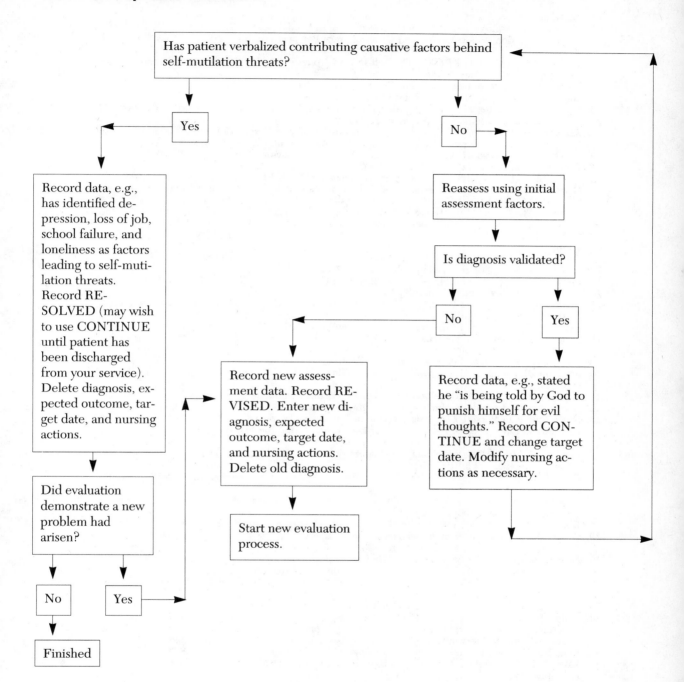

References

1. Le Mone, P: Analysis of a human phenomenon: Self-concept. Nurs Diag 2:126, 1991.
2. Turner, R: The self-conception in social interaction. In Gordon, C and Gergen, KJ (eds): The Self in Social Interaction, Vol 1, Classic and Contemporary Perspectives. John Wiley & Sons, New York, 1968.
3. Gordon, C and Gergen, KJ (eds): The Self in Social Interaction, Vol 1, Classic and Contemporary Perspectives. John Wiley & Sons, New York, 1968.
4. James, W: The self. In Gordon, C and Gergen, KJ (eds): The Self in Social Interaction, Vol 1, Classic and Contemporary Perspectives. John Wiley & Sons, New York, 1968.
5. Mead, GH: The genesis of self. In Gordon, C and Gergen, KJ (eds): The Self in Social Interaction, Vol 1, Classic and Contemporary Perspectives. John Wiley & Sons, New York, 1968.
6. Sullivan, HS: Beginnings of the self-system. In Gordon, C and Gergen, KJ (eds): The Self in Social Interaction, Vol 1, Classic and Contemporary Perspectives. John Wiley & Sons, New York, 1968.
7. Bruch, H: Interpersonal theory: Harry Stack Sullivan. In Burton, A (ed): Operational Theories of Personality. Brunner-Mazel, New York, 1968.
8. Perry, HS and Gawel, ML: The Interpersonal Theory of Psychiatry. Norton, New York, 1953.
9. Glasersfeld, EV: Cybernetics, experience and the concept of self. In Gergen, KJ & Davis, RE (eds): The Social Construction of the Person. Springer-Verlag, New York, 1985.
10. Watts, A: The Book: On the Taboo against Knowing Who You Are. Random House, New York, 1966.
11. Jourard, S: Healthy personality and self-disclosure. In Gordon, C & Gergen, KJ (eds): The Self in Social Interaction, Vol 1, Classic and Contemporary Perspectives. John Wiley & Sons, New York, 1968.
12. Dufault, K and Martocchio, B: Hope: Its spheres and dimensions. Nsg Clinics of NA 20:379, 1985.
13. Vaillot, M: Hope: The restoration of being. AJN 70:268, 1970.
14. McGee, R: Hope: A factor influencing crisis resolution. Adv in Nsg Sc 7:34, 1968.
15. Miller, J: Inspiring hope. AJN 85:22, 1985.
16. Watson, J: Nursing: The Philosophy and Science of Caring. Colorado Associated University Press, Boulder, 1985.
17. Evans, R: The Making of Psychology. Knopf, New York, 1976.
18. Lynch, WF: Image of Hope: Imagination as Healer of the Hopeless. University of Notre Dame Press, Notre Dame, IN, 1974.
19. Bateson, G: Steps to an Ecology of Mind. Ballantine, New York, 1972.
20. Erickson, H, Tomling, E, and Swain, MA: Modeling and Role-Modeling. Prentice-Hall, Englewood Cliffs, NJ, 1983.
21. Santrock, JW: Life Span Development, ed 4. WC Brown, Dubuque, IA, 1992.
22. Eliopoulos, C: A Guide to Nursing of the Aging. Williams & Wilkins, Baltimore, 1987.
23. North American Nursing Diagnosis Association: Taxonomy I: Revised 1990. Author, St. Louis, 1990.
24. Bull, M and Lawrence, D: Mother's use of knowledge during the first postpartum weeks. J Obstet Gynecol Neonatal Nurs 14:315, 1985.
25. Reeder, SJ, Martin, LL, and Koniak, D: Maternity Nursing: Family, Newborn and Women's Health Care. JB Lippincott, Philadelphia, 1992.
26. Fogel, CI and Woods, NF: Health Care of Women: A Nursing Perspective. CV Mosby, St. Louis, 1981.
27. Griffith-Kenney, JW: Contemporary Women's Health: A Nursing Advocacy Approach. Addison-Wesley, Menlo Park, CA, 1986.
28. Jacobson, N and Margolin, B: Marital Therapy. Brunner-Mazel, New York, 1989.
29. Drew, B: Differentiation of hopelessness, helplessness, and powerlessness using Erik Erikson's "Roots of Virtue." Arch Psychiatr Nurs 4:332, 1990.
30. Keeney, BP: Aesthetics of Change. Guilford, New York, 1983.
31. Tulman, L and Fawcett, J: Return of functional ability after childbirth. Nurs Res 37:77, 1988.
32. Matteson, MA and McConnell, ES: Gerontological Nursing: Concepts and Practices. WB Saunders, Philadelphia, 1988.
33. Gilliss, C, et al: Toward a Science of Family Nursing. Addison-Wesley, Menlo Park, CA, 1989.
34. Miller, JF: Coping with Chronic Illness: Overcoming Powerlessness. FA Davis, Philadelphia, 1983.
35. Burnside, IM: Nursing and the Aged: A Self-Care Approach, ed 3. McGraw-Hill, New York, 1988.
36. Norris, J: Nursing intervention for self-esteem disturbances. Nurs Diagn 3:48, 1992.
37. King, KS, Dimond, M, and McCance, KL: Coping with relocation. Geriatr Nurs 8:258, 1987.
38. Valente, S: Deliberate self-injury: Management in a psychiatric setting. J Psychosoc Nurs Ment Health Serv 29:19, 1991.
39. Gallop, R: Self-destructive and impulsive behavior in the patient with a borderline personality disorder: Rethinking hospital treatment and management. Arch Psychiatr Nurs 6:178, 1992.
40. Reeder, D: Cognitive therapy of anger management: Theoretical and practical considerations. Arch Psychiatr Nurs 5:147, 1991.

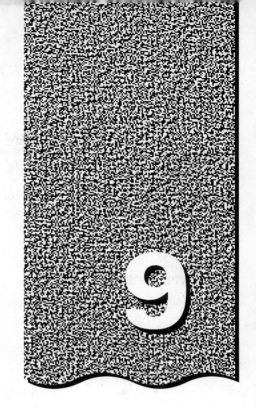

Role-Relationship Pattern

PATTERN INTRODUCTION
Pattern Description

The Role-Relationship Pattern is concerned with how a person feels he or she is performing the expected behavior delineated by the self and others. Each of us has several roles we fulfill during our daily life, and with these roles come related responsibilities. Included in our roles are family, work, and social relationships. Disruption in these roles, relationships, and responsibilities can lead a patient to seek assistance from the health care system. Likewise satisfaction with the roles, relationships, and responsibilities are patient strengths that can be used in planning care for other health problem areas.

Pattern Assessment

1. Is the client exhibiting distress over a potential loss?
   a. Yes (Anticipatory Grieving)
   b. No
2. Is the client denying a potential loss?
   a. Yes (Anticipatory Grieving)
   b. No
3. Is the client exhibiting distress over an actual loss?
   a. Yes (Dysfunctional Grieving)
   b. No
4. Is the client denying an actual loss?
   a. Yes (Dysfunctional Grieving)
   b. No
5. Is the client making verbal threats against others?
   a. Yes (High Risk for Violence)
   b. No
6. Is the client exhibiting increased motor activity?
   a. Yes (High Risk for Violence)
   b. No
7. Can the patient speak English?
   a. Yes
   b. No (Impaired Verbal Communication)
8. Does the patient demonstrate any difficulty in talking?
   a. Yes (Impaired Verbal Communication)
   b. No
9. Does the client verbalize difficulty with social situations?
   a. Yes (Impaired Social Interaction)
   b. No
10. Does the client indicate strained relationships with his or her family or others?
    a. Yes (Impaired Social Interaction)
    b. No
11. Does the patient have family or significant others visiting or calling?
    a. Yes
    b. No (Social Isolation)

12. Is the patient uncommunicative and withdrawn or avoiding eye contact?
    a. Yes (Social Isolation)
    b. No
13. Does the client indicate admission might impact role (family, work, leisure)?
    a. yes (Altered Role Performance)
    b. No
14. Does family or significant other verbalize admission might impact patient's role (family, work, leisure)?
    a. Yes (Altered Role Performance)
    b. No
15. Does the child show signs and symptoms of physical or emotional abuse?
    a. Yes (Altered Parenting)
    b. No
16. Do parents indicate difficulty in controlling the child?
    a. Yes (Altered Parenting)
    b. No
17. Do parents demonstrate attachment behaviors?
    a. Yes
    b. No (High Risk for Altered Parenting)
18. Do parents make negative comments about the child?
    a. Yes (High Risk for Altered Parenting)
    b. No
19. Does the family demonstrate ability to meet the child's physical needs?
    a. Yes
    b. No (Altered Family Process)
20. Does the family demonstrate ability to meet the child's emotional needs?
    a. Yes
    b. No (Altered Family Process)
21. Do the parents express concern about ability to meet the child's physical or emotional needs?
    a. Yes (Parental Role Conflict)
    b. No
22. Do parents frequently question decisions about the child's care?
    a. Yes (Parental Role Conflict)
    b. No

Nursing Diagnoses in This Pattern

1. Caregiver Role Strain: High Risk for and Actual (page 699)
2. Family Process, Altered (page 710)
3. Grieving, Anticipatory (page 720)
4. Grieving, Dysfunctional (page 732)
5. Parenting, Altered: High Risk for, Actual, and Parental Role Conflict (page 742)
6. Relocation Stress Syndrome (page 756)
7. Role Performance, Altered (page 763)
8. Social Interaction, Impaired (page 772)
9. Social Isolation (page 781)

10. Verbal Communication, Impaired (page 791)
11. Violence, High Risk for: Self-Directed or Directed at Others (page 801)

Conceptual Information

The social connotation for role performance and relationships is a major premise for the intended use of this pattern. A role is a comprehensive pattern of behavior that is socially recognized, provides a means of identifying, and places an individual in a society. Role is the interaction point between the individual and society. It also serves as a means of coping with recurrent situations. The term "role" is borrowed from the theater; it emphasizes the distinction between the actor and the part. A role remains relatively stable even though a variety of persons may play it; however, the expectations of the script, other players, and the audience all influence role enactment.[1] The importance of each of these factors varies with the context. In our personal roles, the script is equivalent to the societal "norms" and our audience can be real or imagined. Uniqueness of style may exist within the boundaries of the role as determined by society.

Because roles are such an integral part of our lives they are seldom analyzed until they become a problem to one's internal or external adaptation to life's demands. Roles that are often associated with stages of development serve as society's guides for meaningful and satisfying relationships in life by facilitating an orderly method for transferring knowledge, responsibility, and authority from one generation to the next.

During the childhood years, an individual will have numerous contacts with different individuals of differing values. The child learns to internalize the values of those significant in his or her life as personal goals are actualized. When the goals are realistic, consistent, and attainable, the individual is assisted in developing a sense of self-esteem as these various roles are mastered. Each new role carries with it the potential for gratification and increased ego identity if the role is acquired. If the role is not mastered, poor self-esteem and role confusion may ensue. The potential for role mastery is diminished with multiple role demands and the absence of suitable role models. Additionally, role acquisition depends on adequate patterns of cognitive-perceptual ability and a healthy sense of self.

Although all roles are learned within the context of one's culture, specific roles are delineated in two ways: acquired and achieved. Acquired roles are those roles with variables over which the individual has no control, such as gender or race. Achieved roles allow for some personal choice; the individual may purposefully select and earn—for example, that of a professional nurse.

Many roles are not clearly defined as being either acquired or achieved, but rather are a combination of the two. Roles are not mutually exclusive, but are interdependent. The roles an individual assumes usually blend well; however, the roles that a person achieves or acquires may not always make for a harmonious blend. Role conflicts may occur at the most internalized personal level or at a generalized societal level.

Roles may be influenced by a multitude of factors, including economics, family dynamics, institutional changes, and changing expectations. Roles can be mediated through role-playing skills and self-conceptions. It is hoped that with the increased demands on the individual, society will continue to value human dignity with respect for life itself. Roles should allow for self-actualization.

One of the more recent eclectic theories of personality development encompassing role theory is that of symbolic interaction. In this orientation, social interaction has symbolic meaning to the participants in relation to the roles assigned by society. (For further related conceptual information, refer to Chapter 8, Self-Perception and Self-Concept Pattern.)

Symbolic interaction encompasses the roles assumed by humans in their constant interaction with other humans, communicating symbolically in almost all they do. This interaction has meaning to both the giver and the receiver of the action, thus requiring both persons to interact symbolically with themselves as they interact with each other. Symbolic interaction involves *interpretation*—ascertaining the meaning of the actions or remarks of the other person—and *definition*—conveying indication to another person as to how he or she is to act. Human association consists of a process of such interpretation and definition. Through this process the participants fit their own acts to the ongoing acts of others and guide others in doing so.[2]

To further explore how relationships develop, we offer a brief overview of kinship. A kinship system is a structured system of relationships in which individuals are bound to one another by complex, interlocking relationships. These relationships are commonly referred to as families. It is not so much the family form in which one lives as how that family form functions that defines whether there is a cohesive family structure:

> An ideal family environment consists of a family that has many routines and traditions, provides for quality time between adults and children, has regular contact with relatives and neighbors, lives in a supportive and safe neighborhood, has contact with the work world and has adult members who model a harmonious and problem-solving relationship.[3:505-506]

The 1980s saw great change in family structures, with an explosion of individualized living arrangements and life-styles requiring new definitions of the family.[3-6] Fewer families consisting of husband, wife, and children exist today, and this is no longer the only acceptable form for family life. Some of the different family forms identified in today's society are:[3-6]

Nuclear family: Husband, wife, and children living in a common household sanctioned by marriage
Nuclear dyad: Husband and wife alone; childless or children have left home
Single-parent family: One head of household, mother or father, as a result of divorce, abandonment, or separation
Single adult alone: Either by choice, divorce, or death of a spouse
Three-generation family: three generations or more in a single household
Kin network: Nuclear households or unmarried members living in close geographical proximity
Institutional family: Children in orphanages or residential schools
Homosexual family: Homosexual couples with or without children

Despite the differences in family forms and cultural differences, primary relationships within various family structures reveal markedly similar characteristics in all societies. These relationships were described in 1949[7] and still exist in the various family forms cited today.

Husband and wife: Economic specialization and cooperation; sexual cohabitation; joint responsibility for support, care, and upbringing of children; well-defined reciprocal rights with respect to property, divorce, and spheres of authority

Father and son: Economic cooperation in masculine activities under leadership of the father; obligation of material support vested in father during childhood of son and in son during old age of father; responsibility of father for instruction and discipline of son; duty of obedience and respect on part of son, tempered by some measure of comradeship

Mother and daughter: Relationship parallel to that between father and son, but with more emphasis on child care and economic cooperation and less of authority and material support; however, strong relationships in the development of mothering skills and parenting techniques lead to obligations of emotional support and caretaking activities vested in the mother during the childhood of daughter and in daughter during old age of mother

Father and daughter: Responsibility of father for protection and material support prior to marriage of daughter; economic cooperation, instruction, and discipline appreciably less prominent than in father-son relationship; playfulness common in infancy of daughter, but normally yields to a measure of reserve with the development of a strong incest taboo

Mother and son: Relationship parallel to mother and daughter, but with more emphasis on financial and emotional support in later life of mother

Elder and younger brother: Relationship of playmates, developing into that of comrades; economic cooperation under leadership of elder; moderate responsibility of elder for instruction and discipline of younger

Elder and younger sister: Relationship parallel to that between elder and younger brother but with more emphasis on physical care of the younger sister

Brother and sister: Early relationship of playmates, varying with relative age; gradual development of an incest taboo, commonly coupled with some measure of reserve; moderate economic cooperation; partial assumption of parental role, especially by the elder sibling

The nurse must exercise great sensitivity to the individual meaning attached to various roles and the way in which these roles are perceived and assumed. With the current societal and economic changes, the individual's roles are being impacted on a daily basis even without the added stress of a health problem.

Developmental Considerations

INFANT

The newborn period is especially critical for the development of the first attachment, which is so vital for all future human relationships. Attachment behavior includes crying, smiling, clinging, following, and cuddling. The infant is dependent on its mother and father for basic needs of survival. This is often demanding and requires parents to place self-needs secondary to the needs of the infant. This makes for a potential role-relationship alteration.

Although dependent on others, the infant is an active participant in role-relationship pattern development from conception on. The infant is capable of influencing the interactions of those caring for him or her. Reciprocal interactions also influence the maternal-paternal-infant relationship. Positive interactions will be greatly influenced by infant-initiated behavior at well as maternal-paternal responses and the reciprocal interaction of all involved. The state of the infant as well as the state of the parent interacting within the infant must be considered as critical.

It is important to note than any alteration in health status of the mother, the neonate, or both has the potential of interfering with the establishment of the maternal-infant relationship. This may not necessarily be the case, but it is often critical that the potential risk be acknowledged early so that residual secondary problems can be prevented with appropriate nursing intervention. It is also important to keep in mind that the infant is taking in all situational experiences and that as learning occurs through interaction with the environment, a gradual evolution of role-relationship patterns occurs.

By approximately 12 months of age, the infant shows fear of being left alone and will search for the parents with his or her eyes. The infant will avoid and reject strangers. There is an obvious increasing interest in pleasing the parent. In protest the infant cries, screams, and searches for the parent. In despair the infant is listless, withdrawn, and uninterested in the environment. In detachment or resignation a superficial "adjustment" occurs in which the infant appears interested in surroundings, happy, and friendly for short periods of time. The infant is emotionally changeable from crying to laughing with a beginning awareness of separation from the environment. Still, the infant uses mother as a safe haven from which to explore the world. The infant will have a favorite toy, blanket, or other object which serves to comfort him or her in times of stress. (Sucking behavior may also serve to calm the infant, and eventually the infant will develop self-initiated ways of dealing with the stressors of life, such as thumb sucking versus the actual taking of formula or milk).

The infant receives cues from significant others and primary caregivers regarding grief responses such as crying, with a preference for the mother. Depending on age and situational status, the infant may protest by crying for mother. In a weakened state, the infant may show little preference for one caregiver over another.

According to family structure, the neonate or infant will adapt to usual socialization routines within reasonable limits. Actual social isolation for the infant could occur if the primary caregiver could not exercise usual role-taking behavior for socialization for example, the mother has a chronic disease that limits her social activities. If this behavior is arrested for marked periods of time, there is a potential for developmental delays secondary to the lack of appropriate social stimulation.

The newborn period is especially critical for the development of future human relationships. During this period the infant must depend on others for care and basic needs. This is often a demanding situation for parents, who must sacrifice their own needs to best meet the needs of their infants.

The infant is dependent on others for all care ranging from food to appropriate sensory and social stimulation. In the absence of a stable, well-functioning family unit, the infant may be at risk for failure to thrive or developmental delay. Ultimately, rather than developing a sense of trust that the world is a place in which one's needs are met, the infant will doubt and mistrust others. This in turn places the infant at risk for an abnormal pattern of development.

Crying serves as the primitive verbal communication for the neonate and infant. As the infant begins to understand and respond to the spoken word, the world should be symbolized as comforting and safe. With time, basic attempts at verbalization are noted in imitation of what is heard. There is a correlation between parental speech stimulation and the actual development of speech in young children, suggesting a positive effect for early stimulation. Echolalia (the often pathological repetition of what is said by other people, as if echoing them) and attempts at making speech are most critical to note during this time.

Individuals unable to deal with the usual role-relationship patterns may lash out at the crying infant or even become violent. The infant is unable to defend itself. Therefore, any suspected abusive or negligent behavior must be reported. At particular risk are infants with feeding or digestive disorders, premature or small-for-gestational-age infants who require feedings every 2 hours, or others perceived as "demanding" or "irritable." Also at risk are infants with congenital anomalies or disfigurement.

TODDLER AND PRESCHOOLER

The toddler has an increasing sense of identity and knows himself or herself as a separate person. The toddler treats other children as if they were objects and gradually becomes involved in parallel play, which then leads to a more interactive play with peers. Toddlers should not be expected to share possessions yet. The toddler begins to formulate a sense of right and wrong and has the ability to conform to some social demand, as exemplified by the capacity for self-toileting. The toddler can begin to work through problems of family relations with other children while playing.

The preschool child talks and plays with an imaginary playmate as a projection. What is offered may be what the child views as bad in himself or herself. The preschooler may have some friends of the same sex, and opportunities for socialization serve critical functions. The preschool child lives in the here and now and is capable of internalizing more and more of society's norms. There is a sense of morality and conscience by this age. A strong sense of family exists for the preschooler.

The toddler may be unusually dependent on mother, objects of security, and routines. He or she is capable of magical thinking and may believe in animation of inanimate objects, such as believing an x-ray machine is really a mean monster. Toddlers may be fearful of seeing blood. These fears may be unrelated to actual situations.

The preschooler may be critical of himself or herself and may blame himself or herself for a situation with some attempt at viewing the current situation as punishment for previous behavior or thoughts. He or she will tolerate brief separation from parents in usual functioning. Play or puppet therapy that is appropriate to the situation will help the preschooler in expressing feelings.

The toddler must have room to safely explore; a sense of autonomy evolves in the ideal situation. If social isolation limits these opportunities, the toddler will be limited in role-relationship exposure. This will often result in either social isolation or a form of forced precocious role taking in which the toddler is perceived as being able to satisfy the companionship needs of adults. The toddler may misinterpret socialization opportunities as abandonment or punishment, so short intervals of parallel play with one peer are best to begin with. Toddlers who are denied opportunities for peer interaction are at risk for role-relationship problems.

The child of the preschool age group may experience alteration in socialization attempts if overpowered by peers, if there are too many rigid or unrealistic rules, or if the situation places the child in a situation that present values greatly different from those of the child and his or her family. If the child at this age experiences prolonged social isolation or rejection, there could be marked potential for difficulty in forming future relationships. If things do not go well regarding socialization, the child at this age may blame himself or herself.

The toddler will seek out opportunities to explore and interact with the environment, provided there is a safe haven to return to as represented by the family. When this facilitative factor is not present, the toddler may regress and become dependent on primary caregivers or others or manifest frustration via extremes in demanding behavior. The child's subsequent development may also be affected by family process alteration.

The preschool child is able to verbalize concerns regarding changes in family process but is unable to comprehend dynamics. It is critical to attempt to view the altered process through the eyes of the preschooler, who may blame himself or herself for the change or crisis or think magically and have fears that may be unrelated to the situation. Subsequent development may be altered by family process dysfunction, with regression often occurring.

At this age it is important to stress the need for ritualistic behavior as a means of mastering the environment with adequate anticipatory safety. This period allows for knowing "self" as a separate entity. The toddler is capable of attempting to conform to social demands but lacks the ability for self-control.

The importance of setting limits must be stressed with regard to safety and disciplinary management. At this age the child begins to resist parental authority. Methods of dealing with differences or rules from one setting to another must be simple and appropriate to the situation.

For the toddler this time can prove frustrating because of the need to be understood despite a limited vocabulary. Jargon and gestures may be misinterpreted, with resultant frustration for child and parent. Patience and understanding go far with a child of this age. Pictures and story telling serve as means of enhancing speech as well as instilling an appreciation for reading and speech. Feelings may also be expressed verbally. The child is able to refer to the self as "I" or "me" or by name.

By preschool age, the child is able to count to 10, define at least one word, and name four or five colors. Speech now serves as a part of socialization in play with peers. Wants should be expressed freely as the child broadens his or her contact with persons other than primary family members. The preschooler enjoys stories and television programs and attempts to tell stories of his or her own creation.

If the toddler is unable to meet the expectations of parents or caregivers, there is risk of abuse. Toilet training often becomes a battleground, placing the toddler in a target population for abuse. At this age the toddler may be unable to verbally express hostility or anger, so temper tantrums are a common occurrence. The toddler who resists parental authority and cannot meet the demands of the parents is at risk for violence.

SCHOOL-AGE CHILD

Learning social roles as male or female is a major task for the school-age child, who generally prefers spending time with friends of the same sex rather than the family. The school-age child is capable of role taking and values cooperation and fair play. Morality may be viewed in strict black-and-white terms, with no room for gray areas. The school-age child enjoys simple household chores, likes a reward system, and has the capacity for expressing feelings. Fear of disability and concern for missing school are typical concerns for this age group.

Illness may impose separation from the peer group. Although independent of parents in health, the school-age child may require a close parental relationship in illness or crisis. Loss of control and fear of mutilation and death are real concerns.

The school-age child may fear disgracing parents if loss of control such as crying occurs. He or she is aware of the severity of his or her prognosis and may even deal with reality better than parents or adults might. The school-age child may use art as a means of expressing his or her feelings.

This child is at risk of social isolation if a situation is different from previous socialization opportunities. He or she may experience value conflict and question the rules. He or she may also be afraid to express desires or concerns regarding socialization needs for fear of punishment. Peer involvement is a vital component in assisting the school-age child to formulate views of acceptable social behavior.

The school-age child may try to assume the role of a parent if the family dysfunction relates to the same-sex parent. This may be healthy, with appropriate acknowledgment of limitations. At this age, the child is concerned with what other friends may think about the family with some stigma attached in certain cultures to divorce, homosexuality, and altered life-styles. It would be critical for the school-age child to have a close friend who shares the cultural views of his or her own family to best endure the altered family process.

Allowance for increasing interests outside the home should be made with a sensitivity to parental approval or disapproval. The child may rebel against parental authority in an attempt to be like peers.

Confidence in self and a general sense of well-being will promote adequacy in communication development. The child of this age continues to learn vocabulary and takes pride in his or her ability to demonstrate appropriate use of words. At this age jokes and riddles serve as a means of encouraging peer interaction with speech. Reading is a leisure activity for the school-age child.

The child will usually enjoy school and consider peer interaction an enjoyable part of life. In instances in which the child feels inferior, there may be a risk for violence or abusive behavior as a cover-up for poor self-image or low self-esteem. Often there will be related role-relationship alterations as well. The family serves as a means of valuing the interaction that should foster the appropriate enjoyment of friendships. Children with learning disabilities or handicaps, parental conflicts, or related role-relationship alteration are at risk.

ADOLESCENT

Vacillation between dependence and independence is a common occurrence for the adolescent who is attempting to establish a sense of identity. The adolescent questions traditional values, especially those of parents. There is a gradual trend to independent functioning, which allows the adolescent to assume roles of adulthood, including the development of intensive relationships with members of the opposite sex.

The adolescent will be constantly weighing self-identity versus perceived identity expressed via peers. He or she may be fearful of expressing true feelings or concerns for fear of rejection by peers, parents, or significant others. Isolation from peers will place the adolescent at risk for altered self-identity as well as altered role-relationship patterns.

The adolescent is able to assist within the family during times of altered process. It is important to stress that in more and more dual-career or single-parent families, young adolescents spend more and more time alone. Nonetheless, adolescents should still have opportunities for peer interaction and socialization according to the family's needs.

There may be marked vacillations as the adolescent strives to find self-identity and work out dependence-independence issues. Even more marked rebellion against parental wishes may be manifest at this time as peer approval is sought.

Factors that interfere with usual speech patterns may prove especially difficult for the adolescent. This may include braces, the eruption of 12-year molars, and impacted wisdom teeth—any of which may be painful and result in altered self-image. Expressed wit is valued in this age group, as might be special colloquial expressions to qualify for group or peer identity. Difficulty in expression of self may prove most difficult for this individual. Respect for times of reflection and estrangement should be maintained.

The adolescent may be caught in an emotional crossfire around dependence-independence issues. For this group it is paramount that self-control be attained in order to develop the meaningful relationships so critical for appropriate role-relationship patterns. Often those adolescents who have not acquired appropriate socialization skills resort to drugs or alcohol as a means of feeling better and escaping the reality of life. This may also foster loss of control as reality is distorted. In many instances there may be related juvenile delinquency with resultant law-breaking.

Additionally, any adolescent who is assuming a role that stresses or negates the usual development of self-identity is at risk for violence as a means of coping; for example, young teenagers attempting to parent when they themselves still require parenting.

YOUNG ADULT

Although biophysical and cognitive skills reach their peak during the adult years, the young adult is still in a period of growth and development. Striving for an education, job security, and meaningful intimate relationships with others and establishing a family are the primary focuses of the young adult. While young adults usually have achieved independence, they find themselves learning socially relevant behavior and settling into specific acquired roles within a chosen profession or occupation. They begin to adopt some of the values of the group to which they belong and to assume assured roles, such as marriage and parenting.

Cognitively, young adults have reached their peak level of intellectual efficiency, and they are able to think abstractly and to synthesize and integrate their ideas, experiences, and knowledge. Thinking for the adult usually involves reasoning, taking into consideration past experiences, education, and the possible outcomes of a situation more realistically and less egocentrically than the adolescent.

Young adulthood is still a time of great adjustment. The individual is expected to look at self in relation to society, learning how to deal with personal needs and desires as opposed to the needs and desires of others, and managing the economic and physical needs of life. Sexual activity focuses on the development of a single, intimate, meaningful relationship and the establishment of a family. In the parenting role, young adults often fall back on the parenting patterns and behavior of their own parents.

The young adult begins to assume the responsibility of providing for a family. Most young adults are members of dual-career families and thus face the stresses of multiple roles. Many of these young adults become single parents, and the stresses of multiple responsibilities and roles are greater both at home and at work. Just as during adolescence, the negation of development of self-identity can lead to crises, role strain, and conflict in the young adult, resulting in developmental crises and failure.

As the adult acquires full role responsibility, there may be difficulties related to role diffusion, role confusion, role strain, or related assumption of appropriate roles. Also, the ultimate developmental need for assumption of accountability for self may be unresolved. Men and women alike may be forced to assume a wide variety of roles that were once clearly assigned to either men or women alone; for example, the roles of primary breadwinner and primary nurturer may be assumed by either sex. This challenge also brings the potential for growth and fulfillment in self-actualizing individuals.

MIDDLE-AGE ADULT

Middle age, or "middlescence," is often considered the busiest period of an individual. Persons in this age group are usually secure in a profession or career, in the middle of raising a family, and often responsible for aging parents.

As biological changes occur there is a concurrent adaptation of the cognitive and physical activities of the individual. The body ages in varying stages or degrees, and young middle-age adults usually retain the body structure and activity level they established as young adults. Middle-age adults, with more sedentary life-styles, must establish exercise programs to retain their youthful figures. The greatest changes facing both men and women during this time are those associated with the climacteric and the loss of reproductive capabilities. These biologic and physical changes can affect sexual life-styles either positively or negatively, depending on the perception and orientation of the individual.

Most middle-age adults function well and learn to gradually accept the changes of aging; with proper nutrition, exercise, and a healthy life-style they can experience excellent health and a productive middlescence. Middle-age persons usually begin to face more accidents, illness, and death; they begin to deal with their own aging process and death, as well as that of their parents. There is often a role reversal, with the middle-age adult assuming the role of parent.

This is the time of life when individuals usually review their goals and aspirations, sometimes to find that they did not reach the potential they once dreamed of. Most middle-age adults begin to feel that there is not enough time to accomplish all they want to accomplish, and they begin to adjust to the fact that they may not reach all of the goals they set in their youth. This can result in a loss of self-esteem, or it can be a motivation to develop previously untapped reservoirs, which can lead to self-actualization and personal satisfaction.

OLDER ADULT

With aging, individuals may have fewer demands placed upon them, thus leaving more time and fewer potential opportunities for role performance. This may also be a time when one is able to fulfill volunteer roles and those of choice versus those of demand. A critical factor may be the freedom one feels as basic needs are met. If health is satisfactory and one has children or grandchildren to enjoy, financial stability, and the ability to pursue fulfillment via role engagement, this time may be one of self-actualization. On the other hand, if one's health fails, few meaningful family supports exist, and financial needs arise, self-actualizing role performance is potentially threatened.

The older adult must deal with decreasing function, with resultant decreasing socialization potential. This is a time for retrospection and a need to ponder the past with sincere concerns regarding the future and death. In some instances full functional level is possible, whereas for others life is lived vicariously. Role-modeling opportunities for the elderly still exist in many cultures. For these individuals the aging process is welcomed and enjoyed as the fullest potential is actualized for role-relationship patterning, namely the generation of values in the young in society. In those instances where aging is accompanied by loss in whatever form, the potential exists for the individual to become dependent. This dependency may range from minor to major, with total dependence on others. The onset of dependency may be gradual or sudden. In either instance, the nurse must recognize the impact of the loss for the patient according to the values of the patient and family.

APPLICABLE NURSING DIAGNOSES

Caregiver Role Strain: High Risk for and Actual

DEFINITION

High Risk for: A caregiver is vulnerable for the felt difficulty in performing the family caregiver role

Actual: A caregiver's felt difficulty in performing the family caregiver role[8]

NANDA TAXONOMY: RELATING 3.2.2.1, 3.2.2.2

DEFINING CHARACTERISTICS[8]

1. High Risk for Caregiver Role Strain:
   a. The risk factors also serve as the defining characteristics.
2. Caregiver Role Strain:
   Caregivers report they
   a. Do not have enough resources (time, emotional strength, physical energy, help from others) to provide the care needed.
   b. Find it hard to do specific caregiving activities such as bathing, cleaning up after incontinence, managing behavior problems, and managing pain.
   c. Worry about such things as the care receiver's health and emotional state, having to put the care receiver in an institution, and finding someone to care for the care receiver if something should happen to the caregiver.
   d. Feel that caregiving interferes with other important roles in their lives, such as being a worker, parent, spouse, or friend.
   e. Feel loss because the care receiver is like a different person compared to before caregiving began or, in the case of a child, that the care receiver was never the child the caregiver expected.
   f. Feel family conflict around issues of providing care because other family members do not do their share in providing care to the care receiver, or because not enough appreciation is shown for what the caregiver does.
   g. Feel stress or nervousness in their relationship with the care receiver.
   h. Feel depressed.

RELATED FACTORS[8]

1. High Risk for Caregiver Role Strain
   Risk factors include the following:
   a. Pathophysiological:
      (1) Illness severity of the care receiver
      (2) Addiction or codependency
      (3) Premature birth or congenital defect
      (4) Discharge of family member with significant home care needs
      (5) Caregiver health impairment
      (6) Unpredictable illness course or instability in the care receiver's health
      (7) Caregiver is female
      (8) Psychological or cognitive problems in care receiver
   b. Developmental:
      (1) Caregiver is not developmentally ready for caregiver role: for example, a young adult needing to provide care for middle-age parent
      (2) Developmental delay or retardation of the care receiver or caregiver
   c. Psychological:
      (1) Marginal family adaptation or dysfunction prior to the caregiving situation
      (2) Marginal caregiver's coping patterns
      (3) Past history of poor relationship between caregiver and care receiver
      (4) Caregiver is spouse
      (5) Care receiver exhibits deviant, bizarre behavior
   d. Situational:
      (1) Presence of abuse or violence
      (2) Presence of situational stressors which normally affect families: significant loss, disaster, or crisis; poverty or economic vulnerability; major life events, such as birth, hospitalization, leaving home, returning home, marriage, divorce, employment, retirement, or death
      (3) Duration of caregiving required
      (4) Inadequate physical environment for providing care, for example, housing, transportation, community services, or equipment
      (5) Family or caregiver isolation
      (6) Lack of respite and recreation for caregiver
      (7) Inexperience with caregiving
      (8) Caregiver's competing role commitments
      (9) Complexity or amount of caregiving tasks
2. Caregiver Role Strain
   The related factors for this diagnosis are the same as the risk factors for the High Risk diagnosis.

RELATED CLINICAL CONCERNS

1. Any chronic, debilitating illness, for example, Alzheimer's disease, cancer, or rheumatoid arthritis
2. Severe mental retardation
3. Chemical abuse
4. Closed head injury
5. Schizophrenia
6. Personality disorders

HAVE YOU SELECTED THE CORRECT DIAGNOSIS?

Ineffective Individual Coping This diagnosis and Caregiver Role Strain are very close; however, the differentiating factor is whether the individual is involved in a caregiver role or not. If significant caregiving is a part of the individual's role, then initial interventions should be directed toward resolving the problems with caregiving role. (See page 892.)

Impaired Adjustment Certainly needing to assume a caregiving role would require some adjustment. However, this diagnosis relates to an individual adjusting to his or her own illness or health problem, not to someone else's illness or health problem. (See page 861.)

Ineffective Family Coping (Compromised; Disabling) These diagnoses could be companion diagnoses to Caregiver Role Strain. If the family cannot adapt to a change in a member's condition and assigns the caregiver role to just one family member, then both Ineffective Family Coping and Caregiver Role Strain are likely to develop. (See page 874.)

EXPECTED OUTCOME

1. The caregiver will implement a plan to reduce strain by (date) and/or
2. The caregiver will verbally describe decreased strain by (date)

TARGET DATE

A target date of 5 days would be the earliest date to begin evaluation of progress toward meeting the expected outcome.

NURSING ACTIONS AND INTERVENTIONS WITH RATIONALES

Adult Health

Actions/Interventions	Rationales
• Encourage patient to talk about caregiver role by active listening, reflection, open-ended questions, acceptance of feelings for 15 minutes twice a day at (times).	Decreases anxiety when allowed to ventilate positive and negative feelings in nonthreatening, empathetic environment.
• Teach stress management techniques such as relaxation, meditation, deep breathing. Have patient return-demonstrate techniques for 5 minutes every 4 hours while awake at (times).	Relieves stress, identifies alternative coping strategies, and decreases depression.
• Identify community support groups such as Mother's Day Out, day-care centers, housekeeping services, home health aides, hospice, or respite care prior to discharge.	Provides alternatives for coping and resources to support in short-term and long-term problems.

Continued

Actions/Interventions	Rationales
Also cooperative arrangement could be made with friends and neighbors for release time from care activities.	
• Encourage family conferences to discuss role expectations, role conflict, role strain, and role negotiation for 1 hour every other day.	Opens communication and promotes cooperative problem solving.
• Refer to psychiatric nurse specialist as needed. (See Mental Health nursing actions.)	Collaboration promotes holistic health care; interventions may require expertise of specialist.

Child Health

Actions/Interventions	Rationales
• Monitor for contributing factors with a focus on high-risk populations:	Unrealistic demands of parenting or care provision increase the likelihood of role strain.
○ Excessive demands secondary to a child requiring extensive care, for example, several small children in family with one child requiring extensive assistance with physical or mental problems	
○ A patient who has a total self-care deficit	
○ Caregiver indicates inability to carry out usual routines	
• Schedule a daily conference with caregiver of at least 30 minutes.	Allows identification of current perception of role strain by encouraging ventilation of feelings; provides teaching opportunity; assists in identification of needed referrals.
• Explore with parent or caregiver, during conference, options available to assist with the demands of the situation. Encourage caregiver to provide time for self on a daily basis through such means as seeking outside help, for example, visiting nurse, housekeeping assistance, respite care, or temporary or permanent institutionalization.	Support from others serves as a means of preventing further demise of desired role taking while also considering long-term needs. Time for self will enhance coping abilities and, ultimately, self-esteem.
• Identify, during conference, available community resources, especially parenting support groups.	Provides long-term support and information; encourages sharing of concerns with others in the same situation.
• Schedule family conference, as needed, to focus on family's willingness to provide assistance in caregiving.	Assists in delineating roles for each family member and providing relief for primary caregiver on a more regular basis.
• Determine via an ongoing assessment any unresolved guilt regarding role demands,	Unresolved conflict increases the likelihood of little change in behavior.

"less-than-perfect child," or related aspects of situation. (See Dysfunctional Grieving.)

- Assist caregiver and significant others to explore inevitabilities and realities associated with the care situation.
- Preserve the effective functioning of the caregiver through teaching and support in conferences.

Expectations may be unrealistic; clarification of expectations and reality assist in problem solving.

The likelihood of secondary and tertiary alterations for the caregiver increase when primary needs of rest and own physical self are not met.

Women's Health

Actions/Interventions	Rationales
• Assist new mother in developing realistic plans for infant care. Have mother review plans for self-care and care of the infant in the home.	Provides time for assessment and planning for home care. Affords opportunity to teach and give realistic feedback regarding the impact a newborn makes on former lifestyle.
• Include significant other in plans for care of new mother and infant after discharge from the hospital. Encourage discussion by mother and significant other of various role changes in the family that will occur as the new infant is incorporated into the household; for example, roles of sibling, wife, husband, grandparents.	
• Encourage discussion of the new role of mother and father and its effect on the husband and wife roles.	
• Assist with development of plan to save time, such as learning to sleep when the infant sleeps, turning telephone off when trying to rest, putting sign on front door when sleeping.[10]	Assists in reducing fatigue, which is a significant contributor to the development of caregiver role strain.
• Identify areas in which the significant other can assist the new mother and help reduce fatigue; for example, if breast-feeding, let father get the infant, change the diaper, and bring the infant to the mother for feeding during the night.[10]	
• Plan meals for the family before leaving for the hospital, cook and freeze them so that there will be only a need to thaw and microwave or warm during the first few weeks at home.[10]	

NOTE: The nursing actions for the teenage parent will be the same as above, with the following additions.

Continued

Actions/Interventions	Rationales
• Refer the young couple or teenager to young parents groups in the community for social and personal support.	Provides long-term support and an information source.[11]
• Give the young couple telephone hotlines they can call for assistance and support: hospital nursery, young parent services, YWCA, and so on.	
• Assist the young parent to get into or stay in school by giving references for child care.	Promotes long-range planning and reduces the likelihood of strain for the young parents.
• Encourage the young couple to express their feelings about the new responsibilities they face.	

Mental Health

> NOTE: For information related to the caregivers of those clients with a medical diagnosis of dementia, refer to the section on Gerontic Health. As used in this discussion, "caregiver" can mean one person or an extended family system.

Actions/Interventions	Rationales
• Spend (number) minutes (number) times per week interacting with primary caregiver.	Promotes the development of a trusting relationship.

• Provide a role model for effective communication by:
  ○ Seeking clarification
  ○ Demonstrating respect for individual family members and the family system
  ○ Listening to expression of thoughts and feelings
  ○ Setting clear limits
  ○ Being consistent
	Family problem solving is improved when family members can effectively communicate with one another and the health care team.[12]

• Include caregiver in weekly treatment planning meetings with the client. Note time for this meeting and persons responsible for providing the information here.	Assists in providing information to the caregiving group so that they can better cope with the uncertainty of a psychiatric diagnosis.[12, 13]
• Spend (number) minutes (number) times per week educating the primary caregiver about the client's diagnosis. Provide both written and verbal information.	Provides caregiver with an increased understanding of the diagnosis and assists in the development of a home care plan. When anxiety is high, caregivers may have difficulty remembering information provided only in verbal form. Increases the stability in the living environment by decreasing caregiver's anxiety.

- Communicate understanding of the difficulty of the caregiver role by:
  - Answering questions honestly
  - Providing time to interact with the caregivers when they visit
  - Inquiring about the caregivers' self-care activities
  - Encouraging the caregiver to use the time the client is in the hospital to rest and meet personal needs
  - Providing time for the caregiver to express feelings related to the client and the hospitalization

Promotes the development of a trusting relationship and assists the caregiver in the process of working through feelings related to the client.

- Normalize caregivers' feelings of guilt and/or ambivalence by informing them that these are normal feelings for anyone who assumes the level of responsibility they have.

Promotes a positive orientation and enhances self-esteem.

- Have caregivers identify areas where they feel a need for support on a daily basis and assist them in networking community resources to meet these needs. This should be a process that allows the nurse to teach caregivers the skills necessary to accomplish this networking on their own after discharge.

Promotes caregivers' sense of control and provides positive reinforcement when they can accomplish the task, thus enhancing self-esteem.

- Spend (number) minutes (number) times per week discussing their self-care activities. This could include planning time away from the client, inviting friends to visit, going for a walk, arranging to get uninterrupted sleep, and so on. Inform caregivers that if they do not care for themselves, they will eventually not have the energy to care for the client. A specific plan should be developed and noted here.

Gives permission to the caregivers to care for themselves. Promotes the caregivers' strengths.

- Before the client is discharged, meet with the client and caregivers to review
  - Information about the diagnosis and hospital course
  - Special treatments the client is to receive
  - Client's medications
  - Anticipated problems
- A specific plan should be developed for coping with anticipated problems. This plan should be written down and given to both the client and the caregivers.

Anxiety can decrease an individual's ability to process information during hospitalization. A specific coping plan provides direction during times of crisis and prevents reliance on ineffective patterns of coping. These actions increase the caregivers' repertoire of strategies to deal with the problems.[14]

Gerontic Health

Actions/Interventions	Rationales
• Monitor for signs of increasing strain in caregiver, such as an increase in episodes of illness.	The stresses of caregiving have a negative effect on the caregiver's immune system.[15]
• Assist caregiver in discussing feelings about caregiving. For example, encourage sharing by use of statements such as, "Often people in your situation say they feel angry/ helpless/guilty/depressed."	Provides opportunity for ventilation of feelings about caregiving; this assists in reducing stress.
• Determine caregiver's knowledge of support services in the community such as adult day care, respite services, family support groups.	Assists in identifying actual or potential resources based on the individual's current knowledge of services. Expands options available to caregiver.
• Discuss with caregiver stress management techniques such as imagery, deep breathing, exercise. What has been tried? How helpful was it?	
• Encourage caregiver to use a journal to evaluate stresses, prioritizing stresses and noting his or her usual response. Are there specific times, days, or circumstances when stress is especially high?	Provides database to use in planning interventions to reduce stress.
• If needed, consult with social services for increased support in home care.	Highlights attention to caregiver; realistic planning serves to reduce stress.
• Discuss with caregiver, prior to patient discharge, plans for maintaining self-health and coping abilities.[16]	

Home Health

> NOTE: See section on Mental Health for additional interventions.

Actions/Interventions	Rationales
• Monitor for factors contributing to Caregiver Role Strain.	Provides database for early recognition and intervention.
• Involve client and family in planning, implementing, and promoting reduction or elimination of caregiver role strain: ○ *Family conference*: Clarify expected role performance of all family members. Discuss each member's perception of the situation. ○ *Mutual goal setting*: Decide on short-term goals to relieve caregiver strain. Specify tasks and roles for each member.	Family involvement enhances effectiveness of intervention.

- ○ *Communication*: Establish open, direct communication with positive feedback.
- Assist client and family in making required life-style adjustments: Long-term changes in behavior require support and education.
  - ○ Institutionalization of care receiver
  - ○ Respite for care provider
  - ○ Family relationships
  - ○ Treatment of physical or emotional disability in caregiver and care receiver
  - ○ Stress management
  - ○ Development and use of support networks
  - ○ Requirements for redistribution of family tasks
  - ○ Education and practice if special treatments are required
  - ○ Safe and supportive environment
- Consult with community resources as indicated. (See Appendix B.)   Promotes efficient use of existing resources. A psychiatric nurse clinician, family therapist, day-care or respite center, and support groups can enhance the treatment plan.

FLOW CHART EVALUATION
Flow Chart Expected Outcome 1

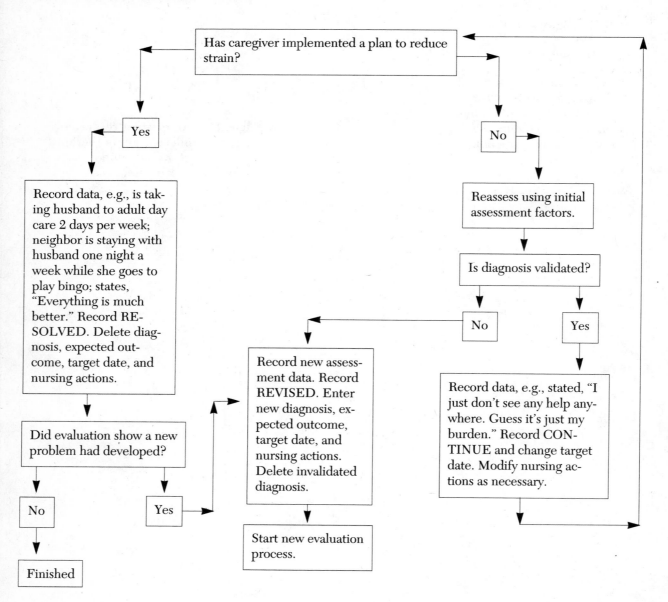

Flow Chart Expected Outcome 2

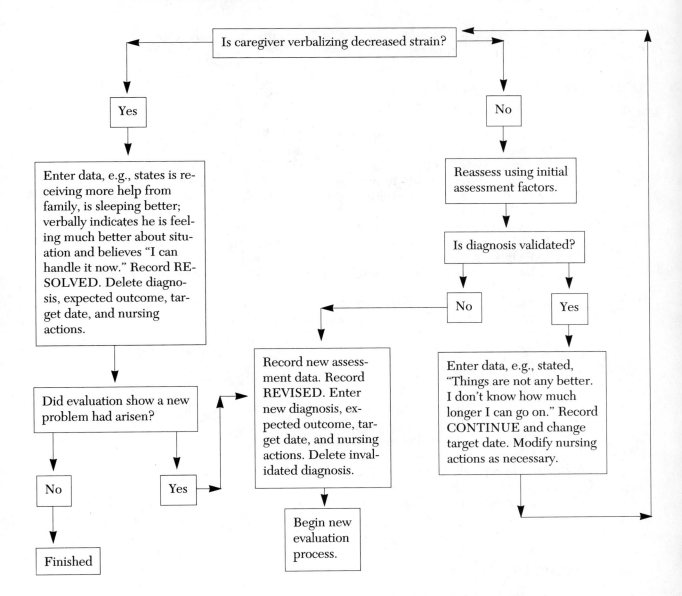

Family Process, Altered

DEFINITION

The state in which a family that normally functions effectively experiences a dysfunction.[17]

NANDA TAXONOMY: RELATING 3.2.2

DEFINING CHARACTERISTICS[17]

1. Major defining characteristics:
   a. Family system unable to meet physical needs of its members
   b. Family system unable to meet emotional needs of its members
   c. Family system unable to meet spiritual needs of its members
   d. Parents do not demonstrate respect for each other's views on child-rearing practices
   e. Inability to express or accept wide range of feelings
   f. Inability to express or accept feelings of members
   g. Family unable to meet security needs of its members
   h. Inability of the family members to relate to each other for mutual growth and maturation
   i. Family uninvolved in community activities
   j. Inability to accept or receive help appropriately
   k. Rigidity in function and roles
   l. Family not demonstrating respect for individuality and autonomy of its members
   m. Family unable to adapt to change or deal with traumatic experience constructively
   n. Family failing to accomplish current or past developmental task
   o. Unhealthy family decision-making process
   p. Failure to send and receive clear messages
   q. Inappropriate boundary maintenance
   r. Inappropriate or poorly communicated family rules, rituals, and symbols
   s. Unexamined family myths
   t. Inappropriate level and direction of energy
2. Minor defining characteristics:
   None given

RELATED FACTORS[17]

1. Situation transition and/or crises
2. Developmental transition and/or crisis

RELATED CLINICAL CONCERNS

1. Surgery
2. Trauma
3. Mental retardation
4. Chronic illness

(See page 874.)

HAVE YOU SELECTED THE CORRECT DIAGNOSIS?

Ineffective Family Coping This diagnosis indicates a history of destructive patterns of behavior. For the diagnosis of Altered Family Process to be applicable, there would be evidence that the usual adequacy in coping is altered in relation to a specific crisis. (See page 874.)

EXPECTED OUTCOMES

1. Will verbalize increased satisfaction with family interactional pattern by (date) and/or
2. Will describe specific plan to cope with (specific stressor) by (date)

TARGET DATE

Five to seven days would be the earliest acceptable target date. Even after the expected outcome has initially been met, there may be other precipitating events that will again alter family processes; therefore, a long-term date should be designated.

NURSING ACTIONS/INTERVENTIONS WITH RATIONALES

Adult Health

Actions/Interventions	Rationales
• Promote a trusting therapeutic relationship during interaction with patient and family by being empathetic, listening actively, accepting feelings and attitudes, and being nonjudgmental.	Provides comfort and aids in crisis resolution.
• Promote open, honest communications among the family members by facilitating group interaction. Encourage the patient and family to express feelings regarding current family process by spending (specific time) each shift, while awake, for this purpose.	Promotes verbalization of feelings and shared understanding of problems. Assists the family to acknowledge and accept the problem. Promotes a common definition of the problem and assists in identifying ways to cope with the problem.
• Allow the family to grieve by providing time, giving permission, referring to clergy and/or bereavement group.	Assists in crisis intervention and provides extra coping mechanisms.
• Monitor readiness to learn; then teach family about the precipitating situation, its implications, and the expected response to treatment.	Provides knowledge base to assist in problem solving; decreases anxiety.
• Allow family members to participate in patient care as possible.	

Continued

Actions/Interventions	Rationales
• Help the family to identify its strengths and weaknesses in dealing with the situation during family conference.	Identifies existing resources for crisis resolution and areas to strengthen; provides positive feedback for strengths that already exist.
• Help family organize to continue usual family activities.	Decreases sense of overwhelming loss of everything; adds stability to activities.
• Refer to community resources. (See Appendix B.)	Provides long-term support and effective use of existing resources.
• See Mental Health section for more detailed interventions.	Collaboration promotes more holistic care; many need specific interventions by a specialist.

Child Health

Actions/Interventions	Rationales
• Promote sibling participation in patient's hospitalization and plans for discharge; for example, allow visitation during game time.	Inclusion of siblings fosters a sense of family concern, and need for support is met for all involved. Undue prolonged separations increase stress on the siblings and family relationships.
• Provide for cultural preferences when possible, including diet, religious needs, and plans for health care.	Attention to preferences demonstrates valuing of and sensitivity for the family.
• Provide reinforcement to appropriately value caretaking behavior.	Reinforcement of desired behaviors serves to offer positive learning with increased likelihood of compliance.

Women's Health

Actions/Interventions	Rationales
• Assist patient and significant others in establishing realistic goals related to changes in role due to newborn; for example, sharing of tasks, parenting skills.	Assists family with role changes during a normal but often unexpected amount of role change. Provides basis for planning necessary changes.
• Provide positive reinforcement for parenting tasks.	Provides motivation and enhances likelihood of effective parenting.
• Assist parents in identifying infant behavior patterns, such as crying and fussing, and understanding how they allow the infant to communicate with them.	Assists in reducing stress and promotes positive parenting.
• Assist patient in verbalizing her perceptions of the infant's growth and development,	Provides database that allows more effective teaching and planning for effective parenting.

individual and family needs, and the stresses of being a new parent.

• Identify support groups such as Mother's Day Out, parenting groups, family, friends.	Promotes planning and allows early intervention in potential stress areas.
• Encourage open communication between mother and father on household tasks, discipline, fears and anxieties about the less-than-perfect baby.	
• Help develop a plan for sharing household tasks and child care activities: ○ Bathing ○ Feeding ○ Care of siblings ○ Spending quality time with older children	Reduces stress-provoking events.
• Allow older children to assist with newborn care (even the smallest child can do this with parental supervision): ○ Bringing a diaper to parent ○ Pushing baby in stroller ○ Holding baby (while sitting on couch is best)	
• Follow up with home visits after discharge from hospital to physically monitor the infant, monitor family interactions, provide support and referrals to the proper agencies. (See Appendix B.)	Provides long-term support.
• Teach and reinforce methods of caring for and coping with the emotional and physiologic needs of the infant, siblings, parents, and other relatives such as grandparents.	Provides measures and preplanning to cope with potential stressful events.

Mental Health

Actions/Interventions	Rationales
• Provide a role model for effective communication by: ○ Seeking clarification ○ Demonstrating respect for individual family members and the family system ○ Listening to expression of thoughts and feelings ○ Setting clear limits ○ Being consistent ○ Communicating with the individual being addressed in a clear manner	Communication skills provide a framework for effective problem solving.

Continued

Actions/Interventions	Rationales

○ Encouraging sharing of information among appropriate system subgroups
• Demonstrate an understanding of the complexity of system problems by:
  ○ Not taking sides in family disagreements
  ○ Providing alternative explanations of behavior that recognizes the contributions of all persons involved with the problem, including health care providers as appropriate
  ○ Requesting the perspective of multiple family members on a problem or stressor
	Outcome improves when psychosocial problems are treated from a systems perspective.[18]

• Include all family members in the first interview.	Provides opportunity to assess all family members' perceptions of the problem and identify problem-solving strategies that are acceptable to more family members.
• Have each member provide his or her perspective on the current difficulties. • Assist the family in defining a problem that can be resolved. For example, rather than defining the problem as "We don't love each other any more," the problem can be defined as "We do not spend time together in family activities." This definition evolves from the family members' description of what they mean by the more general problem description.	

• Assist family in developing behavioral short-term goals by:
  ○ Asking what they would see happening in the family if the situation improved
  ○ Having them break the problem into several parts that combine to form the identified stressor
  ○ Asking them what they could do in a week to improve the situation (this should include a response from each family member)
	Setting achievable goals increases the opportunities for success, which increases the motivation to continue to work toward problem resolution.

• Maintain the nurse's role of facilitator of family communication by:
  ○ Having family members discuss possible solutions among themselves
  ○ Having each family member talk about how he or she might contribute to both the problem and the problem's resolution
• Provide the family with the information necessary for appropriate problem solving.
	Maintains a context that enhances and supports the family's problem-solving skills.

- Answer all questions in an open, direct manner.
- Support the expression of affect:
  - Have family members share feelings with one another.
  - Normalize the expression of emotion; for example, "Most persons experience anger after they have experienced a loss."
  - Provide a private environment for this expression.
- Maintain and support functional family roles; for example, allow parents private time alone, allow children to visit parents, present problems to the "family leader."
- Schedule a time with the family to discuss how the current situation affects family roles and possible changes that may be necessary.
- Have family identify those systems in the community that could support them during this time, and assist family in contacting these systems. Note here systems to be contacted and how they will assist the family.
- Provide positive verbal reinforcement for the family's accomplishments.
- Assist family in identifying patterns of interaction that interfere with successful problem resolution. For example, the husband frequently asks his wife close-ended questions, which discourages her from sharing her ideas; the children interrupt the parents when their level of conflict increases to a certain level; the wife walks out of the room when the husband brings up issues related to finances.
- Assist family in planning fun activities together. This could include time to play together, exercise together, or engage in a shared project.
- Teach family methods of anxiety reduction; establish a practice schedule and a schedule for discussing how this method could be used on a daily basis in the family. The selected method along with the schedule for discussion and practice should be listed here.
- Include family in discussions related to planning care and sharing information about the client's condition.

Promotes a trusting relationship.

Promotes communication among family members while developing a positive expectational set.

Provides positive reinforcement for functional interactions and serves to encourage this behavior while enhancing self-esteem.

Promotes and develops family's strengths.

Positive reinforcement encourages behavior and enhances self-esteem.
Facilitates the development of more appropriate coping behaviors.

Families in crisis often limit their emotional experiences.

Relaxation response inhibits the activation of the autonomic nervous system's fight-or-flight response. Repeated practice of a behavior internalizes and personalizes the behavior.

Support system involvement in problem solving increases the opportunities for a more positive outcome.

Continued

Actions/Interventions	Rationales
• Assist family in developing a specific plan when the client is scheduled for a pass or discharge. Note that plan here, including the assistance needed from the nursing staff for implementation.	Promotes client's sense of control. Planned coping strategies facilitate the enactment of new behaviors when stress is experienced. This increases the opportunities for successful coping and enhances self-esteem.

Gerontic Health

See Adult Health and Mental Health sections.

Home Health

NOTE: See Mental Health section for detailed psychosocial interventions.

Actions/Interventions	Rationales

• Teach client and family appropriate information regarding the care of family members:
  ○ Discipline strategies appropriate for developmental level
  ○ Normal growth and development
  ○ Expected family life-cycles, for example, child rearing, grandparenting
  ○ Coping strategies for family growth
  ○ Care of health deviations
  ○ Developing and using support networks
  ○ Safe environment for family members
  ○ Anticipatory guidance regarding growth and development, discipline, family functioning, responses to illness, role changes, and so on.
	Basic knowledge that contributes to successful family functioning.

• Involve client and family in planning and implementing strategies to decrease or prevent alterations in family process:
  ○ Family conference to ascertain perspective of members on current situation and to identify strategies to improve situation
  ○ Mutual goal setting to identify realistic goals, with evaluation criteria and specific activities for each family member
  ○ Clear, consistent, and honest communication with positive feedback
  ○ Distribution of family tasks so that all members are involved in maintaining family based on developmental capacity
	Family involvement enhances effectiveness of intervention.

- Assist client and family in life-style adjustments that may be required:
  - Separation or divorce
  - Temporary stay in community shelter
  - Family therapy
  - Communication of feelings
  - Stress reduction
  - Identification of potential for violence
  - Providing safe environment
  - Therapeutic use of anger
  - Seeking and providing support for family members
  - Coping with catastrophic or chronic illness
  - Requirements for redistributing family tasks
  - Changing role functions and relationships
  - Financial concerns
- Consult with or refer to community resources as required. (See Appendix B.)

Permanent changes in behavior and family roles require support.

Provides efficient use of existing resources. Support groups, psychiatric nurse clinicians, and teachers can enhance the treatment plan.

FLOW CHART EVALUATION
Flow Chart Expected Outcome 1

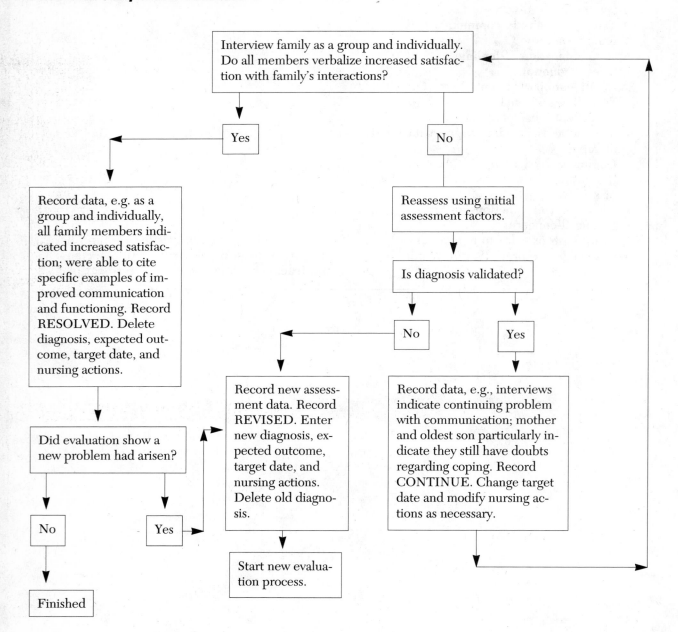

Flow Chart Expected Outcome 2

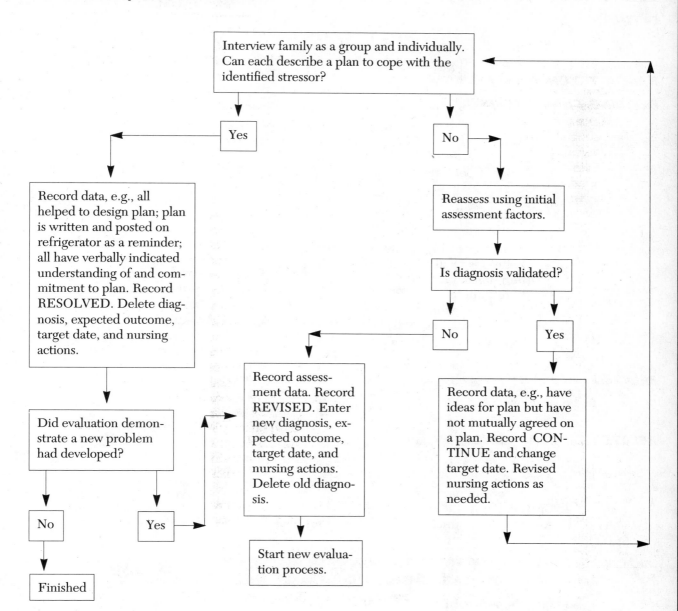

Grieving, Anticipatory

DEFINITION

None given

NANDA TAXONOMY: FEELING 9.2.1.2

DEFINING CHARACTERISTICS[17]

1. Major defining characteristics:
   a. Potential loss of significant object
   b. Expression of distress at potential loss
   c. Denial of potential loss
   d. Guilt
   e. Anger
   f. Sorrow
   g. Choked feelings
   h. Changes in eating habits
   i. Alterations in sleep patterns
   j. Alterations in activity level
   k. Altered libido
   l. Altered communication patterns
2. Minor defining characteristics:
   None given

RELATED FACTORS[17]

To be developed.

RELATED CLINICAL CONCERNS

1. Cancer
2. Amputation
3. Spinal cord injury
4. Birth defects
5. Any diagnosis which family has been told has a terminal prognosis

HAVE YOU SELECTED THE CORRECT DIAGNOSIS?

Sensory-Perceptual Alteration   This diagnosis will be identified according to the patient's change in capacity to exercise judgment or think critically with appropriate sensory-perceptual functioning. This may well be related to Anticipatory Grieving. (See page 562.)

Anxiety; Fear   Anxiety is the response the individual has to a threat that is for the most part unidentified. Fear is the response to an identified threat. When the patient is faced with the thought of death, loss of a limb, loss of functioning, or loss of a loved one, Anxiety and Fear may arise as parallel diagnoses with Anticipatory Grieving. (See pages 605 and 628.)

> **Ineffective Individual Coping** This is the appropriate diagnosis if the individual is not making the necessary adaptations to deal with the threatened loss. This diagnosis can be a companion diagnosis to Anticipatory Grieving. (See page 892.)
>
> **Spiritual Distress** When faced with a devastating loss, the client may well express Spiritual Distress. This quite often is a companion diagnosis to Anticipatory Grieving. (See page 923.)

EXPECTED OUTCOMES

1. Will verbalize feelings about impending loss by (date) and/or
2. Will identify at least two support systems by (date)

TARGET DATE

A target date ranging from 2 to 4 days would be appropriate in evaluating progress toward achievement of the expected outcome.

NURSING ACTIONS/INTERVENTIONS WITH RATIONALES

Adult Health

See Mental Health section.

Child Health

Actions/Interventions	Rationales

• Spend at least 30 minutes every 8 hours (or as situation dictates) to address specific anticipated loss:
  ○ Encourage patient and family to express perception of current situation (may be facilitated by age and developmentally appropriate intervention such as drawing, play or puppet therapy, or the like).
  ○ Provide active listening in a quiet, private environment.
  ○ Offer clarification of procedures, treatment, or plans for patient and family.
  ○ Revise plan of care to honor preferences when possible.
  ○ Discuss and identify impact of anticipated loss.
	A structured discussion places value on the importance of grieving and provides critical data for the plan of care.

• Collaborate with appropriate health care professionals to meet needs of patient and	Appropriate collaboration and the coordination of efforts results in more holistic

Continued

Actions/Interventions	Rationales
family in realistically anticipating loss. (See Appendix B.)	versus fragmented care at a time of special need. A sense of support remains long after the event itself.

• Encourage patient and family to realistically develop coping strategies to best prepare for anticipated loss:
  ○ Engage in diversional activities of choice.
  ○ Reminisce about times spent with loved one or associated with anticipated loss.
  ○ Identify support groups.
	Fostering coping strategies provides an opportunity for growth with minimal support from others, thereby increasing empowerment for the family.

• Encourage optimal function for as long as possible, with identification of need for proper attention to rest, diet, and health of all family members at this time of stress.	Participation in usual daily activities provides a sense of normalcy despite impending loss and provides validation of life.

• Promote parental and sibling participation in care of infant or child according to situation:
  ○ Feedings and selection of menu
  ○ Comfort measures such as holding, backrubs, and so on
  ○ Diversional activities, quiet games, stories
  ○ Decisions regarding life-support measures and resuscitation
	Maintenance of family input and participation in care aids in continuation of the family unit at a time when unity can serve to positively influence daily coping for all.

• Reassure infant or child that he or she is loved and cared for by providing ample opportunities to answer questions regarding specific anticipated loss, whether related to self or others. According to age and developmental status, provide reassurance that patient is not cause of situation.	Reassurance lessens the likelihood of guilt while demonstrating there is no need for assignment of blame to any member of the family.
• Remember that hearing is one of the last of the senses to remain functional. Exercise opportunities for loved ones and staff to continue to address patient even though patient may be unable to answer or respond.	Speaking can serve to reassure child of worth; urge caution in conversations because child may well be able to hear.
• Provide for appropriate safety and maintenance related to physical care of patient.	Standard practice requires safety maintenance; special attention is required when the infant or child is comatose or cannot respond regarding sensations, especially for pressure areas, heat, cold, and so on.

Women's Health

Actions/Interventions	Rationales

• Obtain a thorough obstetric history, including previous occurrences of fetal demise.
• Ascertain if there were any problems conceiving this pregnancy or any attempts to terminate this pregnancy.
• Assess and record mother's perception of cessation of fetal movements.
• Monitor and record fetal activity or lack of activity.
• Inform mother and significant others of antepartal testing and why it is being ordered, and explain results:
  ◦ Nonstress testing
  ◦ Oxytocin challenge test
  ◦ Ultrasound
	Provides essential database needed to plan for effective interventions.

• Be considerate and honest in keeping patient and significant others informed. Share information as soon as it becomes available.	Promotes trusting relationship and provides support during a very difficult time.
• Allow mother and family to express feelings and begin grieving process.	Provides support and care to patient and family, who are unable to begin real grieving because death is not yet real to them while they are going through a '"normal" birthing process.
• With collaboration of physician, facilitate necessary laboratory tests and procedures: blood tests such as complete blood count (CBC), type and crossmatch, and so on; DIC screening and coagulation studies; real time or ultrasound; amniotomy. • Provide emotional support for the couple during labor and birth process. • Closely monitor labor. • Explain the procedure of induction of labor and the use of pitocin, IVs, and the uterine contraction pattern.	In instances where fetal death has been ascertained, labor is induced to prevent further complications.
• Watch for nausea, vomiting, and diarrhea. • Provide comfort measures: analgesics, tranquilizers, and medications for side effects or prostaglandins as ordered. • Change patient's position at least every 2 hours on the (odd/even) hour. • Observe for full bladder. Record intake and output every 8 hours.	

Continued

Actions/Interventions	Rationales

• Provide ice chips for dry mouth, lip balm or petroleum jelly for dry lips.
• Monitor vital signs every 2 to 4 hours at (times).
• Use breathing and relaxation techniques with patient for comfort.
• Inform physician of mother's wishes for use of anesthetic for birth — awake and aware, sedated, or asleep.
• Prepare infant for viewing by mother and significant others:
  ○ Clean infant as much as possible.
  ○ Use clothing to hide gross defects, such as a hat for head defects and a T-shirt or diapers for trunk defects.
  ○ Wrap in soft, clean baby blanket (allow mother to unwrap infant if she desires).
	Initiates the grieving process in a supportive environment; demonstrates respect for and understanding of the family's emotional state.

• Provide private, quiet place and time for parents and family to:
  ○ See and hold infant
  ○ Take pictures
	Provides essential support for family during time of grief; provides reality by letting parents hold infant.

• Provide a certificate for recording footprints, handprints, lock of hair, armbands, date and time of birth, weight of infant, and name of infant. • Contact religious or cultural leader as requested by mother or significant other. Provide for religious practices such as baptism. • Explain need for autopsy or genetic testing of infant.	

• In instances of infertility, assist in realistic planning for future:
  ○ Possible extensive testing
  ○ Fear
  ○ Economics
  ○ Uncertainty
  ○ Embarrassment
  ○ Surgical procedures
  ○ Feelings of inadequacy
  ○ Life without children
  ○ Adoption
	Provides database that can be used in assisting couple to cope with situation and initiate realistic planning for the future.

Mental Health

NOTE: It may take clients anywhere from 6 months to a year to complete the process of grief. This should be taken into consideration when developing evaluation dates. In a short-stay hospitalization, a reasonable set of goals would be to assist the client system in beginning a healthy grieving process. It is also important to note the anniversary date, since grief can be experienced past the 1-year period noted above.

Actions/Interventions	Rationales
• Assign client a primary care nurse and inform client of this decision. (This nurse must be comfortable discussing issues related to loss and grief.)	Promotes the development of a trusting relationship.
• Primary nurse will spend 30 minutes once a shift with client discussing his or her perceptions of the current situation. These discussions could include: ○ His or her perceptions of the loss ○ His or her values or beliefs about the lost "object" ○ Client's past experiences with loss and how these were resolved ○ Client's perceptions of the support system and possible support system responses to the loss	Promotes the development of a trusting relationship; provides a supportive environment for the expression of feelings, which facilitates a healthy resolution of the loss.
• Primary nurse will schedule 30-minute interactions with client and support system to assist them in discussing issues related to the loss and answering any questions they might have. (Note time and date of this interaction here.)	
• Primary nurse will discuss with client and family role adjustments and other anticipated changes related to the loss.	Anticipatory planning facilitates adaptation.
• If necessary after the first interaction, primary nurse will schedule follow-up visits with the client and his or her support system. (Note schedule for these interactions here.)	
• Spend (number) minutes with client each hour. (This should begin as 5-minute times and increase to 10 minutes as client needs and unit staffing permit.) If client does not desire to talk during this time, it can be used to give a massage (backrub) or sit with client in silence. Inform client of these times, let him or her know if for some reason this schedule has to be altered, and develop a new time for the visit. Inform client that the purpose of this time is for him or her to use as he or she sees fit. The	Promotes the development of a trusting relationship and client's sense of control.

Continued

Actions/Interventions	Rationales
nurse should be seated during this time if he or she is not providing a massage.	
• Provide positive verbal and nonverbal reinforcement to expressions of grief from both the client and the support system. This would include remaining with the client when he or she is expressing strong emotions.	Positive reinforcement encourages the behavior and enhances self-esteem.
• Once the client and the support system are discussing the loss, assist them in scheduling time when they can be alone.	Facilitates healthy resolution of the loss.
• Answer questions in an open, honest manner.	Promotes the development of a trusting relationship and promotes the client's sense of control.
• If the client expresses anger toward the staff and this anger appears to be unrelated to the situation, accept it as part of the grieving process and support the client in its expression by: ○ Not responding in a defensive manner ○ Recognizing the feelings that are being expressed; for example, "It sounds like you are very angry right now" or "It can be very frustrating to be in a situation where you feel you have little control"	Expression of anger is a normal part of the grieving process, and it is "safer" to be angry with members of the health care team than with the family.
• Recognize that stages of grief can progress at individual rates and in various patterns. Do not force a client through stages or express expectations about what the "normal" next step should be.	Supports the client's perception of control and strengths.
• If the client is in denial related to the loss, allow this to happen and provide client with information about the loss at the client's pace. If the client does not remember information given before, simply provide the information again.	Serves as a way for client to protect self from information he or she is not ready to cope with. As coping behaviors are strengthened, clients will be able to accept and respond to this information.
• Allow client and support system to participate in decisions related to nursing care. Those areas in which client decision making is to be encouraged should be noted here, along with the client's decisions.	Promotes client's sense of control and enhances client's strengths.
• Normalize client's and support system's experience of grief by telling client that his or her experience is normal and by discussing with him or her potential future responses to loss.	Promotes the client's sense of control and a positive orientation, which enhance self-esteem.
• Recognize that this is an emotionally	Encourages expression of feelings and

painful time for the client and the support system, and share this understanding with the client system.

- Assist client in obtaining the spiritual support needed.
- Monitor the use of sedatives and tranquilizers. Consult with the physician if overuse is suspected.

Extensive use of these medications may delay the grieving process.

- Monitor the client system's use of alcohol and nonprescription drugs as a coping method. Refer to Ineffective Individual Coping (Chapter 11) if this is assessed as a problem.

These are symptoms of ineffective coping and interfere with the normal grieving process.

- Have client and support system develop a list of concerns and problems and assist them in determining those they have the ability to change and those they do not.

Promotes the client's strengths.

- When they have a list of workable problems, have client system list all of the solutions they can think of for a problem, and encourage them to include those solutions that they think are impossible or just fantasy solutions. Do this one problem at a time.

Facilitates creative problem solving by assisting the family to try new methods of problem solving.

- Assist client in evaluating solutions generated. Solutions can be combined, eliminated, or altered. From this list the best solution is selected. It is important that the solution selected is the client's solution.

Promotes the development of creative problem solving.

- Assist client in developing a plan for implementing this solution. Note any assistance needed from the nursing staff here.

Planned coping strategies facilitate the enactment of new behaviors when the client is experiencing stress.

- Observe client for signs and symptoms of dysfunctional grieving.

Early intervention promotes positive outcome.

- Monitor client's nutritional pattern, and refer to appropriate nursing diagnoses if a problem is identified.

Nutritional status impacts the individual's ability to cope.

- Develop an exercise plan for the client. Consult with physical therapist as needed. Develop a reward schedule for the accomplishment of this plan. Note schedule for plan here. This can also include the support system.

Exercise increases the production of endorphins, which contribute to feelings of well-being.

- Provide support for the support system:
  ○ Have them develop a schedule for rest periods.
  ○ Provide snacks for them and schedule periods of high nursing involvement with the client at a time when support persons

facilitates progression through the grieving process.

Support system reactions can impact the client.

Continued

Actions/Interventions	Rationales
can obtain meals; this can reassure the support person that client will not be alone while he or she is gone. ○ Assist support system in finding cafeteria and transportation. ○ Suggest that support persons rest or walk outside or around hospital while client is napping. ○ Help support persons discuss their feelings with client.	

Gerontic Health

Actions/Interventions	Rationales
• Provide information to patient regarding what is occurring as well as expected or anticipated changes. • Discuss with the individual the grieving process, what can be anticipated, and how each person grieves in his or her own way.	This intervention is viewed by survivors as especially helpful during the dying process.[19] Provides information on common responses to loss and what emotions are commonly experienced by grieving people. Promotes grieving process and reassures survivor that he or she is coping well.

Home Health

NOTE: See Mental Health section for detailed interventions.

Actions/Interventions	Rationales
• Teach client and family appropriate monitoring of signs and symptoms of anticipatory grief: ○ Crying, sadness ○ Alterations in eating and sleeping patterns ○ Developmental regression ○ Alterations in concentration ○ Expressions of distress at loss ○ Denial of loss ○ Expressions of guilt ○ Labile affect ○ Grieving beyond expected time ○ Preoccupation with loss ○ Hallucinations	Provides database for early recognition and intervention.

- ○ Violence toward self or others
- ○ Delusions
- ○ Prolonged isolation
- Involve client and family in planning and implementing strategies to reduce or cope with anticipatory grieving:
  - ○ *Family conference*: Develop list of concerns and problems; identify those concerns that family can control.
  - ○ *Mutual goal setting*: Set realistic short-term goals and evaluation criteria. Specify role of each family member.
  - ○ *Communication*: Discuss loss in supportive environment.

Family involvement in planning enhances effectiveness of plan.

- Assist client and family in life-style adjustments that may be required:
  - ○ Provide realistic hope.
  - ○ Identify expected grief pattern in response to loss.
  - ○ Recognize variety of accepted expressions of grief.
  - ○ Help client develop and use support networks.
  - ○ Encourage client to communicate feelings.
  - ○ Provide a safe environment.
  - ○ Discuss therapeutic use of denial.
  - ○ Identify suicidal potential or potential for violence.
  - ○ Note therapeutic use of anger.
  - ○ Explore meaning of situation.
  - ○ Promote stress reduction.
  - ○ Promote expression of grief.
  - ○ Discuss decision making for future.
  - ○ Promote family cohesiveness.

Permanent changes in behavior and life-style and facilitated by knowledge and support.

- Assist client and family in setting criteria to determine when intervention of health care professional is required; for example, client is threat to self or others or client is unable to perform activities of daily living.

Provides data for early intervention.

- Consult and/or refer to community resources as indicated. (See Appendix B.)

Provides efficient use of existing resources. Self-help groups, religious counselor, or psychiatric nurse clinician can enhance the treatment plan.

Role-Relationship Pattern

FLOW CHART EVALUATION
Flow Chart Expected Outcome 1

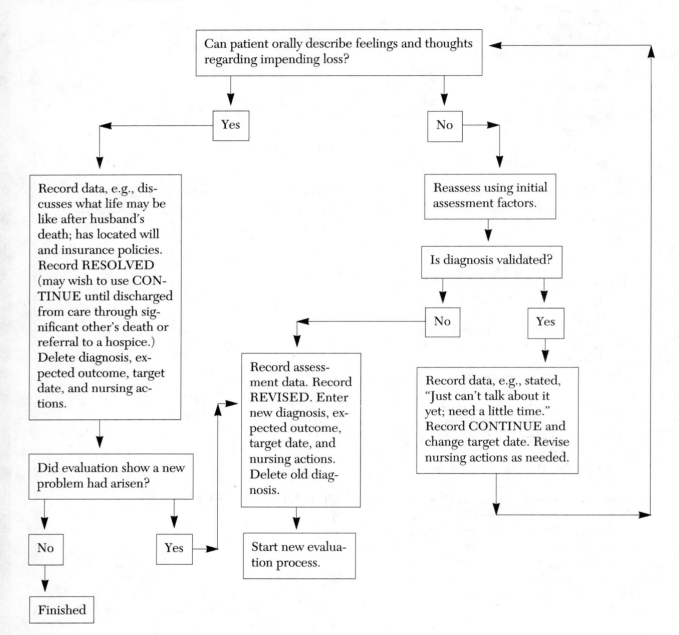

Flow Chart Expected Outcome 2

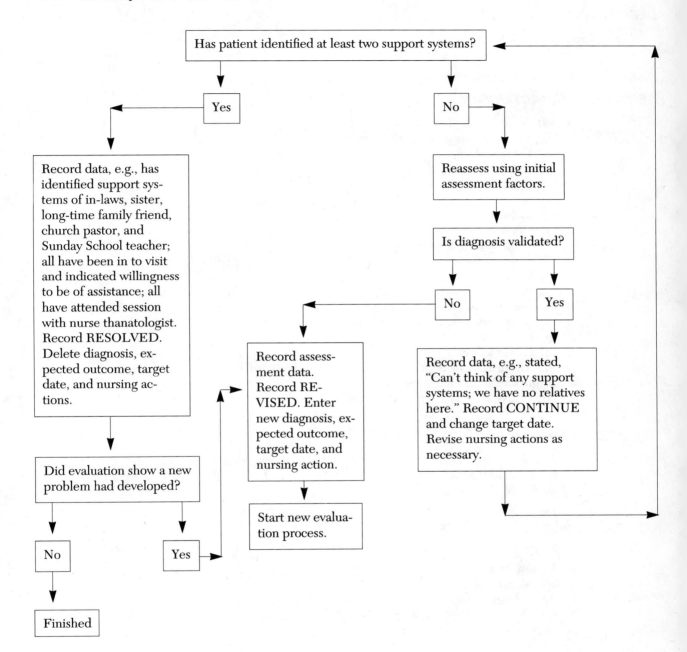

Grieving, Dysfunctional

DEFINITION

None given.

NANDA TAXONOMY: FEELING 9.2.1.1

DEFINING CHARACTERISTICS[17]

1. Major defining characteristics:
   a. Verbal expression of distress at loss
   b. Denial of loss
   c. Expression of guilt
   d. Expression of unresolved issues
   e. Anger
   f. Sadness
   g. Crying
   h. Difficulty in expressing loss
   i. Alterations in eating habits, sleep patterns, dream patterns, activity level, libido
   j. Idealization of lost object
   k. Reliving of past experiences
   l. Interference with life functioning
   m. Developmental regression
   n. Labile affect
   o. Alterations in concentration and/or pursuits of tasks
2. Minor defining characteristics:
   None given

RELATED FACTORS[17]

1. **Actual or perceived object loss**: Object loss is used in the broadest sense and may include people, possessions, a job, status, home, ideals, parts and processes of the body.

RELATED CLINICAL CONCERNS

1. Cancer
2. Amputation
3. Spinal cord injury
4. Birth defects
5. Any diagnosis that family has been told has a terminal prognosis
6. Sudden infant death syndrome (SIDS)
7. Stillbirth
8. Infertility

STOP **HAVE YOU SELECTED THE CORRECT DIAGNOSIS?**

Sensory-Perceptual Alteration This diagnosis will be identified according to the patient's change in capacity to exercise judgment or think critically with appropriate sensory-perceptual functioning. This may well be related to Dysfunctional Grieving. (See page 562.)

Anxiety, Fear Anxiety is the response the individual has to a threat that is for the most part unidentified. Fear is the response made by an individual to an identified threat. When the patient has experienced a loss, it is not a threat but an actual event. Therefore, the diagnoses of Anxiety and Fear would not be appropriate. (See pages 605 and 628.)

Ineffective Individual Coping This can be an appropriate diagnosis if the individual is not making the necessary adaptations to deal with crises in his or her life; however, if a real loss has occurred, the most appropriate diagnosis is Dysfunctional Grieving. (See page 892.)

Spiritual Distress When faced with a devastating loss, the client may well express Spiritual Distress. Quite often, this is a companion diagnosis to Dysfunctional Grieving. (See page 923.)

EXPECTED OUTCOME

1. Will verbalize grief feelings by (date) and/or
2. Will identify at least (number) ways to appropriately cope with grief by (date)

TARGET DATE

Grief work should begin within 1 to 2 days after the nurse has intervened; the complete process of grief may take 6 months to a year.

NURSING ACTIONS/INTERVENTIONS WITH RATIONALES

Adult Health

See Mental Health section.

Child Health

NOTE: It is difficult to make general assumptions as to how each child views death, but according to previous patterns of behavior, including communication, it would be necessary to allow for developmental patterns previously attained. In young children there may be manifestations of obsessive, ritualistic behavior related to the loss or activities surrounding loss. For example, if a loved one dies, young children may think that if they fall asleep they may also die. In the event of grieving, regardless of the precipitating event, the child must be allowed to respond in keeping with developmental capacity. At times when the child is in danger of self-injury or injuring others, the risk for violence must be considered.

Actions/Interventions	Rationales
• Provide opportunities for expression of feelings related to loss or grief according to developmental capacity; for example, puppets or play therapy for toddlers.	Expression of feelings helps to deal with sense of loss and provides a database for intervention. Expression of grief reduces uncontrolled outbursts.
• In the event of a family member's death, offer support in understanding deceased family member's relationship to patient and status for family, with special attention to siblings and their reactions. Identify impact grief has for family dynamics via assessment of same.	Provides database for more accurate intervention in dealing with loss.
• Allow for cultural and religious input in plan of care, especially related to care of dying patient and care of patient at time of death.	Demonstrates valuing of these beliefs to family and decreases stress for family.
• Collaborate with professionals and paraprofessionals to aid in resolution of grief according to family preferences. (See Appendix B.)	Collaboration offers the most comprehensive plan of care and avoids fragmentation of care.
• Identify support groups to assist in resolution of grief, such as Compassionate Friends Organization.	Support groups offer validation of feelings and a sense of hope as similar concerns are shared.
• Assist family members in identification of coping strategies needed for resultant role-relationship changes.	Provides for support during the adjustments that are required because of the loss of a loved one.
• Assist family members to resolve feelings of loss via reminiscing about loved one, positive aspects of situation, or personal growth potential presented. (Remember, behavior often serves as the most effective communication for the toddler or young child.)	Reminiscing about and valuing past experiences will offer an opportunity to project the impact for the present and future.
• Allow family members time and space to face reality of situation and ponder meaning of loss for self and family.	Time and readiness promote the willingness to discuss feelings after the major emotional shock has diminished.
• Direct family to appropriate resources regarding positive methods of acknowledging loved one through memorials or related processes.	A sense of fulfillment may be derived from the sharing of time, talent, or money in the honor of the loved one. This helps to resolve some of the guilt or emptiness associated with the loss.
• Assist in referral to appropriate resources for funeral planning and arrangements if needed.	In times of emotional duress, objective decisions may be difficult. Providing assistance will offer empowerment and a sense of coping.
• In the event of SIDS, provide an opportunity, through a scheduled conference, for verbalization of:	

- How infant's death occurred
- Police investigation
- Sense of guilt
- Feelings of powerlessness
- Questions
- Anger
- Disbelief
- Fears for future pregnancies and births
- Identify the impact the death or grief has on other family members, the relationship of the couple, and the couple's attitude toward having other children.

Provides the essential database to assist in planning that will offset the development of dysfunctional grieving.

Women's Health

Actions/Interventions	Rationales
• Schedule a 30-minute daily conference with couple and focus on: ○ Expression of grief, anger, guilt, frustration ○ The couple's, the relatives', and society's expectations regarding children • Provide factual information on SIDS, stillbirth, or abortion (whichever diagnosis is appropriate). • Encourage couple to share feelings with each other honestly. • During conference, encourage couple to ask questions through open-ended questions, reflection, and so on.	Initiates expression of emotions that allows gradual progress through the grief process. Allows clarification of issues related to a pregnancy that has not resulted in a healthy infant.
• During hospitalization, monitor for signs and symptoms of depression, anger, frustration, and impending crisis. • Encourage couple to seek professional help as necessary to deal with continued concerns, such as their sexual relationship, conflicts, anxieties, parenting, and coping mechanisms that can be used to deal with the loss of fertility.	Provides the database necessary to permit early intervention and prevention of more serious problems during this crisis. Fetal demise, SIDS, and the decision to have an abortion all have long-term effects; therefore, long-term support will be required.
• Assist couple, through teaching and provision of written information, to realize grief may not be resolved for over a year.	Avoids unrealistic expectations regarding grief resolution.

Mental Health

Actions/Interventions	Rationales
• Monitor source of the interference with the grieving process.	Early recognition and intervention can facilitate the grieving process.
• Monitor client's use of medications and the effects this may have on the grieving process. Consult with physician regarding necessary alterations in this area.	Sedatives and tranquilizers may delay the grieving process.
• Assign a primary care nurse to the client.	Facilitates the development of a trusting relationship.
• Provide a calm, reassuring environment.	Excessive environmental stimuli can increase the client's confusion and disorganization.
• When client is demonstrating an emotional response to the grief, provide privacy and remain with the client during this time.	Encourages appropriate expression of feelings.
• Primary nurse will spend 15 minutes twice a day with the client at (times). These interactions should begin as nonconfrontational interactions with the client. The goal is to develop a trusting relationship so the client can later discuss issues related to the grieving process.	Facilitates the development of a trusting relationship.
• Monitor level of dysfunction and assist client with activities of daily living as necessary. Note type and amount of assistance here.	Facilitates the development of a trusting relationship.
• Monitor nutritional status and refer to Altered Nutrition (Chapter 3) for detailed care plan.	Alterations in nutrition can impact coping abilities.
• Monitor significant others' response to the client. Have primary nurse set a schedule to meet with them and the client every other day to answer questions and facilitate discussion between the client and the support system. Note schedule for these meetings here.	Support system understanding facilitates the maintenance of new behaviors after discharge.
• Provide the spiritual support that the client indicates is necessary. Note here the type of assistance needed from the nursing staff.	Clients may find answers to their questions about life and loss through spiritual expression.
• Allow client to express anger and assure him or her that you will not allow harm to come to anyone during this expression.	Violent behavior can evolve from unexpressed anger. Appropriate expression of anger promotes the client's sense of control and enhances self-esteem.
• Provide client with punching bags and other physical activities that assist with the expression of anger. Note tools and specific activities that assist the client with this expression here.	Assists client in developing appropriate coping behaviors, thus enhancing self-esteem.

• Remind staff and support system that client's expressions of anger at this point should not be taken personally, even though they may be directed at specific persons.	Support system understanding facilitates the maintenance of new behaviors after discharge.
• Answer questions directly and openly.	Promotes the development of a trusting relationship.
• Provide time and opportunity for client to participate in appropriate religious rituals. Note assistance needed from nursing staff here.	Rituals provide clarity and direction for the grieving process.
• Sit with client while he or she is talking about the lost object.	The presence of the nurse provides positive reinforcement. Positive reinforcement encourages the behavior.
• When client's verbal interactions increase with the primary nurse to the level that group interactions are possible, schedule client to participate in a group that allows expression of feelings and feedback from peers. Note schedule of group here.	Provides opportunities for peer feedback and peer assistance in problem solving.
• Assign client appropriate tasks in unit activities. Note type of tasks assigned here. These should be based on the client's level of functioning and should be at a level that the client can accomplish. Note type of tasks to be assigned to client here.	Successful accomplishment of tasks enhances self-esteem.
• If delusions, hallucinations, phobias, or depression are present, refer to Ineffective Individual Coping (Chapter 11) and Altered Thought Process (Chapter 7).	
• Primary nurse will engage client and the support system in planning for life-style changes that might result from the loss. Note schedule for these interactions here along with the specific goals.	Planned coping strategies facilitate the enactment of new behaviors when the client is experiencing stress, thus enhancing self-esteem.

Gerontic Health

See Adult Health and Mental Health sections.

Home Health

NOTE: See the section on Mental Health for detailed interventions.

Actions/Interventions	Rationales
• Teach client and family appropriate monitoring of signs and symptoms of dysfunctional grief:	Provides database for early recognition and intervention.

Continued

Actions/Interventions	Rationales

○ Crying, sadness
  ○ Alterations in eating and sleeping patterns
  ○ Developmental regression
  ○ Alterations in concentration
  ○ Expressions of distress at loss
  ○ Denial of loss
  ○ Expressions of guilt
  ○ Labile affect
  ○ Grieving beyond expected time
  ○ Preoccupation with loss
  ○ Hallucinations
  ○ Violence toward self or others
  ○ Delusions
  ○ Prolonged isolation
• Involve client and family in planning and implementing strategies to reduce or cope with dysfunctional grieving:
  ○ *Family conference*: Identify concerns.
  ○ *Mutual goal setting*: Set realistic goals with evaluation criteria. Specify activities for each family member.
  ○ *Communication*: Engage in open and honest communication with positive feedback. Recognize that anger is common and should not be taken personally.
	Family involvement in designing the plan of care enhances the effectiveness of the interventions.

• Assist client and family in life-style adjustments that may be required, including:
  ○ Providing realistic hope
  ○ Identifying expected grief pattern in response to loss
  ○ Recognizing a variety of accepted expressions of grief
  ○ Developing and using support networks
  ○ Communicating feelings
  ○ Providing a safe environment
  ○ Using denial therapeutically
  ○ Identifying suicidal potential or potential for violence
  ○ Using anger therapeutically
  ○ Exploring meaning of situation
  ○ Employing stress reduction
  ○ Promoting expression of grief
  ○ Promoting family cohesiveness
	Dysfunctional grieving can be a chronic condition. Permanent changes in behavior and family roles require support.

• Assist client and family in setting criteria to help them determine when intervention of	Provides for early recognition and intervention.

health care professional is required; for example, when there is prolonged inability to complete activities of daily living or threat to self or others.

- Consult with or refer to community resources as indicated. (See Appendix B.)

Psychiatric nurse clinician and support groups can enhance the treatment plan.

FLOW CHART EVALUATION
Flow Chart Expected Outcome 1

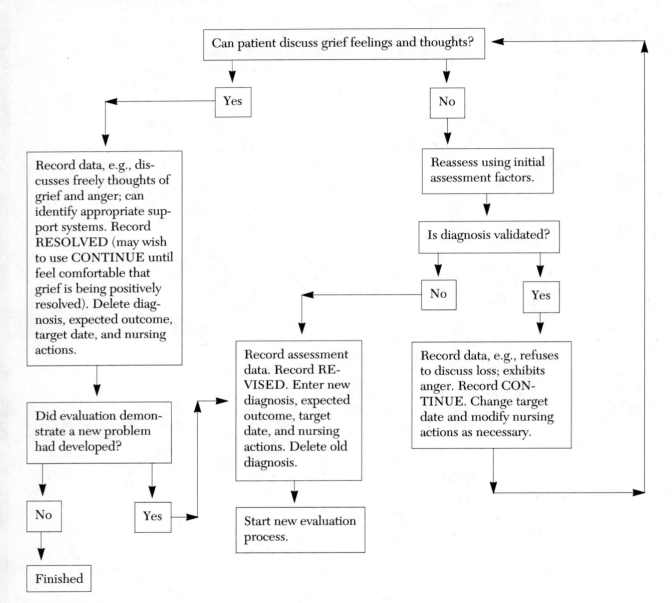

Can patient discuss grief feelings and thoughts?

Yes

No

Record data, e.g., discusses freely thoughts of grief and anger; can identify appropriate support systems. Record RESOLVED (may wish to use CONTINUE until feel comfortable that grief is being positively resolved). Delete diagnosis, expected outcome, target date, and nursing actions.

Reassess using initial assessment factors.

Is diagnosis validated?

No

Yes

Did evaluation demonstrate a new problem had developed?

Record assessment data. Record REVISED. Enter new diagnosis, expected outcome, target date, and nursing actions. Delete old diagnosis.

Record data, e.g., refuses to discuss loss; exhibits anger. Record CONTINUE. Change target date and modify nursing actions as necessary.

No

Yes

Finished

Start new evaluation process.

Flow Chart Expected Outcome 2

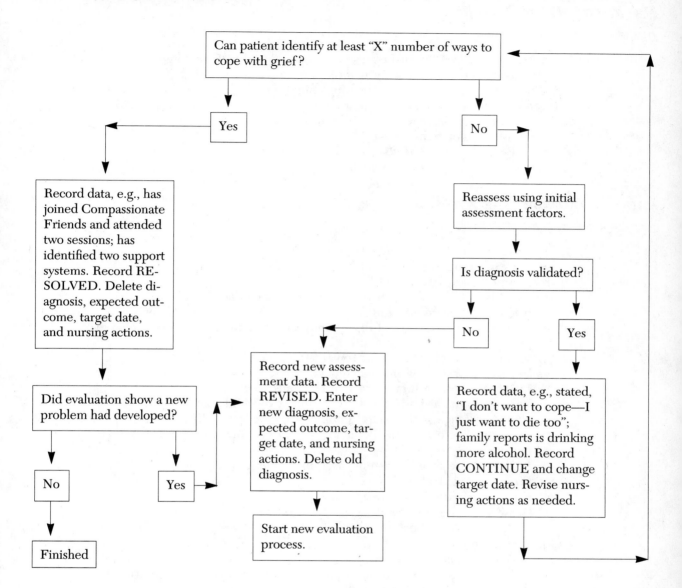

Can patient identify at least "X" number of ways to cope with grief?

Yes

No

Record data, e.g., has joined Compassionate Friends and attended two sessions; has identified two support systems. Record RESOLVED. Delete diagnosis, expected outcome, target date, and nursing actions.

Reassess using initial assessment factors.

Is diagnosis validated?

No

Yes

Did evaluation show a new problem had developed?

Record new assessment data. Record REVISED. Enter new diagnosis, expected outcome, target date, and nursing actions. Delete old diagnosis.

Record data, e.g., stated, "I don't want to cope—I just want to die too"; family reports is drinking more alcohol. Record CONTINUE and change target date. Revise nursing actions as needed.

No

Yes

Start new evaluation process.

Finished

Parenting, Altered: High Risk for, Actual, and Parental Role Conflict

DEFINITIONS

High Risk for Altered Parenting: The state in which a nurturing figure is at risk of experiencing an inability to create an environment that promotes the optimum growth and development of another human being.*

Altered Parenting: The state in which a nurturing figure experiences an inability to create an environment that promotes the optimum growth and development of another human being.*

Parental Role Conflict: The state in which a parent experiences role confusion and conflict in response to crisis.[17]

NANDA TAXONOMY: RELATING 3.2.1.1.2, 3.2.1.1.1, 3.2.3.1

DEFINING CHARACTERISTICS[17]

1. Risk factors for High Risk for Altered Parenting:
   a. Lack of parental attachment behaviors
   b. Inappropriate visual, tactile, or auditory stimulation
   c. Negative identification of infant's or child's characteristics
   d. Negative attachment of meaning to infant's or child's characteristics
   e. Constant verbalization of disappointment in gender or physical characteristics of the infant or child
   f. Verbalization of resentment toward the infant or child
   g. Verbalization of role inadequacy
   h. Inattentiveness to infant's or child's needs (*critical*)
   i. Verbal disgust at body functions of infant or child
   j. Noncompliance with health appointments for self and/or infant or child
   k. Inappropriate caretaking behaviors (toilet training, sleep and rest, feeding) (*critical*)
   l. Inappropriate or inconsistent discipline practices
   m. Frequent accidents
   n. Frequent illness
   o. Growth and development lag in the child
   p. History of child abuse or abandonment by primary caretaker (*critical*)
   q. Verbalization of desire to have child call caretaker by first name versus traditional cultural tendencies
   r. Child receives care from multiple caretakers without consideration for the needs of the infant or child
   s. Compulsive seeking of role approval from others
2. Altered Parenting:
   a. Major defining characteristics:
      (1) Abandonment
      (2) Runaway
      (3) Verbalization that he or she cannot control child

---

*It is important to state as a preface to this diagnosis that adjustment to parenting in general is a normal maturational process that elicits nursing behaviors of prevention of potential problems and health promotion.

        (4) Incidence of physical and psychological trauma

        (5) Lack of parental attachment behaviors

        (6) Inappropriate visual, tactile, or auditory stimulation

        (7) Negative identification of infant's or child's characteristics

        (8) Negative attachment of meanings to infant's or child's characteristics

        (9) Constant verbalization of disappointment in gender or physical characteristics of the infant or child

      (10) Verbalization of resentment toward the infant or child

      (11) Verbalization of role inadequacy

      (12) Inattentive to infant's or child's needs (*critical*)

      (13) Verbal disgust at body functions of infant or child

      (14) Noncompliance with health appointments for self and/or infant or child

      (15) Inappropriate caretaking behaviors (toilet training, sleep and rest, feeding) (*critical*)

      (16) Inappropriate or inconsistent discipline practices

      (17) Frequent accidents

      (18) Frequent illness

      (19) Growth and development lag in the child

      (20) History of child abuse or abandonment by primary caretaker (*critical*)

      (21) Verbalizes desire to have child call caretaker by first name versus traditional cultural tendencies

      (22) Child receives care from multiple caretakers without consideration for the needs of the infant or child

      (23) Compulsively seeking role approval from others

   b. Minor defining characteristics:

   None given

3. Parental Role Conflict:

   a. Major defining characteristics:

      (1) Parent expresses concerns or feelings of inadequacy about providing for child's physical and emotional needs during hospitalization or in the home

      (2) Existence of demonstrated disruption in caretaking routines

      (3) Parent expresses concerns about changes in parental role, family functioning, family communication, family health

   b. Minor defining characteristics:

      (1) Parent expresses concern about perceived loss of control over decisions relating to the child

      (2) Parent is reluctant to participate in usual caretaking activities even with encouragement and support

      (3) Parent verbalizes or demonstrates feelings of guilt, anger, fear, anxiety, and/or frustration about effect of child's illness on family process

RELATED FACTORS[17]

1. High Risk for and Altered Parenting:

   a. Lack of available role model

   b. Ineffective role model

   c. Physical and psychosocial abuse of nurturing figure

    d. Lack of support between or from significant others
    e. Unmet social or emotional maturation needs of parenting figures
    f. Interruption in bonding process—maternal, paternal, or other
    g. Unrealistic expectation for self, infant, or partner
    h. Perceived threat to own physical and emotional survival
    i. Mental and/or physical illness
    j. Presence of stress (financial, legal, recent crisis, cultural move)
    k. Lack of knowledge
    l. Limited cognitive functioning
    m. Lack of role identify
    n. Lack of or inappropriate response of child to relationship
    o. Multiple pregnancies
2. Parental Role Conflict:
    a. Separation from child due to chronic illness
    b. Intimidation with invasive or restrictive modalities (for example, isolation, intubation)
    c. Specialized care center policies
    d. Home care of a child with special needs (for example, apnea monitoring, postural drainage, hyperalimentation)
    e. Change in marital status
    f. Interruptions of family life owing to home care regimen (treatments, lack of respite for caregivers)

RELATED CLINICAL CONCERNS

1. Birth defect
2. Multiple birth
3. Chronically ill child
4. Substance abuse
5. Parental chronic illness
6. Major depressive episode
7. Manic episode
8. Phobic disorders
9. Dissociative disorders
10. Organic mental disorders
11. Schizophrenic disorders

HAVE YOU SELECTED THE CORRECT DIAGNOSIS?

Family Process, Altered   This diagnosis indicates dysfunctioning on part of the entire family, not just the parents. If the entire family is indicating difficulties dealing with current problems or crises, then Altered Family Process is a more correct diagnosis than one of the parenting diagnoses. (See page 710.)

Family Coping, Ineffective   This diagnosis usually arises from the client's perception that his or her primary support is no longer fulfilling this role. If the problem relates to parents and their children, then one of the parenting diagnoses is the most appropriate diagnosis. (See page 874.)

EXPECTED OUTCOMES

1. Will demonstrate appropriate parental role of (specify: feeding, medication administration, and so on) behavior by (date) and/or
2. Will verbalize realistic expectations of self as parent and for child by (date)

TARGET DATE

The diagnosis will require a lengthy amount of time to be totally resolved. However, progress toward resolution could be evaluated within 7 days.

NURSING ACTIONS/INTERVENTIONS WITH RATIONALES

Adult Health

Actions/Interventions	Rationales
• Provide information relative to normal growth and development of self and child by sitting and talking with patient for 30 minutes twice a day at (times).	Provides knowledge base and helps patients to know that some of the things they are experiencing are normal.
• During conference time, assist parent to recognize when stress is becoming distress; for example, irritability turns to rage and/or verbal or physical abuse, sleeplessness, altered thought process, tunnel perception of situation.	Prevents a crisis situation; promotes self-knowledge.
• Teach stress management and parenting techniques; for example, relaxation, deep breathing, Mother's Day Out, safety precautions, toileting process, and so on.	Provides alternative strategies for coping and provides database for dealing with growth and development of child.
• Provide opportunities for parent to participate in child's care.	Gives opportunity to practice parenting skills and obtain feedback in supportive environment.
• Discuss disciplinary methods other than physical: grounding, taking away privileges, positive reinforcement and verbal praise for "good" behavior, and so on.	Physical discipline can lead to abuse; sends wrong message to child.
• Encourage patient to allow time for own needs.	Own needs must be met to decrease stress and facilitate meeting needs of others.
• Encourage use of support groups. (See Appendix B.) Initiate referrals as needed.	Provides an outlet for parents with other parents in similar situations; provides long-term support and assistance.

Actions/Interventions	Rationales
• Review current level of knowledge regarding parenting of infant or child, including: ○ Parental perception of infant or child ○ Parental views of expected development of infant or child ○ Health status of infant or child ○ Current needs of infant or child ○ Infant or child communication (remember, behaviors reveal much about feelings) ○ Normal infant or child responsiveness ○ Family dynamics (for example, who offers support for emotional needs, child's view of mother and father)	Provides database needed to more accurately plan care.
• Determine needs for specific health or developmental intervention from other health care providers as needed. (See Appendix B.)	Needs may be identified with assistance from experts in multidisciplinary domains. Collaboration is essential to avoid fragmentation of care.
• Observe parental readiness and encourage caretaking in a supportive atmosphere in the following ways as applicable: ○ Feeding ○ Bathing ○ Anticipatory safety measures ○ Clarification of medical or health maintenance regimen ○ Play and developmental stimulations for age and capacity ○ Handling and carriage of infant or child ○ Diapering and dressing of infant or child ○ Social interaction appropriate for age and capacity ○ Other specific measures according to patient's status and needs	Provides data needed to plan teaching and to provide individualization of the plan of care.
• Schedule a daily conference of at least 1 hour with parents, and encourage parents to verbalize perceived parenting role, both current and desired.	Provides teaching opportunity; verbalization reveals thoughts and data needed to more accurately plan care.
• Allow parents to gradually assume total care of infant within hospital setting at least 48 hours before dismissal. If more time is required to validate appropriate parenting success, collaborate with pediatrician regarding extending child's stay for 24 hours.	Provides opportunity for practice of needed skills or roles; fosters growth and confidence in parenting.
• During conference, assist parents to identify ways of coping with infant and parental demands, including family, community, and health care professional support.	Provides growth for parents; provides long-term support.

Women's Health

Actions/Interventions	Rationales

• Through monthly conferences, assist patient in completing the tasks of pregnancy by encouraging verbalization of:
○ Fears
○ Mother's perception of marriage
○ Mother's perception of "child within" her
○ Mother's perception of the changes in her life as a result of this birth:
  (1) Relationship with partner
  (2) Relationship with other children
  (3) Effects on career
  (4) Effects on family
• Allow mother to question pregnancy: "Now" and "Who, me?"[20]
	Acceptance of pregnancy and working through the tasks of pregnancy provide a strong basis for positive parenthood and appropriate attachment and bonding.

• Assist mother in realizing existence of child by encouraging mother to: ○ Note when infant moves ○ Listen to fetal heart tones during visit to clinic ○ Discuss body changes and their relationship to infant ○ Verbalize any questions she may have • Assist in preparation for birth by: ○ Encouraging attendance at childbirth education classes ○ Providing factual information regarding the birthing experience ○ Involving significant others in preparation for birthing process • Assist patient in preparing for role transition to parenthood by encouraging: ○ Economic planning; physician, hospital, prenatal testing fees ○ Social planning; changes in life-style	Provides basis for appropriate attachment behaviors and coping skills for transition to maternal role.
• Assist patient in identifying needs related to family's acceptance of the newborn: ○ Mother's perceived level of support from family members ○ Stressors present in family: economics, housing, level of knowledge regarding parenting • Monitor for following behaviors: ○ Refuses to plan for infant ○ No interest in pregnancy or fetal progress ○ Overly concerned with own weight and appearance	Assists in identifying patients at high risk for the development of this diagnosis.

Continued

Actions/Interventions	Rationales
○ Refuses to gain weight (diets during pregnancy)	
○ Negative comments about "what this baby is doing to me!"	
Postpartum	
• Assist patient and significant others in establishing realistic goals for integration of baby into family.	
• Provide positive reinforcement for parenting tasks:	Promotes realistic planning for new baby as well as bonding and attachment.
○ Encourage use of birthing room—labor, delivery, and recovery (LDR) room and labor, delivery, recovery, and postpartum (LDRP) room—for birth to allow active participation in birth process by both parents.	
○ Allow mother and partner time with infant following delivery. (Do not remove to nursery if stable.)	
○ Provide mother-baby care to allow maximum continuity of mother-infant contact and nursing care.	
• Assist parents in identifying different kinds of infant behavior and understanding how they allow the infant to communicate with them:	Provides the parents with essential information they need to care for infant.
○ Perform gestational age assessment with parents and explain significance of findings.	
○ Perform Brazelton neonatal assessment with parents and explain significance of findings.	
○ Demonstrate how to hold infant for maximum communication.	
○ Explain infant reflexes—rooting, Moro—and the importance of understanding them.	
• Assist parents in identifying support systems:	
○ Friends from childbirth classes	
○ Parents and parents-in-law	
○ Siblings	
○ Nurse specialists	
• Encourage parents to reminisce about birthing experience.	
• Assist patient in identifying needs related to family functioning	Provides database needed for planning to offset factors that would result in ineffective parenting.
• Identify negative maternal behavior:	
○ No interest in new baby	
○ Talks *excessively* to friends on phone	

- ○ Is more interested in TV than in feeding infant
  - ○ Refuses to listen to infant teaching
  - ○ Asks no questions
  - ○ *Extraordinary* interest in self-appearance:
    - (1) *Severe* dieting to gain prepregnancy figure
    - (2) *Overutilization* of exercise to gain prepregnancy figure
  - ○ Crying, moodiness
  - ○ Lack of interest in family and other children
  - ○ Failure to perform physical care for infant
  - ○ Noncompliance: Breaks appointments with health care providers for self and infant
- Identify negative paternal behavior:
  - ○ Refusal to support wife by:
    - (1) Not assisting in child care
    - (2) Not sharing household tasks
    - (3) Keeping "his" social contacts and going out while wife remains at home with child
  - ○ Not providing financial support
  - ○ Abandonment
- Assist patient in identifying methods of coping with stress of newborn in family:
  - ○ Seek professional help from nurse specialist, physician (obstetrician or pediatrician), or psychiatrist.
  - ○ Identify support system in family or among friends.
  - ○ Refer to appropriate community or private agencies.

Provides long-term support.

Mental Health

Actions/Interventions	Rationales
• Monitor the degree to which drugs and alcohol interfere with the parenting process. If this is a factor, discuss a treatment program with the client.	Early intervention and treatment increase the likelihood of a positive outcome.
• Ask client who is caring for children while he or she is hospitalized and assess his or her level of comfort with this arrangement. If a satisfactory arrangement is not present,	Early intervention and treatment increases the likelihood of a positive outcome.

Continued

Actions/Interventions	Rationales
refer to social services so arrangements can be made.	
• Discuss with the client expectations and problem perception.	Promotes the client's sense of control.
• Have client identify support systems, and gain permission to include these persons in the treatment plan as necessary. This could include spouse, parents, close friends, and so on.	Support system understanding facilitates the maintenance of behaviors after discharge.
• If client desires to maintain parenting role, arrange to have children visit during hospitalization. Assign a staff member to remain with the client during these visits. The staff person can serve as a role model for the client and facilitate communication between the child and the client. Note here schedule for these visits and the staff person responsible for the supervision of these interactions.	A continuous relationship between parent and child is necessary for the normal development of the child.[21]
• Answer client's questions in a clear, direct manner.	Promotes the development of a trusting relationship.
• Spend 15 minutes twice a day at (times) with the client discussing his or her perception of the parenting role and his or her expectations for self and children.	Promotes the development of a trusting relationship and provides information about the client's worldview that can be utilized in constructing interventions.
• Arrange 30 minutes a day for interaction between the client and one member of the support system. A staff member is to be present during these interactions to facilitate communication and focus the discussion on parenting issues.	Supports the maintenance of these relationships and provides opportunities for the nurse to do positive role modeling.
• Provide client with information on normal growth and development and normal feelings of parents.	Provides information that will assist the client in making appropriate parenting decisions, thus enhancing self-esteem.
• Assist client in developing a plan for disciplining children. This plan should be based on behavioral interventions, and the primary focus should be on positive social rewards.[22]	Facilitates the development of positive coping behaviors and promotes a positive expectational set.
• Teach client ways of interacting with child that reduce levels of conflict, for example, by providing child with limited choices, spending scheduled time with the child, or listening carefully to the child.	Promotes positive orientation and enhances self-esteem.
• Encourage client to maintain telephone contact with children by providing a telephone and establishing a regular time	Assists in maintaining these important relationships, making the transition home easier.

for the client to call home or have the children call the hospital.

- Encourage support system to continue to include client in decisions related to the children by having them bring up these issues in daily visits and by assisting client and support system to engage in collaborative decision making regarding these issues.

  Assists in maintaining client's role functioning, thus enhancing self-esteem.

- Have client identify parenting models and discuss the effect these persons had on their current parenting style.

  Children can be triangled into parental conflicts in an unconscious effort to preserve the marital relationship.[23]

- Observe interaction between parents to assess for problems in the husband-wife relationship that may be expressed in the parenting relationship. If this appears to be happening, refer to family therapy.

- Have client develop a list of problem behavior patterns, and then assist him or her in developing a list of alternative behavior patterns. For example, "*Current*: When I get frustrated with my child, I spank him with a belt. *New*: When I get frustrated with my child, I arrange to send him to the neighbors for 30 minutes while I take a walk around the block to calm down."

  Promotes client's sense of control and begins the development of alternative, more adaptive coping behaviors.

- Role-play with client those situations that are identified as being most difficult, and provide opportunities to practice more appropriate behavior. This should be done daily in 30-minute time periods. Note schedule for this activity here; list time periods and those situations that are to be practiced. It would be useful to include spouse.

  Behavioral rehearsal provides opportunities for feedback and modeling of new behaviors by the nurse.

- Have client attend group sessions where feelings and thoughts can be expressed to peers and the thoughts and feelings of peers can be heard. Note schedule for the group here.

  Assists client to experience personal importance to others while enhancing interpersonal relationship skills. Increasing these competencies can enhance self-esteem and promote positive orientation.

- Assist client in identifying personal needs and in developing a plan for meeting these needs at home; for example, parents will exchange babysitting time with neighbors so they can have an evening out once a month. Note this plan here.

  Assists parents to develop strategies for coping with role strain.

- Monitor staff attitudes toward client, and allow them to express feelings, especially if child abuse is an issue with this client.

  Negative attitudes of staff can be communicated to the client, decreasing the client's self-esteem and increasing the client's defensiveness.

Continued

Actions/Interventions	Rationales

• Assist client with grieving separation from child and refer to section on Anticipatory Grieving for detailed nursing actions.
• Provide client with positive verbal support for positive parenting behavior and for progress on behavior change goal; for example, "You demonstrate a great deal of concern for your child's welfare" or "You have taught your child to be very sensitive." Make sure these comments are honest and fit the client's awareness of the situation.
• Assist client in developing stress reduction skills by:
  ○ Teaching deep muscle relaxation and practicing this with client 30 minutes a day at (time).
  ○ Discussing with client the role physical exercise plays in stress reduction and developing a plan for exercise (note plan and type of exercise here). Have staff member remain with the client during these exercise periods. Note time for these periods here.
• When client's level of tension or anxiety is rising on the unit, remind him or her of the exercise or relaxation technique and work through one of these with him or her.
• Assist client in identifying the symptoms he or she has of rising tension so that he or she can implement the stress reduction activity when client notices this alteration in his or her feelings and behavior.
	Positive reinforcement encourages behavior and enhances self-esteem.
	
	Provides parents with positive coping strategies for dealing with role strain.

Gerontic Health

This would be an unusual diagnosis for the gerontic patient, but it might develop if the grandparents had to take grandchildren into their home because of a family crisis. In that instance, the nursing actions would be the same as those given in Adult Health and Child Health.

Home Health

Actions/Interventions	Rationales
• Act as role model through use of positive attitude when interacting with the child and parents.	Role modeling provides example for parenting skills.
• Report child abuse and neglect to the appropriate authorities.	Satisfies legal requirements and provides for intervention.

• Teach client and family appropriate information regarding the care and discipline of children:
  ○ Cultural norms
  ○ Normal growth and development
  ○ Anticipatory guidance regarding psychosocial, cognitive, and physical needs for children and parents
  ○ Expected family life-cycles
  ○ Development and use of support networks
  ○ Safe environment for family members
  ○ Nurturing environment for family members
  ○ Special needs of child requiring invasive or restrictive treatments
	Knowledge is necessary to provide appropriate child care.

• Involve client and family in planning and implementing strategies to decrease or prevent alterations (risk for or actual) in parenting:
  ○ *Family conference*: Identify each member's perspective on the situation.
  ○ *Mutual goal setting*: Develop short-term, realistic goals with evaluation criteria.
  ○ *Communication*: Encourage open, honest communication with positive feedback.
  ○ *Family tasks*: Have family members perform developmentally and physically appropriate tasks.
  ○ *Parent's self-esteem*: Promote positive support of existence and positive parenting skills.
	Involvement of family in planning enhances the effectiveness of the interventions.

• Assist client and family in life-style adjustments that may be required:
  ○ Development of parenting skills
  ○ Use of support network
  ○ Establishment of realistic expectations of children and spouse
	Long-term behavioral changes require support.

• Refer to appropriate community resources. (See Appendix B.)	Support groups, family therapist, school nurse, and teachers can enhance the treatment plan.

FLOW CHART EVALUATION
Flow Chart Expected Outcome 1

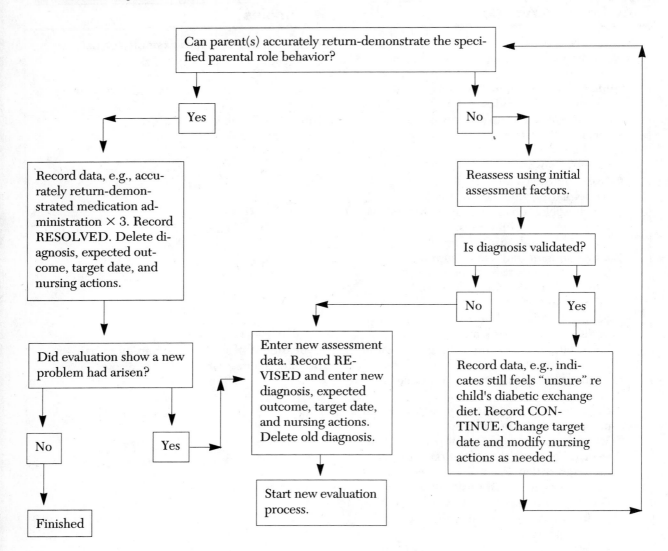

Flow Chart Expected Outcome 2

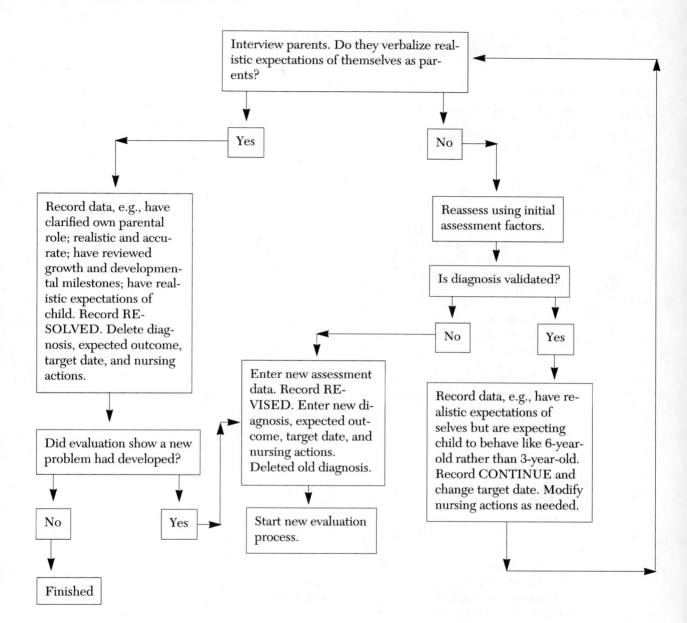

Relocation Stress Syndrome

DEFINITION

Physiological and/or psychosocial disturbances as a result of transfer from one environment to another.[8]

NANDA TAXONOMY: MOVING 6.7

DEFINING CHARACTERISTICS[8]

1. Major defining characteristics:
   a. Anxiety
   b. Apprehension
   c. Increased confusion (elderly)
   d. Depression
   e. Loneliness
2. Minor defining characteristics:
   a. Verbalization of unwillingness to relocate
   b. Sleep disturbance
   c. Change in eating habits
   d. Dependency
   e. Gastrointestinal disturbances
   f. Increased verbalization of needs
   g. Insecurity
   h. Lack of trust
   i. Restlessness
   j. Sad affect
   k. Unfavorable comparison of pretransfer and posttransfer staff
   l. Verbalization of being concerned or upset about transfer
   m. Vigilance
   n. Weight change
   o. Withdrawal

RELATED FACTORS[8]

1. Past, concurrent, and recent losses
2. Losses involved with decision to move
3. Feeling of powerlessness
4. Lack of adequate support system
5. Little or no preparation for the impending move
6. Moderate to high degree of environmental change
7. History and types of previous transfers
8. Impaired psychosocial health status
9. Decreased physical health status

RELATED CLINICAL CONCERNS

1. Any diagnosis which would require transfer of the patient to a long-term care facility
2. A chronic disease that would require the older adult to move in with his or her children

HAVE YOU SELECTED THE CORRECT DIAGNOSIS?

Ineffective Individual Coping This diagnosis and Relocation Stress Syndrome do sound similar in some ways; however, the differentiating factor is whether the individual is being or has recently been involved in a transfer from one care setting to another. If such a transfer is being considered or has occurred, initial interventions should be directed toward resolving the problems associated with relocation of the patient. (See page 892.)

Impaired Adjustment Certainly any move requires some adjustment. However, this diagnosis relates to an individual's adjusting to his or her own illness or health problem, not adjustment to a change in the health care setting. (See page 861.)

EXPECTED OUTCOMES

1. The patient will verbalize increased satisfaction with new environment by (date) and/or
2. The patient will demonstrate a decrease in the major defining characteristics for Relocation Stress Syndrome by (date)

TARGET DATE

An initial target date of 7 days would be reasonable to assess for progress toward meeting the expected outcome.

NURSING ACTIONS/INTERVENTIONS WITH RATIONALES

Adult Health

Actions/Interventions	Rationales
• Encourage verbalization of feelings, both positive and negative, by active listening, reflection, or open-ended questions about relocation. Schedule 30 minutes twice a day at (times) to focus on this topic.	Brings feelings out into the open, clarifies emotions, and makes them easier to cope with.
• Determine any previous experience with relocation and the strategies used to cope with the experience during discussions with the patient.	Provides understanding of problem and information to further develop interventions; determines previously used coping strategies, which ones were successful or unsuccessful, and what alternative strategies may be tried.
• Allow patient to control his or her environment to the extent possible.	Increases self-confidence and decreases feeling of powerlessness.
• Provide consistency in daily care: same primary nurse, daily routines, or environment.	Provides security, thus facilitating adjustment.

Continued

Actions/Interventions	Rationales
• Explain all procedures prior to implementation.	Decreases anxiety.
• Teach stress management techniques such as relaxation, meditation, deep breathing, exercise, diversional activities. Have patient return-demonstrate technique for 15 minutes twice a day at (times).	Decreases anxiety so that energy can be used to implement effective coping strategies.
• Consult with other health care professionals as necessary. (See Appendix B.)	Collaboration promotes care that incorporates physiologic and psychosocial interventions that may be needed as a result of relocation stress.
• Help patient maintain former relationships by providing letter-writing materials or a telephone.	Decreases feelings of isolation and depression.
• Provide patient with a list of organizations and community services available for newcomers; for example, Welcome Wagon, senior citizens groups, churches, singles groups.	Assists patient to develop new relationship and may hasten adjustment.

Child Health

Actions/Interventions	Rationales
• Assess, to the degree possible, the emotional stability of the patient and family. (Use Chess-Thomas Temperament Scale.[24])	Adaptability to change is determined to a large degree by temperament and previous coping.

• Schedule at least a 1-hour family conference daily and focus on:
  ○ Feelings of patient and family regarding move
  ○ Aspects of relocation that are problematic: school, friends, and so on
  ○ Potential benefits and growth the relocation might offer
	Provides support to cope with changes caused by relocation.

• Encourage plans for maintaining desired relationships despite physical move by means of letters, telephone calls, and visits.	

Women's Health

See Adult Health and Gerontic Health.

Mental Health

See Adult Health and Gerontic Health.

Gerontic Health

NOTE: These actions apply to patient entering an acute care facility.

Actions/Interventions	Rationales
• Establish whether the patient is at high risk for Relocation Stress Syndrome. In older adults this may include those with no confidante (social support), those who perceive themselves as worriers, those in poor health, and those with low self-esteem.[25]	Early identification of high-risk patients can mean earlier intervention and a possible decrease in the negative consequences of relocation.
• Assist patient in realistic perception of event: what has occurred, reasons for transfer based on physical needs, changed health status.	May assist in accepting need for relocation.
• Provide supportive care as the situation requires, such as answering questions regarding the routines in the hospital or expected course of treatment.	Allows responses that are tailored to the individual's expressed needs.
• Discuss possible occurrence of syndrome with significant others.	Provides anticipatory information that avoids undue stress on family.
• Discuss with the patient and significant others the patient's usual coping skills.	Provides database to build on prior to discharge from acute care facility.
• Discuss transfer with patient and family.	Provides time to question and promotes positive adjustment to the change in location.
• If not returning to prehospitalization location, discuss with the patient his or her proposed plans, reasons for transfer, and response to proposal.	Allows time for ventilation of feelings related to the relocation.

Home Health

NOTE: See Mental Health for additional interventions.

Actions/Interventions	Rationales
• Monitor for signs of Relocation Stress Syndrome.	Provides database for early recognition and intervention.
• Involve client and family in planning, implementing, and promoting reduction or elimination of relocation stress: ○ *Family conference*: Discuss each member's	Family involvement enhances effectiveness of interventions. If client is moving into a family member's residence, entire family will experience change.

Continued

Actions/Interventions	Rationales
perception of the situation. Clarify potential responses to move. ○ *Mutual goal setting*: Identify goals and evaluation criteria. Specify tasks and roles for each member. ○ *Communication*: Encourage open, direct communication with positive feedback. • Assist client and family in life-style adjustments that may be required: ○ Adjustment to changing role functions and relationships ○ Requirements for redistribution of family tasks ○ Redistribution of space in the household ○ Preparation for the move ○ Orientation to new surroundings ○ Provision of selected items that are meaningful to the client ○ Preparation for potential responses; for example, interruption of usual sleep and eating routines, sleep and eating ○ Provision of any special treatments or equipment ○ Changes in financial situation • Consult with or refer to community resources as indicated. (See Appendix B.)	Social services, support groups, and a psychiatric nurse clinician can enhance the treatment plan.

FLOW CHART EVALUATION
Flow Chart Expected Outcome 1

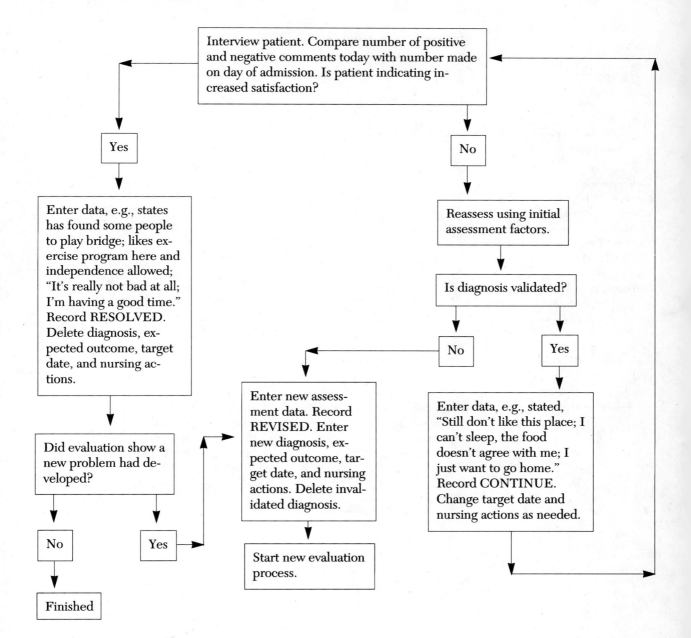

Interview patient. Compare number of positive and negative comments today with number made on day of admission. Is patient indicating increased satisfaction?

Yes

No

Enter data, e.g., states has found some people to play bridge; likes exercise program here and independence allowed; "It's really not bad at all; I'm having a good time." Record RESOLVED. Delete diagnosis, expected outcome, target date, and nursing actions.

Reassess using initial assessment factors.

Is diagnosis validated?

No

Yes

Did evaluation show a new problem had developed?

No

Yes

Enter new assessment data. Record REVISED. Enter new diagnosis, expected outcome, target date, and nursing actions. Delete invalidated diagnosis.

Enter data, e.g., stated, "Still don't like this place; I can't sleep, the food doesn't agree with me; I just want to go home." Record CONTINUE. Change target date and nursing actions as needed.

Finished

Start new evaluation process.

Flow Chart Expected Outcome 2

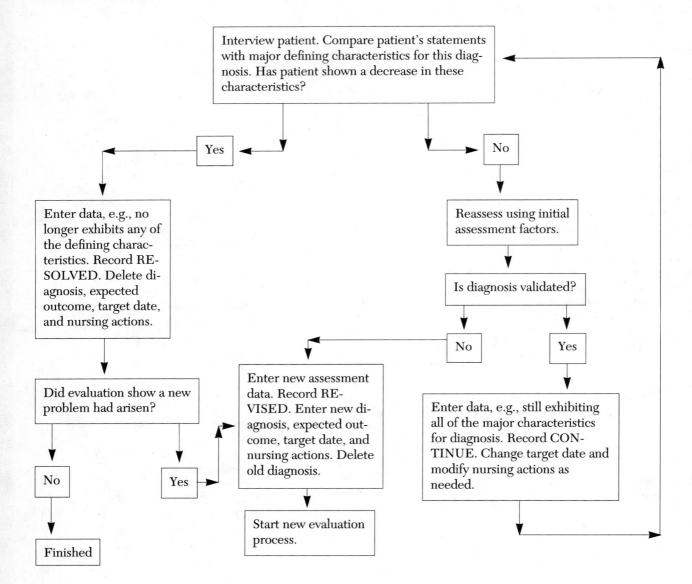

Role Performance, Altered

DEFINITION

Disruption in the way one perceives one's role performance.[17]

NANDA TAXONOMY: RELATING 3.2.1

DEFINING CHARACTERISTICS[17]

1. Major defining characteristics:
   a. Change in self-perception of role
   b. Denial of role
   c. Change in others' perceptions of role
   d. Conflict in roles
   e. Change in physical capacity to resume role
   f. Lack of knowledge of role
   g. Change in usual patterns of responsibility
2. Minor defining characteristics:
   None given

RELATED FACTORS[17]

To be developed.

RELATED CLINICAL CONCERNS

1. Any major surgery
2. Any chronic disease
3. Any condition resulting in hemiplegia, paraplegia, or quadriplegia
4. Chemical abuse
5. Cancer

HAVE YOU SELECTED THE CORRECT DIAGNOSIS?

Social Isolation This diagnosis is related to the patient who, because of physical, communicative, or social problems, chooses to be alone or perceives that he or she is alone and therefore isolated from society. This diagnosis deals mainly with the individual who cannot or will not perform any role. (See page 781.)

Altered Family Process This diagnosis refers to an entire family that must in one way or another alter the processes that go on within the family. Many times this will involve altered role performances of individual family members; however, the overall focus is on the alteration within the family and not on the individual members of the family. (See page 710.)

EXPECTED OUTCOMES

1. Will list at least (number) factors contributing to disturbance in role performance by (date) and/or
2. Will implement plan to offset factors contributing to disturbance in role performance by (date)

TARGET DATE

Target dates for this diagnosis will have to be highly individualized according to each situation. A minimum target date would be 5 days to allow time to identify impinging factors and methods to cope with those factors.

NURSING ACTIONS/INTERACTIONS WITH RATIONALES

Adult Health

Actions/Interventions	Rationales
• Encourage patient to express his or her perception of role responsibilities by active listening, reflection, open-ended questions, acceptance of feelings, and nonjudgmental attitude.	Relieves stress and helps patient to clarify feelings in a safe environment.
• Help patient and significant others realistically negotiate role responsibilities by assisting in the problem-solving process: What is the role? What are its responsibilities? How can responsibilities be shared? What are outcomes expected of the role? Have patient and significant others meet together for 1 hour every other day.	Facilitates problem solving; promotes cooperation among involved persons.
• Teach patient about role: parent, caregiver, breadwinner, and so on. Allow time for discussion, return-demonstrations, and questioning prior to discharge.	Clarifies misconceptions and provides realistic role expectations.
• Help patient identify community resources to assist in role responsibilities prior to discharge. (See Appendix B.)	Provides support for short-term and long-term problem solving.
• Refer to psychiatric nurse clinician as needed. (See section on Mental Health for more detailed interventions.)	Collaboration promotes holistic plan of care, and problem may need specialized interventions.

Child Health

Actions/Interventions	Rationales
• Determine how child and parents perceive the expected role for the child.	Provides essential database necessary to plan care.
• Identify confusion or diffusion of role according to child's and parents' expectations versus actual role.	Problem identification serves to establish common areas to be further explored in role performance.
• Determine value the child has in the family.	The value a child has for each family is critical to expectations for all involved.
• Determine child's self-perception.	Self-perception provides insight into how one evaluates one's own performance.
• Identify ways to alleviate role-performance alteration according to actual cause. If child is temporarily unable to participate in certain physical activities, explore other nonphysical ways the child can participate.	Alleviation of one or more role-performance alterations may prevent further deterioration in role functioning, with a greater appreciation for the value of all roles.
• Allow for ventilation of feelings by child via puppetry, art, or other age-appropriate methods. Schedule at least 30 minutes during each 8-hour shift for this activity. Note times here.	Feelings are most critical in exploring one's role performance. Appropriate aids in communication serve to foster focused play or behaviors to reveal thoughts of the child who is unable to express himself or herself.
• Provide patient and parents with options to best facilitate needs for future implications of compromised role performance; for example, shared experiences with peers who have temporarily had to forsake physical activities due to illness—how they kept up with the team, and so on.	Vicarious involvement allows for shared activities and the sense of maintaining closeness with the desired groups or person.
• Allow for family time and support for choices to uphold role needs; for example, visitation by peers.	Shared time with family and friends is especially important in times of role stress to maintain value of self.
• Provide for safety needs of child and family.	Standard care includes safety. The tendency is to relax concerns in times of less stressful activity.
• Assist in follow-up plans with appropriate appointments for psychiatric or pediatric care.	Arrangements for follow-up promote valuing of follow-up and increase the likelihood for compliance.
• Provide support in identification of risk to normal actualization of potential of child.	Early identification of primary or secondary risks may prevent or minimize tertiary risks for the child and family.

Women's Health

Actions/Interventions	Rationales
• Allow patient to describe her perception of her role as a mother, wife, and working woman. • Identify sources of role stress and strain that contribute to role conflict and fatigue. • Assist in developing a schedule that manages time well, both at home and at work.	Provides database to initiate care planning.

• Involve significant others in planning methods of reducing role stress and strain at home by:
  ○ Assisting with child care
  ○ Assisting with household duties
  ○ Sharing car-pooling and children's activities
• Encourage patient to use time at work for "work activities" and time at home for "home activities"; that is, do not take work home.
• Look at possibility of job sharing or part-time employment while children are at home.
• Plan home activities in advance, such as shopping and cooking meals in advance and freezing them for later use.
• Encourage division of work load by exchanging child care activities with friends or other families in the neighborhood.
	Encourages patient to identify various roles she is currently fulfilling, and provides support that allows planning of coping strategies and techniques.

Mental Health

Actions/Interventions	Rationales
• Sit with client (number) minutes (number) times per day to discuss client's feelings about self and role performance. • Answer questions honestly.	Provides information about client's perceptions and expectations that can be utilized in developing specific interventions. Promotes the development of a trusting relationship.

• Provide feedback to client about nurse's perceptions of client's abilities and appearance by:
  ○ Using "I" statements
  ○ Using references related to the nurse's relationship to the client
  ○ Describing the nurse's feelings in relationship
	Assists the client in realistically evaluating his or her perceptions.

- Provide positive reinforcement. List those things that are reinforcing for the client and when they are to be used; also list those things that have been identified as nonreinforcers for this client. Include social rewards.

  Positive reinforcement encourages behavior and enhances self-esteem.

- Provide group interaction with (number) persons (number) minutes three times a day at (times). This activity should be gradual and within client's ability. For example, on admission client may tolerate one person for 5 minutes. If the interactions are brief, the frequency should be high; 5-minute interactions should occur at 30-minute intervals.

  Assists client to experience personal importance to others while enhancing interpersonal relationship skills. Increasing these role competencies can enhance self-esteem and promote a positive orientation.

- Reflect back to negative self-statements made by the client. This should be done with a supportive attitude in a manner that will increase client's awareness of these negative evaluations of self.

  This will increase the client's awareness of these statements and facilitate the development of alternative cognitive patterns.

- Set achievable goals for the client.

  Achievement of goals provides positive reinforcement, which encourages the behavior and enhances self-esteem.

- Provide activities that the client can accomplish and that the client values. (Care should be taken not to provide tasks that the client finds demeaning; this could reinforce client's negative self-evaluation.)

  Accomplishment of valued tasks provides positive reinforcement, which encourages behavior and enhances self-esteem.

- Provide verbal reinforcement for the achievement of steps toward a goal.

  Promotes a positive orientation.

- Have client develop a list of strengths and potentials.

- Define the client's lack of goal achievement or failures as simple mistakes that are bound to occur when one attempts something new; "Learning comes with mistakes; if one does not make mistakes one does not learn."

  Promotes a positive orientation.

- Define past failures as the client's best attempts to solve a problem; "If the client had known a better solution, he or she would have used it; one does not set out to fail."

- Make necessary items available for the client to groom self.

  Appropriate grooming improves the client's self-evaluation.

- Spend (number) minutes at (time) assisting the client with grooming, providing necessary assistance and positive reinforcement for accomplishments.

  The nurse's presence can provide positive reinforcement, which encourages positive behavior.

Continued

Actions/Interventions	Rationales
• Focus client's attention on the here and now.	Past happenings are difficult for the nurse to provide feedback on.
• Present the client with opportunities to make decisions about care, and record these decisions on the chart.	Promotes client's sense of control and enhances self-esteem.
• Develop with the client alternative coping strategies.	Promotes the development of more adaptive coping behaviors, and increases the client's role competence.
• Practice new coping behavior with client (number) minutes at (time).	Repeated practice of a behavior internalizes and personalizes the behavior.
• Discuss with the client ideal versus current perceptions of role performance.	Assists client in a cognitive appraisal of perceptions to eliminate unrealistic or irrational beliefs.
• Discuss with the client those factors that are perceived to be interfering with role performance.	Assists client in cognitive evaluation of perception of role performance.
• Have the client develop a list of alternatives for resolving interfering factors. (This list should be noted here.)	Facilitates the development of alternative coping behaviors.
• Establish an appointment with significant others to discuss their perceptions of the client's role performance and their perceptions of the various roles involved in the identified situations. (Date and time of this meeting should be written here.)	Assists in establishing agreement on the performance of role pairs to decrease role conflict and strain. This is of primary importance, since roles occur in interactions.
• Discuss with the client and significant others alterations in role that will facilitate successful performance. (Date and time of this meeting should be written here.)	
• Develop a specific list of necessary changes, and provide the client system with a written copy.	
• Role-play altered role situations with the client system for 1 hour once a day at (time). This would include opportunities for clients to practice those areas of role performance that may be new or unique.	Repeated practice of a behavior internalizes and personalizes the behavior.

• If client and client system cannot achieve agreement on the problematic role, refer to:
  ○ Psychiatric mental health clinical nurse specialist
  ○ Family therapist
  ○ Social worker
	Interactions with the health care system involve role pairs with the role expectations that are present in any social situation. As in any interaction, there can be differing expectations about role performance, which can lead to role conflict and strain.

• If problematic roles involve interactions between client and members of the health care team (nurses, physicians, and so on), request consultation with psychiatric mental health clinical nurse specialist or mental	

health specialist with experience in the area of resolving system problems, that is, family therapists or social workers.

Gerontic Health

Actions/Interventions	Rationales
• Discuss with the patient how he or she perceives his or her role performance has altered.	Provides opportunity to gain patient's exact perspective on situation; provides database need for most effective planning.
• Discuss with patient potential role modifications or substitutions, such as foster grandparenting, friendly visitor at a long-term care facility, participant in intergenerational programs, or telephone reassurance visitor or caller.	Depending on the patient's interests and abilities, these measures would provide an alternate method to achieve role satisfaction.

Home Health

Actions/Interventions	Rationales
• Monitor for factors contributing to disturbed role performance.	Provides database for early recognition and intervention.
• Involve client and family in planning, implementing, and promoting reduction or elimination of disturbance in role function:	Family involvement in planning increases the likelihood of effective intervention.
○ *Family conference*: Clarify expected role performance of all family members.	
○ *Mutual goal setting*: Set realistic goals and evaluation criteria. Identify tasks for each family member.	
○ *Communication*: Promote open, direct communication with positive feedback.	
• Assist client and family in life-style adjustments that may be required:	Long-term behavioral changes require support.
○ Treatment of physical or emotional disability	
○ Stress management	
○ Adjustment to changing role functions and relationships	
○ Development and use of support networks	
○ Requirements for redistribution of family tasks	
• Consult with community resources as indicated. (See Appendix B.)	Utilization of existing services is efficient use of resources. Psychiatric nurse clinician, occupational and physical therapists, and support groups can enhance the treatment plan.

FLOW CHART EVALUATION
Flow Chart Expected Outcome 1

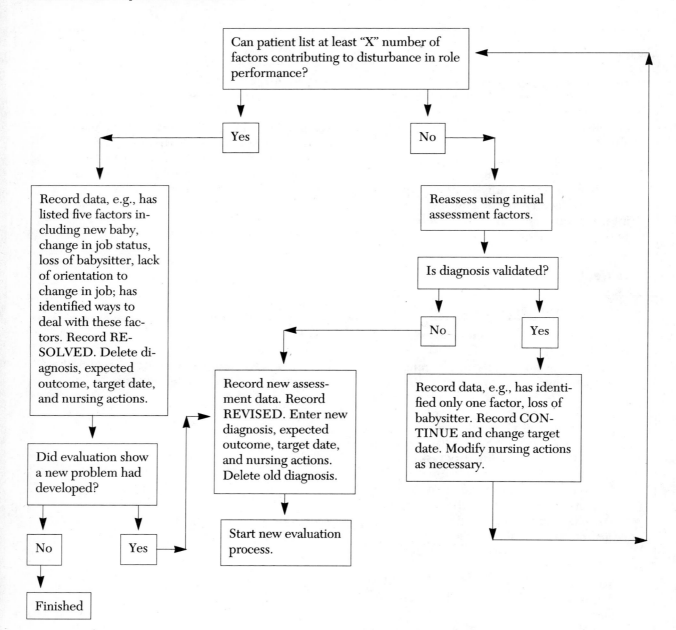

Flow Chart Expected Outcome 2

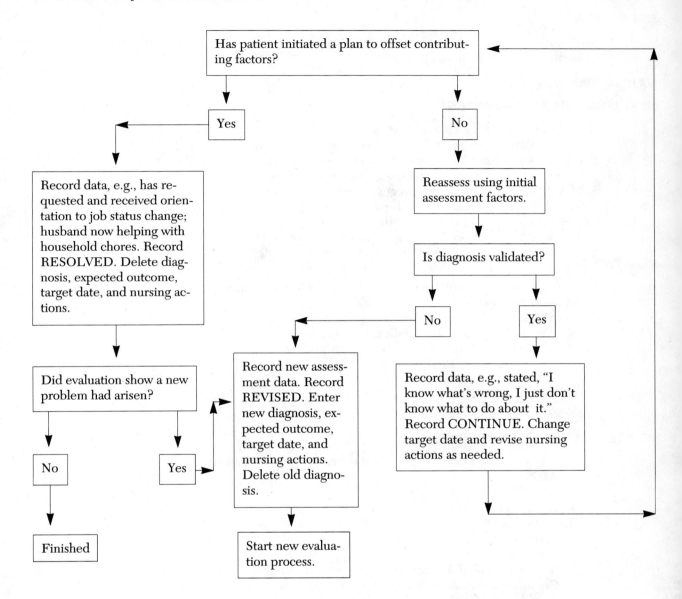

Social Interaction, Impaired

DEFINITION

The state in which an individual participates in an insufficient or excessive quantity or ineffective quality of social exchange.[17]

NANDA TAXONOMY: RELATING 3.1.1

DEFINING CHARACTERISTICS[17]

1. Major defining characteristics:
   a. Verbalized or observed discomfort in social situations
   b. Verbalized or observed inability to receive or communicate a satisfying sense of belonging, caring, interest, or shared history
   c. Observed use of unsuccessful social interaction behaviors
   d. Dysfunctional interaction with peers, family, and/or others
2. Minor defining characteristics:
   a. Family report of change of style or pattern of interaction

RELATED FACTORS[17]

1. Knowledge or skill deficit about ways to enhance mutuality
2. Communication barriers
3. Self-concept disturbance
4. Absence of available significant others or peers
5. Limited physical mobility
6. Therapeutic isolation
7. Sociocultural dissonance
8. Environmental barriers
9. Altered thought process

RELATED CLINICAL CONCERNS

1. Any condition causing paraplegia, hemiplegia, or quadriplegia
2. AIDS
3. Alzheimer's disease
4. Cancer of the larynx
5. Mental retardation
6. Substance abuse
7. Communicable disease
8. Altered physical appearance secondary to disease or trauma
9. Psychiatric disorders, for example, major depression, borderline personality disorder, schizoid personality disorder

HAVE YOU SELECTED THE CORRECT DIAGNOSIS?

Knowledge Deficit This diagnosis, particularly as related to mutuality, would be the most appropriate alternate diagnosis if the individual verbalized or demonstrated an inability to attend to significant others' social actions in the context of independent and dependent aspects of their role. (See page 536.)

Impaired Verbal Communication This would be the most appropriate diagnosis if the individual is unable to receive or send communication. Certainly Impaired Verbal Communication could relate to Impaired Social Interaction and would be the primary problem that has to be resolved. (See page 791.)

Social Isolation This would be the more appropriate diagnosis when the individual is placed in or chooses isolation due to physiologic, sociologic, or emotional concerns. Further assessment is required to completely delineate the exact problem when self-isolation is chosen as the diagnosis. (See page 781.)

EXPECTED OUTCOMES

1. Will verbalize satisfaction with quantity and quality of social interactions by (date) and/or
2. Will demonstrate (increased/decreased) involvement in social interactions by (date)

TARGET DATE

Assisting the patient to modify social interactions will require a significant amount of time. A target date ranging between 7 and 10 days would be appropriate for evaluating progress.

NURSING ACTIONS/INTERVENTIONS WITH RATIONALES

Adult Health

Actions/Interventions	Rationales
• Encourage patient to express how he or she feels or what he or she fears in a social situation by scheduling at least 10 minutes twice a day at (times) to focus on this topic.	Assists patient to examine social experience and verbalize feelings; encourages therapeutic relationship.
• Listen to patient's communication skills and help him or her to find alternative ones during interactions with patient.	Improves communication skills.
• Help patient obtain a realistic perception of self by focusing on and enhancing strengths during conferences with patient.	Helps patient to see that no one is perfect, and improves self-concept.
• Role-play social interactions with patient. Allow patient to choose which social interactions he or she wishes to role-play for 10 minutes twice a day at (times).	Promotes self-confidence in social situations by allowing practice in a safe environment.
• Help patient participate in group interactions; use crutches, wheelchair, or stretcher to get patient out of his or her room at least twice per shift, while awake, at (times).	Increases social skills by providing social contact.

Continued

Actions/Interventions	Rationales
• Involve patient in daily care; help the patient to make decisions about own care.	Improves self-concepts; increases motivation; decreases feeling of powerlessness.
• If patient is in isolation, spend at least 10 minutes every hour with the patient.	Avoids feeling of total isolation for patient.
• Consult with patient's minister, priest, or rabbi as patient desires.	Provides reinforcement for self-worth.
• Initiate referrals to support groups prior to discharge. (See Appendix B.)	Puts patient in contact with community groups to interact with patient and decrease social isolation.

Child Health

Actions/Interventions	Rationales
• Monitor for contributory factors to altered social interaction pattern; for example, role-play with puppets.	Provides database needed to plan appropriate care.
• Determine the effect the altered social interaction has on the child, parent, family, and school.	Provides data needed to accurately plan intervention.
• Develop a plan of care to best meet child's potential for succeeding with appropriate social interaction. *Note*: this will be highly qualified by social class and values.	Individual family values will dictate the way in which social interaction is dealt with.
• Determine if conflict exists between parent's and child's desired social interaction.	Conflict may prevent appropriate attention to actual social interaction, but must be dealt with as it will remain a critical component. This may be true particularly at times of authority issues, for example, during adolescence.
• If conflict exists regarding social interaction, deal with this as needed in values or beliefs pattern.	Values and beliefs may be in conflict, and some resolution of the problem is essential to prevent further long-term effects.
• Assist child, parents, and family in ventilation of feelings regarding social interaction impairment, including actual consequences of same.	Ventilation of feelings serves to help patient reduce anxiety and initiate problem resolution.
• Make referrals as appropriate to professionals best able to assist in dealing with problem; for example, psychiatric nurse, clinical specialist, play therapist, or family therapist.	Referral serves to best deal with problems according to a match of needs and resources.
• Identify local support groups to appropriately match needs: parent-child support groups for the handicapped, United	Resource groups provide vital support through provision of a common shared sense of concern, coping, and empowerment.

Cerebral Palsy Association, Spina Bifida Association, and so on.

• If impaired social interaction also relates to school, include teacher and essential school personnel in plans for resolving the impairment and for best follow-up.	Valuing the importance of school and the need to provide the best for the child and family in the development of positive social interaction shows respect for the patient and family.
• Identify follow-up appointment needs and ways to monitor progress for child and family; for example, stickers as incentives to reinforce desired behavior.	Provides reinforcement and attaches value to follow-up.
• Anticipate discrepant or unrealistic expectations by child's parents. Monitor for potential child abuse.	Unrealistic demands or expectations are risk indicators for abuse.

Women's Health

See Adult Health.

Mental Health

Actions/Interventions	Rationales
• If delusions or hallucinations are present, refer to Sensory-Perceptual Alteration for detailed interventions.	Promotes the development of a trusting relationship.
• Assign primary care nurse to client.	
• Primary nurse will spend (number) minutes twice a day at (times) with client. The focus of this interaction will change as a relationship is developed. Initially, the nurse should model for the client how to develop a relationship through his or her behavior in developing this relationship with the client. This modeling should include demonstrating respect for the client; consistency in interaction; congruence between thoughts, feelings, and actions; and empathy.	Promotes the development of a trusting relationship, and provides opportunities for the client to observe the nurse in appropriate interpersonal interactions.
• Have client identify those persons in the environment who are considered family, friends, and acquaintances. Then have client note how many interactions per week occur with each person. Have client identify his or her thoughts, feelings, and behavior about these interactions.	Assists the client in testing the belief that he or she is having difficulty with interpersonal relationships.
• Provide appropriate confrontation with client about his or her behavior patterns	Assists client in developing alternative coping behaviors that are adaptive.

Continued

Actions/Interventions	Rationales
that inhibit interaction in relationships with the nurse.[13]	
• Observe client in interactions with others on the unit, and identify patterns of behavior that inhibit social interaction.	Facilitates the provision of feedback to the client on methods he or she could use to improve interpersonal effectiveness. Positive reinforcement encourages behavior.
• Develop a list of those things the client finds rewarding, and provide these rewards as client successfully completes progressive steps in treatment plan.	
• When client is demonstrating socially inappropriate behavior, keep interactions to a minimum and escort client to a place away from activities.	Continuing the interaction could provide positive reinforcement and encourage an inappropriate behavior.
• When inappropriate behavior stops, discuss the behavior with the client and develop a list of alternative kinds of behavior for the client to use in situations where the inappropriate behavior is elicited. Note those kinds of behavior that are identified as problematic here with the action to be taken if they are demonstrated; for example, client will spend time out in seclusion and away from group activity.	Promotes the client's sense of control, and begins the development of alternative, more adaptive coping behaviors. Social isolation assists in decreasing behaviors.
• Develop a schedule for gradually increasing time client spends in group activities. For example, client will spend (number) minutes in the group dining hall during mealtimes or will spend (number) minutes in a group game. Note client's specific activities here.	Social interaction can provide positive reinforcement and opportunities for the client to practice new behaviors in a supportive environment.
• Primary nurse will spend 30 minutes a day with client exploring thoughts and feelings about social interactions and in assisting with reality testing of social interaction; for example, what others might mean by silence and other nonverbal responses.	
• Identify with client areas of social skill deficit and develop a plan for improving these areas. This could include: ○ Assertiveness training. ○ Role-playing difficult situations. ○ Teaching client relaxation techniques to reduce anxiety in social situations. (Note plan and schedule for implementation here. This should be a progressive plan, with rewards for accomplishment of each step.)	Promotes the client's sense of control and begins the development of alternative, more adaptive coping behaviors by increasing role competence.
• Consult with occupational therapist if client needs to learn specific skills to facilitate	Increasing behavioral repertoire increases role competence, which enhances self-esteem.[1]

social interactions; for example, cooking skills so friends can be invited to dinner or craft skills so client can join others in social interactions around these activities.

- Include client in group activities on the unit. Assign client activities that can be easily accomplished and that will provide positive social reinforcement from other persons involved in the activities.

Positive reinforcement encourages behavior and enhances self-esteem.

- When client demonstrates tolerance for groups interactions, schedule time for the client to participate in a group therapy that provides opportunities for feedback about relationship behavior from peers and for listening to the thoughts and feelings of peers.

Disconfirms the client's sense of aloneness; assists client in experiencing personal importance to others while enhancing interpersonal relationship skills. Increasing these competencies can enhance self-esteem and promote positive orientation.

- Discuss with support system ways in which they can facilitate client interaction.
- Have client identify those activities in the community that are of interest and would provide opportunities for interaction. List those activities here and develop a plan for client to develop necessary skills to ensure opportunities for interactional success during these activities; for example, practicing a card game or table tennis while in the hospital.

Support system understanding facilitates the maintenance of new behaviors after discharge. Increases the client's ability to successfully perform these roles, which provides positive reinforcement, thus encouraging the behavior and enhancing self-esteem.

- When client reports problems in an interaction, review his or her perceptions of the interaction and an evaluation of when the problems began.

Assists clients with reality testing of his or her perceptions.

- Limit amount of time client can spend alone in room. This should be a gradual alteration and done in steps that can easily be accomplished by the client. Note specific schedule for client here. Have staff person remain with client during these times until client demonstrates an ability to interact with others.

Successful accomplishment of a task provides positive reinforcement and promotes a positive orientation.

- Have referral source make contact with client before discharge, and schedule a postdischarge meeting.

Promotes the development of a trusting relationship while the client is in a safe environment.

Gerontic Health

See Adult Health and Mental Health.

Home Health

Actions/Interventions	Rationales
• Monitor for factors contributing to the impaired social interaction: psychologic, physical, economic, spiritual, and so on.	Provides database for early recognition and intervention.
• Involve client and family in planning, implementing, and promoting reduction or elimination of impaired social interaction: ○ *Family conference*: Identify perspective of each member. ○ *Mutual goal setting*: Set consistent rules and behavior, and provide support for care providers. Identify tasks for each member.	Family involvement enhances the effectiveness of the interventions.
• Assist patient and family in lifestyle adjustments that may be required: ○ Safe environment ○ Support networks ○ Changes in role functions ○ Prescribed treatments: medications, behavioral interventions, and so on ○ Assistance with self-care activities ○ Possible hospitalization or placement in halfway house ○ Treatment of drug or alcohol abuse ○ Development and practice of social skills ○ Independent living skills ○ Finances ○ Stress management ○ Suicide prevention	Permanent changes in behavior and family roles require support.
• Assist client and family to develop criteria to determine when crisis exists and professional intervention is necessary: ○ Violence ○ Sudden change in ability to care for self ○ Hallucinations or delusions	Provides database for early recognition and intervention.
• Consult with or refer to community resources as indicated. (See Appendix B.)	Promotes efficient use of existing resources. Respite care and support groups can enhance the treatment plan.

FLOW CHART EVALUATION
Flow Chart Expected Outcome 1

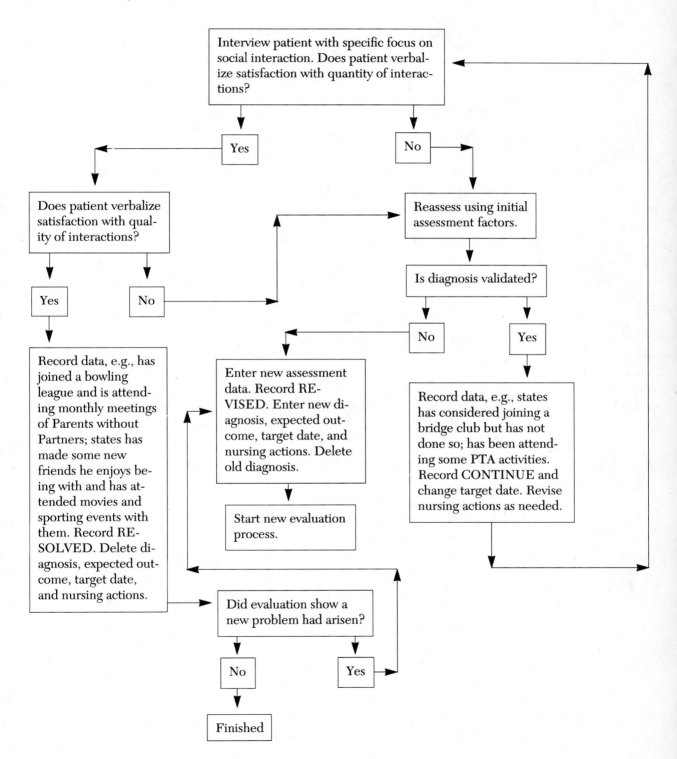

Flow Chart Expected Outcome 2

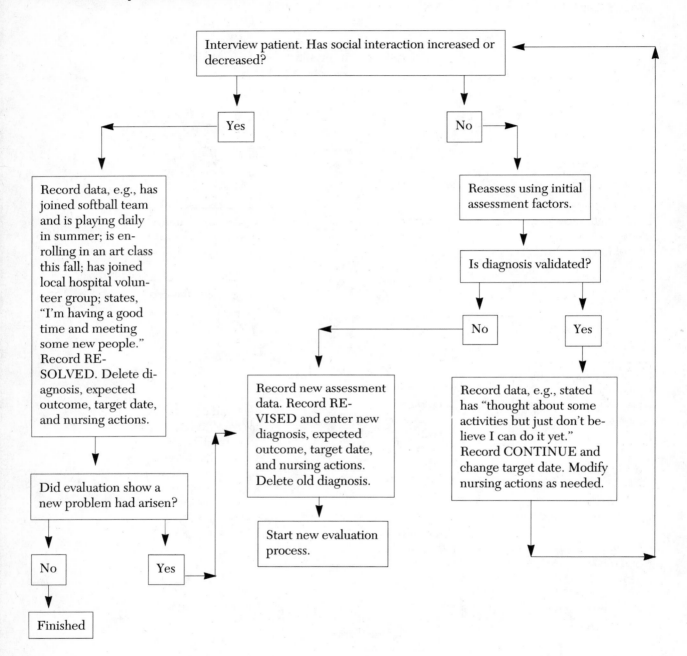

Social Isolation

DEFINITION

Aloneness experienced by the individual and perceived as imposed by others and as a negative or threatened state.[17]

NANDA TAXONOMY: RELATING 3.1.2

DEFINING CHARACTERISTICS[17]

1. Objective:
   a. Absence of supportive significant others (family, friends, group) (*critical*)
   b. Sad, dull affect
   c. Inappropriate or immature interests or activities for developmental age or stage
   d. Uncommunicative, withdrawn, no eye contact
   e. Preoccupation with own thoughts or with repetitive meaningless actions
   f. Projects hostility in voice and behavior
   g. Seeks to be alone or exists in a subculture
   h. Evidence of physical or mental handicap or altered state of wellness
   i. Shows behavior unacceptable by dominant cultural group
2. Subjective:
   a. Expresses feelings of aloneness imposed by others (*critical*)
   b. Expresses feelings of rejection (*critical*)
   c. Experiences feelings of difference from others
   d. Inadequacy in or absence of significant purpose in life
   e. Inability to meet expectations of others
   f. Insecurity in public
   g. Expresses values acceptable to the subculture but unacceptable to the dominant cultural group
   h. Expresses interests inappropriate to the developmental age or stage

RELATED FACTORS[17]

Factors contributing to the absence of satisfying personal relationships such as:

1. Delay in accomplishing developmental tasks
2. Immature interests
3. Alterations in physical appearance
4. Alterations in mental status
5. Unaccepted social behavior
6. Unaccepted social values
7. Altered state of wellness
8. Inadequate personal resources
9. Inability to engage in satisfying personal relationships

RELATED CLINICAL CONCERNS

1. Any condition which has resulted in scarring
2. Alzheimer's disease
3. AIDS

4. Tuberculosis
5. Any condition causing impaired mobility
6. Psychiatric disorders such as major depression, schizophrenic disorders, paranoid disorders, or conduct disorders

HAVE YOU SELECTED THE CORRECT DIAGNOSIS?

Knowledge Deficit This diagnosis, particularly as related to mutuality, would be the most appropriate alternate diagnosis if the individual verbalized or demonstrated an inability to attend to significant others' social actions in the context of independent and dependent aspects of their role. (See page 536.)

Impaired Verbal Communication This would be the most appropriate diagnosis if the individual is unable to receive or send communication. Certainly Impaired Verbal Communication could relate to Impaired Social Interaction and would be the primary problem that has to be resolved. (See page 791.)

Impaired Social Interaction Impaired Social Interaction can be either too much or too little in terms of social activity and is more focused on the individual's choice. In Social Isolation the patient sees this problem as being caused by others. (See page 772.)

EXPECTED OUTCOMES

1. Will identify at least (number) ways to increase social interaction by (date) and/or
2. Will participate in social activities at least weekly by (date)

TARGET DATE

A target date of 2 to 7 days would be acceptable, depending on the exact social interaction chosen.

NURSING ACTIONS/INTERVENTIONS WITH RATIONALES

Adult Health

Actions/Interventions	Rationales
• Encourage patient to verbalize feelings of isolation and aloneness by visiting patient every hour and scheduling a discussion for at least 10 minutes each shift while awake.	Promotes a therapeutic relationship where patient can verbalize in a nonthreatening environment.
• Provide positive feedback and support for social interactional skills as appropriate.	Increases self-confidence; decreases anxiety in social situations.
• Encourage patient to use assistive or corrective devices such as artificial vocal cords; limb, eye, or breast prostheses; special makeup. Have patient perform self-care management activities at least daily.	Increases self-esteem and self-confidence.

- Encourage visits from family and significant others daily.
- Encourage patient to participate in diversional activities, especially those involving groups, daily.
- Encourage patient to identify and use community support systems and groups prior to discharge. (See Appendix B.)

Increases social contacts and interactional skills.

Increases social contacts and interactional skills.

Increases social contacts; promotes assistance with short-term and long-term goals.

Child Health

Actions/Interventions	Rationales
• Provide opportunities for expression of feelings about desired social activity by spending 15 to 20 minutes per shift, during waking hours, at (times) with patient and family.	Ventilation allows for insight into patient's thinking and assists in reducing anxiety.
• Determine what obstacles are perceived by patient and family in pursuit of desired social activities by asking both direct and open-ended questions, for example, "What do you think prevents you from doing what you want to?"	Directed inquiry into obstacles which prevent the patient from engaging in desired social interaction increases the likelihood of a more complete database that will allow more individualized planning.
• Identify what realistic patterns for socialization are applicable for patient and family in collaboration with the patient and family.	Realistic goals are more likely to bring about the desired changes for more effective social interaction.
• Collaborate with other health care professionals to meet realistic goals for patient and family socialization. (See Appendix B.)	Appropriate use of resource personnel ensures optimal likelihood for goal attainment.
• Monitor for contributory related factors to best consider social activity pattern.	All factors must be considered to provide a holistic plan of care.
• Identify support groups to assist in realization of desired social activities.	Support groups provide a sense of sharing and empowerment.
• Monitor patient's and family's perceptions of the effect desired social activities might have on current role-relationship pattern.	Roles are closely impacted by patterns of social interaction.
• Provide appropriate opportunities for assessment of young child's perceptions of situational needs and how he or she views self.	The child's view of self in relationship to social patterns is vital to planning the most effective interventions.
• Assist patient to develop schedule for consideration of desired social activities at least 2 days before dismissal from hospital.	Appropriate planning serves to increase success with desired activities.
• Provide for appropriate follow-up appointment as needed prior to dismissal from hospital.	Follow-up plans attach value to long-term care for the patient.

Women's Health

The following nursing actions apply to the social isolation experienced by the patient who has a sexually transmitted disease such as herpes genitalia, syphilis, chlamydia, gonorrhea, or AIDS.

Actions/Interventions	Rationales

• Assure patient of confidentiality.
• Refer for counseling and/or treatment to:
  ○ Support groups
  ○ Professionals, for example, public health clinic, nurse specialists, physician
• Provide a nonjudgmental atmosphere to encourage verbalization of concerns:[26]
  ○ Recurrent nature of disease, especially herpes and chlamydia
  ○ Lack of cure for disease (AIDS)
  ○ Economics in treating disease
  ○ Social stigma associated with disease
  ○ Opportunity for entrance into health care system
• Encourage honesty in answers to such questions as:
  ○ Multiple sexual partners (identify contacts)
  ○ Describing sexual behavior
• Encourage honest communication with sexual partners.
	Promotes sharing of information by patient. Provides long-term support and care for patient.
	
	Provides database needed to provide appropriate care and teaching.
	
	Sexual partners will need to seek health care also.

Mental Health

Actions/Interventions	Rationales
• If delusions and/or hallucinations are present, refer to Sensory-Perceptual Alteration for detailed interventions. • If social isolation is related to client's feelings of powerlessness, refer to Powerlessness (Chapter 8) for detailed interventions. • Discuss with client his or her perception of the source of the social isolation, and have him or her list those ways he or she has tried to resolve the situation. • Have client list those persons in the environment who are considered family, friends, and acquaintances. Then have client note how many interactions per week	Assists in understanding the client's worldview, which facilitates the development of client-specific interventions. Facilitates the client's reality testing of his or her perception of being socially isolated.

occur with each person. Have client identify what interferes with feeling connected with these persons. This activity should be implemented by the primary nurse. Note schedule for this interaction here.

- When contributing factors have been identified, develop a plan to alter these factors. This could include:
  - Assertiveness training.
  - Role-playing difficult situations.
  - Teaching client relaxation techniques to reduce anxiety in social situations. (Note plan and schedule for implementation here.)

Facilitates the development of alternative coping behaviors, which enhances role performance.

- Develop a list of those things the client finds rewarding, and provide these rewards as client successfully completes progressive steps in treatment plan. This schedule should be developed with the client. Note schedule for rewards and the kinds of behavior to be rewarded here.

Positive reinforcement encourages behavior and enhances self-esteem.

- Consult with occupational therapist if client needs to learn specific skills to facilitate social interactions, such as cooking skills so friends can be invited to dinner, craft skills or dancing so client can join others in these social activities.

Increases the client's competence and thus enhances role performance and self-esteem.

- Provide client with those prostheses necessary to facilitate social interactions, for example, hearing aids, eyeglasses. Note here assistance needed from nursing staff in providing these to client. Also note where they are to be stored while not in use.

- Include client in group activities on the unit; assign client activities that can be accomplished easily and that will provide positive social reinforcement from other persons involved in the activities. This could include things like having client assume responsibility for preparing part of a group meal or for serving a portion of a meal.

Successful accomplishment of a valued task can provide positive reinforcement, which encourages behavior.

- Role-play with client those social interactions identified as most difficult. This will be done by primary nurse. Note schedule for this activity here.

Repeated practice of a behavior internalizes and personalizes the behavior.

- Discuss with client those times it would be appropriate to be alone, and develop a plan for coping with these times in a positive

Promotes the client's sense of control while facilitating the development of alternative coping behaviors.

Continued

Actions/Interventions	Rationales
manner; for example, client will develop a list of books to read and music to listen to.	
• When client is demonstrating socially inappropriate behavior, keep interactions to a minimum and escort to a place away from group activities.	Lack of positive reinforcement decreases a behavior.
• When inappropriate behavior stops, discuss the behavior with the client and develop a list of alternative kinds of behavior for the client to use in situations where the inappropriate behavior is elicited. Note those kinds of behavior that are identified as problematic here, with the action to be taken if they are demonstrated; for example, client will spend time out in seclusion or sleeping area.	Promotes client's sense of control while facilitating the development of alternative coping behaviors.
• Develop a schedule of gradually increasing time for client to spend in group activities; for example, client will spend (number) minutes in the group dining hall during mealtimes or will spend (number) minutes in a group game twice a day. Note specific goals for client here.	Provides client with opportunities to practice new behaviors in a safe, supportive environment.
• Primary nurse will spend 30 minutes once a day with client at (time) discussing client's reactions to social interactions and assisting client with reality testing of social interactions; for example, what others might mean by silence, or various nonverbal and common verbal expressions. This time can also be used to discuss role relationships and client's specific concerns about relationships.	
• Assign client a room near areas with high activity.	Facilitates client's participation in unit activities.
• Assign one staff person to the client each shift, and have this person interact with client every 30 minutes while awake.	Decreases the client's opportunities for socially isolating self.
• Be open and direct with client in interactions, and avoid verbal and nonverbal behavior that requires interpretation by client.	Promotes a trusting relationship.
• Have client tell staff his or her interpretation of interactions.	Assists client in reality testing of perceptions that might inhibit social interactions.
• Have client identify those activities in the community that are of interest and would provide opportunities for interactions with others. List client's interests here.	Promotes the client's sense of control.

- Develop with the client a plan for making contact with the identified community activities before discharge.
- When client demonstrates tolerance for group interactions, schedule time for the client to participate in a therapy group that provides opportunities for feedback about relationship behavior from peers and for listening to the thoughts and feelings of peers.
- Arrange at least 1 hour a week for client to interact with support system in the presence of the primary nurse. This will allow the nurse to assess and facilitate these interactions.
- Discuss with support system ways in which they can facilitate client interaction.
- Model for support system and for client those kinds of behavior that facilitate communication.[27,28]
- Limit the amount of time client can spend alone in room. This should be a gradual alteration and should be done in steps that can easily be accomplished by client. Note specific schedule for client here; for example, client will spend 5 minutes per hour in day area. Have staff person remain with client during these times until client demonstrates an ability to interact with others.
- Refer client to appropriate community agencies. (See Appendix B.)

Promotes the client's sense of control, and begins the development of adaptive coping behaviors.
Disconfirms the client's sense of aloneness and helps client to experience personal importance to others while enhancing interpersonal relationship skills. Increasing these competencies can enhance self-esteem and promote positive orientation.

Support system understanding facilitates the maintenance of new behaviors after discharge.

Provides opportunities for client to practice new role behaviors in a safe, supportive environment.

Gerontic Health

Actions/Interventions	Rationales
- Discuss with patient what efforts he or she has made to increase social contacts and what results have been obtained.	Assists in determining what interventions may result in positive outcomes.
- Ask patient to identify hobbies and activities that have been a part of his or her adult life.	Provides information on preferred activities, and guides the nurse in seeking resources that match the patient's interests.
- Ask patient to identify barriers to continuing with the hobbies and activities he or she enjoyed in the past.	Barriers may be indicators of need for use of specific resources such as adaptive equipment or transportation.
- Assist patient in identifying and contacting community support services.	In many areas, initial contact with support services can entail numerous telephone calls to reach the appropriate resource.

Home Health

NOTE: See Mental Health nursing actions for detailed interventions.

Actions/Interventions	Rationales

• Involve client and family in planning and implementing strategies to reduce social isolation:
  ○ *Family conference*: Discuss perceptions of source of social isolation, and list possible solutions.
  ○ *Mutual goal setting*: Set realistic goals with evaluation criteria. Set specific tasks for each family member.
  ○ *Communication*: Encourage positive feedback.
	Family involvement in planning enhances the effectiveness of interventions.

• Assist family and patient with life-style adjustments that may be required:
  ○ Promote social interaction.
  ○ Provide transportation.
  ○ Provide activities to keep busy during lonely times.
  ○ Provide communication alternatives for those with sensory deficits.
  ○ Assist with disfiguring illness; employ enterostomal therapist or prosthesis manufacturer.
  ○ Control incontinence or provide absorbent undergarments when socializing.
  ○ Promote self-worth.
  ○ Promote self-care.
  ○ Develop and utilize support groups.
  ○ Use pets.
  ○ Establish regular telephone contact.
  ○ Inform patient of volunteer programs in community that person could work for.
	Permanent changes in behavior and family roles require support.

• Consult with or refer to community resources as indicated. (See Appendix B.)	Provides efficient use of existing resources. Self-help groups, occupational therapists, and homebound programs can enhance the treatment plan.

FLOW CHART EVALUATION
Flow Chart Expected Outcome 1

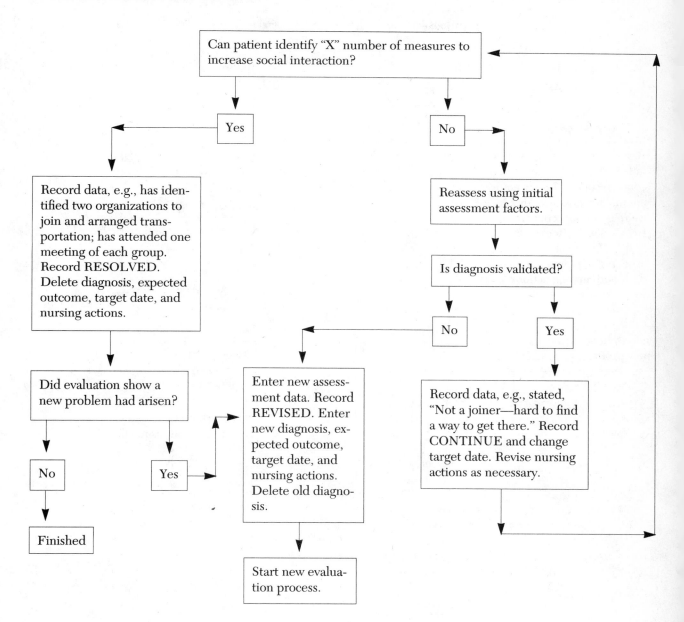

Can patient identify "X" number of measures to increase social interaction?

Yes

No

Record data, e.g., has identified two organizations to join and arranged transportation; has attended one meeting of each group. Record RESOLVED. Delete diagnosis, expected outcome, target date, and nursing actions.

Reassess using initial assessment factors.

Is diagnosis validated?

No

Yes

Did evaluation show a new problem had arisen?

Enter new assessment data. Record REVISED. Enter new diagnosis, expected outcome, target date, and nursing actions. Delete old diagnosis.

Record data, e.g., stated, "Not a joiner—hard to find a way to get there." Record CONTINUE and change target date. Revise nursing actions as necessary.

No

Yes

Finished

Start new evaluation process.

Flow Chart Expected Outcome 2

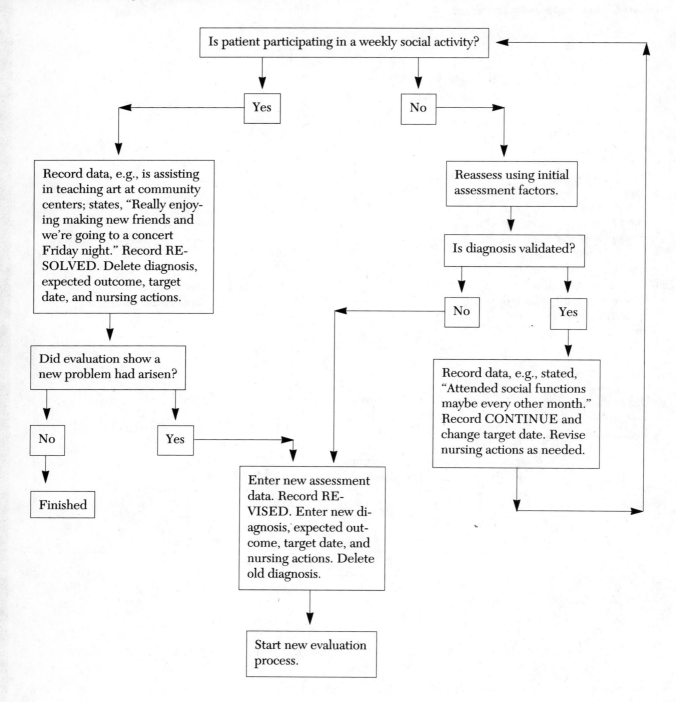

Verbal Communication, Impaired

DEFINITION

The state in which an individual experiences a decreased or absent ability to use or understand language in human interaction.[17]

NANDA TAXONOMY: COMMUNICATING 2.1.1.1

DEFINING CHARACTERISTICS[17]

1. Major defining characteristics:
   a. Unable to speak dominant language (*critical*)
   b. Speaks or verbalizes with difficulty (*critical*)
   c. Does not or cannot speak (*critical*)
   d. Stuttering
   e. Slurring
   f. Difficulty forming words or sentences
   g. Difficulty expressing thoughts verbally
   h. Inappropriate verbalization
   i. Dyspnea
   j. Disorientation
2. Minor defining characteristics:
   None given

RELATED FACTORS[17]

1. Decrease in circulation to brain
2. Brain tumor
3. Physical barrier (tracheostomy, intubation)
4. Anatomical defect, cleft palate
5. Psychologic barriers (psychosis, lack of stimuli)
6. Cultural difference
7. Developmental or age-related

RELATED CLINICAL CONCERNS

1. Laryngeal cancer
2. Cleft lip, cleft palate
3. Cerebrovascular accident
4. Facial trauma
5. Respiratory distress
6. Late-stage Alzheimer's disease
7. Tourette disorder
8. Psychiatric disorders such as schizophrenic disorders, delusional disorders, psychotic disorders, delirium
9. Autism

HAVE YOU SELECTED THE CORRECT DIAGNOSIS?

Social Isolation   Social Isolation can occur because of the reduced ability or inability of an individual to use language as a means of communication. The primary diagnosis would be Impaired Verbal Communication, since resolution of the problem would assist in alleviating Social Isolation. (See page 781.)

Sensory-Perceptual Alteration (Auditory)   If the individual has difficulty in hearing, then he or she will also reflect Impaired Verbal Communication. The primary problem is the auditory difficulty, since correcting this deficit will help improve communication. (See page 562.)

EXPECTED OUTCOMES

1. Will verbalize satisfaction with communication process by (date) and/or
2. Will communicate in a clear manner via (state specific method: orally, esophageal speech, computer, and so on) by (date)

TARGET DATE

The target date for resolution of this diagnosis will be long-range. However, 7 days would be appropriate for initial evaluation.

NURSING ACTIONS/INTERVENTIONS WITH RATIONALES

Adult Health

Actions/Interventions	Rationales
• Maintain a patient, calm approach by: ○ Allowing adequate time for communication ○ Not interrupting the patient or attempting to finish his or her sentences ○ Asking questions that require short answers or a nod of the head ○ Anticipating needs	Avoids interfering with patient's communication attempts.
• Provide materials that can be used to assist in communication: magic slate, flash cards, pad and pencil, "speak-and-spell" computer toy, pictures, letter board.	Provides alternative methods of communication; decreases anxiety and feelings of powerlessness and isolation.
• Inform family, significant others, and other health care personnel of the effective ways patient communicates.	Promotes effective communication; avoids frustration for patient.
• Answer call bell promptly rather than using the intercom system.	Decreases stress for patient by not straining communication resources.
• Assure patient that parenteral therapy does not interfere with patient's ability to write.	Decreases anxiety.
• Initiate referral to speech therapist if appropriate.	Initial teaching regarding speech may require interventions by specialist.

• Initiate referrals to support agencies such as Lost Chord Club or New Voice Club as appropriate.	Groups that experience the same problems can assist in rehabilitation and decrease social isolation; promotes patient's comfort.
• Discuss use of electronic voice box, esophageal speech prior to discharge. Have patient practice using device.	Reduces anxiety, increases self-confidence.
• Encourage patient to have recordings made for reaching police, fire department, doctor, or emergency medical service if impaired verbal communication is a long-term condition.	Promotes safety; increases comfort; decreases anxiety.

Child Health

Actions/Interventions	Rationales
• Monitor patient's potential for speech according to subjective and objective components, including: 　○ Reported or documented previous speech capacity or potential 　○ Health history for evidence of cogntive, sensory, perceptual, or neurologic dysfunction 　○ Actual auditory documentation of speech potential 　○ Assessment done by speech specialist 　○ Patterns of speech of parents and significant others 　○ Cultural meaning attached to speech or silence of children 　○ Any related trauma or pathophysiology 　○ Parental perception of child's status, especially in instances of congenital anomaly such as cleft lip or palate 　○ Identification of dominant language and secondary languages heard or spoken in family	Provides database needed to plan more complete and accurate interventions.
• Assist the patient and parents to understand needed explanations for procedures, treatments, and equipment to be used in nursing care.	Provides teaching opportunity; decreases anxiety, which can interfere with communication.
• Encourage feelings to be expressed by taking time to understand possible attempts at speech. Use pictures if necessary for young children.	Alternative methods of communication and sensitivity to attempts at communication attach value to the patient and serve to reinforce future attempts at communication.

Continued

Actions/Interventions	Rationales
• Encourage family participation in care of patient as situation allows.	Family input provides an opportunity for communication and improves parent-child relationship.
• Assist family to identify community support groups.	Provides long-term support for coping.
• Assist patient and family in determining the impact Impaired Verbal Communication may have on family functioning.	Family functioning relies heavily on communication.
• Provide information for long-term medical follow-up as indicated, especially for congenital anomalies.	Knowledge helps to prepare family for long-term needs and reduce anxiety about unknowns.
• Assist in identification of appropriate financial support for medical needs of child.	Funding by third-party payment may be available, depending on patient's medical status.
• Monitor for changes in role-relationship patterns resulting from Impaired Verbal Communication.	Alterations in communication can affect the role-relationship pattern.
• Monitor for changes in self-concept or coping patterns resulting from Impaired Verbal Communication.	Alterations in communication may impact the patient's self-esteem and should be considered a risk factor.
• Provide appropriate patient and family teaching for care of patient if permanent tracheostomy or related prosthetic is to be used:	Basic standards of care for the patient with a tracheostomy.
○ Appropriate number or size of tracheostomy tube	
○ Appropriate duplication of tracheostomy tube in event of accidental dislodging or loss	
○ Appropriate administration of oxygen via trach adapter	
○ Appropriate sterile and nonsterile suctioning technique	
○ Appropriate list of supplies and how to procure them	
○ Resources for actual care in emergency, with phone numbers of ambulance and nearest hospital	
○ Appropriate indications for notification of physician (these may vary slightly according to physician's plan or actual patient status)	
(1) Bleeding from tracheostomy	
(2) Coughing out or dislodging of tracheostomy	
(3) Difficulty in passing catheter to suction tracheostomy	
(4) Fever above 101°F	

(5) Appropriate daily hygiene of tracheostomy

(6) Caution regarding use of regular gauze or other substances which might be inhaled or ingested through tracheostomy

(7) Need for humidification of tracheostomy

Women's Health

See sections on Adult Health, Mental Health, Gerontic Health, and Home Health.

Mental Health

Actions/Interventions	Rationales
• If impaired communication is related to alterations in physiology or surgical alterations, refer to Adult Health nursing actions.	
• Create a calm, reassuring environment.	Inappropriate levels of sensory stimuli can increase confusion and disorganization.
• Provide client with a private environment if he or she is experiencing high levels of anxiety to assist in focusing on relevant stimuli.	High levels of anxiety decrease the client's ability to process information.
• Communicate with client in clear, concise language: ○ Speak slowly to client. ○ Do not shout. ○ Face client when talking to him or her. ○ Role-model agreement between verbal and nonverbal behavior.	Inappropriate levels of sensory stimuli can increase confusion and disorganization. When verbal and nonverbal behavior are not in agreement, a double-bind or incongruent message may be sent. These incongruent messages place the receiver in a "damned if you do, dmaned if you don't" situation and promote interpersonal ineffectiveness.
• Spend 30 minutes twice a day at (times) with client discussing communication patterns. This time could also include, as the client progresses: ○ Constructive confrontation about the effects of the dysfunctional communication pattern on relationships ○ Role-playing of appropriate communication patterns ○ Pointing out to client the lack of agreement between verbal and nonverbal behavior and context	Promotes the development of a trusting relationship while providing the client with a safe environment in which to practice new behaviors. Behavioral rehearsal helps to facilitate the client's learning new skills through the use of feedback and modeling by the nurse.

Continued

Actions/Interventions	Rationales
○ Helping client to understand purpose of dysfunctional communication patterns ○ Developing alternative ways for client to have needs met	
• With the client's assistance, develop a reward program for appropriate communication patterns and for progress on goals. Note the kinds of behavior to be rewarded and schedule for reward here.	Positive reinforcement encourages behavior while enhancing self-esteem.
• Instruct client in assertive communication techniques, and practice these in daily interactions with the client. Note here those assertive skills client is to practice and how these are to be practiced; for example, each medication is to be requested by the client in an assertive manner.	Assertiveness improves the individual's ability to act appropriately and effectively in a manner that maximizes coping resources.[23]
• Provide the client with positive verbal rewards for appropriate communication.	Positive reinforcement encourages behavior.
• Sit with client while another client is asked for feedback about an interaction.	The nurse's presence provides support while the client receives feedback on interpersonal skills from a peer. Inappropriate levels of sensory stimuli can increase confusion and disorganization.
• Keep interactions brief and goal-directed when client is communicating in dysfunctional manner.	
• Spend an extra 5 minutes in interactions in which client is communicating clearly, and inform client of this reward of time.	Time with the nurse can provide positive reinforcement.
• Reward improvement in client's listening behavior. This can be evaluated by having the client repeat what he or she has just heard. Provide clarification for the differences between what was heard and what was said.	Improved attending skills improve the client's ability to understand communication from others and clarify unclear portions of communication.
• Have support system participate in one interaction per week with the client in the presence of a staff member. The staff member will facilitate communication between the client and the support system. Note time for these interactions here with the name of the staff person responsible for this process.	Behavioral rehearsal provides opportunities for feedback and modeling from the nurse. Support system understanding facilitates the maintenance of new behaviors after discharge.
• Arrange for client to participate in a therapetic group. Note schedule for these groups here.	Provides an opportunity for the client to receive feedback on communication from peers and observe the interactions of peers so that they may increase their requisite variety of responses in a social situation.
• Request that client clarify unclear statements or communications in private language.	Models appropriate communication skills for the client.

- Teach client to request clarification on confusing communications. This may be practiced through role playing.
- Include client in unit activities, and assign appropriate tasks to client. These should require a level of communication the client can easily achieve so that a positive learning experience can occur. Note level of activity appropriate for client here.
- If communication problems evolve from a language difference, have someone who understands the language orient the client to the unit as soon as possible and answer any questions the client might have.
- Use nonverbal communication to interact with client when there is no one available to translate.
- Obtain information about nonverbal communication in the client's culture and about appropriate psychosocial behavior. Alter interactions and expectations to fit these beliefs as they fit the client. Note here information that is important in providing daily care for this client.
- Determine if the client understands English and in what form: written or spoken.
- If client does not understand English, determine if a language other than the one from the culture of origin is spoken. Perhaps a common language for staff and client can be found. For example, few people other than Navajos speak Navajo, but some older Navajos also speak Spanish.
- Do not shout when talking with someone who speaks another language. Speak slowly and concisely.
- Use pictures to enhance nonverbal communication.

- If a staff member does not speak the client's language, arrange for a translator to visit with the client at least once a day to answer questions and provide information. Have a schedule for the next day available so this can be reviewed with the client and information can be provided about complex procedures. Have a staff member remain with the client during these interactions to serve as a resource person for the translator. Allow time for the client to ask questions and express feelings. Note schedule for these visits here with the name of the translator.

Repeated practice of a behavior internalizes and personalizes the behavior.

Provides opportunities for the client to practice new behaviors in a supportive environment.

Decreases the client's sense of isolation and anxiety.

Decreases the client's sense of social isolation, and promotes the development of a trusting relationship.
Decreases the possibilities for misunderstanding.

Promotes the development of a trusting relationship.
Communication facilitates social interaction and increases the client's sense of control.

Inappropriate levels of sensory stimulation can increase confusion and disorganization.

Pictures facilitate communication when the caregiver and client do not share the same language.
Promotes the client's sense of control, and decreases social isolation.

Gerontic Health

See Adult Health and Mental Health.

Home Health

Actions/Interventions	Rationales

• Involve client and family in planning and implementing strategies to decrease, prevent, or cope with impaired verbal communication:
   ○ *Family conference*: Discuss each member's perspective of situation.
   ○ *Mutual goal setting*: Set short-term accomplishable goals with evaluation criteria; specify tasks for each member.
   ○ *Communication*: Identify ways to communicate with client.
	Family involvement enhances effectiveness of interventions.

• Teach client and family appropriate information regarding the care of a person with impaired verbal communication:
   ○ Use of pencil and paper, alphabet letters, head signals, sign language, pictures, flash cards, computer
   ○ Use of repetition
   ○ The importance of facing the person when communicating
   ○ Use of simple, one-step commands
   ○ Allowing time for person to respond
   ○ Use of drawing, painting, coloring, singing, exercising
   ○ Identifying tasks the person with impaired verbal communication can do well
   ○ Decreasing external noise
	Provides knowledge base required to interact with family member who is verbally impaired.

• Assist patient and family in life-style adjustments that may be required:
   ○ Stress management
   ○ Changing role functions and relationships
   ○ Learning a foreign language
   ○ Acknowledging and coping with frustration with communication efforts
   ○ Obtaining necessary supportive equipment: hearing aid, special telephone, artificial larynx
	Life-style changes require long-term behavioral changes. Support enhances permanent changes in behavior.

• Consult with or refer to appropriate community resources as required. (See Appendix B.)	Self-help groups and rehabilitation services can enhance the treatment plans.

FLOW CHART EVALUATION
Flow Chart Expected Outcome 1

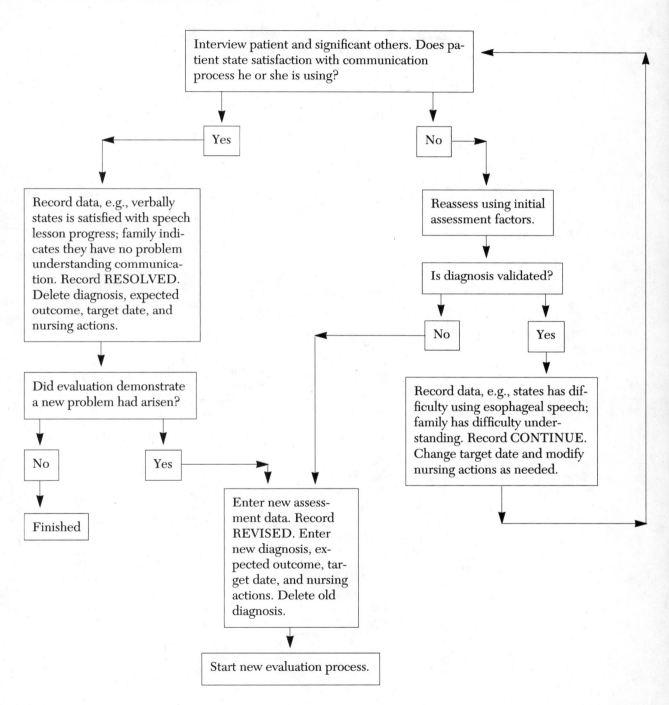

Flow Chart Expected Outcome 2

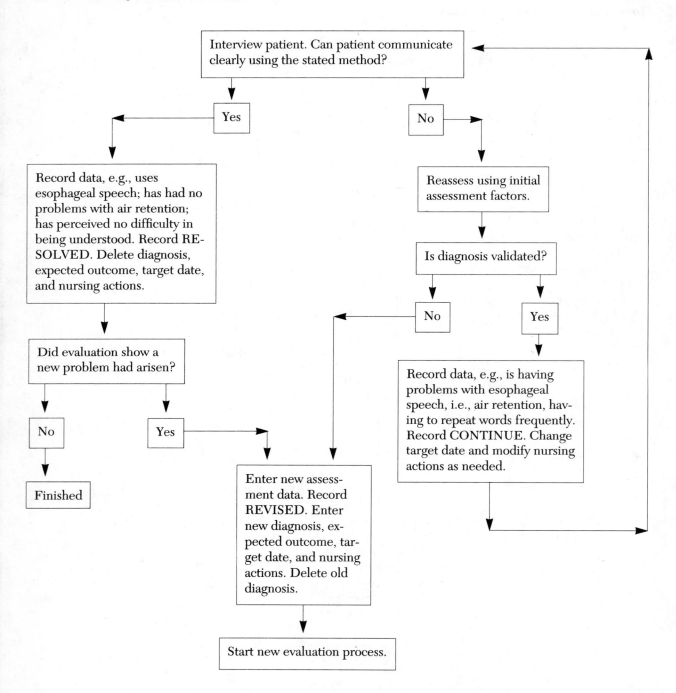

Violence, High Risk for: Self-Directed or Directed at Others

DEFINITION

A state in which an individual experiences behaviors that can be physically harmful either to the self or to others.[17]

NANDA TAXONOMY: FEELING 9.2.2

DEFINING CHARACTERISTICS[17]

1. Risk factors:
   a. Body language: clenched fists, tense facial expression, rigid posture, tautness indicating effort to control
   b. Hostile, threatening verbalizations: boasting of or prior abuse of others
   c. Increased motor activity: pacing, excitement, irritability, agitation
   d. Overt and aggressive acts: goal-directed destruction of objects in environment
   e. Possession of destructive means: gun, knife, or other weapon
   f. Rage
   g. Self-destructive behavior, active aggressive suicidal acts
   h. Suspicion of others, paranoid ideation, delusions, hallucinations
   i. Substance abuse or withdrawal
2. Other possible characteristics:
   a. Increasing anxiety levels
   b. Fear of self or others
   c. Inability to verbalize feelings
   d. Repetition of verbalizations: continued complaints, requests, and demands
   e. Anger
   f. Provocative behavior: argumentative, dissatisfied, overreactive, or hypersensitive
   g. Vulnerable self-esteem
   h. Depression: especially active, aggressive, suicidal acts

RELATED FACTORS[17]

1. Antisocial personality disorder
2. Battered woman
3. Attention-deficit hyperactivity disorder
4. Child abuse
5. Autistic disorder
6. Organic brain syndrome
7. Mania
8. Borderline personality disorder
9. Suicidal behavior
10. Temporal lobe epilepsy
11. Toxic reactions to medication
12. Conduct disorder
13. Paranoid disorder

14. Psychotic disorders
15. Schizophrenic disorders
16. Substance use disorders

RELATED CLINICAL CONCERNS

1. Physical abuse
2. Organic brain syndrome; Alzheimer's disease
3. Attempted suicide
4. Temporal lobe epilepsy
5. Panic episode

HAVE YOU SELECTED THE CORRECT DIAGNOSIS?

Ineffective Family Coping: Disabled or Compromised   This diagnosis relates to the inability of the primary caregiver or caretaker to meet the needs of the patient. No violence is included in this diagnosis. If violence (abuse) has been found, then the diagnosis should be changed. (See page 874.)

Altered Parenting   This diagnosis relates to the relationship between the nurturing figure and the child. Child abuse is included within this diagnosis, but as an actual fact, not as a potential risk. If a risk for abuse exists, then High Risk for Violence is the most appropriate diagnosis. (See page 742.)

EXPECTED OUTCOMES

1. Will demonstrate at least (number) alternative methods for releasing anger by (date) and/or
2. Will identify factors that contribute to risk for violence by (date)

TARGET DATE

For the sake of all concerned, the patient should begin to demonstrate progress within 3 to 5 days. However, the patient must be monitored on a daily basis. Total control of violent behavior may take months.

NURSING ACTIONS/INTERVENTIONS WITH RATIONALES

Adult Health

NOTE: See also Mental Health.

Actions/Interventions	Rationales
• Refer to psychiatric nurse clinician.	Violence or High Risk for Violence requires specific interventions by a specialist in the area of mental health.

- Monitor for signs of anger or distress such as restlessness, pacing, wringing of hands, or verbally abusive behavior.

  Monitors for deterioration of condition, and promotes early intervention.

- Accept anger of patient, but do not participate in it when interacting with patient.

  Anger is an acceptable behavior if appropriately handled, but escalation of anger is to be avoided.

- Remain calm; set limits on patient's behavior; reduce environmental stimuli.

  Decreases sensory stimuli; decreases anxiety and violence-provoking situations.

- Encourage patient to verbalize angry feelings or physically demonstrate them in constructive ways, such as punching a bag, banging a trash can, taking a walk, and so on. Schedule 30 minute twice a day at (times) to confer with patient regarding this topic.

  Promotes an acceptable alternative strategy for dealing with anger.

- Let the patient know that he or she has control of own actions; he or she is responsible for own actions. Help patient identify situations that interfere with his or her control.

  Reinforces reality, and maintains limits on behavior.

- Provide a safe environment by removing clutter, breakables, or potential weapons. Restrain or seclude patient as needed.

  Promotes safety, and reduces risk of harm to patient or others.

- At least once an hour, observe for indications of suicidal behavior, for example, withdrawal, depression, planning and organizing for attempt.

  Prevents self-inflicted violence.

- Give medications (tranquilizer, sedative, and so on) as ordered, and monitor effects of medication.

  Determines effectiveness of medication as well as monitoring for unwanted side effects.

Child Health

Actions/Interventions	Rationales
• Assist patient and family to describe usual patterns of role-relationship activities.	Insight into role relationships is basic in determining the risk for violence.
• Monitor for precipitating or triggering events that seem to recur as the pattern for violence is explored.	Risk indicators can be identified as assessment for repeated violence is considered.
• Help the patient and family to describe own perceptions of the actual or potential violence pattern.	Insight of patient or parents reveals basic data about the violence pattern and assists in accurate intervention.
• Provide opportunities for expression of emotions related to the violence appropriate for age and developmental capacity; for example, with a toddler, use dolls, puppets, or other noninvasive methods.	Expression of thoughts and feelings in a directive, age-appropriate manner helps to clarify the impact of the violence and assists in reducing anxiety for the child.

Continued

Actions/Interventions	Rationales
• Provide appropriate collaboration for long-term follow-up regarding appropriate intervention. (See Appendix B.)	Valuing long-term follow-up fosters compliance and shows sensitivity to the patient's needs for long-term support. Safety is also at risk. In many instances, legal mandates will dictate exact protocols to be enforced.
• Provide for role taking by parents in a supportive manner when possible.	Supportive role modeling provides a safe and nonjudgmental milieu for parents to practice parenting and appropriate behaviors with child. It also allows for observation of behaviors to follow reciprocity of parent-infant dyad or triad.
• Provide consistency in caregivers to best develop a trust for nursing staff during hospitalization.	Consistency increases trust in caregivers.
• Provide for confidentiality and privacy.	These standards are too often overlooked.
• Ensure that discussions regarding child and family be carried out with objectivity.	Objective dialogues are less threatening for all involved.
• Identify appropriate authorities as needed for protection of child and family members, including police or others according to institutional policy.	Appropriate child-protective measures must be taken.
• Provide support in determining how usual coping patterns may be enhanced to deal with altered role-relationship pattern of violence.	Support in coping and dealing with violence will help reduce likelihood of increasing violence and assist in reducing anxiety.
• Assist in plans for placement, transitional placement, or discharge.	Appropriate planning for changes in care and the environment lessens the emotional trauma of these changes.
• Assist in identification of specific resources for long-term planning as appropriate.	Follow-up ensures attention to long-term needs and attaches value to follow-up care.
• Maintain objectivity in documentation of parent-child interactions.	Documentation, in nursing records, in an objective manner ensures appropriate standards for the legal and ethical issues involved in the care of the patient.

Women's Health

NOTE: These actions relate specifically to the abused or battered woman.[26,27,29–31]

Actions/Interventions	Rationales
• Be alert for cues that might indicate battering:[26,27,29–31] ○ Hesitancy in providing detailed information about injury and how it occurred	Provides database necessary to accurately assess the true causative factor.

○ Inappropriate affect for the situation
○ Delayed reporting of symptoms
○ Types and sites of injuries, such as bruises to head, throat, chest, breast, or genitals
○ Inappropriate explanations
○ Increased anxiety in presence of the batterer

- Provide a quiet, secure atmosphere to facilitate verbalization of fear, anger, rage, guilt, and shame.

Provides emotional support to patient; fosters security for patient in realizing she is not alone or the only person to have had this experience.

- Provide information on options available to patient; women's shelters, Legal Aid, and so on.

Provides basic information needed by the patient for future planning.

- Assist the patient in raising her self-esteem by:[26,27,29-31]
  ○ Asking permission to do nursing tasks
  ○ Involving patient in decision making
  ○ Providing patient with choices
  ○ Encouraging patient to ask questions
  ○ Assuring patient of confidentiality

Provides the information, long-range support, and essentials for resolving the problem.

- Assist patient in reviewing and understanding family dynamics.
- Encourage and assist in planning for economic and financial needs such as housing, job, child care, food, clothing, school for the children, and legal assistance.
- Refer to social services for immediate financial assistance for shelter, food, clothing, and child care.
- Assist patient in identifying life-style adjustments that each decision could entail.
- Encourage development of community and social network systems. (See Appendix B.)

Mental Health

Actions/Interventions	Rationales
- Introduce self to client and call client by name.	Conditions that make people feel anonymous facilitate aggressive behavior.[32]
- If aggressive behavior is resulting from toxic substances, consult with physician for medication and detoxification procedure.	Staff and client safety is of primary concern.
- Observe client every 15 minutes during detoxification, assessing vital signs and mental status until condition is stable.	Client safety is of primary concern.

Continued

Actions/Interventions	Rationales
• Place client in quiet environment for detoxification.	Inappropriate levels of sensory stimuli can increase confusion and disorganization.
• Eliminate environmental stimuli that affect client in a negative manner. This could include staff, family, and other clients. Establish balance between being in control and being controlling.	Inappropriate levels of sensory stimuli can increase confusion and disorganization, increasing the risk for violent behavior.
• Provide a calm, reassuring environment. Respect client's requests for quiet time alone.	
• Protect client from harm by:	Provides basic client safety.
○ Removing sharp objects from environment	
○ Removing belts and strings from environment	
○ Providing a one-to-one constant interaction if risk for self-harm is high	
○ Checking on client's whereabouts every 15 minutes	
○ Removing glass objects from environment	
○ Removing locks from room and bathroom doors	
○ Providing a shower curtain that will not support weight	
○ Checking to see if client swallows medication	
• Observe client's use of physical space, and do not invade client's personal space.	Encroachment on the client's personal space may be perceived as a threat.[33]
• If it is necessary to have physical contact with the client, explain this need to the client in brief, simple terms before approaching.	Clarifies role of staff to client so that the intent of these interactions can be framed in a positive manner.
• Remove unnecessary clutter and excess stimuli from the environment.	Inappropriate levels of sensory stimuli can increase the client's confusion and disorganization, thus increasing the risk for violent behavior.
• Talk with client in calm, reassuring voice.	
• Do not make sudden moves.	
• Remove persons that irritate the client from the environment. Remember, the best intervention for violent behavior is prevention. Observe client carefully for signs of increasing anxiety and tension.	
• Do not assume physical postures that are perceived as threatening to the client.	
• If increase in tension is noted, talk with client about feelings.	Assists client in developing coping behaviors.
• Help client attach feelings to appropriate persons and situations; for example, "Your boss really made you angry this time."	Assists client in developing coping behaviors that are appropriate to the situation. Promotes the client's sense of control.[33]

- Suggest to client alternative behavior for releasing tension; for example, "You really seem tense right now; let's go to the gym so you can use the punching bag" or "Let's go for a walk."

Assists client in releasing physical tension associated with high levels of anger.

- Provide medication as ordered, and observe client for signs of side effects, especially orthostatic hypotension.

Provides the least restrictive way of assisting client to control behavior.

- Answer questions in an open, direct manner.

Promotes the developing of a trusting relationship and promotes consistency in interventions.[33]

- Orient client to reality in interactions. Use methods of indirect confrontation that do not pose a personal threat to client. Do not agree with delusions; for example, "I do not hear voices other than yours or mine" or "This is the mental health unit at (name) Hospital."

Direct confrontations could be perceived as a threat to the client and precipitate violent behavior.[34]

- Refer to Altered Thought Process (Chapter 7) for detailed interventions for delusions and hallucinations.

Promotes the development of a trusting relationship. In crisis, clients are more likely to respond positively to someone with whom they have a trusting relationship. Increases consistency in interventions.[33]

- Assign one primary caregiver to the client to facilitate the development of a therapeutic relationship.

- Inform client before making any attempts at physical contact in the process of normal provision of care; for example, explain to client you would like to assist him or her with dressing, and ask if this will be all right.

Clients who are prone to violence need increased personal space. Intrusions could provoke violent behavior.[33]

- Assist client in identifying potential problem behavior by providing feedback about his or her behavior.

Promotes client's sense of control, which decreases risk for violent behavior.[33]

- Have client talk about angry feelings toward self and others.

Assisting client to understand the reasons for the anger can defuse the situation.[33]

- Contract with client to talk with staff member when he or she feels an increase in internal tension or anger.

Promotes client's sense of control by assuring the client that if he or she can no longer maintain control, the staff has a specific plan to assist with this.[33]

- Set limits on inappropriate behavior, and discuss these limits with the client. Note these limits here as well as the consequences for these kinds of behaviors. This information should be very specific so that the intervention is consistent from shift to shift. Present these limits as choices.

- If conflict occurs between client and someone else, sit with them as they resolve

Staff presence can reinforce use of appropriate problem-solving skills.

Continued

Actions/Interventions	Rationales
the conflict in an appropriate manner. The nurse will serve as a facilitator during this interaction.	
• Discuss tension reduction techniques with client; develop a plan for client to learn these techniques and apply them in difficult situations. Note the plan here.	Promotes the client's sense of control. Repeated practice of a behavior internalizes and personalizes the behavior.
• Develop with the client a reward system for appropriate behavior. Note reward system here.	Positive reinforcement encourages behavior.
• Talk with client about the differences between feelings and behavior. Role-play with client, attaching different kinds of behavior to feelings of anger.	Promotes the client's sense of control by establishing limits around feelings in the cognitive realm. Repeated practice of a behavior internalizes and personalizes the behavior.
• Help client in determining if the feeling being experienced is really anger. Explain that at times of high stress we can misinterpret feelings and must be very careful not to express the wrong feeling. Anger may be relabeled anxiety, frustration, and so on.	Placing other names on the feeling may open new behavior possibilities to the client while promoting a positive orientation; for example, if this were anger, lashing out would be appropriate, but since it is anxiety, it is more appropriate to relax.
• When client is capable, assign to group in which feelings can be expressed and feedback can be obtained from peers. Note schedule for group activity here.	Promotes the client's sense of control by providing role models for alternative ways of coping with feelings.
• Review with client consequences of inappropriate behavior, and assess the gains of this behavior over the costs.	Assesses the possibility for secondary gain in inappropriate behavior.
• Accept all threats of aggressive behavior as serious.	Client and staff safety are of primary importance.
• Remind staff not to take aggressive acts personally even if they appear to be directed at one staff member.	As the nurse's level of arousal increases, judgment decreases, making the nurse less effective when working with the client who is experiencing difficulty.[33]
• Provide client with positive verbal feedback about positive behavior changes.	Positive feedback encourages behavior.
• Do not place client in frustrating situations without a staff member to support client during the experience.	Frustration can increase the risk for aggression.[32]
• If client is suicidal, place in a room with another client.	Decreases the amount of time the client is alone.
• Provide client with opportunities to regain self-control without aggressive interventions by giving client choices that will facilitate control; for example, "Would you like to take some medication now or spend some time with a staff member in your room" or	Promotes the client's perception of control while supporting self-esteem.

"We can help you into seclusion, or you can walk there on your own."
- Provide client with opportunities to maintain dignity.
- Assure client that you will not allow him or her to harm self or someone else.
- Reinforce this by having more staff present than necessary to physically control client if necessary. Persons from other areas of the institution may be needed in these situations. If others are used, they should be trained in proper procedures.

Client and staff safety are of primary concern.

- If potential for physical aggression is high:[33,34]
  - Place one staff member in charge of the situation.

    Promotes consistency in intervention and decreases inappropriate levels of sensory stimulation.

  - As primary person attempts to talk client down, other staff member should remove other clients and visitors from the situation.

    Client and staff safety are of primary concern.

  - Other staff members should remove potential weapons from the environment in an unobtrusive manner. This could include pool cues and balls, chairs, flower vases, books, and so on.

    Assists in reducing levels of emotion.

  - Avoid sudden movements.
  - Never turn back on client.
  - Maintain eye contact (this should not be direct, for this can be perceived as threatening to the client) and watch client's eyes for cues about potential targets of attack.

    Assists in assessing the client's intentions without appearing threatening.

  - Do not attempt to subdue client without adequate assistance.

    Client and staff safety are of primary concern.

  - Put increased distance between client and self.

    Clients who have a potential for violent behavior need more personal space.

  - Tell client of the concern in brief, concise terms.

    Maintains appropriate levels of sensory stimuli.

  - Suggest alternative behavior.

    Promotes the client's sense of control.

  - Help client focus aggression away from staff.

    May prevent the need for more restrictive interventions.

  - Encourage client to discuss concerns.

    Assists in reducing levels of emotion and deescalation of behavior.

- If talking does not resolve the situation:
  - Have additional assistance prepared for action (at least four persons should be present).

    Client and staff safety are of primary concern.

  - Have those who are going to be involved in the intervention remove any personal

Continued

Actions/Interventions	Rationales
items that could harm client or self; glasses, guns, long earrings, necklaces, bracelets, and so on. ○ Have seclusion area ready for client, remove glass objects and sharp objects, and open doors for easy entry. ○ Briefly explain to client what is going to happen and why. ○ Use method practiced by intervention team to place client in seclusion or restraints. ○ Protect self with blankets, arms bent in front of body to protect head and neck. ○ Be prepared to leave the situation and be aware of location of exits. • See Impaired Physical Mobility (Chapter 5) for care of client in seclusion or restraints. • Discuss the violent episode with the client when control has been regained. Answer questions client has about the situation, and provide client with opportunities to express thoughts and feelings about the episode. • Inform client of the behavior that is necessary to be released from seclusion or restraints. • Process situation with client after incident. • Assess milieu for "organizational provocation."	Client and staff safety and coordination are of primary concern. Contains the client's body and blocks the client's vision if it is necessary to disarm the client.[34] Client and staff safety are of primary concern. Debriefing diminishes the emotional impact of the intervention and provides an opportunity to clarify the need for the intervention, offer mutual feedback, and promote client's self-esteem.[35] Promotes the client's sense of control and enhances self-esteem.

Gerontic Health

Actions/Interventions	Rationales
• In cases of dementia, discuss with the caregiver if there is a usual pattern of violence; for example, does startling or speaking in loud tones or having several people speaking at once usually result in a violent outburst by the patient?	Awareness of violence triggers provider guidelines to adjust environment and staff behaviors.

Home Health

Actions/Interventions	Rationales
• Teach client and family appropriate monitoring of signs and symptoms of the High Risk for Violence: ○ Substance abuse ○ Increased stress ○ Social isolation ○ Hostility ○ Increased motor activity ○ Disorientation to person, place, and time ○ Disconnected thoughts ○ Clenched fists ○ Throwing objects ○ Verbalizations of threats to self or others	Provides database for early recognition and intervention.
• Assist client and family in life-style adjustments that may be required: ○ Recognition of feelings of anger or hostility ○ Developing coping strategies to express anger and hostility in acceptable manner: exercise, sports, art, music, and so on ○ Prevention of harm to self and others ○ Treatment of substance abuse ○ Management of debilitating disease ○ Coping with loss ○ Stress management ○ Decreasing sensory stimulation ○ Provision of safe environment: removal of weapons, toxic drugs, and so on ○ Development and use of support network ○ Restriction of access to weapons, especially handguns[36]	Permanent changes in behavior require support.
• Involve patient and family in planning and implementing strategies to reduce the risk for violence: ○ Family conference ○ Mutual goal setting ○ Communication	Provides for early intervention.
• Help client and family to determine when intervention of law enforcement officials or health professionals is required, for example, when there is a threat to self or others.	
• Consult with or refer to community resources as appropriate. (See Appendix B.)	Provides efficient use of existing resources. Psychiatric nurse clinician and support groups can enhance the treatment plan.

FLOW CHART EVALUATION
Flow Chart Expected Outcome 1

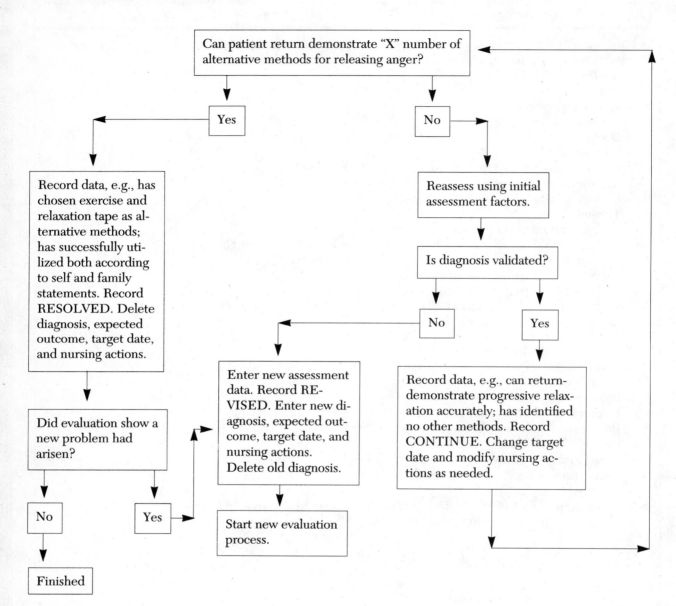

Flow Chart Expected Outcome 2

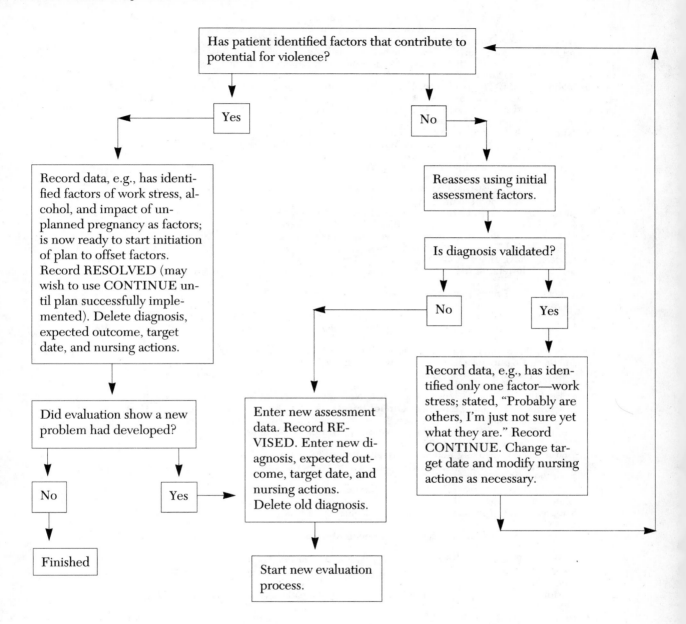

References

1. Turner, J: The Structure of Sociological Theory, ed 3. Dorsey Press, Homewood, IL, 1982.
2. Shibutani, R: Human Nature and Collective Behavior: Papers in Honor of Herbert Blumer. Prentice-Hall, Englewood Cliff, NJ, 1970.
3. Johnson, GB: American families: Changes and challenges. Fam Soc 72:502, 1991.
4. Clemen-Stone, S, Eigsti, DG, and McGuire, SL: Comprehensive Family and Community Nursing. CV Mosby, St. Louis, 1991.
5. Mallinger, KM: The American family: History and development. In Nurses and Family Health Promotion: Concepts, Assessment, and Interventions. Williams & Wilkins, Baltimore, 1989.
6. Stanhope, M and Lancaster, J: Community Health Nursing: Process and Practice for Promoting Health. CV Mosby, St. Louis, 1988.
7. Murdock, G: Social Structure. Macmillan, New York, 1949.
8. North American Nursing Diagnosis Association: Proposed New Nursing Diagnoses: NANDA'S 10th Annual Conference. Author, St. Louis, 1992.
9. Gennaro, S: Postpartal anxiety and depression of mothers of term and preterm infants. Nurs Res 37:82, 1988.
10. Weiss, ME and Armstrong, M: Postpartum mothers' preferences for nighttime care of the neonate. J Obstetr Gynecol Neonatal Nurs 20:290, 1991.
11. Reeder, SJ, Martin, LL, and Koniak, D: Maternity Nursing: Family, Newborn and Women's Health Care. JB Lippincott, Philadelphia, 1992.
12. Chafetz, L and Barnes, L: Issues in psychiatric caregiving. Arch Psychiatr Nurs 3:61, 1989.
13. Wilson, H and Kneisl, C: Psychiatric Nursing, ed 4. Addison-Wesley, Redwood City, CA, 1992.
14. Anderson, CM, Hogarty, GE, and Reiss, DJ: The psychoeducational family treatment of schizophrenia. In Goldstein, M (ed): New Directions for Mental Health Services. Jossey-Bass, San Francisco, 1981.
15. Baldwin, BA: Family caregiving: Trends and forecasts. Geriatr Nurs 11:172, 1990.
16. Gaynor, S: When the caregiver becomes the patient. Geriatr Nurs 10:120, 1989.
17. North American Nursing Diagnosis Association: Taxonomy I: Revised 1990. Author, St. Louis, 1990.
18. Leahey, M and Wright, L: Families and Psychosocial Problems. Springhouse Corp, Springhouse, PA, 1987.
19. Richter, JM: Support: A resource during crisis of role loss. J Geront Nurs 13:18, 1987.
20. Rubin, R: Cognitive style in pregnancy. AJN 3:502, 1970.
21. Gilliss, C, et al: Toward a Science of Family Nursing. Addison-Wesley, Menlo Park, CA, 1989.
22. Patterson, G: Families. Research Press, Champaign, IL, 1971.
23. Haber, J, et al: Comprehensive Psychiatric Nursing, ed 4. CV Mosby, St. Louis, 1992.
24. Whaley, L and Wong, D: Nursing Care of Infants and Children. CV Mosby, St. Louis, 1991.
25. King, KS, Dimond, M, and McCance, KL: Coping with relocation. Geriatr Nurs 8:258, 1987.
26. Griffith-Kenney, JW: Contemporary Women's Health: A Nursing Advocacy Approach. Addison-Wesley, Menlo Park, CA, 1986.
27. Smitherman, C: Nursing Actions for Health Promotion. FA Davis, Philadelphia, 1981.
28. Watzlawick, P, Beavin, JH, and Jackson, DP: Pragmatics of Human Communication. WW Norton, New York, 1967.
29. Parker, B and McFarlane, J: Identifying and helping battered pregnant women. MCH Am J Matern Child Nurs 16:161, 1991.
30. Sampselle, CM: The role in preventing violence against women. J Obstet Gynecol Neonatal Nurs 20:481, 1991.
31. Campbell, JC: A test of two explanatory models of women's responses to battering. Nurs Res 38:18, 1989.
32. Zimbardo, P: Interview. In Evans, R (ed): The Making of Psychology. Knopf, New York, 1976.
33. Stevenson, S: Heading off violence with verbal de-escalation. J Psychosoc Nurs Ment Health Serv 29:6, 1991.
34. Morton, P: Staff roles and responsibilities in incidents of patient violence. Arch Psychiatr Nurs 1:280, 1987.
35. Norris, M and Kennedy, C: The view from within: How patients perceive the seclusion process. J Psychosoc Nurs Ment Health Serv 30:7, 1992.
36. Loftin, C, McDowell, D, Wiersema, B, and Cotey, T: Effects of restrictive licensing of handguns and homicide and suicide in the District of Columbia. N Engl J Med 325:1615, 1991.

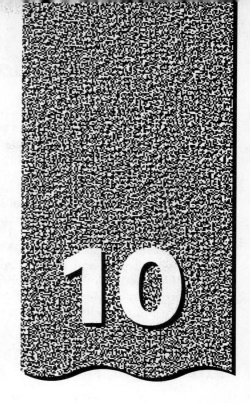

10

Sexuality-Reproductive Pattern

PATTERN INTRODUCTION

Pattern Description

This pattern focuses on the sexual and reproductive aspects of individuals over the entire life span. Sexuality patterns involve sex-role behavior, gender identification, physiologic and biologic functioning, as well as the cultural and societal expectations of sexual behavior. An individual's anatomic structure identifies sexual status, which determines the social and cultural responses of others toward the individual and, in turn, the individual's responsive behavior toward others.

Reproductive patterns involve the ability to procreate, actual procreation, and the ability to express sexual feelings. The success or failure of psychologically and physically expressing sexual feelings and procreating can affect an individual's life-style, health, and self-concept.

The nurse may care for clients who, because of illness, violence, or life-styles, experience alterations or disturbances in their sexual health that affect their sexuality and reproductive patterns.

Pattern Assessment

1. Following a rape, is the patient experiencing multiple physical symptoms?
   a. Yes (Rape Trauma Syndrome: Compound Reaction)
   b. No
2. Following a rape, is the patient indicating severe emotional reactions?
   a. Yes (Rape Trauma Syndrome: Compound Reaction)
   b. No
3. Is the client using alcohol or drugs to cope following a rape?
   a. Yes (Rape Trauma Syndrome: Compound Reaction)
   b. No
4. Has the client changed her relationship with males?
   a. Yes (Rape Trauma Syndrome: Silent Reaction)
   b. No
5. Does client indicate increased anxiety in follow-up counseling?
   a. Yes (Rape Trauma Syndrome: Silent Reaction)
   b. No
6. Does client verbalize any problems related to sexual functioning?
   a. Yes (Sexual Dysfunction)
   b. No
7. Does client exhibit any indications of physical or psychosocial abuse?
   a. Yes (Sexual Dysfunction)
   b. No
8. Does client relate any changes in sexual behavior?
   a. Yes (Altered Sexuality Patterns)
   b. No
9. Does client report any difficulties or limitations in sexual behavior?
   a. Yes (Altered Sexuality Patterns)
   b. No

Nursing Diagnoses in This Pattern

1. Rape Trauma Syndrome: Compound Reaction or Silent Reaction (page 821)
2. Sexual Dysfunction (page 833)
3. Altered Sexuality Patterns (page 844)

Conceptual Information

Gender development and sexuality are closely entwined with biologic, psychologic, sociologic, spiritual, and cultural aspects of human life. The biologic sex of an individual is decided at the time of conception, but sexual patterning is influenced from the moment of birth by the actions of those surrounding the individual. From this moment, males and females receive messages about who they are and what it means to be masculine or feminine.[1]

The sexuality of an individual is composed of biologic sex, gender identity, and gender role. The biologic and psychologic perspectives of culture and society determine how an individual develops sexually, particularly in one's sense of being male or female (gender identity). Biologic identity begins at the moment of fertilization, when chromosomal sex is determined, and becomes even more defined at 5 to 6 weeks of fetal life. At this time the undifferentiated fetal gonads become ovaries (XX, female chromosomal sex) or testes (XY, male chromosomal sex); hormones finalize the genital appearance between the 7th and 12th weeks. Fetal androgens (testicular hormones) must be present for male reproductive structures to develop from the Wolffian ducts. If fetal androgens are not present the fetus will develop female reproductive structures. By the 12th week of fetal life biologic sex is well established.[1,2]

Reactions by others begin the moment the biologic sex of the fetus or infant is known. The parents and those about them prepare for either a boy or a girl by buying clothes and toys for a boy (color blue, pants, shirts, football) or a girl (color pink, frilly dresses, dolls). They speak to the infant differently according to sex. Girls are usually spoken to in a high, sing-song voice: "Oh, isn't she cute!"; boys are spoken to in a low-pitched, matter-of-fact voice: "Look at that big boy—he will really make a good football player one of these days!" These actions contribute to the infant's gender identity and perception of self. Behavioral responses from the infant are elicited by the parents based on their views of what roles a boy or girl should fulfill.

Gender role is determined by the kinds of sex behavior that are performed by individuals to symbolize to themselves and others that they are masculine or feminine.[3] Early civilizations assigned roles according to who performed what tasks for survival. Women were relegated to specific roles because of the biologic nature of bearing and raising children and gathering food. The men were the hunters and soldiers. Advanced technologies, changing mores, birth control, and alternative methods of securing food and raising children have led to changes in roles based on gender in Western society. Gender roles are influenced by cultural, religious, and social pressures. Schuster and Ashburn[4] define gender-role stereotypes as "culturally assigned clusters of behaviors or attributes covering everything from play activities and personal traits to physical appearance, dress and vocational activities."

As in gender identity, researchers have noticed gender role-play in children as young as 13 months. Schoolchildren are particularly exposed and pressured into gender-role stereotyping by parents, teachers, and peers, who demand rigid behavior patterns according to the sex of the child. Girls and boys are often treated differently and gradually molded into different gender roles. Little girls are usually handled gently as infants; caregivers may fuss with the baby's hair and tell her how pretty she is. Little boys are usually roughhoused and told "What a big boy you are." Sex directional training is also accomplished by such verbalizations as "Where's Daddy's girl?" and "Big boys don't cry; be a man."[5]

North American society is moving toward a blending of male and female roles; however, stereotyping still exists. According to Schuster and Ashburn,[4] stereotyping is not all bad, as it can help "reduce anxiety arising from gender differences and may aid in the process of psychic separation from one's parents." Therefore, they conclude that stereotypes can either provide structure and facilitate development or restrict development by being too rigid, thus interfering with a child's potential.

One's sexuality develops over a lifetime, changing as one matures and progresses through the life-cycle. It is impossible to separate an individual's sexuality from his or her development, as sexuality combines the interaction of the biophysical and psychosocial elements of the individual.

According to a recent national research study,[6] rape in the United States occurs far more often than previously recognized. This study found that 683,000 American women were raped in 1990—a far higher number than had been estimated. Almost 62 percent of these women stated they were minors when they were raped, and about 29 percent stated they were younger than 11 when the rape occurred. This indicates rape is most definitely a traumatic event for our young in America. Of the rapists, 75 percent were known to the victim and included such persons as neighbors, friends, relatives, boyfriends, ex-boyfriends, husbands, or ex-husbands. Only 22 percent of the rapists were strangers to the victim. In 28 percent of the cases, the victim sustained injuries beyond the rape itself. Sadly, only 16 percent of the victims tell police about the attack; many of the victims are concerned about the family finding out, being blamed by others for the attack, and having others know about the attack. These concerns have decreased in victims raped in the past 5 years; however, in this group, there were increased concerns about having their name become public, getting AIDS and other sexually transmitted diseases, and becoming pregnant. Name confidentiality is a high priority for these victims.

Developmental Considerations

INFANT

Erikson defines the major task of infancy as the development of trust versus mistrust. The parents' nurturing and caretaking activities allow the infant to begin to experience various pleasures and physical sensations such as warmth, pleasure, security, and trust,[1] and it is through these acts of nurturing that the infant begins to develop a sense of masculinity or femininity (gender identity). The infant is further molded by the parents' perceptions of sex-appropriate behavior through reward and punishment. Female infants tend to be less aggressive and develop more sensitivity because girls are usually rewarded for "being good." Male infants develop more aggressively and learn to be independent; boys are told that "big boys don't cry," so they learn to comfort themselves. By the age of 13 months sexual behavior patterns and differences are in place,[1,4] and core gender identity is probably formed by 18 months.[7] "These early behaviors are so critical to one's core gender-identity that children who experience gender reassignment after the age of 2 years are high-risk candidates for psychotic disorders."[4:321]

Infants who are sexually abused are usually physically traumatized and often they die. These children often experience developmental delays: failure to thrive, low or no weight gain, lethargy, and flat affect.

TODDLER AND PRESCHOOLER

Neuromuscular control allows toddlers to explore their environment, interact with their peers, and develop autonomy and independence.[1,4,7] Genital organs continue to increase in size but their function does not change. Their vocabulary increases, they distinguish between male and female by recognizing clothing and body parts, and they develop pride in their own bodies, especially the genital area, as they become aware of elimination or excretory functions. They need guidance and require parents to set limits as they learn to "hold on" or "let go" in order to achieve a sense of autonomy.[4] By the age of 3, they have perfected verbal terms for the sexes, understand the meaning of gender terms and the roles associated with those terms (girl is a sister or mother, and boy is a brother or father),[1] and receive pleasure from kissing and hugging.[7]

The preschooler is busy developing a sense of socialization and purpose. Learning suitable behavior for girls and boys or sex-role behavior is the major task during the preschool years. Preschoolers will often identify with the parent of the same sex while forming an attachment to the parent of the opposite sex. Preschoolers are inquisitive about sex and are often occupied in exploration of their own and their friends' bodies. This will often be exhibited in group games such as "doctor/nurse," urinating "outside," or masturbating.[7] Children's concept of their bodies, not as a whole but as individual parts, changes when, as preschoolers, they begin to develop "an awareness of themselves as individuals, and become more concerned about body integrity and intactness."[4]

It is important to note that 6-year-olds are the age group most subjected to sexual abuse.[8] How a child handles this experience and his or her future developmental and psychologic growth depends largely on the reactions and actions of the significant adult in the child's life.[7] Rape in early childhood may simply be acknowledged by the child as part of the experience of growing up and may have no long-term effects if it is not repeated. Usually counseling during this developmental age has great effect. All claims of abuse by a child should be investigated and should be handled with someone who has the experience and knowledge to deal with the child and his or her parents in a professional and understanding manner.

SCHOOL-AGE CHILD

Play is the most important work of children: It allows them to be curious and investigate social, sexual, and adult behavior. "Through play children learn how to get their needs met and how to meet the needs of others."[4] Different socialization of boys and girls tends to become apparent in play during the school years; boys engage in aggressive team play, while girls engage in milder play and form individual friendships. These activities can lead to stereotyping and exaggeration of gender difference.

At school children begin to be more independent and form peer groups of the same sex. Although the peer group becomes very important to them, they need adult direction in learning socially acceptable forms of sexual behavior. If they do not receive the information they are seeking, negative feelings and apprehension about sexuality may develop.[1]

Great trauma can occur when rape occurs during these years. It is very damaging to the value systems which are being formed. Sexual identity can be disturbed, and sexual confusion can occur.

ADOLESCENT

Puberty, the period of maturation of the reproductive system, causes profound changes in the individual's sexual anatomy and physiology and is a major developmental crisis for the adolescent. Secondary sex characteristics appear: breasts, pubic hair, and menstruation in girls; testicular and penile enlargement, pubic hair, ejaculation, and growth of muscle mass in boys. The configuration, contour, and function of the body change rapidly, dramatically highlighting sexual differences and the onset of adulthood. These changes bring new feelings, including role confusion and increased awareness of sexual feelings. "The major task of adolescence is the establishment of identity in the face of role confusion."[1]

Peer groups have an important influence on the young adolescent (12 to 15 years), but during late adolescence (16 to 19 years), peer group influence lessens and more intimate relationships with the opposite sex develop.[7] These relationships can involve a wide range of exploratory sexual behavior, sometimes resulting in pregnancy. Exploring behavior can be with the opposite sex (foreplay and intercourse), the same sex (homosexuality), or the self (masturbation). How the teenager views himself or herself sexually will depend on the reassurance and guidance he or she receives from a significant adult in his or her life. The greatest misunderstandings of teenagers involve homosexuality, masturbation, and conception and contraception; how these issues are approached can influence adult sexuality.[1,7]

It is during adolescence, when new sexual experiences take place, that questions about maleness or femaleness arise. Adolescents must evaluate their masculinity and femininity, question and then decide on their gender identity, gender orientation, and gender preference. The adolescent not only deals with physical changes but also integrates past experiences and role models with new experiences and new role models into his or her own gender identity.

Violent sexual occurrences during this period of life can devastate a person for the rest of his or her life. Adolescents are dealing with sexual confusion and identification; rape can stop, slow, or change this process. Fear and loss of self-esteem can dictate actions and influence sexual identity and gender expression.

YOUNG ADULT

The young adult, in his or her twenties and early thirties, is concerned with obtaining an education, selecting a vocation, completing military service, choosing a partner, building a career, and establishing an intimate relationship. This is a period of maximal sexual self-consciousness, commitment to a relationship, and social legitimization of sexual experiences.[1,4,7] Young adults are concerned with marriage and parenting.

Rape can slow or stop normal sexual relationships during the adult years. Fear can become the greater part of life for the victim. These years are ones for forming lasting relationships with the opposite sex, marrying, and beginning families. Rape can cause withdrawal from any interaction with the opposite sex; relationships can break up, not only because of the reaction of the victims of rape, but also because of the reactions of the families and spouses of the victim.

ADULT

Demands placed on adults by their careers and raising children may interfere with their sexual interest and activity.[1] The major task of this period of life is to accent one's own life-style and decisions rather than feeling frustrated and disappointed. "Social pressures and expectations, feedback from significant others and finally self-perception all influence how one evaluates the success of one's life."[1]

Although the adult is at the peak of his or her career, physiologic changes begin to influence the adult's life-style. The aging process, illnesses, and midlife change (both male and female) cause changes in life-style and everyday activities. Sexual activities can be altered by these physical and physiologic changes; however, the adult who lives a healthy life-style, eats right, exercises, and has an optimistic outlook usually feels good and functions well sexually. Often, middle-age adults, just as they have finished raising their children, are faced with the task of caring for their elderly parents which may place a strain on marital relationships at a time when the couple was looking forward to having time for each other.

OLDER ADULT

As in adolescence, dramatic body changes begin in late middle age and continue into old age. There is no reason that healthy men and women cannot continue to enjoy their sexuality into old age. Women must deal with menopause and postmenopause, and men must often deal with impotence; however, with an interested sexual partner, good, healthy sexuality can continue.

Older women are viewed by rapists as easy victims. Slowing of physical reactions and disabilities of old age (seeing, hearing, slow gait) keep them from being alert to danger and from reacting quickly. More important, the older woman often views herself as inferior, and this contributes to her own victimization.[9] Because most women outlive men and face changes in life-style and economic status, they are reluctant, and often cannot afford, to leave familiar older parts of cities, which often change and deteriorate. This may expose them to the accompanying increase in crime rates.[9]

APPLICABLE NURSING DIAGNOSES
Rape Trauma Syndrome: Compound Reaction and Silent Reaction

DEFINITION

Forced, violent sexual penetration against the victim's will and consent. The trauma syndrome that develops from this attack or attempted attack includes an acute phase of disorganization of the victim's life-style and a long-term process of reorganization of life-style. This syndrome includes the following three components: Rape Trauma Syndrome, Rape Trauma with Compound Reaction, and Rape Trauma with Silent Reaction.[10]

NANDA TAXONOMY: FEELING 9.2.3.1, 9.2.3.1.1, 9.2.3.1.1.2

DEFINING CHARACTERISTICS[10]

1. Rape Trauma Syndrome:
   a. Acute phase:
      (1) Emotional reactions (anger, embarrassment, fear of physical violence and death, humiliation, revenge, self-blame)
      (2) Multiple physical symptoms (gastrointestinal irritability, genitourinary discomfort, muscle tension, sleep pattern disturbance)
   b. Long-term phase:
      (1) Changes in life-style (change in residence, dealing with repetitive nightmares and phobias, seeking family support, seeking social network support)
2. Rape Trauma: Compound Reaction:
   a. Acute phase:
      (1) Emotional reaction (anger, embarrassment, fear of physical violence and death, humiliation, revenge, self-blame)
      (2) Multiple physical symptoms (gastrointestinal irritability, genitourinary discomfort, muscle tension, sleep pattern disturbance)
      (3) Reactivated symptoms of previous conditions, for example, physical illness, psychiatric illness, reliance on alcohol and/or drugs
3. Rape Trauma: Silent Reaction:
   a. Major defining characteristics:
      (1) Abrupt changes in relationships with men
      (2) Increase in nightmares
      (3) Increased anxiety during interview, for example, blocking of associations, long periods of silence, minor stuttering, physical distress
      (4) Pronounced changes in sexual behavior
      (5) No verbalization of the occurrence of rape
      (6) Sudden onset of phobic reactions
   b. Minor defining characteristics:
      None given

RELATED FACTORS[10]

Included in definition of diagnosis.

RELATED CLINICAL CONCERNS

Not applicable.

HAVE YOU SELECTED THE CORRECT DIAGNOSIS?

Sexual Dysfunction   Rape can be the cause of sexual dysfunction in a patient who cannot learn to put into perspective or deal with the rape experience. Rape Trauma is always the result of a violent act and must be dealt with according to the individual situation. Although Sexual Dysfunction can occur as the result of rape, the nurse must assist the patient to deal with the trauma of the rape in order to assist with the sexual dysfunction. (See page 833.)

EXPECTED OUTCOMES

1. Will identify and use at least (number) support systems by (date) and/or
2. Will verbalize (number) positive self-statements related to personal response to the incident by (date)

TARGET DATES

Owing to the varied physical and emotional impact of rape, a target date of 3 days would not be too soon to evaluate for progress.

NURSING ACTIONS/INTERVENTIONS WITH RATIONALES

Adult Health

Actions/Interventions	Rationales
• Explore your own feelings about rape prior to initiating patient care. Maintain nonjudgmental attitude. Actively listen when survivor wants to talk about event. Encourage verbalization of thoughts, feelings, and perceptions of the event. Explore basis for and reality of thoughts, feelings, and perceptions.	The nurse's feelings can be sensed by the survivor and can influence the survivor's coping and sense of self.
• Attend to physical and health priorities such as lacerations or infection with appropriate explanations and preparation.	Prompt attention to physical needs provides comfort and facilitates a trusting relationship.
• Promote trusting, therapeutic relationship by spending at least 30 minutes every 4 hours (while awake) at (times) with survivor.	Promotes expression of feelings and validates reality.
• Use calm, consistent approach when interacting with survivor. Respect survivor's rights.	Assists in reducing anxiety.
• Be supportive of survivor's values and beliefs.	Survivor's sexuality is intimately linked to her value or belief system.
• Explain need for medical and legal procedures, procedures to assess for sexually transmitted diseases, prophylactic medications, and postcoital contraception medications before performing procedures. Refer to section on Women's Health for specifics about procedures.	Enlists survivor's cooperation, and prepares her for events if charges are filed against the alleged rapist.
• Provide for appropriate privacy and health teaching as care is administered. Allow survivor to see own anatomy if this seems appropriate as part of health teaching.	Avoids perpetuating survivor's fear; examination and treatment in the same body area involved in the rape could promote a sensation of rape recurrence.
• Assist survivor in activities of daily living (ADLs) after examination.	Promotes a slight sense of return to normalcy; emotional shock may render survivor temporarily unable to perform basic ADLs.

Continued

Actions/Interventions	Rationales

• Determine to what degree or extent symptoms of physical reactions exist, such as:
  ○ Pain, body soreness
  ○ Sleep disturbances
  ○ Altered eating patterns
  ○ Anger
  ○ Self-blame
  ○ Mood swings
  ○ Feelings of helplessness
	Basic database needed to plan for long-term effects of rape.

• Administer medications as ordered to alleviate pain, anxiety, or inability to sleep, and teach survivor how to safely take such medications.	Allows time for survivor to process event in a way that maintains self-integrity and self-esteem.
• Recognize that survivor will proceed at own rate in resolving rape trauma when interacting with survivor. Do not rush or force survivor.	
• Identify available support systems, for example, rape crisis center, and involve significant other as appropriate.	Support systems that know signs and symptoms of Rape Trauma Syndrome can provide help for both short-term and long-term interventions; promotes effective coping for the survivor.
• Monitor coping in survivor and significant other until discharged from hospital.	Monitors for adaptive and maladaptive coping strategies. Provides opportunity to assist survivor and significant other to practice alternative coping strategies.
• Assist survivor to identify own strengths in dealing with the rape.	Helps to build survivor's self-esteem and overcome self-blame.
• Provide anticipatory guidance about the long-term effects of rape. Promote self-confidence and self-esteem through positive feedback regarding strengths, plans, reality.	Helps to prepare for expected and unexpected reactions in self, friends, and significant others.
• Provide for appropriate epidemiologic follow-up in cases of venereal disease.	Required by law.
• Collaborate with other health care professionals as needed.	Promotes holistic approach and more complete plan of care.
• Arrange for appropriate long-term follow-up before dismissal from hospital, for example, counseling.	Provides for long-term support.

Male Rape Victim

• Provide same considerations as with female survivor. (Most, but not all, reported cases are children and early adolescents.)	The act of rape is an act of violence regardless of the gender of the patient and requires the same type of care and concern.
• Refer to trained male counselor at rape crisis center.	

Child Health

Actions/Interventions	Rationales
• Encourage collaboration among health professionals to best address patient's needs. (See Appendix B.)	Specialist will be required to deal with the unique needs of the young child enduring rape. There is a strong likelihood that the rapist and the victim are closely related.
• Try to establish trust as dictated by age and circumstances related to rape trauma (with nurse being same sex as patient). *Do not* leave the child alone. Be gentle and patient. ○ *Infants and toddlers*: Ensure continuity of caregivers. Explain procedures with dolls and puppets. ○ *Preschoolers*: Ensure continuity of caregivers. Allow patient to perform self-care as ability presents. Use art and methods that deal with general view of what happened, clarifying that the child is not the "cause" of this incident. ○ *School-age children*: Maintain continuity of caregivers. Assist patient to express concerns related to incident. Use appropriate techniques in interviewing to determine extent of sexual dysfunction or potential threat to future functioning. ○ *Adolescents*: Maintain continuity of caregivers. Encourage patient to express how this experience affects own self-identity and future sexual activities. Encourage psychiatric assistance in resolving this crisis for any patients of this age group. Look for signs of growth of secondary sex characteristics.	
• Follow up with appropriate documentation and coordination of child protective service needs. Assist parents or guardians in signing proper release forms. Determine if situation involves incest.	Appropriate protocols for documentation and reporting of rape or incest must be followed according to state and federal guidelines.
• Assist patient to deal with residual feelings, such as guilt for revealing or identifying assailant by allowing at least 30 minutes per shift (while awake) at (times). (This often involves dealing with members of immediate family or extended family.) Use simple language when dealing with child.	Resolution of unresolved guilt or feelings about the event must be dealt with as soon as patient's condition permits.
• Encourage family members to assist in care and follow-up of patient's reorganization plans:	Risk behaviors serve as cues to alert the family or caregiver to monitor the child's progress in resolving the crisis.

Continued

Actions/Interventions	Rationales
○ Be alert for signs of distress such as refusing to go to school, bad dreams or nightmares, or verbalized concerns. ○ Identify ways to gradually resume normal daily schedule. ○ Assist family to identify how best to resolve and express feelings about the incident. • Carry out appropriate health teaching regarding normal sexual physiology and functioning according to age and developmental capacity.	Normalcy is afforded as attempts are realistically made to resolve any aspects of rape trauma.
Incest	
• Monitor for inappropriate sexual behavior among family members. • Monitor for children who know more about the actual mechanics of sexual intercourse than their developmental age indicates. • Monitor for girls who seem to have taken over the mother's role in the home. • Monitor for mothers who have withdrawn from the home, either emotionally or physically.	Provides database needed to accurately assess for incest.

Women's Health

Actions/Interventions	Rationales
• Assist the survivor through the procedures for provision of necessary health care treatment. Explain each phase of examination to survivor. Remain with the survivor at all times. • Take a complete history, noting the following: ○ Previous venereal diseases ○ Previous pelvic infections ○ Any injuries that were present before attack ○ Obstetric and menstrual history • Assist in gathering information to provide proper health and legal care. • Secure survivor's description of any objects used in the attack and how these objects were used in the attack.	Provides database necessary for intervention; secures chain-of-evidence procedure; assists in reducing client anxiety.

- Follow correct sequence and procedures for collection and storage of evidence:
  - Label each specimen as follows:
    (1) Survivor's name and hospital number
    (2) Date and time of collection
    (3) Area from which specimen was collected
    (4) Collector's name
  - Ensure proper storage and packaging of specimens:
    (1) Clothing and items that are wet with blood or semen should be put in paper, not plastic, bags. (Plastic bags will cause molding of wet items.)
    (2) Specimens obtained on microscopic slides or swabs need to be air-dried before packaging.
  - Comb pubic hair for traces of attacker's pubic hair or other evidence:
    (1) Submit paper towel placed under victim to catch combings, as well as the comb used and pubic hair.
    (2) Pluck (do not cut) 2 to 3 pubic hairs from the patient, and label properly. These are used for comparison.
  - Record transfer of evidence to police correctly. Include:
    (1) Signatures of individuals transferring and receiving the evidence
    (2) Complete list of evidence transferred
    (3) Date and time
  - Take photographs of injuries or torn clothing.
  - Have survivor sign forms for release of information to authorities.
  - Provide medical treatment and follow-up for:
    (1) Injuries
    (2) Sexually transmitted diseases, for example, AIDS, gonorrhea, syphilis
    (3) Pregnancy
- Report to proper authorities any suspicion of family violence.

  Initiates long-range support for patient.

- Evaluate for increased rate of changing residences, repeated nightmares, and sleep pattern disturbance.

  Provides database that allows accurate interpretation of long-range impact. Provides information needed to plan long-term care.

- Encourge patient to discuss phobias, frustrations, and fears.
- Be available and allow patient to express

  Provides long-term essential support.

Continued

Actions/Interventions	Rationales
difficulties in establishing normal activities of daily living and redescribe attack as needed.	
• Assist patient in developing a plan of reorganization of activities of daily living.	Promotes realistic planning for problem while avoiding continued denial of problem.

Mental Health

Actions/Interventions	Rationales
• Assign a primary care nurse to client. This nurse should be the same sex as the client demonstrates most comfort with at the current time.	Promotes the development of a trusting relationship.
• Primary care nurse will remain with the client during the orientation to the unit.	Promotes the development of a trusting relationship.
• Limit visitors as client feels necessary.	Promotes the client's sense of control while meeting security needs.
• Answer client's questions openly and honestly.	Promotes the development of a trusting relationship.
• Primary care nurse will be present to provide support for client during medical or legal examinations if the client has not identified another person.	Promotes the development of a trusting relationship while meeting the client's security needs.
• Assist client in identifying a support person, and arrange for this person to remain with the client as much as necessary. Note the name of this person here.	Promotes the client's sense of control while meeting security needs.
• Provide information to the client's support system as the client indicates is needed.	Enhances ability of support system to support the client in a constructive manner.
• Allow client to talk about the incident as much as is desired. Sit with client during these times and encourage expression of feelings.	Facilitates the confrontation of the memories of the event and attachment of meaning to the situation in a way that will promote a sense of control.[11]
• Communicate to client that his or her response is normal. This could include expressions of anger, fear, discomfort with persons of the opposite sex, discomfort with sexuality, personal blame, and so on.	Normalization of the client's feelings without diminishing the experience enhances self-esteem and helps client to move from a position of victim to that of a survivor.[12]
• Inform client that rape is a physical assault rather than a sexual act, and that rapists choose victims without regard for age, physical appearance, or manner of dress.	Promotes the client's resolution of guilt and feelings of responsibility.
• Assist client in developing a plan to return to activities of daily living. The plan should begin with steps that are easily	Promotes the client's sense of control and inhibits the tendency toward social isolation.[12]

accomplished so that the client can regain a sense of personal control and power. Note the steps of the plan here.

- Provide positive social rewards for the client's accomplishment of established goals. Note here the kinds of behavior that are to be rewarded and the rewards to be used.

Positive reinforcement encourages behavior while enhancing self-esteem.

- Provide the client with opportunities to express anger at the assailant in a constructive manner, for example, talking about fantasies of revenge, using punching bag or pillow, physical activity, and so on.

Assists client in moving from a position of powerless victim to a position of survivor.

- When client can interact with small groups, arrange for client's involvement in a therapeutic group that provides interaction with peers. Note time of group meetings here.

Provides the client opportunities to resolve feelings of being different while decreasing social isolation. Promotes consensual validation of experience with others in similar situations, thus enhancing self-esteem and emotional resources available for coping.[12]

- Involve client in unit activities. Assign client activities that can be easily accomplished. Note client's level of functioning here along with those tasks that are to be assigned to the client.

Prevents social isolation. Task accomplishment enhances self-esteem with positive reinforcement. Also provides opportunities to test reality of self-perceptions against those of peers on the unit.

- Primary nurse will spend (number) minutes with client twice a day at (times) to focus on expression of feelings related to the rape. Encourage client not to close these feelings off too quickly. Assist client in reducing stress in other life situations while healing emotionally from the rape experience. Begin to facilitate client's use of cognitive coping resources by logically assessing various aspects of the situation.

Promotes reality testing of feelings related to the rape, and inhibits the development of self-blame and guilt, which often occur in survivors.

- Assist client in developing a plan to reduce life stressors so emotional healing can continue. Note this plan here with the support needed from the nursing staff in implementing this plan.

Promotes the client's sense of control and provides a positive orientation.

- Primary nurse will meet with client and primary support person once a day to facilitate discussion of the rape. If the client is involved in an ongoing relationship, such as a marriage, this interaction is very important. The support person should be encouraged to express his or her thoughts and feelings in a constructive manner. If it is assessed that the rape has resulted in potential long-term relationship difficulties such as rejection or sexual problems, refer to couples therapy.

Support system understanding and acceptance facilitate the client's coping and the maintenance of these relationships.

Continued

Actions/Interventions	Rationales
• Refer client to appropriate community support groups, and assist with contacting these before discharge. (See Appendix B.)	Promotes the client's reintegration into the community and inhibits the isolating behavior often exhibited by these clients.[12]

Gerontic Health

Actions/Interventions	Rationales
• In the event of the rape being secondary to elder abuse, refer the patient to adult protective services.	Provides a resource for the older adult to explore options and prevent recurrence of problem.

Home Health

Actions/Interventions	Rationales
• During the acute phase, be sure that appropriate assessment, law enforcement involvement, and treatment of physical injuries or sexually transmitted diseases are provided.	Early and accurate intervention decreases sequelae and provides documentation for any legal action.
• Assist client and family in life-style changes that may be needed: ○ Treatment for physical injuries or sexually transmitted disease ○ Testimony in court ○ Protection ○ Coping with terror, nightmares, or fear ○ Coping with alterations in sexual response to significant other ○ Development and use of support networks ○ Stress management ○ Changing phone number or moving ○ Traveling with companion ○ Strategies for prevention of rape	Provides support and enhances recovery.
• Assist client and family in planning and implementing strategies for resolution of rape trauma syndrome: ○ Open discussion of feelings of family members ○ Mutual sharing and trust ○ Strategies to reduce possibility of future attacks	Crimes of violence upset the family equilibrium and require support to correct. Involvement of client and significant others is important to ensure successful resolution.
• Consult with or refer to community resources as appropriate. (See Appendix B.)	Use of existing resources and expertise provides high-quality care and makes effective use of available resources.

FLOW CHART EVALUATION
Flow Chart Expected Outcome 1

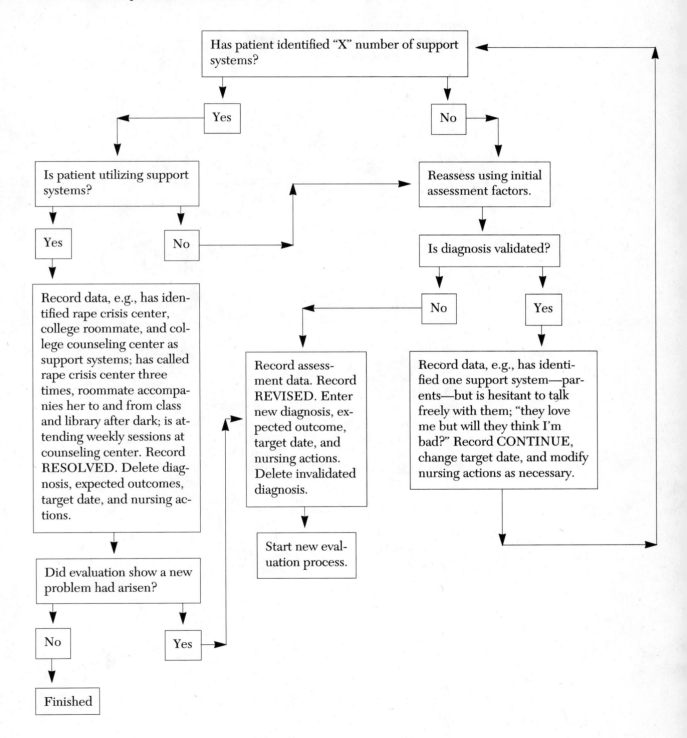

Flow Chart Expected Outcome 2

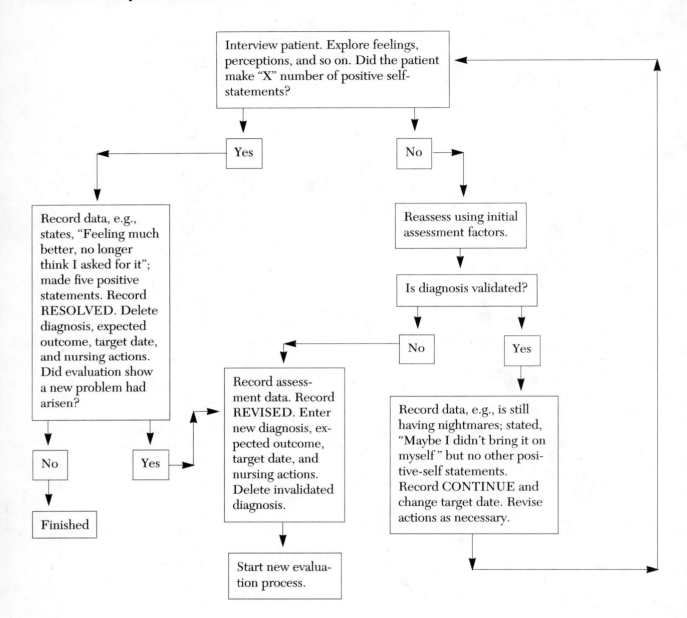

Sexual Dysfunction

DEFINITION

The state in which an individual experiences a change in sexual function that is viewed as unsatisfying, unrewarding, or inadequate.[10]

NANDA TAXONOMY: RELATING 3.2.1.2.1

DEFINING CHARACTERISTICS[10]

1. Major defining characteristics:
   a. Verbalization of problem
   b. Alterations in achieving perceived sex role
   c. Actual or perceived limitation imposed by disease and/or therapy
   d. Conflicts involving values
   e. Alteration in achieving sexual satisfaction
   f. Inability to achieve desired satisfaction
   g. Seeking confirmation of desirability
   h. Alteration in relationship with significant other
   i. Change of interest in self and others
2. Minor defining characteristics:
   None given

RELATED FACTORS[10]

1. Biopsychosocial alteration of sexuality
2. Ineffectual or absent role models
3. Physical abuse
4. Psychosocial abuse, for example, harmful relationships
5. Vulnerability
6. Values conflict
7. Lack of privacy
8. Lack of significant others
9. Altered body structure or function (pregnancy, recent childbirth, drugs, surgery, anomalies, disease process, trauma, radiation treatment)
10. Misinformation or lack of knowledge

RELATED CLINICAL CONCERNS

1. Endocrine, urological, neuromuscular, and skeletal disorders
2. Genital trauma
3. Agoraphobia
4. Pelvic surgery
5. Malignancies of the reproductive tract
6. Female circumcision[13]
7. Psychiatric disorders such as mania, major depression, dementia, borderline personality disorder, substance abuse, anxiety disorder, and schizophrenia

HAVE YOU SELECTED THE CORRECT DIAGNOSIS?

Altered Sexuality Pattern In this diagnosis, the individual is expressing concern about his or her sexuality. This diagnosis could be a result of Sexual Dysfunction but does not mean that it is necessarily a problem to the patient. Altered Sexuality Pattern can be compatible with the patient's life-style for whatever reason and create no overwhelming problems for the patient. (See page 844.)

Rape Trauma Syndrome This diagnosis could result in Sexual Dysfunction because of the patient's inability to deal with the violence, trauma, and life-style changes as a result of rape. It is absolutely essential for the nurse to ascertain the cause of the Sexual Dysfunction and to determine if it is the result of the patient's perception of sexuality in general, pathophysiology, or trauma. (See page 821.)

EXPECTED OUTCOMES

1. Will have decreased complaints of sexual dysfunction by (date) and/or
2. Will report return, as near as possible, to previous levels of sexual functioning by (date)

TARGET DATE

Depending on the patient's perception of the sexual dysfunction, target dates may range from 1 week to several months.

NURSING ACTIONS/INTERVENTIONS WITH RATIONALES

Adult Health

Actions/Interventions	Rationales
• Facilitate communication between patient and partner by providing at least (number) minutes per day for privacy to communicate.	Promotes identification of issues involved in sexual dysfunction.
• Encourage patient and partner to talk about concerns and problems during conference.	Sexual behavior includes verbal, nonverbal, genital, and nongenital activities.
• Talk with patient and partner about alternate ways to attain sexual satisfaction and express sexuality, for example, hugging, touching, kissing, masturbation, hand holding, and use of sexual aids. Provide factual informational material.	
• Clarify misconceptions about sexual activity after a heart attack, among older people, or after hysterectomy.	Misinformation and myths contribute to sexual dysfunction.
• Be nonjudgmental in your attitudes.	Sexuality is a highly personal experience; nonjudgmental attitudes reduce anxiety and open the way for therapeutic communication.

• Respect patient's values and attitudes about sexuality and sexual functioning.	Sexual behavior is intimately linked to the value and belief system; demeaning these values and beliefs will cause anxiety in patient.
• Provide accurate information about effects of medical diagnosis or treatment on sexual functioning.	Clarify misconceptions; provide information on changes or modifications in sexual activities that may need to occur due to disease process.
• Implement measures to improve self-concept, for example, positive self-talk, assertiveness, new hairdo, new clothes, new social surroundings.	How one feels about self is important in perception of sexuality.
• Provide privacy for expressing sexuality through masturbation or sexual intercourse (particularly when patient has been hospitalized for a significant length of time or has been separated from significant other for a significant length of time).	Expression of sexuality may be inhibited by hospitalization, but the need exists.
• Teach patient importance of adequate rest before and after sexual activity.	Sexual activity increases basal metabolic rate and initiates the sympathetic nervous system, inducing a high level of stress.

• If dyspareunia is a problem, teach patient and significant other to:
  ○ Use adequate amounts of water-soluble lubricant.
  ○ Use vaginal steroid cream.
  ○ Take sitz baths.
	Increases comfort and reduces trauma; eases dryness and avoids irritation.

• If impotence is a problem, advise patient to:
  ○ Get a complete physical examination.
  ○ Consult with sex therapist.
  ○ Consider penile prosthesis.
	Discover underlying causes of impotence. Provides an alternative method of penile erection to find satisfaction in intercourse.

Child Health

This diagnosis is not appropriate for a child.

Women's Health

NOTE: Very little information is found in the literature on Sexual Dysfunction of lesbian women, as they often conceal their sexual orientation when they receive health care and some choose not to receive health care if there is a danger of exposure.[14] The following actions refer to those who have a heterosexual relationship.

Actions/Interventions	**Rationales**
• Obtain detailed sexual history. • Determine who the patient is: ○ Female	Provides database needed to plan accurate intervention.

Continued

Actions/Interventions	Rationales

◦ Male
   ◦ Couple or partners
   ◦ Review communication skills between partners.
• Ascertain couple's knowledge of:
   ◦ Sexual performance
   ◦ Female and male anatomy and physiology
   ◦ Orgasm in men and women
   ◦ Anticipatory performance anxiety
   ◦ Unrealistic romantic ideas
   ◦ Rigid religious conformity
   ◦ Negative conditioning in formative years
   ◦ Erection and ejaculation
   ◦ Stimulation
   ◦ Arousal
   ◦ Sexual anxiety
   ◦ Fear of failure
   ◦ Demand for performance
   ◦ Fear of rejection	

• Dispel sexual myths and fallacies or misinformation about sexuality by:
   ◦ Allowing patient to talk about beliefs and practices in a nonthreatening atmosphere
   ◦ Providing correct information
   ◦ Answering questions in an honest manner
   ◦ Referring to the appropriate agencies or health care providers
	Provides basic information and support that can assist patient in long-term care.

• Obtain description of current problem:
   ◦ Psychologic
   ◦ Physical
   ◦ Social
	Provides essential database to permit narrowing of focus for intervention.

• Determine type of sexual dysfunction:
   ◦ General
   ◦ Lack of erotic feeling
   ◦ Lack of sexual responses
   ◦ No pleasure in sexual act
   ◦ Consider it an ordeal
   ◦ Avoidance
   ◦ Frustration
   ◦ Disappointment
   ◦ Fear
   ◦ Disgust
   ◦ Orgasmic difficulties
• If client is sexually responsive but cannot complete sexual response cycle, determine if this is:
   ◦ *Situational*: client is inhibited, disappointed, or uninterested.	

- ○ *Physiologic*: resulting from lack of lubrication, impotence, or interference with sexual response cycle.
  - ○ *Psychologic*: ambivalence, guilt, or fear are present.
- If vaginismus (tight closing of vaginal muscle with any attempt at penetration) is present, determine if this results from:
  - ○ Fear of vaginal penetration
  - ○ Spasm of vaginal muscles
  - ○ Frustration
  - ○ Fear of inadequacy
  - ○ Guilt
  - ○ Pain
  - ○ Prior sexual trauma
  - ○ Strict religious code
  - ○ Rape
  - ○ Dyspareunia
- Discuss consequences of sexual acts and situations in an honest and nonthreatening manner.
- Collaborate with appropriate therapists.

Initiates intervention in a supportive environment.

Provides the long-term care and support that is needed to resolve the basic problem.

Mental Health

NOTE: If sexual dysfunction is related to physiologic limitations, loss of body part, or impotence, refer to Adult Health care plan. If dysfunction is related to ineffective coping or poor social skills, initiate the following actions.

Actions/Interventions	Rationales
• Set limits on the inappropriate expression of sexual needs. Note the kinds of behavior to be limited and the consequences for inappropriate behavior here; for example, when client approaches staff member with sexually provocative remarks, the staff member will use constructive confrontation and discontinue the interaction.[15] Inform client of these limits.	Promotes client's sense of control while maintaining the safety of the milieu.
• Assign primary care nurse to client on each shift. The primary nurse will spend 15 minutes with the client twice per shift at (times) to develop a relationship and then begin to explore with the client the effects this behavior has on others and the needs that are being met by the behavior.	Promotes the development of a trusting relationship.

Continued

Actions/Interventions	Rationales
• Assist client in identifying environmental stimuli that provoke sexual behavior and in developing alternative responses when these stimuli are present in inappropriate situations.	
• Develop with the client a list of alternative kinds of behavior to meet the need currently being met by the sexual behavior. (Note alternative behavior patterns here with plan for implementing them.)	Promotes the client's sense of control.
• Provide client with information about appropriate sexual behavior: "normal" sexual expressions, appropriate ways to meet sexual needs (intercourse with appropriate person or masturbation at suitable time in an appropriate place), and so on.	Facilitates the development of appropriate coping behaviors.
• Role-play with client those social situations that have been identified as problematic. These could include setting limits on others' inappropriate behavior toward the client or situations in which the client needs to practice appropriate social responses.	Behavioral rehearsal provides opportunities for feedback and modeling of new behaviors by the nurse.
• Assist client in appropriate labeling of feelings and needs; for example, anxiety may be inappropriately labeled as sexual tension.	Promotes the client's sense of control, and facilitates the development of adaptive coping behaviors.
• Plan a private time and place for client. Inform client that this can be used for appropriate sexual expression. Note this here.	Social isolation inhibits inappropriate behavior by removing social rewards.
• If client begins inappropriate sexual behavior while involved in group activities, remove client from group to a private place and explain to client purpose of this. Inform client that he or she may return to the group when (the limit set by the care team will be noted here).	
• If sexual behavior results from anxiety, refer to Anxiety (Chapter 8, page 605) for detailed care plan.	Promotes the development of adaptive interpersonal skills in an environment that provides supportive feedback from peers.
• Assign client tasks in unit activities that are appropriate for client's level of comfort with group interaction; for example, if client is uncomfortable with persons of opposite sex, assign a task that requires involvement with a same-sex group or	

involvement with an opposite-sex staff member who can begin a relationship.

- Recognize and support client's feelings; for example, "You sound confused."

Promotes the development of a trusting relationship. Models for the client appropriate expressions of feelings in a supportive environment. Helps the client to learn to talk about feelings rather than act on them.

- Engage client in a socialization group once a day at (time). This should provide the client with an opportunity to interact with peers in an environment that provides feedback to the client in supportive manner.

Decreases social isolation and provides the client with an opportunity to practice interpersonal skills in a supportive environment.

- Arrange a consultation with occupational therapist to assist client in developing needed social skills, for example, cooking skills or skills at games that require socialization.

Increases the client's interpersonal competence and enhances self-esteem.

- Provide an environment that does not stimulate inappropriate sexual behavior. For example, staff member should avoid indirectly encouraging client's behavior with dress or verbal comments; other clients should not be allowed to interact with client in a sexual manner.

Promotes an environment that increases the opportunities for the client to succeed with new behaviors. This success serves as positive reinforcement, which encourages behavior and enhances self-esteem.

- Sit with client (number) minutes once a shift at (time) to discuss nonsexual-related information.

Nurses' interactions can provide social reinforcement for the client's appropriate interactions. Provides opportunity for the client to practice new behaviors in a supportive environment. Success in this situation provides positive reinforcement, which encourages behavior and enhances self-esteem.

- Provide positive social rewards for appropriate behavior. (The rewards as well as the kinds of behavior to be rewarded should be noted here.)

Positive reinforcement encourages behavior and enhances self-esteem.

- Evaluate the effects of the client's current medication on sexual behavior, and consult with physician as needed for necessary alterations.

Basic monitoring of medication efficiency.

- Develop a structured daily activity schedule for the client, and provide client with this information.

Assists the client in focusing away from issues of sexuality and engaging in socially appropriate activity.

- Schedule time for client to engage in physical activity. This activity should be developed with the client's assistance and could include walking, jogging, basketball, cycling, dancing, "soft" aerobics, and so on. A staff member should participate with the

Physical activity decreases anxiety and increases the production of endorphins, which increase the client's feelings of well-being.[16] Provides opportunities for the client to learn alternative ways of coping with anxiety in a supportive environment.

Continued

Actions/Interventions	Rationales
client in these activities to provide positive social reinforcement. Note schedule and type of activity here.	

Gerontic Health

Actions/Interventions	Rationales
• Monitor for use of medications that may induce sexual dysfunction. Male impotency may be related to antihypertensive medications.	Identifies correctable source of impotency.
• Determine individual patient's knowledge of facts and myths regarding sexual changes in aging.	Knowledge of expected aging changes may encourage the individual to discuss changes experienced and seek treatment for dysfunction.
• Identify resources for assistance with sexual dysfunction, such as Impotents Anonymous groups.[17]	Provides an information source and support for individuals with a common problem. Impotence, regardless of etiology, shows marked increase beyond age 65.
• Provide resources for patients with chronic illnesses, such as chronic obstructive pulmonary disease or arthritis, that address and assist in problem solving regarding disease-related sexual difficulties.[18]	
• Provide uninterrupted time for couples, particularly in long-term care settings, where it may be difficult to maintain or attain privacy.	Assists patients in maintaining sexuality as long as possible.

Home Health

Actions/Interventions	Rationales

• Involve client and significant other in planning and implementing strategies for reducing sexual dysfunction and enhancing sexual relationship. Develop:
  ○ *Communication*: open discussion of concerns and ideas for intervention
  ○ *Mutual sharing and trust*
  ○ *Problem solving*: identification of specific strategies with defined roles, such as
	Sexual dysfunction affects and is affected by relationships. Involvement of significant people in strategies is vital to enhance the potential for success.

second honeymoon or specific sexual arousal exercises
- Assist patient and significant other with life-style adjustments that may be required:
  - ○ Provide accurate and appropriate information regarding contraception.
  - ○ Teach stress management.
  - ○ Provide information regarding sexuality, and clarify myths regarding sexuality.
  - ○ Explore strategies for coping with disabling injury or disease.
  - ○ Use massage.
  - ○ Use touch.
  - ○ Treat substance abuse.
  - ○ Exercise regularly.
  - ○ Cope with changes in role functions and role relationships.
  - ○ Use water-soluble lubricants.
  - ○ Obtain treatment for physical problems: vaginal infections, penile discharge, and so on.
  - ○ Teach changes accompanying pregnancy.
  - ○ Teach side effects of medication.
- Consult with or refer to community resources as indicated. (See Appendix B.)

Life-style changes require permanent behavior changes. Support and self-evaluation can improve the probability of successful change.

Provides for quality care and effective use of existing services.

FLOW CHART EVALUATION
Flow Chart Expected Outcome 1

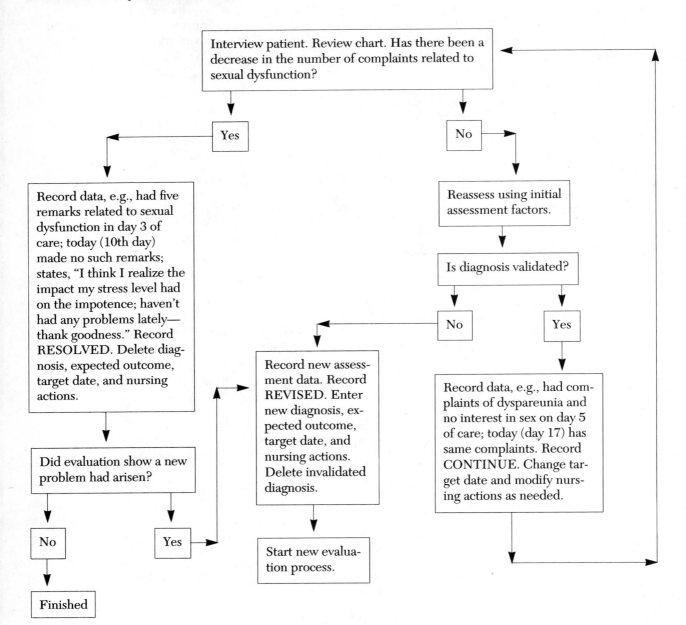

Interview patient. Review chart. Has there been a decrease in the number of complaints related to sexual dysfunction?

Yes

No

Record data, e.g., had five remarks related to sexual dysfunction in day 3 of care; today (10th day) made no such remarks; states, "I think I realize the impact my stress level had on the impotence; haven't had any problems lately—thank goodness." Record RESOLVED. Delete diagnosis, expected outcome, target date, and nursing actions.

Reassess using initial assessment factors.

Is diagnosis validated?

No

Yes

Did evaluation show a new problem had arisen?

Record new assessment data. Record REVISED. Enter new diagnosis, expected outcome, target date, and nursing actions. Delete invalidated diagnosis.

Record data, e.g., had complaints of dyspareunia and no interest in sex on day 5 of care; today (day 17) has same complaints. Record CONTINUE. Change target date and modify nursing actions as needed.

No

Yes

Start new evaluation process.

Finished

Flow Chart Expected Outcome 2

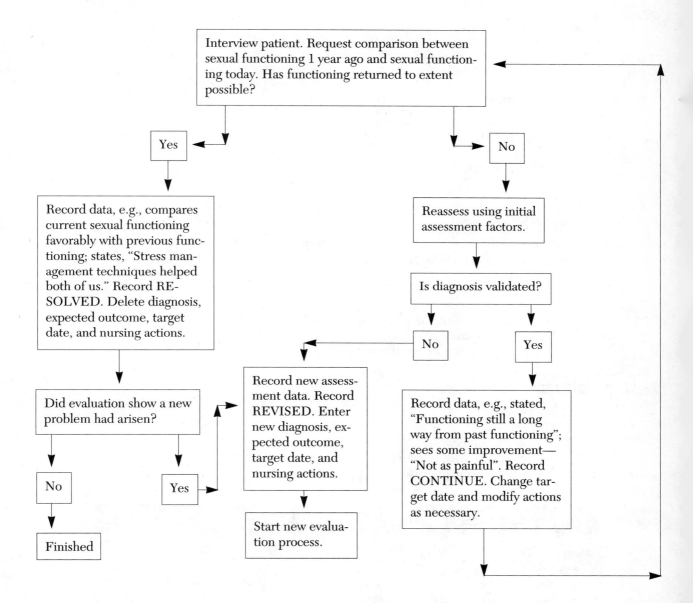

Sexuality Patterns, Altered

DEFINITION

The state in which an individual expresses concern regarding his or her sexuality.[10]

NANDA TAXONOMY: RELATING 3.3

DEFINING CHARACTERISTICS[10]

1. Major defining characteristics:
   a. Reported difficulties, limitations, or changes in sexual behaviors or activities
2. Minor defining characteristics:
   None given

RELATED FACTORS[10]

1. Knowledge or skills deficit about alternative responses to health-related transitions, altered body function or structure, illness or medical problem
2. Lack of privacy
3. Lack of significant others
4. Ineffective or absent role models
5. Conflicts with sexual orientation or variant preferences
6. Fear of pregnancy or of acquiring a sexually transmitted disease
7. Impaired relationship with a significant other

RELATED CLINICAL CONCERNS

1. Mastectomy
2. Hysterectomy
3. Cancer of the reproductive tract
4. Any condition resulting in paralysis
5. Sexually transmitted disease: syphilis, gonorrhea, AIDS, and so on.

HAVE YOU SELECTED THE CORRECT DIAGNOSIS?

Sexual Dysfunction Sexual Dysfunction indicates there are problems in sexual functioning. Altered Sexual Patterns refers to concerns about sexuality but does not necessarily mean an overwhelming problem. In some instances this may involve a life-style different from heterosexual norms. (See page 833.)

Rape Trauma Syndrome Certainly a traumatic event such as a rape could result in Altered Sexuality Patterns. The nurse would focus, however, on assisting the patient to deal with the rape trauma first. Resolving this problem would assist in resolving the Altered Sexuality Patterns. (See page 821.)

Other Diagnoses Many other nursing diagnoses can impact sexual feelings and functioning in both men and women. Examples are Body Image Disturbance, Pain, Chronic Pain, Fear, Anxiety, Dysfunctional Grieving, and Altered Role Performance.

EXPECTED OUTCOME

1. Will identify at least (number) factors contributing to Altered Sexual Patterns by (date) and/or
2. Will verbalize fewer complaints regarding Altered Sexual Patterns by (date)

TARGET DATE

Because of the extremely personal nature of sexuality, the patient may be reluctant to express needs or problems in this area. For this reason, a target date of 5 to 7 days would be acceptable.

NURSING ACTIONS/INTERVENTIONS WITH RATIONALES

Adult Health

Actions/Interventions	Rationales
• Establish therapeutic and trusting relationship with patient and significant other.	Promotes therapeutics and open communication.
• Address other primary nursing needs, especially those related to physiology and self-image.	Meeting these needs promotes resolution of Altered Sexuality Patterns.
• Actively listen to patient's and significant other's efforts to talk about fears or changes in body image affecting sexuality or altered sexual preferences. Assist patient and family to identify how the desired sexual function may be attained.	Promotes open and therapeutic communication.
• Help patient and significant other to understand that sexuality does not necessarily mean intercourse.	Misinformation and myths may create unrealistic expectations about sexuality and the sexual experience.
• Discuss alternate methods for expressing sexuality, including masturbation.	Sexuality includes verbal, nonverbal, genital, and nongenital sexual activities.
• Do not be judgmental with patient or significant other.	Sexuality is a highly personal behavior; the nurse's attitude can create guilt feelings and stress in the patient.
• Provide privacy and time for patient and significant other to be alone if so desired.	Allows for sexual expressions.
• Administer medications as ordered, and monitor for potential side effects.	
• Monitor for contributory causative components, and provide appropriate education and follow-up.	Permits a more fully developed and accurate plan of care; provides for long-term support.

Child Health

Actions/Interventions	Rationales
• Encourage child and family to verbalize perception of altered sexual functioning, for example, undescended testicle.	Provides the database necessary to accurately plan intervention.
• Assist patient and family to identify how the desired sexual function may be attained.	Specific plans for goals of sexual function desired will help determine treatment, for example, surgery for future procreation.
• Include appropriate collaboration with other health care team members as needed. (See Appendix B.)	Specialist may best meet the unique needs represented by altered sexual functioning.
• Provide attention to developmentally appropriate role modeling for age and situation.	Opportunities appropriate for age with role models serve as valuable learning modes.
• Encourage peer support during hospitalization as appropriate.	Peer support fosters sense of self, which is also a composite of sexuality.
• Plan for potential long-term nursing follow-up.	The chronic nature of many physiologic components will necessitate serial rechecks and treatment over time as the child grows and matures.

Women's Health

Actions/Interventions	Rationales
• Assist the patient to describe her sexuality and understanding of sexual functioning as it relates to her life-style and life-style decisions.	Provides database needed to plan for successful interventions.
• Allow patient time to discuss sexuality and sex-related problems in a nonthreatening atmosphere. Obtain a complete sexual history, including current emotional state.	
• Assist patient in listing life-style adjustments that need to be made, for example, different methods of achieving sexual satisfaction in the presence of mutilating surgery.	
• Identify significant others in patient's life and involve them, if so desired by patient, in discussion and problem-solving activities regarding sexual adjustments.	

• Provide atmosphere that allows patient to discuss freely:
  ○ Partner choice
  ○ Sexual orientation
  ○ Sexual roles
	Assists patient in planning coping strategies for various life situations, and provides information the patient needs for planning.

- Assist patient in identifying life-style adjustments to each different cycle of reproductive life:
  - Puberty
  - Pregnancy
  - Menopause
  - Postmenopause
- Discuss pregnancy and the changes that will occur during pregnancy:
  - Sexuality
  - Mood swings

Provides essential information needed by patient to offset concerns regarding maintaining sexuality during pregnancy.

- Discuss alternative methods of intercourse during pregnancy
  - Positions
  - Frequency
  - Effects on baby
  - Effects on pregnancy
  - Fears about sexual changes
- Assist patient facing surgery or body structure changes in identifying life-style adjustments that may be necessitated by ileostomy, colostomy, mastectomy, hysterectomy, and so on.
- Allow patient to grieve for loss of body image.
- Reassure patient that she can still participate in sexual activities.

Provides support to patient who is questioning continuance of sexuality.

- Assure confidentiality for patient with sexually transmitted diseases.

Promotes sharing of information necessary to plan care.

- Encourage verbalization of concerns about sexually transmitted diseases:

Provides the database need to most accurately plan care.

  - Recurrent nature of disease, especially herpes and chlamydia
  - Lack of cure for disease (AIDS)
  - Economics in treating disease
  - Social stigma associated with disease
- Encourage honesty in answers to such questions as:
  - Multiple sex partners
  - Descriptions of sexual behavior
- Encourage honest communication with sexual partners.

Sexual partners will require health care.

Mental Health

NOTE: If alteration is related to altered body function or structure or illness, refer to Adult Health.

Actions/Interventions	Rationales
• Assign primary care nurse who is comfortable discussing sexually related material with client.	Promotes the development of a trusting relationship.

• Primary care nurse will spend (number) minutes (number) times a day with client discussing issues related to diagnosis. These discussions will include:
  ○ Client's thoughts and feelings about alteration
  ○ Other stressors and concerns in the client's life that could affect sexual patterns
  ○ Client's perceptions of partner's responses
  ○ Client's perceptions of self as a sexual person without a partner
  ○ Client's perceptions of social or cultural expectations
  ○ Client's thoughts and feelings about sexuality
	Expression of feelings and perceptions in a supportive environment facilitates the development of alternative coping behaviors.

• If alteration is related to lack of information, develop a teaching plan and note teaching plan here.	Provides guide to ensure client gets accurate and consistent information.
• When client identifies *specific* difficulties that contribute to the concern, develop specific action plan to cope with these and note the plan here.	Promotes the client's sense of control and enhances self-esteem.
• If alteration is related to problems with the significant other, arrange a meeting with client and significant other to discuss the perceptions each has about the problem. If these difficulties are related to a lack of information, develop a teaching plan and note it here. If alteration is related to long-term relationship or if alteration is only one of several problems, refer to marriage and family therapist or clinical nurse specialist.	Provides opportunity for nurse to facilitate communication between the partners and for the partners to communicate their relationship needs as well as personal needs in a nonthreatening environment.
• Arrange private time for client and partner to discuss relationship issues, including sexuality. Note time and place arranged for this discussion here.	Provides recognition and support for this relationship.
• During interactions with client and significant other, have them express feelings about their relationship. These should be both positive and negative feelings.	Promotes the development of a positive expectational set. Positive feelings enhance self-esteem and personal psychologic resources for coping with the difficult aspects of the relationship.

Gerontic Health

> See Adult Health.

Home Health

Actions/Interventions	Rationales
• Monitor for factors contributing to Altered Sexuality Patterns by (date).	Provides database for early identification and intervention.
• Involve appropriate family members (significant others or parents of child) in planning, implementing, and promoting reduction or elimination of Altered Sexuality Patterns:	Sexual behavior can affect the entire family. Involvement of family in problem identification and intervention enhances the probability of successful intervention.
○ *Communication*: open discussion of values and sexual mores	
○ *Mutual sharing and trust*	
○ *Problem solving*: identification of strategies acceptable to all involved, with the role of each person identified	
○ *Sex education*: clarification of any misconceptions regarding sexual behavior and sexuality	
• Assist client and family with life-style adjustments that may be required:	Provides knowledge and support necessary for permanent behavioral change.
○ Accurate and appropriate information regarding sexuality and contraception	
○ Time and privacy for development and improvement of sexual relationship	
○ Stress management	
○ Coping with loss of sexual partner	
○ Accurate and appropriate information regarding sexually transmitted diseases	
○ Accurate and appropriate information regarding sexual orientation: homosexuality, heterosexuality, transsexuality, and so on.	
○ Coping with physical disability	
○ Side effects of medical treatment	
• Consult with community resources as indicated. (See Appendix B.)	Specialized counseling may be indicated. Use of existing resources provides effective use of resources.

FLOW CHART EVALUATION
Flow Chart Expected Outcome 1

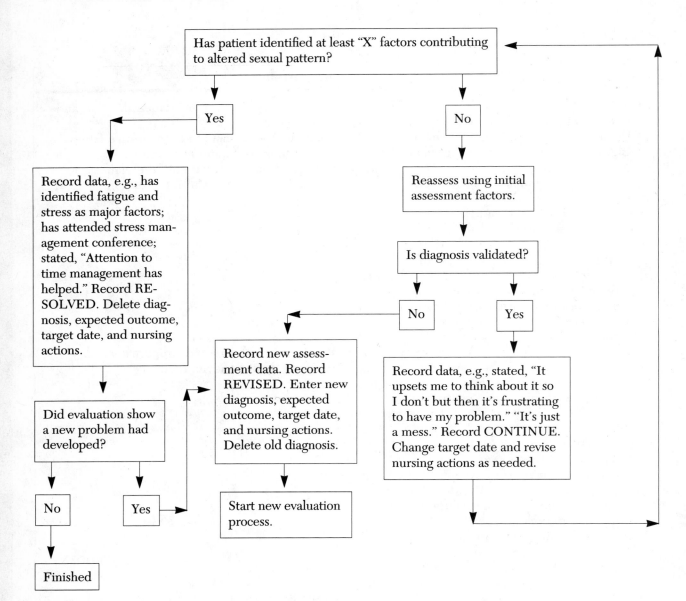

Has patient identified at least "X" factors contributing to altered sexual pattern?

Yes

No

Record data, e.g., has identified fatigue and stress as major factors; has attended stress management conference; stated, "Attention to time management has helped." Record RESOLVED. Delete diagnosis, expected outcome, target date, and nursing actions.

Reassess using initial assessment factors.

Is diagnosis validated?

No

Yes

Did evaluation show a new problem had developed?

No

Yes

Record new assessment data. Record REVISED. Enter new diagnosis, expected outcome, target date, and nursing actions. Delete old diagnosis.

Record data, e.g., stated, "It upsets me to think about it so I don't but then it's frustrating to have my problem." "It's just a mess." Record CONTINUE. Change target date and revise nursing actions as needed.

Start new evaluation process.

Finished

Flow Chart Expected Outcome 2

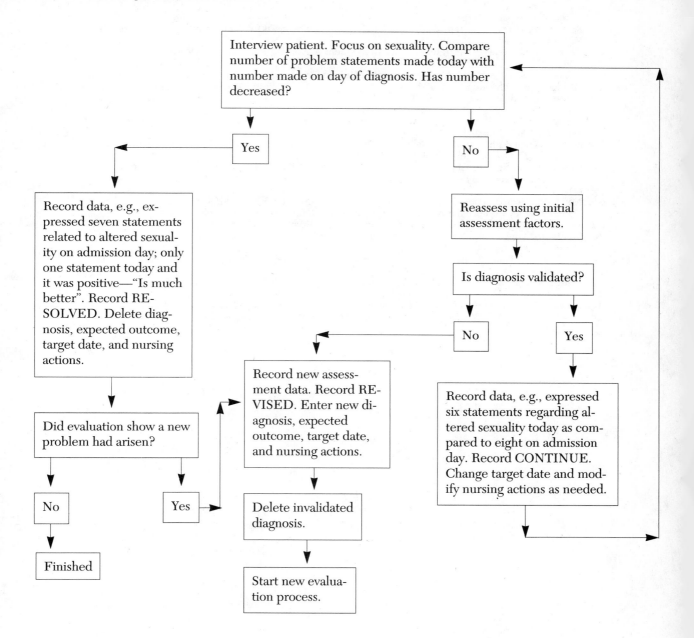

References

1. Wood, NF: Human Sexuality in Health and Illness, ed 3. CV Mosby, St. Louis, 1984.
2. Speroff, L, Glass, RH, and Kase, NG: Clinical Gynecologic Endocrinology and Infertility, ed 3. Williams & Wilkins, Baltimore, 1989.
3. Fogel, CI and Woods, NF: Health Care of Women: A Nursing Perspective. CV Mosby, St. Louis, 1981.
4. Schuster, CS and Ashburn, SS: The Process of Human Development: A Holistic Life-Span Approach. JB Lippincott, Philadelphia, 1992.
5. Biddle, BJ and Thomas, EJ: Role Theory: Concepts and Research. Robert E. Drieger, Huntington, NY, 1979.
6. Associated Press: Study finds greater number of rape victims than supposed. Lubbock Avalanche Journal 70:A-11, April 24, 1992.
7. Molcan, KL and Fickley, BS: Sexuality and the life cycle. In Poorman, SG (ed): Human Sexuality and the Nursing Process. Appleton & Lange, Norwalk, CT, 1988.
8. Ames, LB and Ilg, FL: Child Behavior. Dell, New York, 1976.
9. Warner, CG: Rape and Sexual Assault: Management and Intervention. Aspen Systems, Germantown, MD, 1980.
10. North American Nursing Diagnosis Association. Taxonomy I: Revised 1990. Author, St. Louis, 1990.
11. Haber, J, et al: Comprehensive Psychiatric Nursing, ed 4. CV Mosby, St. Louis, 1992.
12. McArthur, M: Reality therapy with rape victims. Arch Psychiatr Nurs 4:360, 1990.
13. Lightfoot-Klain, H and Shaw, E: Special needs of ritually circumcised women patients. J Obstet Gynecol Neonatal Nurs 20:102, 1991.
14. Hitchcock, JM and Wilson, HS: Personal risking: Lesbian self-disclosure of sexual orientation to professional health care providers. Nurs Res 41:178, 1992.
15. Wilson, HS and Kneisl, CR: Psychiatric Nursing, ed 4. Addison-Wesley, Redwood City, CA, 1992.
16. Dossey, B et al: Holistic Nursing. Aspen, Rockville, MD, 1988.
17. Buczny, B: Impotence in older men: A newly recognized problem. J Geront Nurs 18:25, 1992.
18. Elioupoulas, C: A Guide to the Nursing of the Aging. Williams & Wilkins, Baltimore, 1987.

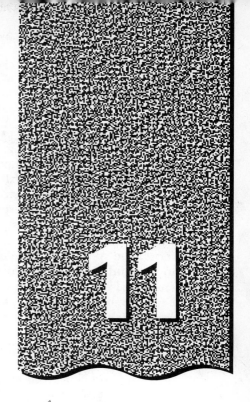

Coping – Stress
Tolerance Pattern

PATTERN INTRODUCTION
Pattern Description

Stress has been defined as the response of the body or the system to any demand made on it.[1] This response can be both physiologic and psychosocial. Since demands are synonymous with living, stress has been defined as "life itself."[1] The system's (individual, family, or community) ability to respond to these demands has an effect on the well-being of the system. Stress tolerance pattern refers to the system's usual manner of responding to stress or to the amount of stress previously experienced. This includes the stress response history of the individual, family, or community.[2] Coping has been defined as "efforts to master condition of harm, threat, or challenge when a routine or automatic response is not readily available."[3] Thus, coping pattern is the system's pattern of responding to nonroutine threats. The client's ability to respond to stress is affected by a complex interaction of physical, social, and emotional well-being. Assessment of this pattern focuses on gaining an understanding of the interaction of these factors within the system. Interventions are related to maximizing the system's well-being.[1,3]

Pattern Assessment

1. Does client verbalize inability to cope?
   a. Yes (Ineffective Individual Coping)
   b. No
2. Does client demonstrate inability to problem solve?
   a. Yes (Ineffective Individual Coping)
   b. No
3. Does client deny problems or weaknesses in spite of evidence to the contrary?
   a. Yes (Defensive Coping)
   b. No
4. Is client projecting blame for current situation on other persons or events?
   a. Yes (Defensive Coping)
   b. No
5. Did patient delay seeking health care assistance to detriment of his or her health?
   a. Yes (Ineffective Denial)
   b. No
6. Does patient downplay condition?
   a. Yes (Ineffective Denial)
   b. No
7. Does patient verbalize nonacceptance of health status change?
   a. Yes (Impaired Adjustment)
   b. No
8. Is patient moving toward independence?
   a. Yes
   b. No (Impaired Adjustment)
9. Is client's primary caregiver denying the severity of the client's problem?
   a. Yes (Ineffective Family Coping: Disabling)
   b. No

10. Does client demonstrate indications of neglect?
    a. Yes (Ineffective Family Coping: Disabling)
    b. No
11. Does client state concerns about care being received from primary care-giver?
    a. Yes (Ineffective Family Coping: Compromised)
    b. No
12. Can primary caregiver verbalize understanding of care requirements?
    a. Yes
    b. No (Ineffective Family Coping: Compromised)
13. Does family indicate physical and emotional support for client?
    a. Yes (Family Coping: Potential for Growth)
    b. No
14. Does family or primary caregiver indicate interest in a support group?
    a. Yes (Family Coping: Potential for Growth)
    b. No
15. Does patient reexperience traumatic events (flashbacks, nightmares)?
    a. Yes (Posttrauma Response)
    b. No
16. Does patient exhibit vagueness about traumatic event?
    a. Yes (Posttrauma Response)
    b. No

Nursing Diagnoses in This Pattern

1. Adjustment, Impaired (page 861)
2. Family Coping, Ineffective: Compromised and Disabling (page 874)
3. Family Coping: Potential for Growth (page 885)
4. Individual Coping, Ineffective; Defensive Coping; and Ineffective Denial (page 892)
5. Posttrauma Response (page 908)

Conceptual Information

To understand coping one must first understand the concept of stress; coping is the system's attempt to adapt to stress. An understanding of these concepts and their relationship is crucial for the promotion of well-being. Research has clearly demonstrated that undue stress can be related to major health problems if inappropriate coping is present.[1]

Stress has been defined as the body's nonspecific response to any demand placed upon it.[1] These demands can be any situation that would require the system to adapt. For the individual this could include anything from getting out of bed in the morning to experiencing the loss resulting from a major environmental disaster. Stress is life.

The body's physiologic response to stress involves activation of the autonomic nervous system. The symptoms of this activation can include sweating, tachycardia, tachypnea, nausea, and tremors. This process has been labeled the general adaptation syndrome (GAS)[4] and occurs in three stages. These stages are alarm reaction, resistance, and exhaustion. The alarm stage mobilizes the system's defense forces by initiating the autonomic nervous system response. The system is prepared for fight or flight. In the resistance stage, the system fights back and adapts, and normal functioning returns. If the stress continues and all attempts of the system to adapt fail, exhaustion occurs and the system is at risk for experiencing major disorganization.

Four levels of psychophysiologic stress responses have been described.[4] Level 1 comprises the day-to-day stressors that all systems experience as a part of living. This stress calls upon the self-regulating processes of the system for adaptation. Intrasystem coping mechanisms are used, and the system does not require assistance from outside sources to adapt. Level 2 comprises less routine or new experiences encountered by the system. The system experiences a mild alarm reaction that is not prolonged. The individual system might experience a mild increase in heart rate, sensations of bladder fullness and increased frequency of urination, temporary insomnia, tachypnea, anxiety, fear, guilt, shame, or frustration. Some outside assistance may be necessary to facilitate adaptation. This assistance could be identifying stressors and strengths or encouraging the individual to solve problems. Level 3 consists of the moderate amount of stress that occurs when a persistent stress is encountered or when a new situation is perceived as threatening. Emergency adaptation processes are activated. The individual would experience tachycardia, palpitations, tremors, weakness, cool pale skin, headache, oliguria, vomiting, constipation, and increased susceptibility to infections. This level of stress usually requires assistance from a professional helper. This assistance can include identifying problems and coping strengths, teaching, performing tasks for the client, or altering the environment to facilitate coping. When the system cannot adapt to a stressful situation with assistance, a severe degree of stress is experienced. This is labeled Level 4. This occurs when all coping strategies are exhausted. Intervention at this level requires the assistance of professionals who have the skills to assist with the development of unique coping strategies.

Since stress is life itself, adaptation to reduce the effects of stress on the system is imperative. To begin this process it is important to understand those factors that can influence the system's ability to respond to stress. Stress can arise from biophysical, chemical, psychosocial, and cultural sources. The basic health of the affected system improves the ability to respond to these stressors. Response to the biophysical and chemical stressors can be improved by improving the condition of the biological system. This would include proper nutrition, appropriate amounts of rest, appropriate levels of exercise, and reduced exposure of the system to toxic chemicals.[1]

The literature[1] indicates that a great deal of psychosocial and cultural stress evolves from a philosophy of life that is impossible to fulfill. This would indicate that a great deal of stress arises from the perception of events, not the events themselves. This is compounded by the social and cultural influences on the system. The sociocultural influences could include cultural attitudes about age, body appearance, and family roles as well as the social approaches to assistance for working mothers, advancement in employment status, and so on. The system's beliefs about these sociocultural stressors can affect the degree to which the stressors affect the system. If the stressor is perceived as unnatural or impossible to adapt to, the system's stress level will be increased. Response to the psychosocial and cultural stressors can be improved with attitude assessment and interventions that reduce the physiologic response to psychosocial stressors.

Coping has been defined as behavior (conscious and unconscious) that a system uses to change a situation for the better or to manage the stress-resultant emotions.[5] These kinds of behavior can occur on the biologic, psychologic, and social levels. Effective coping uses biologic, psychologic, and social resources in attempts to manage the situation.

A coping model has been presented[3] that addresses the biologic, psychologic, and sociocultural aspects of this process. The model indicates that systems have generalized resistance resources (GRRs) to facilitate coping.

GRRs are those characteristics of the system that can facilitate effective tension management. Genetic characteristics that provide increased resistance to the effects of stressors are considered physical and biochemical GRRs. These GRRs can include levels of immunity, nutritional status, and the adaptability of the neurologic system. Valuative and attitudinal GRRs describe consistent features of the system's coping behavior. This could include personality characteristics and the system's perception of the stressor. The more flexible, rational, and long-term these are, the more effective they are as GRRs. Interpersonal-relational GRRs include social support systems and can provide an important resource in managing stress. Finally, those cultural supports that facilitate coping are referred to as macrosociocultural GRRs. Macrosociocultural GRRs could include religions, rites of passage, and governmental structures.

In 1979, Kobasa introduced the concept of hardiness to the literature on coping.[6,7] She described hardy individuals as having three characteristics that provide them with the ability to cope effectively with stress. The first characteristic is *commitment*, or a purpose and involvement in life. *Challenge* is the second characteristic of the hardy individual. Challenge is the belief that the changes in life can be meaningful opportunities for personal growth. The third characteristic is *control*. Control has three components: cognitive control, decisional control, and repertoire of coping skills. Kobasa and other authors[6-8] proposed that the hardy individual would remain healthier and experience less disabling psychological stress.

An understanding of the concept of hardiness can facilitate the nurse's assessment of the client's potential ability to cope with life's stresses. Based on this assessment, the nurse can then develop interventions that support or develop commitment, challenge, and control for the client. These interventions might include providing the client with as much control as possible in the situation, facilitating his or her positive orientation with reframes, and assisting in the development of a variety of coping strategies.[6]

Wagnild and Young[8] have questioned the validity of hardiness as a concept. The concern of these authors evolves from their observation that the tools utilized to measure the various components of hardiness do not provide clear distinctions between the identified concepts and other influencing variables. Wagnild and Young conclude that it is important to continue the research related to a hardiness concept, and until a more precise understanding of what constitutes this concept is developed, it will be difficult to apply it to therapeutic interventions. From a clinical perspective hardiness is a useful concept to consider when interacting with the client system, for it provides a model for understanding client response and presents fertile content for clinical nursing research related to psychosocial aspects of coping.

Effective coping can occur when the system has a strong physiologic base combined with adequate psychosociocultural support. This implies that any intervention that addresses coping behavior should address each of these areas. Interventions that have been applied to this process include therapeutic touch, kinesiology, meditation, relaxation training, hypnosis, family therapy, nutritional counseling, massage, and physical exercise.

Developmental Considerations

The number of resources available to the system greatly affects its ability to cope with stressors. This indicates a need to maximize physical, cognitive, and psychosocial development. Cross-cultural research has identified those characteristics that are common to individuals who are perceived as mature and capable of coping effectively. These characteristics include an ability to anticipate consequences; calm, clear thinking; potential fulfillment; problem solving that is orderly and organized; predictability; purposefulness; realistic thinking; reflectiveness; strong convictions; and implacability.[9] The development of these characteristics is maximized in environments that provide children with a loving, warm environment; respect and acceptance for personal interests, ideas, needs, and talents; stable role models; challenges that foster development of competence and responsibility; opportunities to explore all of their feelings; a variety of experiences as well as opportunities for age-appropriate problem solving and the knowledge that they must live with the consequences of their decisions; opportunities to develop commitments to others; and encouragement in the development of their own standards, values, and goals.[9]

According to developmental stages, there are some specific etiologies and symptom clusters.

INFANT

Interactions with significant others are the primary source of the infant's response to trauma or stress. If the significant other is supportive and consistent, the effects of the event on the infant are minimized. Events that separate infants from their significant others also pose a threat to this age group. Primary symptoms are disruptions in physiologic responses.

Chronic diseases place this age group at special risk. Since the development of coping behavior is limited at this age, the primary caregivers (usually the parents) provide the child with the support to cope. If the caregivers cannot provide the proper supports, then the child is affected. Chronic illness in the child places an extreme stress on the family and can result in divorce. Support for the parents is crucial in supporting the child's coping.

TODDLER AND PRESCHOOLER

Responses of significant others are still the primary supports for the child in this age group. Thus, as for the infant, the response of significant others or separation from these persons can have an effect on the toddler and preschooler. In addition, threats to body integrity pose a special threat to this age group. Traumatic events that inflict physical damage on these children place the child at greatest risk. Regression is the primary symptom and coping behavior. This can be frustrating to caregivers who expect the child to assist in a time of crisis with age-appropriate developmental behavior when the child may regress to a very dependent stage. Other methods used by young children in coping include denial, repression, and projection. Coping may be more difficult because adults may not recognize that young children can experience crisis and will, therefore, not provide assistance with the coping process.[10]

SCHOOL-AGE CHILD

Symptoms include problems with school performance, withdrawal from family and peers, behavioral regression, and physical problems related to anxiety and aggressive behavior to self or others. Coping behavior includes that used by the younger child, only in a more effective manner. This age group may find a great deal of support from siblings during crisis. Situations that can precipitate crisis in this age group include school entry, threats to body image, peer problems, and family stress such as divorce or death of a loved one.[10]

Chronic disease or disability also affects the adjustment of this age group. Again, the primary support for adaptation comes from the primary caregivers, usually the parents.

ADOLESCENT

The adolescent demonstrates more adultlike coping behavior. Symptoms of stress include anxiety, increased physical activity, increased daydreaming, increased apathy, change in mood cycles, alteration in sleeping patterns, aggressive behavior directed at self or others, and physical symptoms associated with anxiety. Crisis-producing situations can include role changes, peer difficulties, threats to body integrity, rapidly changing body functioning, conflict with parents, personal failures, sexual awareness, and school demands.[10]

Response to traumatic events is similar to that of adults. Etiologies of crisis-producing events, for this age group, are also similar to those for adults. Specific events that place this age group at greater risk are those that affect the peer group and could have effects on body image or sexual functioning. Coping behavior is adultlike. This age group may find support from peers especially useful in facilitating coping. Coping may also be affected by limited life experience and impulsive behavior.

Illnesses that threaten body image could result in difficulties in adjustment. Peers again provide a primary support system and can have a great impact on the adolescent's acceptance. Educating significant peers about the client's situation could facilitate their acceptance of the client and in turn facilitate the client's adjustment to the change in health status. Adjustment could also be facilitated by involving the client in a support group composed of peers with similar alterations.

ADULT

Symptoms of problems with coping in the young adult include changes in performance of roles at home and at work, aggressive behavior directed at the self or others, and physical symptoms associated with anxiety and denial. Changes in role performance might include loss of interest in sexual relationships or withdrawal from the community. Situations that might tax the coping abilities of the young adult include balancing increasing role responsibilities; dealing with threats to the self or to body integrity; leaving home; and making career choices.[10]

Alterations in health status that affect the ability of role performance place this age group at risk for impaired adjustment. This could include loss of ability to function in job responsibilities. Behavior can include regression, but this does not necessarily indicate that the client is experiencing impaired adjustment.

Coping resources have broadened for the middle-age adult because of past successful coping experiences and the possible addition of adult children as supports during crisis. Symptoms of difficulties with coping are similar to those of the young adult. Age-related stressors include increased loss, including significant others and physical functioning; role changes such as job loss and the departure of adult children; aging parents; career pressures; and cultural role expectations.[10]

Symptoms of extreme stress in the older adult may be overlooked and attributed to senility. These symptoms include withdrawal, decreased functioning, increased physical complaints, and aggressive behavior. Coping behavior is affected by decreased function of hearing, vision, and mobility as well as loss of support systems and other resources. These problems can be balanced by life experience that has provided the individual with many situations of successful coping to fall back on during stressful times. Situations that place this age group at risk are multiple losses, decreased physical functioning, increased dependence, retirement, relocation, and loss of respect owing to cultural attitudes.

The effects of multiple losses related to alteration in health status and the loss of support systems place the older adult at risk for impaired adjustment. In the absence of illness affecting cognitive functioning, the older adult can assume responsibility for making decisions related to alterations in health status. This ability combined with life experience can facilitate creative problem solving with the support of health care personnel.[11]

The following is a presentation of the developmental framework of the family life-cycle as described by Carter and McGoldrick.[12]

Between families: The process of the unattached young adult is to accept parent-child separation. The individual must separate from family of origin and develop intimate peer relationships and a career.

The joining of families through marriage: The process of the newly married couple involves commitment to a new system. The individuals form a marital system and realign relationships with extended families and friends to include spouse.

The family with young children: The task is to accept a new generation of members into the system. The marital system adjusts to make space for the child(ren) and assumes parent roles. Another realignment takes place to include parenting and grandparenting roles.

The family with adolescents: The family task is to increase flexibility of family boundaries to include children's independence. The parent-child relationship shift to allow the adolescents to move in and out of the system. The parents refocus on midlife marital and career issues, and there is a beginning shift toward concerns for the older generation.

The family in later life: Accepting the shifting of generational roles is the task of this stage. The system maintains individual and couple functioning and interests in conjunction with physiologic decline. There is an exploration of new role options, with more support for a more central role for the middle generation. The system also makes room for the wisdom and experience of the elderly and support of the older generation without overprotecting them. This stage will also include coping with the deaths of significant others and preparation for death.

Specific problems can arise in family coping when the family developmental cycle or expectations do not correspond with the developmental tasks of individual family members. There are three stages that are nodal points in family development.

The joining of families through marriage requires a commitment to a new system. If the separation from the parents is not successful, then the new family does not have an opportunity to form its own identity, combining the experiences both bring into this new relationship. Symptoms of unsuccessful resolution of this stage could result in the marital partners returning home to their parents when conflict arises or an ongoing struggle over loyalties to families of origin.

The second major shift occurs when children enter the system. The new role of parent is assumed and the couple boundaries must be opened to accept the child. Unsuccessful resolution of this stage could result in physical or emotional abuse of the child. If there is a developmental delay in the parents and they are not ready to assume the responsibilities that accompany parenthood, family dysfunction can occur.

A family with adolescents is faced with the task of increasing flexibility to include children's independence. This may require a major shift in family rules. This is also influenced by the parents' perception of the adolescent and the environment. If the adolescent is seen as being competent, and the environment that the adolescent interacts in is seen as safe, then it will be much easier for the family to provide the necessary shifts in relationships. When this stage is not resolved successfully, the adolescent may enhance behavior that highlights his or her differences with the family to force separation, or the frequency and intensity of family conflict may increase. Unsuccessful resolution of this stage may indicate that the family has overly rigid boundaries to the external world and individual boundaries that are overly permeable.

NOTE: For the individual diagnoses in this chapter, the mental health nursing actions serve as the generic nursing actions. This is because the nature of the diagnoses in this chapter basically call for the skills, knowledge, and expertise of a psychiatric or mental health nursing specialist.

APPLICABLE NURSING DIAGNOSES
Adjustment, Impaired

DEFINITION

The state in which the individual is unable to modify his or her life-style or behavior in a manner consistent with a change in health status.[13]

NANDA TAXONOMY: CHOOSING 5.1.1.1.1

DEFINING CHARACTERISTICS[13]

1. Major defining characteristics:
   a. Verbalization of nonacceptance of health status change
   b. Nonexistent or unsuccessful ability to be involved in problem solving or goal setting
2. Minor defining characteristics:
   a. Lack of movement toward independence
   b. Extended period of shock, disbelief, or anger regarding health status change
   c. Lack of future-oriented thinking

RELATED FACTORS[13]

1. Disability requiring change in life-style
2. Inadequate support systems
3. Impaired cognition
4. Sensory overload
5. Assault to self-esteem
6. Altered locus of control
7. Incomplete grieving

RELATED CLINICAL CONCERNS

1. Alzheimer's disease
2. Head injury sequelae
3. Any new diagnosis for the patient
4. Couvade syndrome
5. Postpartum depression, puerperal psychosis
6. Personality disorders
7. Substance use or abuse disorders
8. Psychotic disorders

HAVE YOU SELECTED THE CORRECT DIAGNOSIS?

Ineffective Individual Coping   This diagnosis results from the client's inability to cope appropriately with stress. Impaired Adjustment is the client's inability to adjust to a specific disease process. If the client's behavior is related to the adjustment to a specific disease process, the diagnosis would be Impaired Adjustment; however, if the behavior is related to coping with general life stressors, the diagnosis would be Ineffective Individual Coping. (See page 892.)

Powerlessness   This diagnosis would be appropriate as a primary or codiagnosis if the client demonstrates the belief that personal action cannot affect or alter the situation. Impaired Adjustment may result from Powerlessness. If this is the situation, then the appropriate primary diagnosis would be Powerlessness. (See page 657.)

Sensory-Perceptual Alteration   This diagnosis can affect the individual's ability to adjust to an alteration in health status. If it is determined that perceptual alterations are affecting the client's ability to adapt, then the appropriate primary diagnosis would be Sensory-Perceptual Alteration. (See page 562.)

Altered Thought Process   This diagnosis can inhibit the client's ability to adapt effectively to an alteration in health status. If the inability to adapt to the alteration is related to an alteration in thought processes, then the appropriate primary diagnosis would be Altered Thought Process. (See page 577.)

Dysfunctional Grieving   Grieving can have a strong effect on the client's ability to adjust to an alteration in health status. The differentiation is complicated by the fact that a normal response to an alteration in health status can be grief. If, however, the client is not reporting a sense of loss, then the appropriate diagnosis would be Impaired Adjustment. If the client reports a sense of loss with the appropriate defining characteristics, then the appropriate diagnosis would be Grieving. If the grieving is prolonged or exceptionally severe, then an appropriate codiagnosis with Impaired Adjustment would be Dysfunctional Grieving. (See page 732.)

EXPECTED OUTCOMES

1. Will verbalize increased adaptation to change in health status by (date) and/or
2. Will return-demonstrate measures necessary to increase independence by (date)

TARGET DATE

Adjustment to a change in health status will require time; therefore, an acceptable initial target date would be no sooner than 7 to 10 days following the date of diagnosis.

NURSING ACTIONS/INTERVENTIONS WITH RATIONALES

Adult Health

Actions/Interventions	Rationales
• Establish a therapeutic relationship with patient and significant others by showing empathy and concern for patient, calling patient by name, answering questions honestly, involving patient in decision making, and so on.	A therapeutic relationship promotes cooperation in the plan of care and gives patient a person to talk with.
• Explain the disease process and prognosis to patient.	Knowledge of disease process and limitations are necessary for adjustment.
• Provide opportunities for patient to ask questions about health status, and ask patient to share his or her understanding of the situation.	Increasing knowledge and understanding leads to improved coping and adjustment.
• Encourage patient to express feelings about disease process and prognosis by sitting with the patient for 30 minutes once a shift at (times). Use techniques such as active listening, reflection, open-ended questions, and so on.	Verbalization of feelings leads to understanding and adjustment.
• Identify previous coping mechanisms and help patient to find new ones.	Determines what coping strategies have been successful and provides an opportunity to try new strategies.
• Help patient find alternatives or modification to previous life-style behavior by using assistive devices, changing level of	Helps patient continue to have satisfaction in activities and provides a sense of control in life-style.

Continued

Actions/Interventions	Rationales
participation in activities, learning new behaviors, and so on.	
• Encourage independence in self-care activities by focusing on patient's strengths, rewarding small successes, and so on.	Provides a sense of control and increases self-esteem and adjustment.
• Refer to psychiatric nurse practitioner. (See Mental Health section.)	Collaboration promotes holistic approach to care; problems may need intervention by specialist.

Child Health

Actions/Interventions	Rationales
• Monitor for all possible etiologic factors via active listening as appropriate for child (who, what, where, when) regarding first feeling of not being able to adjust.	Provides the database needed to most accurately plan care.
• Help the child to realize it is normal to need some time and assistance in adjusting to changes; for example, the child will need assistance with ambulation following surgery.	Realistic planning increases the likelihood of compliance and increases sense of success.
• Explore the child's and family's previous coping strategies.	Previous coping strategies serve as critical information in developing interventions for the current status.
• Identify ways the child can feel better about coping with the needed adjustment, including reinforcement of desired behavior.	Effective coping can empower the child and family and thereby afford a positive adjustment.
• Assist the child and family in creating realistic goals for coping.	Realistic goals enhance success.
• Collaborate with related health team members as needed. (See Appendix B.)	Collaboration with specialists serves to meet the unique needs of the patient and family.
• Provide clear and simple explanations for procedures.	Simple and clear instructions promote the child's functioning while in a stress situation.
• Address educational needs related to health care.	Knowledge serves to empower and provide guidelines for compliance with expected behavior.
• Deal with other primary care needs promptly.	Basic primary needs required prompt attention to offer the best likelihood of minimizing adjustment difficulty.
• Provide for posthospitalization follow-up with home care as needed.	Follow-up affords long-term resolution of adjustment.
• Assist patient and family in identification of community resources to offer support. (See Appendix B.)	Identification of resources serves to provide a group for sharing like needs; this will enhance coping skills of both patient and family.

Women's Health

Actions/Interventions	Rationales
• When counseling with expectant fathers, be alert for characteristics of couvade syndrome:[14] ○ Syndrome affects males only. ○ Wives are usually in the 3rd or 9th month of gestation. ○ Symptoms are confined to the gastrointestinal or genitourinary system; notable exceptions are toothache and skin growths. ○ Physical findings are minimal; laboratory and x-ray tests yield normal results. ○ Anxiety and affective disturbances are common. Expectant father constantly expresses worry about labor ("I can't do this" or "I just know I will faint") and/or overmanages arrangements for new baby (painting nursery three times, and so on). ○ Patient makes no connection between his symptoms and his wife's pregnancy.	Provides database that allows early intervention.
• Provide a nonjudgmental atmosphere to allow patient with couvade syndrome to express his concerns: ○ Self-image as a father ○ Relationship with his own father ○ Sense of responsibility ○ Feelings about wife's or partner's pregnancy ○ Concerns about wife's or partner's safety	Encourages patient to talk about feelings and allows planning of how to channel feelings into activities that will assist in preparing for fatherhood.
• Accurately record physical symptoms described by expectant father: ○ Fatigue ○ Weight gain ○ Nausea, vomiting ○ Headaches ○ Backaches ○ Food cravings	Allows more effective interventions and planning.
• Support and guide the expectant father through the changes being experienced.	
• Assure expectant couple that: ○ Expectant fathers can suffer physical symptoms during partner's pregnancy. ○ Pregnancy affects both partners. ○ Fathers also have emotional needs during pregnancy.	Emphasizes that this is not necessarily unusual behavior. Assists with positive actions that support both partners and allow the male to view pregnancy realistically.

Continued

Actions/Interventions	Rationales

• In instances of postpartum depression or puerperal psychosis, encourage patient to express fears about less-than-perfect infant; low-birth-weight infant; wrong sex; fussy infant; complications during pregnancy, delivery, or postpartum; and so on.
• Provide nonjudgmental atmosphere for patient to discuss problematic family situation. Issues may include
  ○ Partner's lack of sexual interest
  ○ Any illnesses or problems with older children
  ○ Marital status
  ○ Planned or unplanned pregnancy
  ○ Disappointment in experience (unexpected cesarean section, medications administered during labor, any unexpected occurrences)
  ○ Isolation during postpartum (unable to return to work immediately, no adults available to talk to during day, unable to complete daily activities owing to fatigue, demands of infant, uncooperative partner, lack of support system, and so on)
	Encourages patient to discuss feelings and verbalize disappointments or problems so that plans for coping with reality of birth experience can be initiated.

Mental Health

Actions/Interventions	Rationales
• Discuss with client his or her perception of the current alteration in health status. This should include information about coping strategies that have been attempted and his or her assessment of what has made them ineffective in promoting adaptation. • Provide client with clocks and calendars to promote orientation and involvement in the environment. • Give client information about the care that is to be provided, including times for treatments, medicines, groups, and other therapy. • Assign client appropriate tasks during unit activities. These should be at a level that	Communicates respect for the client and his or her experience of the stressor, which promotes the development of a trusting relationship. Provides information about the client's strengths that can be utilized to promote coping. Provides the nurse with an opportunity to support these strengths in a manner that promotes a positive orientation. Maintains the client's cognitive strengths in a manner that will facilitate the development of coping strategies.[6] Promotes the client's sense of control. Accomplishment of tasks provides positive reinforcement, which enhances self-esteem,

can be accomplished easily. Provide client with positive verbal support for completing the task. Gradually increase the difficulty of the tasks as the client's abilities increase.

- Sit with client (number) minutes (number) times per day at (times) to discuss current concerns and feelings.

motivates behavior, and helps the client to develop a positive expectational set.

Communicates concern for the client and facilitates the development of a trusting relationship. Promotes the client's sense of control by communicating that his or her ideas and concerns are important.
Promotes the client's sense of control while meeting safety and security needs.

- Provide client with familiar needed objects. These should be noted here. These should assist the client in identifying a personal space over which he or she feels some control. This space is to be respected by the staff, and the client's permission should be obtained before altering this environment.

- Provide client with an environment that will optimize sensory input. This should include compensation for sensory deficit as well as reduction of sensory overload. Specific interventions could include provision of hearing aids, eyeglasses, pencil and paper; noise reduction in conversation areas; appropriate lighting; and so on. The specific interventions for this client should be noted here; for example, "Place hearing aid in when client awakens and remove before bedtime (9:00 p.m.)."

Achieving appropriate levels of sensory input decreases confusion and disorganization, maximizing the client's coping abilities.

- Communicate to client an understanding that all coping behavior to this point has been his or her best effort and that asking for assistance at this time is not failure: a complex problem often requires some outside assistance in resolution.

- Call client by the name he or she has identified as the preferred name with each interaction. Note this name on the chart.

Promotes a positive orientation while enhancing self-esteem.

- Have client dress in street clothing. This should be items of clothing that have been brought from home and in which the client feels comfortable.

Promotes positive orientation and the client's sense of control by supporting normal daily routine and activities.

- Provide client with opportunities to make appropriate decisions related to care at his or her level of ability. This may begin as a choice between two options and then evolve into more complex decision making. It is important that this be at the client's level of functioning so that confidence can be built with successful decision-making

Promotes the client's sense of control and enhances self-esteem when appropriate decisions are made.

Continued

Actions/Interventions	Rationales
experiences. Note those decisions that the client has made here.	
• Provide client with primary care nurse on each shift. Nurse will spend 30 minutes once per shift at (time) developing a relationship with the client. This time could be spent answering client's questions about the hospital, daily routines, and so on or providing the client with a backrub.	Promotes the development of a trusting relationship while promoting the client's sense of control with knowledge about the environment.
• Identify with client methods of anxiety reduction. The specific method selected by the client should be noted here. For the first 3 days, the staff should remain with the client during a 30-minute practice of the selected method. The method should be practiced 30 minutes three times a day at (times). (See Anxiety, Chapter 8, for specific instructions about anxiety reduction methods.)	High levels of anxiety interfere with decision making. Increased control over anxiety promotes the client's sense of control. The presence of the nurse can provide positive reinforcement, which encourages behavior. Behavioral rehearsal internalizes and personalizes the behavior.
• Provide positive social reinforcement and other behavioral rewards for demonstration of adaptation. Those things that the client finds rewarding should be listed here with a schedule for use. The kinds of behavior that are identified by the treatment team as rewarding should also be listed, together with the appropriate reward.	Positive reinforcement encourages behavior and enhances self-esteem.
• Assist client in identifying support systems and in developing a plan for their use. The support systems identified should be noted, along with the plan for their use.	Support systems can support and facilitate the client's coping strategies.
• Schedule a meeting with the identified support system to assist them in understanding alterations in the client's health. Provide time to answer any questions they may have. Note the time for this meeting here and the person responsible for this meeting.	Promotes the development of a trusting relationship and provides the support system with information they can utilize to provide more effective support.
• Provide client with group interaction with (number) persons, (number) minutes, (number) times per day at (times). This activity should be graded with client's ability; for example, on admission client may tolerate one person for 5 minutes. If the interactions are brief, the frequency should be high; for example, 5-minute interactions should occur at 30-minute intervals. If the client is meeting with a	Disconfirms the client's sense of aloneness and helps the client to experience personal importance to others while enhancing interpersonal relationship skills. Increasing these competences can enhance self-esteem and promote positive orientation.

large client group, this may occur only once a day. The larger groups should include persons who are both more advanced and less advanced in adapting to their alterations.

- Make available items necessary for client to groom self. Have these items adapted as necessary to facilitate client use. List those items that are necessary here along with any assistance that is necessary from the nursing staff. Assign one person per day to be responsible for this assistance. Provide positive social reinforcement for client's accomplishments in this area.

Appropriate grooming enhances self-esteem. Positive reinforcement encourages behavior while enhancing self-esteem.

- Set an appointment to discuss with client and significant others effects of the loss or change on their relationship. (Time and date of appointment and all follow-up appointments should be listed here.) Note person responsible for these meetings.

Promotes communication in the system that can serve as the basis for developing coping strategies.

- Monitor nurse's nonverbal reactions to loss or change, and provide client with verbal information when necessary to establish nurse's acceptance of the change.

Promotes the development of a trusting relationship and a positive orientation.

- If nursing staff is having difficulty coping with the client's alterations, schedule a staff meeting where these issues can be discussed. An outside clinical nurse specialist may be useful in facilitating these meetings. Schedule ongoing support meetings as necessary.

Staff thoughts and feelings can be indirectly communicated to the client. This could have a negative effect on the client's ability to develop a positive orientation.

- Utilize constructive confrontation if necessary, including "I" statements, relationship statements that reflect nurse's reaction to the interaction, and responses that will assist client in understanding, such as paraphrasing and validation of perceptions.

Models appropriate communication skills while providing the client with information that facilitates consensual validation.

- When a relationship has been developed, the primary care nurse will spend 30 minutes twice a day at (time) with the client discussing thoughts and feelings related to the alteration in health status. These discussions could include memories that have been activated by this alteration, client's fears and concerns for the future, client's plans for the future before the alteration in health status, client's perceptions of how this alteration will affect daily life, client's perceptions of how

Promotes the development of adaptive coping strategies.

Continued

Actions/Interventions	Rationales
this alteration will affect the lives of significant others, and so on.	
• Provide client with information about care and treatment. Give information in concise terms appropriate to the client's level of understanding. Note here those kinds of information that client needs the most, together with a plan for providing this information.	Promotes the client's sense of control. Inappropriate levels of sensory input can increase the client's confusion and disorganization.
• Do not argue with client while he or she is experiencing an alteration in thought process. (Refer to Altered Thought Process, Chapter 7, for related nursing actions.)	Arguing with these perceptions decreases the client's self-esteem and increases the need to enlist dysfunctional coping behavior.
• Develop with the client a very specific behavioral plan for adapting to the alteration in health status. Note that plan here. This plan should include achievable goals so the client will not become frustrated.	Achievement of a specific plan provides positive reinforcement and enhances self-esteem, which motivates behavior.
• Refer client to occupational therapy to develop the necessary adaptations to the occupational role. Note time for these meetings here.	Successful adaptation to the occupational role enhances self-esteem.
• Schedule time for the client and his or her support system to be together without interruptions. The times for these interactions should be noted here.	Provides opportunities for the support system to maintain normal relationships while the client is hospitalized.
• If client is disoriented, orient to reality as needed and before attempting any teaching activity. Provide client with clocks and calendars, and refer to day, date, and time in each interaction with this client.	Enhances the client's cognitive functioning, improving his or her ability to problem-solve and cope.
• Refer client to appropriate community resources as indicated. (See Appendix B.) Note those referrals here, with the name of the contact person.	Establishes the client's support system in the community.

Gerontic Health

See Adult Health and Mental Health.

Home Health

Actions/Interventions	Rationales
• Monitor for factors contributing to impaired adjustment: psychologic, social, economic, spiritual, environmental, and so on.	Provides database for interventions.
• Involve client and family in planning, implementing, and promoting reduction or elimination of impaired adjustment:	Family involvement enhances effectiveness of interventions.
○ *Family conference*: Discuss feelings and altered roles. Identify coping strategies that have worked in the past.	
○ *Mutual goal sharing*: Establish realistic goals and specify role of each family member in providing a safe environment, supporting self-care, and so on.	
○ *Communication*: Promote clear and honest communication among family members. If sensory impairments exist, corrective interventions such as eyeglasses or hearing aid are needed.	
• Assist client and family in life-style adjustments that may be required:	Family relationships can be altered by impaired adjustment. Permanent changes in behavior and family roles require evaluation and support.
○ Stress management	
○ Development and use of support networks	
○ Treatment for disability	
○ Appropriate balance of dependence and independence	
○ Grief counseling	
○ Change in role functions	
○ Treatment for cognitive impairment	
○ Provision of comfortable and safe environment	
○ Activities to increase self-esteem	
• Consult with or refer to appropriate community resources as indicated. (See Appendix B.)	Promotes efficient use of existing resources, such as occupational therapist, psychiatric nurse clinician, and support groups. This can enhance the treatment plan.

FLOW CHART EVALUATION
Flow Chart Expected Outcome 1

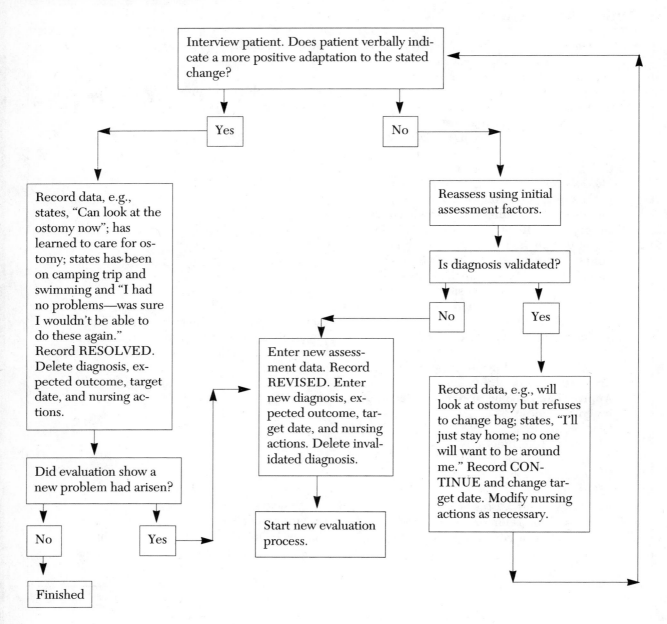

Flow Chart Expected Outcome 2

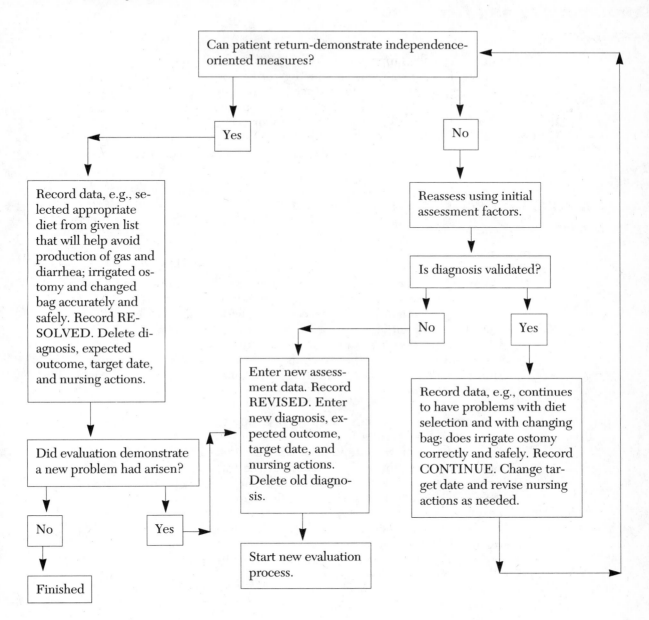

Can patient return-demonstrate independence-oriented measures?

→ Yes

→ No

Record data, e.g., selected appropriate diet from given list that will help avoid production of gas and diarrhea; irrigated ostomy and changed bag accurately and safely. Record RESOLVED. Delete diagnosis, expected outcome, target date, and nursing actions.

Reassess using initial assessment factors.

Is diagnosis validated?

No

Yes

Did evaluation demonstrate a new problem had arisen?

Enter new assessment data. Record REVISED. Enter new diagnosis, expected outcome, target date, and nursing actions. Delete old diagnosis.

Record data, e.g., continues to have problems with diet selection and with changing bag; does irrigate ostomy correctly and safely. Record CONTINUE. Change target date and revise nursing actions as needed.

No

Yes

Finished

Start new evaluation process.

Family Coping, Ineffective: Compromised and Disabling

DEFINITIONS

Compromised: A usually supportive primary person (family member or close friend) is providing insufficient, ineffective, or compromised support, comfort, assistance, or encouragement that may be needed by the client to manage or master adaptive tasks related to his or her health challenge.

Disabling: Behavior of significant person (family or other primary person) that disables his or her own capacities and the client's capacities to effectively address tasks essential to either person's adaptation to the health challenge.[13]

NANDA TAXONOMY: CHOOSING 5.1.2.1.1, 5.1.2.1.2

DEFINING CHARACTERISTICS[13]

1. Compromised:
   a. Subjective:
      (1) Client expresses or confirms a concern or complaint about significant other's response to his or her health problems.
      (2) Significant person describes preoccupation with personal reaction (for example, fear, anticipatory grief, guilt, anxiety) to client's illness, disability, or other situational or developmental crises.
      (3) Significant person describes or confirms an inadequate understanding or knowledge base, which interferes with effective assistive or supportive behaviors.
   b. Objective:
      (1) Significant person attempts assistive or supportive behaviors with less than satisfactory results.
      (2) Significant person withdraws or enters into limited or temporary personal communication with the client at the time of need.
      (3) Significant person displays protective behavior disproportionate (too little or too much) to the client's abilities or need for autonomy.
2. Disabling:
   a. Neglectful care of the client in regard to basic human needs and/or illness treatment
   b. Distortion of reality regarding the client's health problem, including extreme denial about its existence or severity
   c. Intolerance
   d. Rejection
   e. Abandonment
   f. Desertion
   g. Carrying on usual routines, disregarding client's needs
   h. Psychosomaticism
   i. Taking on illness signs of client
   j. Decisions and actions by family that are detrimental to economic or social well-being
   k. Agitation, depression, aggression, hostility

l. Impaired restructuring of a meaningful life for self, impaired individualization, prolonged overconcern for client
m. Neglectful relationships with other family members
n. Client's development of helpless, inactive dependence

RELATED FACTORS

1. Compromised:
   a. Inadequate or incorrect information or understanding by a primary person
   b. Temporary preoccupation by a significant person who is trying to manage emotional conflicts and personal suffering and is unable to perceive or act effectively in regard to client's needs
   c. Temporary family disorganization and role changes
   d. Other situational or developmental crises or situations the significant person may be facing
   e. Little support provided by client for primary person
   f. Prolonged disease or disability progression that exhausts supportive capacity of significant people
2. Disabling:
   a. Significant person with chronically unexpressed feelings of guilt, anxiety, hostility, despair, and so on
   b. Dissonant discrepancy of coping styles for dealing with adaptive tasks by the significant person and client or among significant people
   c. Highly ambivalent family relationships
   d. Arbitrary handling of family's resistance to treatment, which tends to solidify defensiveness as it fails to deal adequately with underlying anxiety

RELATED CLINICAL CONCERNS

1. Alzheimer's disease
2. AIDS
3. Any disorder resulting in permanent paralysis
4. Cancer
5. Any disorder of a chronic nature, for example, rheumatoid arthritis
6. Substances abuse
7. Somatoform disorders

HAVE YOU SELECTED THE CORRECT DIAGNOSIS?

Compromised versus Disabling Coping Compromised dysfunction reflects the family that cannot provide appropriate support to the identified patient. This problem removes a possible support system for the client. If the family dysfunction results in further dysfunction for the identified patient, then the diagnosis is Disabling. Because this diagnosis is used to describe family processes it may be difficult at times to differentiate between Compromised and Disabling because there is not an identified patient or the effects of the family patterns on the client cannot be determined. When this is the situation, the diagnosis can be made as Ineffective Family Coping with no attached label.

Continued

HAVE YOU SELECTED THE CORRECT DIAGNOSIS?—*Continued*

Family Coping: Potential for Growth This diagnosis is appropriate for families that are coping well with current stressors and are in a position to enhance their coping abilities. Ineffective Family Coping describes a family that has a deficit in coping abilities which threatens the family's existence. (See page 885.)

Altered Parenting This diagnosis refers to an inability to fulfill the parenting role. This dysfunction is circumscribed to the parent-child relationship and is time-limited when contrasted with Ineffective Family Coping. (See page 742.)

EXPECTED OUTCOMES

1. Will initiate a plan to cope with (the identified stressor) by (date) and/or
2. Will identify the effects current coping strategies have on the family by (date)

TARGET DATE

The target dates should reflect the complexity and power of the system. Four-week intervals would be appropriate to assess for progress.

NURSING ACTIONS/INTERVENTIONS WITH RATIONALES

Adult Health

Actions/Interventions	Rationales
• Encourage and help family and significant others to verbalize their needs, fears, feelings, and concerns by sitting with patient for 30 minutes per shift at (times) or planning a family conference. Actively listen and facilitate discussion.	Allows for identification of specific stressors and promotes creative problem solving.
• Provide accurate information about the situation.	Clarifies misconceptions and misunderstandings.
• Include family and significant others in decision making and plan of care.	Promotes active participation, motivation, and compliance.
• Help family and significant others to identify and explore alternatives to dealing with the situation: respite care, Mother's Day Out programs, day care centers, and so on.	Promotes creative problem solving.
• Assist family and significant others to identify, prior to discharge, sources of community support that could help them cope with their feelings and supply relief when needed.	Community resources can help strengthen family coping process and prevent isolation of family.

• Encourage family to provide time for themselves on a regular basis.	Reduces stresses and strengthens coping skills.
• Initiate referral to psychiatric clinical nurse specialist as needed.	Problems may need intervention by specialist.

Child Health

Actions/Interventions	Rationales
• Encourage child and family to express feelings and fears by allotting 30 minutes per shift, while wake, for this purpose.	Expression of concerns provides insight into views about problem and the values of the patient and family.
• Review family dynamics previous to crisis.	Knowledge of usual family dynamics is paramount in understanding coping dynamics during times of stress.
• Encourage family members to participate in child's care, including bathing, feeding, comfort, and diversional activity.	Family and patient input ensures individualized plan of care; provides teaching opportunity; increases child's security.
• Provide education to all family members regarding child's illness, prognosis, and special needs as appropriate.	Reduces anxiety, increases likelihood of compliance, empowers family.
• Involve health team members in collaboration for care. (See Appendix B.)	Increases the likelihood of a holistic plan of care for both short-term and long-term goals.
• Provide referral to appropriate community resources for support purposes. (See Appendix B.)	Provides for long-term follow-up and support.
• Provide for home discharge planning at least 5 days prior to discharge.	Allows time for teaching, practice, and return-demonstration.
• Make referral for home health care as needed.	Provides for long-term follow-up and support.

Women's Health

NOTE: This diagnosis would be most likely to relate to the single mother.

Actions/Interventions	Rationales
• Review the physical, mental, social, and economic status of the single mother, taking into account whether she is widowed, divorced, single and a parent by choice, or single and a parent not by choice.	Provides a database that can be used to plan appropriate interventions and locate support systems for patient.
• Identify support system available to the single mother: family, friends, coworkers, formal support groups such as church or community organizations, and so on.	

Continued

Actions/Interventions	Rationales
• Review patient's perception of employment status: educational level and skills, job opportunities, and opportunity for improvement of employment status.	Assists patient in realistically planning for fiscal needs of herself and infant. Allows identification of resources that could assist in improving income status.
• Identify child care requirements, considering the age of children, who has legal custody of children, and child support (financial and emotional).	

• Suggest strategies for exposing children to male role models:[15]
  ○ Assign to classes with male teachers.
  ○ Enlist assistance from brothers or grandparents.
  ○ Involve children in sports (coaches are usually male).
	Provides for male role modeling in the absence of a father figure.

Mental Health

Actions/Interventions	Rationales

• Role-model effective communication by:
  ○ Seeking clarification
  ○ Demonstrating respect for individual family members and the family system
  ○ Listening to expression of thoughts and feelings
  ○ Setting clear limits
  ○ Being consistent
  ○ Communicating with the individual being addressed in a clear manner
  ○ Encouraging sharing of information among appropriate system subgroups
	Models for the family effective communication that can enhance their problem-solving abilities.

• Demonstrate an understanding of the complexity of system problems by:
  ○ Not taking sides in family disagreements
  ○ Providing alternative explanations of behavior patterns that recognize the contributions of all persons involved in the problem, including health care providers if appropriate
  ○ Requesting the perspective of multiple family members on a problem or stressor
	Promotes the development of a trusting relationship while developing a positive orientation.

• Determine risk for physical harm and refer to appropriate authorities (child protective services, battered women's centers, police) if risk is high.	Client safety is of primary concern.

- Assist family in developing behavioral short-term goals by:
  - Asking what changes they would expect to see when the problem is improved
  - Having them break the problem into several parts that combine to form the identified stressor or crisis
  - Setting a time limit of 1 week to accomplish a task; for example, "What could you do this week to improve the current situation?"
- Develop a priority list with family.

Accomplishment of goals provides positive reinforcement, which motivates continued behavior and enhances self-esteem.

- Begin work with the presenting problem and enlist the system's assistance in resolving concerns.
- Include assessment data in determining how to work on the presenting problem; for example, if behavioral controls for a child are requested, the nurse can develop a plan for teaching and implementing them in the home that includes both parents.
- Encourage communication between family members by:
  - Having family members discuss alternatives to the problem in the presence of the nurse
  - Having each family member indicate how he or she might help resolve the problem
  - Having each family member indicate how he or she contributes to the maintenance of the problem or how he or she does not help the identified patient change behavior
  - Spending time having the family members give each other positive feedback
- Support the development of appropriate subgroups by:
  - Presenting problems to the appropriate subsystems for discussion. For example, if the problem involves a discussion of how the sexual functioning of the marital couple will change as a result of illness, this issue should be discussed with the husband and wife.
  - Providing an opportunity for the children to discuss their concerns with their parents.
  - Supporting appropriate generational boundaries, for example, parent's attempts to exclude children from parental roles.

Promotes the family's sense of control and the development of a trusting relationship by communicating respect for the client system. Promotes the development of a trusting relationship while enhancing the client system's sense of control.

Assists the family in developing problem-solving skills that will serve them in future situations.

Promotes healthy family functioning.

Continued

Actions/Interventions	Rationales
• Develop direct interventions that instruct a family to do something different or not to do something. If direct interventions are not successful and reassessment indicates they were presented appropriately, this may indicate the family system is having unusual problems with the change process and should be referred to an advanced practitioner for further care.	Provides information on the family's ability to change at this time while promoting a positive orientation.
• Provide experiences for the family to learn how they can think differently about the problem. For example, a job loss can be seen as an opportunity to reevaluate family goals, focus on interpersonal closeness, and enhance family problem-solving skills.	Promotes a positive orientation while assisting the family in developing problem-solving skills.
• Provide opportunities for the expression of a range of affect; this can mean laughing and crying together. This validates family members' emotions and helps them to identify the appropriateness of their affective responses. This may require that the nurse "push" the family to express feelings with the skills of confrontation or providing feedback.[16,17]	Validates family members' emotions and helps to identify the appropriateness of their affective responses.
• Develop a teaching plan to provide the family with information that will enhance their problem solving.	

• Assist family with interactions with other systems by:
  ○ Providing information about the system
  ○ Maintaining open communication between nurse and other agencies or systems
  ○ Having family identify what their relationship is with the system and how they could best achieve the goals they have for their interactions with this system
	Facilitates the development of support networks in the community that can be called upon in future situations.

• Provide constructive confrontation to the family about problematic coping behavior.[16] Those kinds of behavior identified by the treatment team as problematic should be listed here.	Facilitates the development of functional coping behaviors in a warm, supportive environment.
• Teach family methods to reduce anxiety, and practice and discuss the use of these methods with the family (number) times per week. This should be done at least once a week until family members are using this as a coping method. This could include deep muscle relaxation, physical exercise, family	High levels of anxiety can interfere with adaptive coping behaviors. Repeated practice of a behavior internalizes and personalizes the behavior.

games that require physical activity, cycling, and so on. Those methods selected by the family should be listed here with the time schedule for implementation. The family should be given "homework" related to the practice of these techniques to be performed at home on a daily basis.

- Provide family with the information about proper nutrition that was indicated as missing on the assessment. This should include time spent on discussing how proper nutrition can fit the family life-style. This teaching plan should be listed here. A "homework" assignment related to the necessary pattern change should be given. This should involve all of the family members. Make an assignment that has high potential for successful completion by the family.

Proper nutrition promotes physical well-being, which facilitates adaptive coping. Successful accomplishment of goals provides positive reinforcement and motivates behavior while enhancing self-esteem.

- If a homework assignment is not completed, do not chastise the family. Indicate that the nurse misjudged the complexity of the task, and assess what made it difficult for the family to complete the task. Develop a new, less complex task based on this information. If a family continues to not complete tasks, they may need to be referred to an advanced practitioner for continued care.

Promotes positive orientation.

- Monitor family's desire for spiritual counseling, and refer to appropriate resources. The name of the resource person should be listed here.
- Assist family in identifying support systems and in developing a plan for their use. This plan should be recorded here.
- Refer family to community resources as necessary for continued support. (See Appendix B.)

Community resources can provide ongoing support.

Gerontic Health

Actions/Interventions	Rationales
• Refer to Adult Protective Services if risk of physical harm is high.	Provides means for monitoring patient and family and effective use of resources to reduce risk of harm for patient.

Home Health

NOTE: See Mental Health section for detailed family-oriented interventions.

Actions/Interventions	Rationales

• Involve client and family in planning and implementing strategies to improve family coping:
  ○ *Crisis management*: Identify types of intervention to use in a crisis, for example, removing individuals from situation.
  ○ *Mutual goal setting*: Identify realistic goals, and specify activities for each family member.
  ○ *Communication*: Provide realistic feedback in positive manner.
  ○ *Family conference*: Have each member identify how he or she is involved and identify possible interventions.
  ○ *Support for caregiver*: Identify actions that will support caregiver.
	Family involvement and clarification of roles is necessary to enhance interventions.

• Assist family and client in life-style adjustments that may be required:
  ○ Stress management
  ○ Altering past ineffective coping strategies
  ○ Treatment for substance abuse
  ○ Treatment for physical illness
  ○ Appropriate use of denial
  ○ Avoiding scapegoating
  ○ Activities of daily family living
  ○ Financial concerns
  ○ Change in geographic or sociocultural location
  ○ Identifying potential for violence
  ○ Identifying family strengths
  ○ Obtaining temporary assistance: housekeeper, sitter, temporary placement outside home, and so on.
	Changes in family roles and behaviors require long-term behavioral changes. Support is required to facilitate these life-style changes.

• Consult with and refer to community resources as appropriate. (See Appendix B.)	Promotes efficient use of existing resources. Such resources as family therapists, protective services, psychiatric nurse clinicians, and community support groups can enhance the treatment plan.

FLOW CHART EVALUATION
Flow Chart Expected Outcome 1

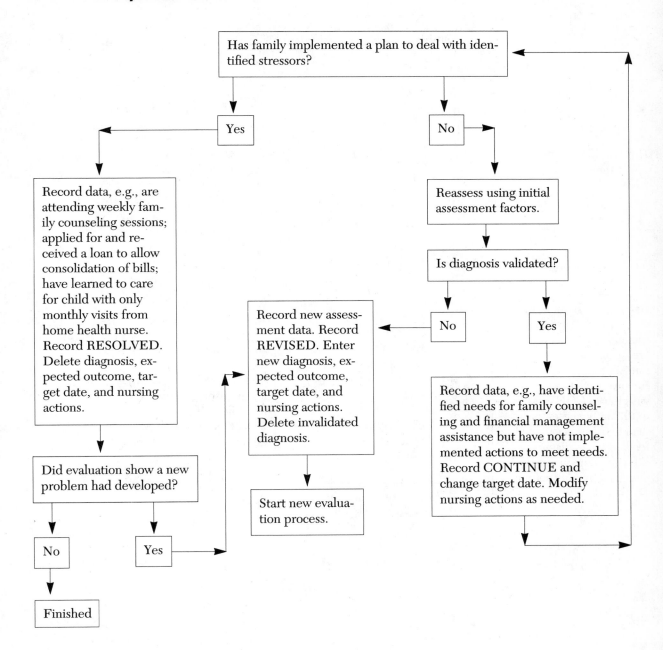

Flow Chart Expected Outcome 2

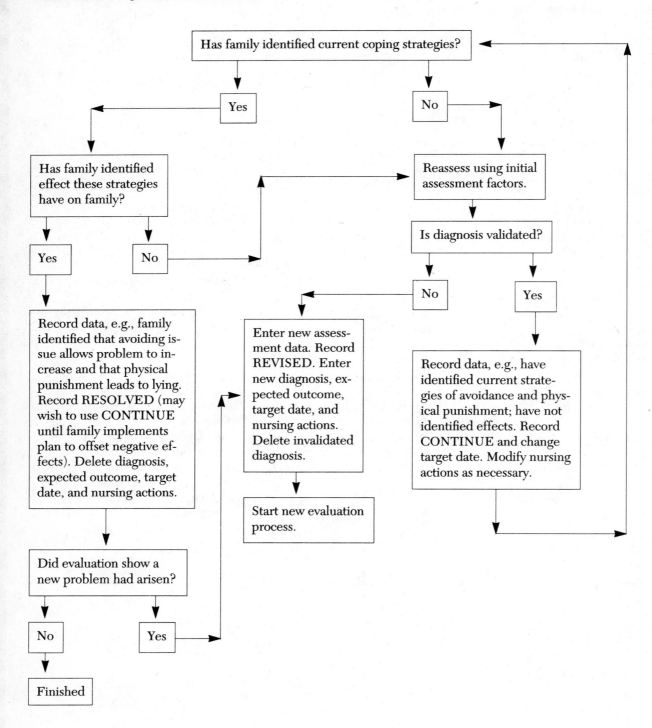

Family Coping: Potential for Growth

DEFINITION

Effective management of adaptive tasks by family member involved with the client's health challenge, who now is exhibiting desire and readiness for enhanced health and growth in regard to self and in relation to the client.[13]

NANDA TAXONOMY: CHOOSING 5.1.2.2

DEFINING CHARACTERISTICS[13]

1. Major defining characteristics:
   a. Family member is attempting to describe growth impact of crisis on his or her own values, priorities, goal, or relationships.
   b. Family member is moving in direction of health-promoting and enriching life-style which supports and monitors maturational processes, audits and negotiates treatment programs, and generally chooses experiences that optimize wellness.
   c. Individual is expressing interest in making contact on a one-to-one basis or through a support group with others who have experienced a similar situation.
2. Minor defining characteristics:
   None given

RELATED FACTORS[13]

1. Needs are sufficiently gratified and adaptive tasks are effectively addressed to enable goals of self-actualization to surface.

RELATED CLINICAL CONCERNS

1. Alzheimer's disease
2. AIDS
3. Any disorder resulting in permanent paralysis
4. Cancer
5. Any disorder of a chronic nature, for example, rheumatoid arthritis

HAVE YOU SELECTED THE CORRECT DIAGNOSIS?

Ineffective Family Coping and Altered Family Process: Family Coping: Potential for Growth addresses the family that is currently handling stresses well and that is in a position to enhance its coping abilities. The other nursing diagnoses related to family functioning address various aspects of family dysfunction. If any dysfunction is present, Family Coping: Potential for Growth would not be the diagnosis of choice. (See pages 710 and 874.)

EXPECTED OUTCOMES

1. Will verbalize satisfaction with current progress toward family goals by (date) and/or
2. Will identify at least (number) community groups that can provide family with useful input and output by (date)

TARGET DATE

Depending on the family size and the commitment of each member to growth, the target date could range from weeks to months. A reasonable initial target date would be 2 weeks.

NURSING ACTIONS/INTERVENTIONS WITH RATIONALES

Adult Health

Actions/Interventions	Rationales
• Provide opportunities for family and significant others to discuss patient's condition and treatment modalities by scheduling at least one family session every other day.	Promotes understanding, open communication, creative problem solving, and growth.
• Include family and significant others in planning and providing care.	Promotes active participation, motivation, and compliance; provides a teaching opportunity and an opportunity for family to practice in a supportive environment.
• Provide instruction as needed in supportive and assistive behavior for patient.	Understanding and knowledge base is needed to adapt to situations; reduces anxiety.
• Answer questions clearly and honestly.	Promotes a trusting relationship.
• Refer family and significant others to support groups and resources as indicated.	Coordination and collaboration organize resources and decrease duplication of services; provide a broader range of networked resources.

Child Health

Actions/Interventions	Rationales
• Identify how the child views the current crisis by using play, puppetry, and so forth.	The impact of the crisis on the child is basic data needed for planning care.
• Identify family's and child's previous and current coping patterns.	Family coping behaviors serve as reference data to understand the child's response and behavior; will also provide needs assessment data for planning of teaching.
• Assist child in identifying ways the current crisis or situation can enhance his or her coping for future needs.	Viewing current situation for beneficial outcomes can assist in a positive outcome.

- Identify appropriate health team members who can assist in providing support for growth potential. (See Appendix B.)
- Offer educational instruction to meet patient's and family's needs related to health care.
- Allow for sufficient time while in hospital to reinforce necessary skills for care; for example, range-of-motion exercises.

Specialists may best assist patient in positive resolution of crisis.

Knowledge serves to empower the patient and family and assists in reducing anxiety.

Learning in a supportive environment provides reinforcement of desired content.

Women's Health

Actions/Interventions	Rationales
• Encourage participation of significant others—spouse, boyfriend, partner, children, in-laws, grandparents, and others that are important to the individual—in birth preparations.	Enhances support system for patient, and promotes positive anticipation of birth.
• Discuss childbirth and the changes that will occur in the family unit.	
• Encourage patient to list family life-style adjustments that need to be made. Involve significant others in discussion and problem-solving activities regarding family adjustments to the newborn: child care, working, household responsibilities, social network, support groups, and so on.	Provides directions for anticipation of birth, and allows more long-range planning that can prevent crises.
• Encourage woman and significant other to attend childbirth education or parenting classes in preparation for the birthing experience.	Provides basic information that assists in easing labor experience; promotes a more positive birth experience and reduces anxiety.

Mental Health

Actions/Interventions	Rationales
• Talk with family members to identify their goals and concerns.	Promotes development of a trusting relationship by communicating respect and concern for the family.
• Assist family in identifying strengths.	Promotes a positive orientation.
• Refer family to appropriate community support groups. (See Appendix B.)	Provides support networks in the community.
• Teach family those skills necessary to provide care to an ill member.	Provides family with an increased repertoire of behavior that they can use to effectively cope with the situation.

Continued

Actions/Interventions	Rationales
• Talk with family about the role flexibility necessary to cope with an ill member and how this may be affecting their family.	Assists family in anticipatory planning for the necessary adjustments that could evolve from the present situation. Anticipatory planning increases their opportunities for successful coping, which enhances self-esteem.
• Provide family with information about normal developmental stages and anticipatory guidance related to these stages.	Promotes sense of control and increases opportunities for successful coping.
• Discuss with family normal adaptive responses to an ill family member, and relate this to their current functioning.	Promotes family's strengths.
• Support appropriate family boundaries by providing information to the appropriate family subgroups.	Promotes healthy family functioning.
• Model effective communication skills for family by using active listening skills, "I" messages, problem-solving skills, and open communication without secrets.	Effective communication improves problem-solving abilities.
• Spend 1 hour with family on a weekly basis providing them with the opportunity to practice communication skills and to share feelings (if this is an identified goal).	Behavioral rehearsal provides opportunities for feedback and modeling of new behaviors by the nurse.
• Arrange 1-hour appointments with client weekly for 1 month to assess progress on the established goals. The need for continued follow-up can be decided at the end of the last scheduled visit.	Provides opportunities for the nurse to give positive reinforcement, and promotes positive orientation.
• Accept family's decisions about goals for care.	Promotes family's sense of control.
• Discuss with family the role nutrition has in health maintenance, and develop a family nutritional plan. Consult with nutritionist as necessary.	Nutrition impacts coping abilities.
• Discuss with family the role exercise has in improving ability to cope with stress, and assist in the development of a family exercise plan. Consult with physical therapist as necessary.	Exercise improves physical stamina and increases the production of endorphins.

Gerontic Health

See Adult Health and Mental Health.

Home Health

NOTE: See Mental Health section for specific family-oriented activities.

Actions/Interventions	Rationales
• Involve client and family in planning and implementing strategies to enhance health and growth: ○ *Family conference*: Identify family strengths. ○ *Mutual goal setting*: Establish family goals, and identify specific activities for each family member. ○ *Communication*: Enhance family discussions and support.	Family involvement in planning enhances growth and implementation of the plan.
• Assist family and client in life-style adjustments that may be required: ○ Provide information related to health promotion. ○ Provide information related to expected growth and development milestones, both individual and family. ○ Assist in development and use of support networks.	Support enhances permanent behavioral changes.
• Consult with and refer to community resources as appropriate. (See Appendix B.)	Community services provide a wealth of resources to enhance growth. Service organizations such as Lion's Club and Altrusa, colleges and universities, and recreational facilities can all offer support.

FLOW CHART EVALUATION
Flow Chart Expected Outcome 1

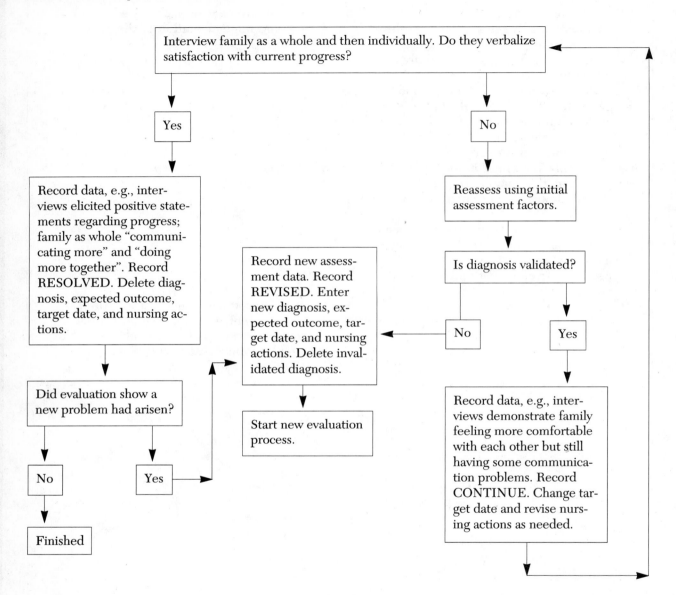

Flow Chart Expected Outcome 2

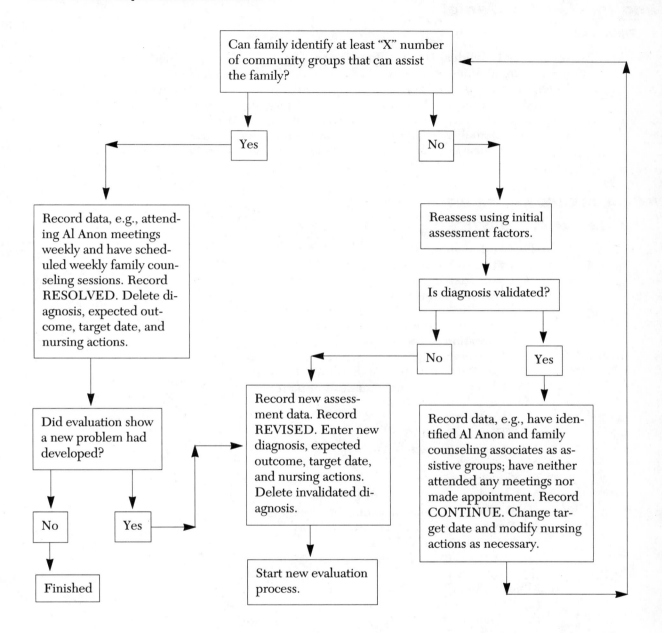

Individual Coping, Ineffective; Defensive Coping; and Ineffective Denial

DEFINITION

Ineffective Individual Coping: Impairment of adaptive behaviors and problem-solving abilities of a person in meeting life's demands and roles.

Defensive Coping: The state in which an individual repeatedly projects falsely positive self-evaluation based on a self-protective pattern that defends against underlying perceived threats to positive self-regard.

Ineffective Denial: A conscious or unconscious attempt to disavow the knowledge or meaning of an event in order to reduce anxiety or fear, to the detriment of health.[13]

NANDA TAXONOMY: CHOOSING 5.1.1.1, 5.1.1.1.2, 5.1.1.1.3

DEFINING CHARACTERISTICS[13]

1. Ineffective Individual Coping:
   a. Major defining characteristics:
      (1) Verbalization of inability to cope or inability to ask for help (*critical*)
      (2) Inability to meet role expectations
      (3) Inability to meet basic needs
      (4) Inability to problem-solve (*critical*)
      (5) Alteration in societal participation
      (6) Destructive behavior toward self or others
      (7) Inappropriate use of defense mechanisms
      (8) Change in usual communication patterns
      (9) Verbal manipulation
      (10) High illness rate
      (11) High accident rate
   b. Minor defining characteristics:
      None given
2. Defensive Coping:
   a. Major defining characteristics:
      (1) Denial of obvious problems or weaknesses
      (2) Projection of blame or responsibility
      (3) Rationalizing of failures
      (4) Hypersensitivity to slight or criticism
      (5) Grandiosity
   b. Minor defining characteristics:
      (1) Superior attitude toward others
      (2) Difficulty establishing or maintaining relationships
      (3) Hostile laughter or ridicule of others
      (4) Difficulty in reality-testing perceptions
      (5) Lack of follow-through or participation in treatment or therapy
3. Ineffective Denial:
   a. Major defining characteristics:
      (1) Delays seeking or refuses health care attention, to the detriment of health
      (2) Does not perceive personal relevance of symptoms or danger

b. Minor defining characteristics:
  (1) Uses home remedies (self-treatment) to relieve symptoms
  (2) Does not admit fear of death or invalidism
  (3) Minimizes symptoms
  (4) Displaces source of symptoms to other organs
  (5) Unable to admit impact of disease on life pattern
  (6) Makes dismissive gestures or comments when speaking of distressing events
  (7) Displaces fear of impact of the condition
  (8) Displays inappropriate affect

RELATED FACTORS[13]

1. Ineffective Individual Coping:
   a. Situational crises
   b. Maturational crises
   c. Personal vulnerability
2. Defensive Coping:
   a. None given
3. Ineffective Denial:
   a. None given

RELATED CLINICAL CONCERNS

1. Eating disorders
2. Substance abuse disorders
3. Psychotic disorder
4. Somatoform disorders
5. Dissociative disorders
6. Adjustment disorders
7. A diagnosis with a terminal prognosis
8. Chronic illnesses or disabilities
9. Any condition that can cause alterations in body image or function

HAVE YOU SELECTED THE CORRECT DIAGNOSIS?

Anxiety Ineffective Individual Coping would be used if the client demonstrates both an inability to cope appropriately and anxiety. If the client is demonstrating anxiety with appropriate coping, then the diagnosis would be Anxiety. Ineffective Individual Coping would only be used if the client could not adapt to the anxiety. (See page 605.)

High Risk For Violence If the aggressive behavior of the client poses the threat of physical or psychologic harm, the most appropriate diagnosis would be High Risk for Violence. If the client's risk for violence is assessed to be very low, then this would be the secondary diagnosis, with Ineffective Individual Coping being the primary diagnosis. In this situation the diagnosis of High Risk for Violence would serve as a reminder to care providers to remain alert to the potential for this behavior. (See page 801.)

Continued

HAVE YOU SELECTED THE CORRECT DIAGNOSIS?—*Continued*

Sensory-Perceptual Alteration   If coping abilities are affected by alterations in sensory input, then Sensory-Perceptual Alteration would be the most appropriate primary diagnosis. (See page 562.)

Altered Thought Process   This diagnosis can affect the individual's ability to cope. If these alterations are present with Ineffective Individual Coping, then the primary diagnosis should be Altered Thought Process. Effective problem solving is inhibited as long as this disruption in thinking is present. (See page 577.)

Dysfunctional Grieving   If the client's behavior can be related to resolving a loss or change, then the appropriate diagnosis is Dysfunctional Grieving. The loss can be actual or perceived. If the client demonstrates an inability to manage this process, then the appropriate diagnosis would be Ineffective Individual Coping. (See page 732.)

Powerlessness   This diagnosis can produce a personal perception that would result in Ineffective Individual Coping. If one perceives that one's own actions cannot influence the situation, then Powerlessness would be the primary diagnosis. (See page 657.)

EXPECTED OUTCOMES

1. Will describe implementation of a plan to cope with the identified stressors by (date) and/or
2. Will return-demonstrate at least (number) new coping strategies by (date)

TARGET DATE

A realistic target date, considering assessment and teaching time, would be 7 days from the date of the diagnosis.

NURSING ACTIONS/INTERVENTIONS WITH RATIONALES

Adult Health

Actions/Interventions	Rationales
• Assist patient to identify specific stressful situations and explore possible alternatives for dealing with the situation by allowing at least 1 hour per shift for interviewing and teaching.	Identification of problem area is first step in problem solving and promotes creative problem solving.
• Help the patient to evaluate the relative success of coping methods he or she has used.	Allows for strengthening of effective coping methods and elimination of ineffective ones. Strengthens and enhances coping skills; increases confidence to risk new coping strategies.
• Monitor for and reinforce behavior suggesting effective coping continuously.	

Actions/Interventions	Rationales
• Maintain consistency in approach and teaching whenever interacting with patient.	Reduces stress; promotes trusting relationship.
• Encourage participation in care by assisting patient to maintain activities of daily living to degree possible.	Promotes self-care, enhances coping, builds self-esteem, increases motivation and compliance.
• Encourage support from family and significant others by allowing participation in care, encouraging questions, and allowing expression of feelings.	Broadens support network; builds self-esteem in support systems.
• Teach relaxation techniques such as meditation, exercise, yoga, deep breathing, imagery. Have patient practice for 10 minutes twice a shift at (times).	Reduces stress and provides alternative coping strategies.
• Assist patient to identify and use available support systems before discharge from hospital.	Broadens support network to reach short-term and long-term goals.
• Initiate referral to psychiatric clinical nurse specialist as needed.	Specialized skills may be needed to intervene in significant problem areas.

Child Health

Actions/Interventions	Rationales
• Establish a trusting relationship with the child and respective family by allowing 30 minutes per shift, while awake, for verbalization of concerns and their perception of the situation.	Promotes communication and allows gathering of data that enhance care planning.
• Identify need for collaboration with related health team members. (See Appendix B.)	Specialist in mental health may best be able to deal with the problem.
• Reinforce appropriate behavior of choosing or coping by verbal praise.	Positive reinforcement will enhance learning of coping mechanisms.
• Assist the patient and family in setting realistic goals.	Realistic goals enhance success, which increases coping ability.
• Provide appropriate attention to primary nursing needs.	Meeting of primary care needs allows patient to focus energy on coping.
• Offer education to provide clarification of information as needed regarding any health-related needs.	Provides basic knowledge needed to avoid future crises; increases options for coping choices.
• Determine appropriate developmental baseline behavior versus actual coping behavior.	Baseline data will be valuable for comparative follow-up.
• Administer medications as ordered, including sedatives.	Relaxation assists in decreasing anxiety and conserves energy to deal with crisis.
• Set aside time each shift (specify) to deal with how child and parents feel about the defensive behavior. This may require art, puppetry, or related expressive dynamics.	Acting out or expression of feelings provides valuable data that increase the likelihood of a successful plan of care.

Continued

Actions/Interventions	Rationales
• Provide feedback with support for progress. When progress is not occurring, provide reflective referral back to child and parent as applicable.	Feedback serves to clarify and allows for review of the specific coping activity, with reteaching as needed.
• Provide ongoing information regarding child's health status that could affect defensive behavior by child or parents.	Factors related to coping may well be influenced by residual effects from illness. Misinformation or lack of information can also be detrimental to positive coping.
• Throughout defensive coping period, monitor and ensure child's safety.	Basic standard of care.
• Determine disciplinary plans for all to abide by, keeping safety in mind.	Structured limit setting will provide security and safety.
• Provide appropriate reality confrontation according to readiness of child and parents.	Reality confrontation helps keep perspective on here-and-now approach to initiate coping with current situation.
• Provide for discharge planning with reinforcement of value of follow-up appointments as needed.	Attaching value to follow-up increases the likelihood of satisfactory attendance at appointments and other follow-up activities.
• Identify, along with patient and family, resources to assist in coping, including support groups.	Support groups provide empowerment and a sense of shared concern.

Women's Health

Actions/Interventions	Rationales
• Identify groups at high risk for ineffective individual coping, for example, single parents, minority women, women with superwoman syndrome, and lesbians.	Provides database that allows for early recognition, planning, and action.
• Identify situations which place patients at risk for ineffective individual coping: unwanted or unplanned pregnancy, unhappy home situation (marriage), demands at work, demands of children or spouse.	
• Assist patient in identifying typical stressors —at home, at work, socially, during an average day.	
• Assist patient in identifying life-style adjustments that may be made to lower stress levels; for example, planning for divorce, planning for job change (either part-time or unemployment for a period of time).	Supports patient in identification and planning of strategies to reduce stress.

- Assist patient in identifying factors which contribute to ineffective coping, for example, depression, guilt (blaming self), assuming helplessness, passive acceptance of traditional feminine role, anger toward self and others (aggressive behavior, suicide threats, substance abuse), failure to make time for self (relaxation, pleasure, self-care).

Identification of factors which contribute to the situation is the first step in learning positive rather than negative skills.

- Assist patient in developing problem-solving skills to modify stressor: using 12-step programs; planning time for self-rewarding activities such as exercise, long quiet bath; and so on.

Assists patient in planning positive actions and in communicating her needs to others.

- Assist patient in identifying negative and positive responses to stressors: pressures at work such as being constantly interrupted, become defensive when challenged, and so on.
- Assist patient in developing an individual plan of stress management: relaxation techniques, assertiveness training.
- Involve significant others in discussion and problem-solving activities.
- Provide a nonjudgmental atmosphere that allows the patient to discuss her feelings about the pregnancy, including such areas as life-style, children, support systems.
- Explore patient's use of contraceptives:[18] birth control pills, intrauterine devices, diaphragm, withdrawal, feminine hygiene products, douching, foams (spermicides), rhythm.

Provides basis for planning life-style options.

- Explore patient's lack of contraceptive use:[19] ignorance; "It won't happen to me" syndrome; guilt ("If I use the pill then I am not good"); desire for spontaneity; excitement created by risk; loneliness; crisis or pressure; uncertainty in sex-role relationships; self-image.

Provides health care personnel information to plan care that enhances likelihood of successful compliance.

Mental Health

Actions/Interventions	Rationales
- Determine client's functional abilities and developmental level for the adaptation of all future interventions. The results of this assessment should be noted here.	Cognitive abilities can impact the client's ability to develop appropriate coping behaviors.

Continued

Actions/Interventions	Rationales
• Discuss with client his or her perception of the current crisis and stressors. This should include information about the coping strategies that the client has attempted and his or her assessment of what has made them ineffective in resolving this stressor or crisis.	Promotes the development of a trusting relationship by communicating respect for the client.
• Assist client in developing an appropriate time frame for the resolution of the situation. Often when experiencing a crisis the individual has the perception that resolution must take place immediately. This could include, as appropriate to the client's situation: ○ Informing client that any difficulty that has taxed his or her resources as much as this one has will take an extended time to resolve because it must be complex. ○ Informing the client that a situation as important as this one is to the client's future deserves a well-thought-out answer, and a decision should not be made hastily. ○ Assisting the client in determining the source of the time pressure and the appropriateness of this time frame. ○ Assisting the client in developing an appropriate perspective on the time frame. One question that could be useful is: "What would be the worst that could happen if this problem is not resolved by (put client's stated time frame here)?"	"Decatastrophizes" the client's perceptions of the situation.[20]
• Provide a quiet, nonstimulating environment or an environment that does not add additional stress to an already overwhelmed coping ability. Potential environmental stressors for this client should be listed here with the plan for reducing them in this environment.	Inappropriate levels of sensory stimuli can increase confusion and disorganization.
• Sit with client (number) minutes (number) times per day at (specify times here) to discuss current concerns and feelings. • Assist client with setting appropriate limits on aggressive behavior. (See High Risk for Violence, Chapter 9, for more detailed nursing actions if this diagnosis develops.)	Communication of concerns in a supportive environment can facilitate the development of adaptive coping behaviors. Continues the development of a trusting relationship. Inappropriate levels of environmental stimuli can increase disorganization and confusion, thus increasing the risk for acting-out behavior.

- ○ Decrease environmental stimulation as appropriate. (This might include a secluded environment.)
- ○ Provide client with appropriate alternative outlets for physical tension (number) times per day at (times) or when increased tension is observed. (This should be stated specifically and could include walking, running, talking with a staff member, using a punching bag, listening to music, or doing a deep muscle relaxation sequence.) These outlets should be selected with the client's input.

Physical activity decreases the tension that is related to anxiety. Appropriate control of behavior promotes the client's sense of control and enhances self-esteem.

- • Orient client to date, time, and place. Provide clocks, calendars, bulletin boards. Make references to this information in daily interactions with the client. The frequency needed for this client should be noted here, for example, every 2 hours, every day, three times a day.

Orientation enhances the client's coping abilities.

- • Provide client with familiar or needed objects. These should be noted here.
- • Provide client with an environment that will optimize sensory input. This could include hearing aids, eyeglasses, pencil and paper, decreased noise in conversation areas, appropriate lighting. These interventions should indicate an awareness of sensory deficit as well as sensory overload. The specific interventions for this client should be noted here; for example, "Place hearing aid in when client awakens and remove before bedtime (9:00 p.m.)."

Promotes the client's sense of control while meeting security needs.
Inappropriate levels of sensory stimuli can increase confusion and disorganization.

- • Provide client with achievable tasks, activities, and goals. (These should be listed here.) These activities should be provided with increasing complexity to give client an increasing sense of accomplishment and mastery.

Accomplishment of these goals provides positive reinforcement and encourages behavior while enhancing self-esteem.

- • Communicate to client an understanding that all coping behavior to this point has been his or her best effort and that asking for assistance at this time is not failure: a complex problem often requires some outside assistance in resolution.

Assists client to maintain self-esteem, diminishes feelings of failure, and promotes a positive orientation.

- • Provide client with opportunities to make appropriate decisions related to care at his or her level of ability. This may begin as a

Continued

Actions/Interventions	Rationales
choice between two options and then evolve into more complex decision making.	
• It is important that this be at the client's level of functioning so confidence can be built with successful decision-making experience.	Promotes the client's sense of control.
• Provide client with a primary care nurse on each shift.	Promotes the development of a trusting relationship.
• When relationship has been developed with primary care nurse, this person will sit with client (minutes) per shift to discuss concerns about sexual issues, fears, and anxieties. Begin with 30 minutes and increase as client's ability to concentrate improves.	Promotes development of a trusting relationship. Discussion of concerns in a supportive environment promotes the development of alternative coping behaviors.
• Provide constructive confrontation for client about problematic coping behavior.[16] Those kinds of behavior identified by the treatment team should be listed here.	Assists client in reality testing of coping behaviors.
• Provide client with information about care and treatment. Give information in concise terms appropriate to the client's level of understanding.	Promotes the client's sense of control. Inappropriate levels of sensory stimuli increase confusion and disorganization.
• Identify with client methods for anxiety reduction. Those specific methods selected should be listed here.	High levels of anxiety decrease the client's coping abilities and interfere with the learning of new behaviors.
• Assist client with practice of anxiety reduction techniques, and remind client to implement these techniques when level of anxiety is increasing.	Repeated practice of a behavior internalizes and personalizes the behavior.
• Provide client with opportunities to test problem solutions either with role-plays or by applying them to graded real-life experiences.	Behavioral rehearsal helps to facilitate the client's learning new skills through the use of feedback and modeling by the nurse.
• Assist client to revise problem solutions if they are not effective. (This will assist learning that no solution is perfect or final and that problem solving is a process of applying various alternatives and revising them as necessary.)	Promotes positive orientation and enhances the client's self-esteem by turning disadvantages into advantages.[20]
• Allow client to discover and develop solutions that best fit his or her concerns. The nurse's role is to provide assistance and feedback and to encourage creative approaches to problem behavior.	Promotes the client's sense of control. Development of new behaviors enhances the client's problem-solving behaviors and improves self-esteem.
• Teach client skills that facilitate problem solving, such as assertive behavior, goal setting, relaxation, evaluation, information	Increases repertoire of coping behaviors and decreases all-or-none thinking.[20]

gathering, requesting assistance, and early identification of problem behavior. Those skills that are identified by the treatment team as being necessary should be listed here with the teaching plan. This should include a schedule of the information to be provided and identification of the person responsible for providing the information.

- Engage client for (number) minutes two times per day at (times) in role playing, problem solving, and implementation of developed solutions. This will be the responsibility of the primary care nurse.

Repeated practice of a behavior internalizes and personalizes the behavior.

- Assist client in identifying those problems he or she cannot control or resolve and in developing coping strategies for these situations. This may involve alteration of the client's perception of the problem.

Increases the client's opportunities for success in early problem-solving attempts. This success provides positive reinforcement, which motivates behavior and enhances self-esteem.

- Monitor client's desire for spiritual counseling and refer to appropriate resources.

Increases the resources available to the client.

- Provide positive social reinforcement and other behavioral rewards for demonstration of adaptive problem solving. (Those things that the client finds rewarding should be listed here with a schedule for use. The kinds of behavior that are to be rewarded should also be listed.)

Positive reinforcement encourages behavior and enhances self-esteem.

- Assist client in identifying support systems and in developing a plan for their use.

Decreases the client's sense of social isolation.

- The following interventions relate to the client who is experiencing problems related to organic brain dysfunction:

Inappropriate levels of sensory stimuli increase confusion and disorganization.

  - Maintain a consistent environment; do not move furniture or personal belongings.
  - Remove hazardous objects from the environment, such as loose rugs or small items on the floor.

Client safety is of primary concern.

  - Provide environmental cues to assist client in locating important places such as the bathroom, own room, or the dining room.
  - Do not argue with client about details of recent past.

The client cannot remember this information. This increases the client's level of frustration, which can precipitate aggressive behavior. Prevention provides the safest approach to aggression.

  - Avoid situations that result in aggressive behavior by redirecting client's attention.
  - Provide a constant daily routine and a homelike atmosphere, to include personal

Appropriate levels of sensory stimuli can increase orientation and organization.

Continued

Actions/Interventions	Rationales
belongings, music, and social mealtimes with assistance with meal preparation. This can often provide appetite cues to the client and stimulate memories.	
○ Provide group experiences that explore current events, seasonal changes, reminiscence, and organizing life experiences.	Promotes the client's orientation and maximizes cognitive abilities.
• The following interventions relate to the client who is experiencing Defensive Coping:	Promotes the development of a trusting relationship.
○ Approach client in a positive, nonjudgmental manner.	
○ Focus any feedback on client's behavior.	Communicates acceptance of the client while providing information on coping behaviors that create problems.
○ Provide an opportunity for client to share his or her perspectives and feelings.	Promotes the development of a trusting relationship by communicating acceptance of the individual. This relationship will decrease the need for Defensive Coping.
○ Use "I" statements; for example, "I feel angry when I see you breaking the window."	Provides modeling of more effective coping behaviors.
○ Develop a trusting relationship with the client before using confrontation or requesting major changes in behavior.[21,22]	Trusting relationship decreases need for Defensive Coping and increases the client's ability to constructively respond to this information.
○ Provide positive reinforcement for client when issues are addressed. (Those things that are reinforcing for this client should be noted here.)	Positive reinforcement encourages behavior while enhancing self-esteem.
○ When client's defenses increase, reduce anxiety in situation. (See Anxiety, Chapter 8, for precise information on anxiety control.)	Anxiety increases the client's use of familiar coping behaviors and makes it difficult to practice new behaviors.
○ Determine the kinds of behavior by staff members that increase client's Defensive Coping, and note them here with a plan to decrease them.	Provides an environment that is supportive of new coping behaviors.
○ Be clear and direct with client.	Inappropriate levels of sensory stimuli can increase confusion and disorganization.
○ If Defensive Coping is related to alteration in self-concept, refer to the appropriate nursing diagnosis for interventions.	High levels of anxiety inhibit the client's ability to learn new behaviors.
○ Reduce or eliminate environmental stressors or threats.	
○ Arrange time for client to be involved in activity that is enjoyed and provides	Promotes positive orientation.

client with positive emotional experiences. Note activity and time for this activity here.

- The following interventions are for the client experiencing Ineffective Denial:
  - Determine if current use of denial is appropriate in the current situations.

    High levels of anxiety increase the client's use of familiar coping behaviors and make it difficult to practice new behaviors.

  - If denial is determined to be inappropriate, initiate the following interventions:

    Communicates acceptance of the client, thus promoting the development of a trusting relationship.

    (1) Provide a safe, secure environment.
    (2) Allow client time to express feelings.
    (3) Provide a positive, nonjudgmental environment.

    Promotes positive orientation.

    (4) Develop a trusting relationship with client before presenting threatening information.

    Trusting relationship decreases the client's need to enlist dysfunctional coping behaviors.

    (5) Present information in a clear, concise manner.

    Inappropriate levels of sensory stimuli can increase the client's confusion and disorganization.

  - Determine which kinds of staff behavior reinforce denial and note them here with alternative behavior.

    Models appropriate coping behavior while decreasing direct threats to the client's self system.

  - Utilize "I" messages and reflect on client's behavior.[17]
  - Present client with information that demonstrates inconsistencies between thoughts and feelings, between thoughts and behavior, and between thoughts about others and their perceptions of the situation.

    Places in question the client's current coping behaviors and facilitates the examining of options and alternatives.[20]

  - Arrange for client to participate in a group that will provide feedback from peers regarding the stressful situation.

    Helps client to experience personal importance to others while enhancing interpersonal relationship skills. Increasing the client's competencies can enhance self-esteem and promote positive orientation.

  - Present client with differences between his or her perceptions and the nurse's perceptions. Use "I" messages.

    Assists client in questioning the evidence that he or she has been using to support ineffective coping behaviors without directly challenging them. This decreases the need for client to use ineffective coping behaviors.[20]

  - Do not agree with client's perceptions that are related to denial.

    Would support and reinforce ineffective coping behaviors.

  - Schedule time for client and support system to discuss issues related to the current problem. Note this time here with the name of the staff person responsible for this session.

    Support system understanding promotes the continuation of new coping behaviors after discharge.

Continued

Actions/Interventions	Rationales
○ Assist support system in learning constructive ways of coping with the client's denial.	Enhances the client's self-esteem and promotes positive orientation.
○ Schedule time for client to be involved in positive esteem-building activity. This activity should be selected with client input.	
○ Provide positive feedback for client, addressing concerns in a direct manner. Note those things that are rewarding for the client here.	Positive feedback encourages behavior and enhances self-esteem.
○ Determine needs that are being met with denial. Establish and present client with alternative kinds of behavior for meeting these needs. Note alternatives here.	

Gerontic Health

Actions/Interventions	Rationales
• Discuss with patient any recent life changes that may have affected his or her coping, such as loss of a loved one, relocation, loss of best friend or a pet.[23]	Recent or multiple losses may significantly impact usual coping skills.

Home Health

NOTE: See Mental Health section for detailed interventions.

Actions/Interventions	Rationales
• Involve client and family in planning and implementing strategies to improve individual coping:	Family involvement enhances effectiveness of interventions.
○ *Family conference*: Identify problem and role each family member plays.	
○ *Mutual goal setting*: Set realistic goals. Specify activities for each family member. Establish evaluation criteria.	
○ *Communication*: Provide accurate and honest feedback in a positive manner.	
• Assist family and client in life-style adjustments that may be required:	
○ Stress management	

    ○ Development and use of support networks
    ○ Alteration of past ineffective coping
       strategies
    ○ Treatment for substance abuse
    ○ Treatment for physical illness
    ○ Activities to increase self-esteem:
       exercise, stress management
    ○ Temporary assistance: babysitter,
       housekeeper, secretarial support, and so
       on.

- Identify signs and symptoms of illness.

         Permanent changes in behavior and family roles require support and accurate information.

- Point out hazards and benefits of home remedies, self-diagnosis, and self-prescribing.
- Consult with and refer to community resources as appropriate. (See Appendix B.)

         Provides efficient use of existing resources. A psychiatric nurse clinician, a family therapist, and support groups can enhance the treatment plan.

FLOW CHART EVALUATION
Flow Chart Expected Outcome 1

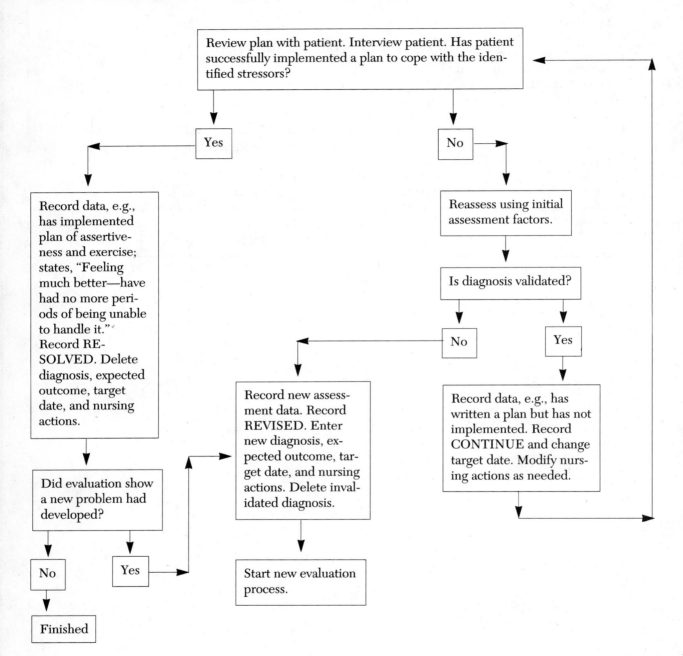

Flow Chart Expected Outcome 2

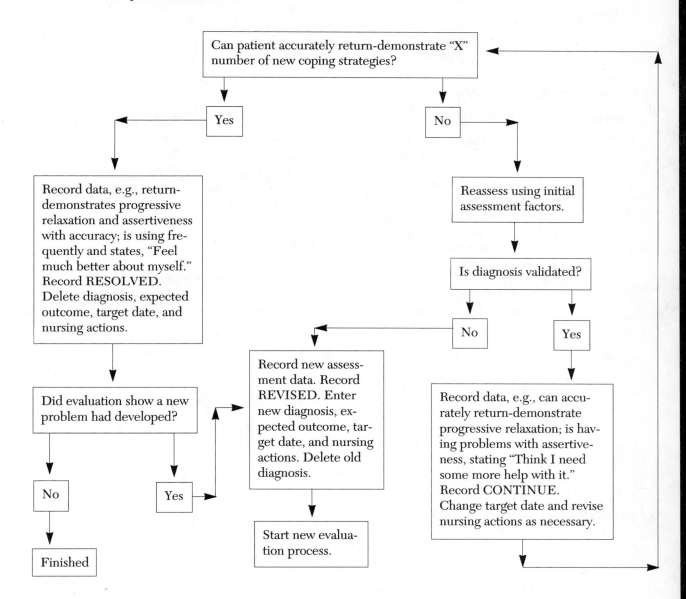

Posttrauma Response

DEFINITION

The state of an individual experiencing a sustained painful response to an overwhelming traumatic event.[13]

NANDA TAXONOMY: FEELING 9.2.3

DEFINING CHARACTERISTICS[13]

1. Major defining characteristics:
   a. Reexperience of the traumatic event through cognitive, affective, and/or sensory motor activities (flashbacks, intrusive thoughts, repetitive dreams or nightmares, excessive verbalization of the traumatic event, verbalization of survival guilt or guilt about behavior required for survival)
2. Minor defining characteristics:
   a. Psychic or emotional numbness (impaired interpretation of reality, confusion, dissociation or amnesia, vagueness about traumatic event, constricted affect)
   b. Altered life-style (self-destructiveness, such as substance abuse, suicide attempt, or other acting-out behavior; difficulty with interpersonal relationships; development of phobia regarding trauma; poor impulse control, irritability, and explosiveness)

RELATED FACTORS[13]

1. Disasters
2. Wars
3. Epidemics
4. Rape
5. Assault
6. Torture
7. Catastrophic illness or accident

RELATED CLINICAL CONCERNS

1. Rape victim
2. Multiple injuries (motor vehicle accident)
3. Victims of assault and torture[24]
4. Posttraumatic stress disorder
5. Multiple personality disorder

HAVE YOU SELECTED THE CORRECT DIAGNOSIS?

Anxiety   This may be the initial diagnosis given to the individual. As the relationship with the client progresses, it may become evident that the source of the anxiety is a traumatic event. If this is the case, then the diagnosis of Posttrauma Response would be added. As long as the symptoms of Anxiety are predominant, this would be the primary diagnosis. (See page 605.)

Altered Thought Process Some of the symptoms of Posttrauma Response are similar to those of Altered Thought Process. If these alterations are present in a client who has experienced a traumatic event, then the primary diagnosis would be Posttrauma Response. If the disruption in thinking persists after intervention has begun for Posttrauma Response, then Altered Thought Process should be reconsidered as a diagnosis. (See page 577.)

Dysfunctional Grieving This is the appropriate diagnosis if the client's behavior is related to resolving a loss or change that is not the result of an overwhelming traumatic event. If it is the result of a traumatic event, then Posttraumatic Response is the most appropriate diagnosis. (See page 732.)

Rape Trauma Syndrome This diagnosis is the correct diagnosis if the individual's symptoms are related to a rape. If the symptoms are related to another overwhelming traumatic event, or if the rape occurred in conjunction with another overwhelming traumatic event, then the appropriate diagnosis would be Posttrauma Response. (See page 821.)

EXPECTED OUTCOMES

1. Will demonstrate return to pretrauma behavior by (date) and/or
2. Will report decrease in signs and symptoms of Posttrauma Response by (date)

TARGET DATE

Owing to the highly individualized and personalized response to trauma, target dates will have to be highly individualized and based on initial assessment. A reasonable initial target date would be 7 days.

NURSING ACTIONS/INTERVENTIONS WITH RATIONALES

Adult Health

Actions/Interventions	Rationales
• Establish a therapeutic relationship by actively listening, calling the person by name, showing empathy and concern, not belittling feelings, and so on.	Promotes trust and open expression of feelings.
• Avoid prolonged waiting periods for patient for routine procedures.	These tactics may have been used by the torturer. Standard care procedures—for example, drawing blood or performing an electrocardiogram—may be perceived as torture because of the memories they evoke.[24]
• Encourage patient to express feelings about the event by actively listening, asking open-ended questions, reflection, and so on.	Provides database for planning interventions.
• Help patient to see the event realistically by clarifying misconceptions and looking at both sides of the situation.	Provides objective view; promotes problem solving.

Continued

Actions/Interventions	Rationales
• Help patient identify, prior to discharge, support groups that have previously experienced the same or similar traumatic events.	Enhances coping methods; promotes use of community resource networks to help meet short-term and long-term goals and advocate for the patient.
• Initiate a psychiatric nursing consultation as needed.	Situation may require specialized skills to intervene.
• Help patient to identify diversional activities to activate when he or she feels he or she is going to reexperience the event.	Provides alternative coping strategy.
• Orient patient to reality as needed.	Helps patient focus on here and now rather than on past events.
• Engage patient in social interactions with nurses or with other support groups as appropriate.	Decreases isolation; encourages communication; provides diversional activity.
• Teach patient relaxation and stress management techniques prior to discharge.	Reduces stress; promotes alternative coping methods.

Child Health

Actions/Interventions	Rationales
• Monitor for details surrounding the incident causing Posttrauma Response.	Circumstances surrounding the event may provide clues as to how the child may be internalizing people, places, and objects as symbols or reminders.
• Allow for developmental needs in encouraging child to express feelings about trauma: ○ Play for infants ○ Puppets or dolls for toddlers ○ Stories or play for preschoolers	Appropriate methods should help to resolve the emotions surrounding the incident and avoid further traumatization.
• Deal appropriately with other primary nursing needs: nutrition, rest, and so on.	Allows focusing of energy on dealing with the crisis.
• Provide for one-on-one care and continuity of staff.	Enhances trust.
• Encourage patient and family to note positive outcomes of experience, for example, being able to deal with crisis.	Potential for growth exists in crisis management.
• Review previous coping skills.	Coping may be enhanced by consideration of previous skills within framework of current situation.
• Address educational needs according to situation; for example, rights of the individual, related follow-up.	Knowledge provides empowerment and enhances decision making.
• Allow for visitation by family and significant others.	Family visitation offers opportunity for reassurance and promotes resumption of daily routines and relationships.

- Refer appropriately for continuity and follow-up after discharge from hospital. (See Appendix B.)
- Provide for diversional activity of child's choice.
- Allow for potential sleep disturbances. Provide favorite toy or security object. Offer adequate comforting by holding infant on waking.
- Provide for follow-up of delayed Posttrauma Response up to 2 years after the trauma.

- Provide reassurance that child is not being punished and is not responsible for trauma.

Continuity and follow-up will foster likelihood of resolution of major conflicts.

Promotes relaxation.

Recurrent nightmares may occur as a result of the trauma.

Delayed response can be noted long after the initial event and must be included in the planning of care.[25]
Depending on the cognitive level and coping ability, the child may associate the event as being caused by something "wrong" he or she did or said.

Women's Health

See Adult Health. Refer also to Rape Trauma Syndrome (Chapter 10) and to the other nursing actions in this section.

Mental Health

Actions/Interventions	Rationales
• Assign a primary care nurse to the client and assign the same staff member to the client each day on each shift.	Promotes the development of a trusting relationship.
• Begin appropriate anxiety-reducing interventions if this is a significant problem for the client. (See Anxiety, Chapter 8, for detailed intervention strategies and assessment criteria.)	Provides the client with increased repertoire of coping behaviors to cope with intense emotional experiences.
• Discuss with client his or her perception of the current situation and stressors. This should include information about the coping strategies that the client has attempted and his or her assessment of what has made them ineffective in resolving this situation.	Promotes the client's sense of control while communicating respect for the client's experience.
• Provide a quiet, nonstimulating environment or an environment that does not add additional stress to an already overwhelmed coping ability. (Potential environmental stressors for this client should be listed here, with the plan for reducing them in this environment.)	Inappropriate levels of sensory stimuli can increase confusion and disorganization.

Continued

Actions/Interventions	Rationales
• Sit with client (number) minutes (number) times a day at (times) to discuss the traumatic event. Person responsible for this activity should be listed here. This should be the nurse who has established a relationship with the client.	Promotes the development of a trusting relationship while providing the client with an opportunity to review and attach meaning to his or her experience.[21]
• Assist client with setting appropriate limits on aggressive behavior. See High Risk for Violence, Chapter 9, for nursing actions.	
○ Decrease environmental stimulation as appropriate. This might include a secluded environment or time out.	Inappropriate levels of sensory stimuli can increase confusion and disorganization, which increases the risk for aggressive behavior. Physical activity decreases physical tension and increases the production of endorphins, which can increase the feeling of well-being. This also provides the client with opportunities to practice new coping behaviors in a supportive environment.
○ Provide client with appropriate alternative outlets for physical tension (number) times per day at (times) or when increased tension is observed. This should be stated specifically and could include walking, running, talking with staff member, using a punching bag, listening to music, doing a deep muscle relaxation sequence. These outlets should be selected with the client's input and should be listed here.	
○ Talk with client about past situations that resulted in loss of control and discuss alternative ways of coping with these situations. Persons responsible for this discussion should be noted here. This will not be accomplished in one discussion; the time and date for the initial discussion should be noted with the times and dates for follow-up discussions.	Increases the client's coping options and assists with cognitive appraisal of past coping behaviors.[20]
• Once the symptoms have been identified and linked to the traumatic event, the primary nurse will sit with the client (number) minutes (begin with 30 minutes and increase as the client's ability to concentrate improves) per shift to discuss the traumatic event. These discussions should include:	Promotes the client's positive orientation.
○ The uniqueness of the situation and the inability to plan for the behavior that might have been needed during this time	
○ Possible inappropriateness of usual moral and ethical standards in evaluating behavior elicited by the unique situation of a traumatic event	Assists the client to evaluate and gain perspective on behavior while moving away from all-or-none thinking.[20]

- ○ Details of the event as the individual remembers them and the thoughts and feelings that occur with these memories
- ○ Meaning of life since the event and the implications this has for the future

Assists the client in attaching meaning to the experience.

- If feelings become extreme, such as rage of despondency, then the client should focus on thoughts rather than feelings about the event.

Promotes positive orientation while assisting the client to review cognitive distortions.[20] Inhibits automatic behavioral responses.[20]

- Provide constructive confrontation for client about problematic coping behavior.[16] Those kinds of behavior identified by the treatment team as problematic should be listed here with the selected method of confrontation.

Assists the client to gain a perspective on the experience and to label cognitive distortions that inhibit effective coping.[20]

- Provide client with information about care and treatment.

Promotes the client's sense of control.

- Provide client with opportunities to make appropriate decisions related to care at his or her level of ability. This may begin as a choice between two options and then evolve into more complex decision making. It is important that this be at the client's level of functioning so confidence can be built with successful decision-making experiences. Those decisions that the client has made should be noted.

Success in this activity provides positive feedback and promotes the client's use of alternative coping behaviors while enhancing self-esteem.

- Provide positive social reinforcement and other behavioral rewards for demonstration of adaptive problem solving and coping. Those things that the client finds rewarding should be listed here, with a schedule for use. Those kinds of behavior that are to be rewarded should also be listed.

Positive reinforcement encourages behavior and enhances self-esteem.

- Assist client in identifying support systems and in developing a plan for their use. This plan should be noted here.

Support system understanding promotes their appropriate support of the client.

- Inform significant others of the relationship between client's behavior and the traumatic event. Discuss with them their thoughts and feelings about the client's behavior. The person responsible for these discussions should be noted here with the schedule for the discussion times. This should also include information about the importance of supporting the client in discussing the event and how this might be facilitated. The concerns the significant others have about their response to this sharing should

Support system understanding promotes their appropriate support of the client.

Continued

Actions/Interventions	Rationales
be discussed, as well as planning for the types of information they might be exposed to.	

• When client develops a degree of comfort discussing the traumatic event, meetings between the client and significant others should be scheduled. Content of these meetings should include:
  ○ Opportunities for the client to share thoughts and feelings about the event
  ○ Opportunities for the significant others to share their thoughts and feelings about client's behavior
  ○ Sharing of thoughts and feelings related to other events in the relationship as they surface as important topics of discussion during the meetings
  ○ Sharing of caring thoughts and feelings with each other
	Promotes the development of adaptive coping within the support system.

• Arrange for client to attend support group meetings with others who have experienced similar traumas.	
• The times and days for these meetings should be noted here, together with any special arrangements needed to facilitate client's attendance, for example, transportation to group meeting place. Groups could include veterans groups, groups of survivors of natural disasters, victim's groups, and so on.	Decreases the sense of social isolation and decreases feelings of deviance. Consensual validation from other group members enhances self-esteem, thus providing increased emotional resources for coping.
• Schedule client involvement in unit activities. Note client responsibilities in these activities here with times the client will be involved in the activity.	Decreases social isolation and provides opportunity to practice new coping skills in a supportive environment.

Gerontic Health

See Adult Health and Mental Health.

Home Health

NOTE: See Mental Health nursing actions for detailed interventions. If family violence is involved, refer to Chapter 9.

Actions/Interventions	Rationales
• Monitor for factors contributing to Posttrauma Response.	Provides database for early recognition and intervention.
• Teach client and family appropriate monitoring of signs and symptoms of Posttrauma Response: ○ Flashbacks ○ Nightmares ○ Survival guilt ○ Confusion ○ Amnesia ○ Constricted affect ○ Substance abuse ○ Suicide attempt ○ Poor impulse control	Permits early intervention.
• Assist client and family in life-style adjustments that may be required: ○ Recognition of feelings ○ Prevention of harm to self or others ○ Treatment of substance abuse ○ Provision of safe environment ○ Development and use of support network ○ Prevention of further trauma ○ Role changes ○ Treatment of injuries	Life-style changes require long-term changes in behavior. Support facilitates these changes.
• Involve client and family in planning and implementing strategies to reduce or eliminate Posttrauma Response: ○ *Family conference*: Identify family member's response to traumatic event. ○ *Communication*: Share caring thoughts and feelings. ○ *Mutual goal setting*: Set realistic goals and specify activities for each individual. Establish evaluation criteria.	Family involvement in planning enhances the effectiveness of the interventions.
• Consult with assistive resources as indicated. (See Appendix B.)	Promotes efficient use of existing resources. Support groups specific to the precipitating event—for example, rape crisis, Vietnam veterans groups—and psychiatric nurse clinicians or family therapists can enhance the treatment plan.

FLOW CHART EVALUATION
Flow Chart Expected Outcome 1

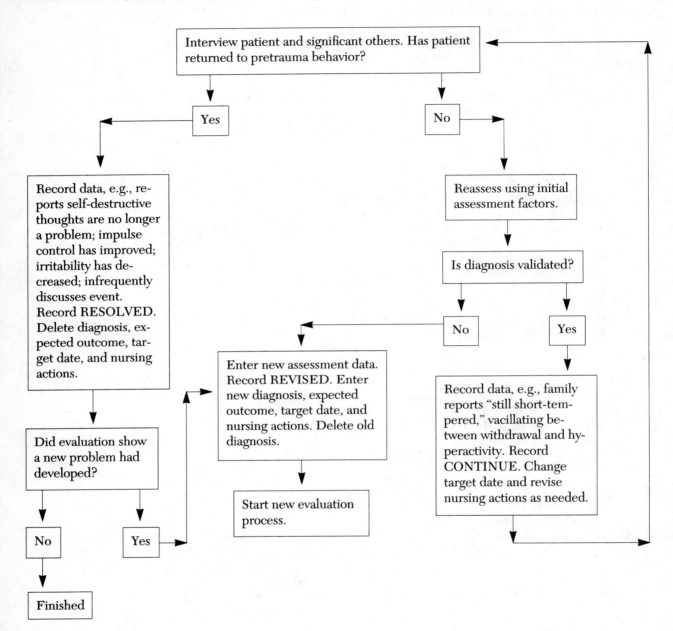

Interview patient and significant others. Has patient returned to pretrauma behavior?

Yes

No

Record data, e.g., reports self-destructive thoughts are no longer a problem; impulse control has improved; irritability has decreased; infrequently discusses event. Record RESOLVED. Delete diagnosis, expected outcome, target date, and nursing actions.

Reassess using initial assessment factors.

Is diagnosis validated?

No

Yes

Enter new assessment data. Record REVISED. Enter new diagnosis, expected outcome, target date, and nursing actions. Delete old diagnosis.

Record data, e.g., family reports "still short-tempered," vacillating between withdrawal and hyperactivity. Record CONTINUE. Change target date and revise nursing actions as needed.

Did evaluation show a new problem had developed?

No

Yes

Start new evaluation process.

Finished

Flow Chart Expected Outcome 2

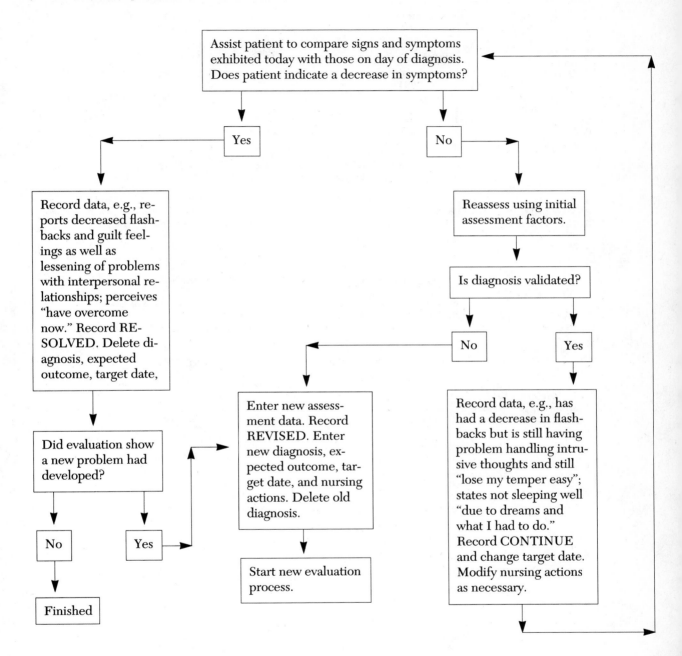

References

1. Sutterly, D: Stress in health: A survey of self-regulation modalities. Top Clin Nurs 1:1, 1979.
2. Gordon, M: Manual of Nursing Diagnosis, 1986–1987. McGraw-Hill, New York, 1987.
3. Ziemer, M: Coping behavior: A response to stress. Top Clin Nurs 4:4, 1982.
4. Frain, M and Valiga, T: The multiple dimensions of stress. Top Clin Nurs 1:43, 1979.
5. Mengel, A: Coping. Top Clin Nurs 4:80, 1982.
6. Davis, L: Hardiness. In Creasia, J and Parker, B (eds): Conceptual Foundation of Professional Nursing Practice. CV Mosby, St. Louis, 1991.
7. Simoni, P: Hardiness and coping approach in the workplace of the nurse. Unpublished manuscript. West Virginia University School of Nursing, Morgantown, WV, 1991.
8. Wagnild, G and Young, H: Another look at hardiness. Image 23:257, 1991.
9. Schuster, CS and Ashburn, SS: The Process of Human Development: A Holistic Life-Span Approach, ed 3. JB Lippincott, Philadelphia, 1992.
10. Smitherman, C: Nursing Actions for Health Promotion. FA Davis, Philadelphia, 1981.
11. Dixon, J and Dixon, JP: An evolutionary-based model of health and viability. Adv Nurs Sc 6:1, 1984.
12. Carter, E and McGoldrick, M (eds): The Family Life Cycle: A Framework for Family Therapy. Gardner Press, New York, 1980.
13. North American Nursing Diagnosis Association: Taxonomy I Revised 1990. Author, St. Louis, 1990.
14. Viken, RM: The modern couvade syndrome. The Female Patient 7:40, 1982.
15. Griffith-Kenney, JW: Contemporary Women's Health: A Nursing Advocacy Approach. Addison-Wesley, Menlo Park, CA, 1986.
16. Wilson, H and Kneisl, C: Psychiatric Nursing, ed 4. Addison-Wesley, Redwood City, CA, 1992.
17. Wright, L and Leahey, M: Nurses and Families: A Guide to Family Assessment and Intervention. FA Davis, Philadelphia, 1984.
18. King, J: Helping patients choose an appropriate method of birth control. MCN Am J Matern Child Nurs 17:91, 1992.
19. Lightfoot-Klain, H and Shaw, E: Special needs of ritually circumcised women patients. J of Obstet, Gynecol Neonatal Nurs 20:102, 1992.
20. Reeder, C: Cognitive therapy of anger management: Theoretical and practical considerations. Arch Psychiatr Nurs 5:147, 1991.
21. Haber, J, et al (eds): Comprehensive Psychiatric Nursing, ed 4. Mosby Year Book, St. Louis, 1992.
22. Stuart, GW and Sundeen, SJ: Principles and Practice of Psychiatric Nursing, ed 4. CV Mosby, St. Louis, 1991.
23. Matteson, MA and McConnell, ES: Gerontological Nursing: Concepts and Practices. WB Saunders, Philadelphia, 1988.
24. Laborde, JM: Torture: A nursing concern. Image 21:31, 1989.
25. Whaley, L and Wong, D: Nursing Care of Infants and Children, CV Mosby, St. Louis, 1991.

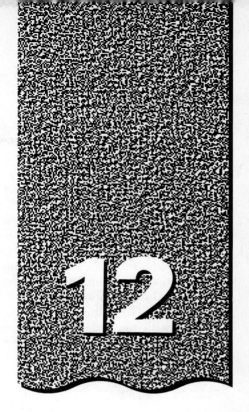

12

Value-Belief Pattern

PATTERN INTRODUCTION
Pattern Description

The nurse may care for patients who, because of health alterations, experience disturbances in their individual value-belief systems. These alterations may take a form ranging from being disturbed to being demolished. These disturbances can be manifested by the inability to practice formal religious directions, such as attending church or following a specific diet, to being totally unable to manage their own spiritual needs and live within a certain spiritual structure. Conversely, religion can affect physical or emotional well-being if the practice of the religion results in spiritual distress. An individual's value-belief system can contribute to alterations in health just as alterations in health can contribute to disturbances in the individual's values and beliefs. The nurse must individualize care to help minimize spiritual distress while meeting the specific needs of the individual patient within his or her value-belief system.

The value-belief pattern looks specifically at how physical illness can interfere with the individual's ability to practice religion and maintain beliefs, values, and spiritual life, as well as how a person's judgment and the meaning of life for himself or herself can affect or interfere with health care practices.

Pattern Assessment

1. Does patient express anger toward a supreme being regarding his or her current condition?
   a. Yes (Spiritual Distress)
   b. No
2. Does patient verbalize conflict about personal spiritual beliefs?
   a. Yes (Spiritual Distress)
   b. No

Nursing Diagnoses in This Pattern

1. Spiritual Distress (Distress of the Human Spirit) (page 923)

Conceptual Information

The faith, belief, or value system of a person can be described as the predominating force (spirituality) that provides the vital direction to that person's existence. This predominating force can be a faith in a supreme being or God, a belief in one's self, or a belief in others. By this, it is conceptualized that each person must find his or her place in the world, in nature, and in relationships with other beings. This faith, belief, or value system is exhibited by the individual in the form of organized religion, attitudes, and actions related to the individual's sense of what is right, cultural beliefs, and the individual's internal motivations.

All persons have some philosophical orientation to life that assists in constructing their reality, regardless of whether or not they practice a formal religion. Spirituality is interwoven into a person's cultural background, beliefs, and individual value system. This spirituality is what gives life meaning and allows the person to function in a more total manner. These beliefs and values influence a person's behavior and attitudes toward what is right and what is wrong as well as the life-style they practice. Many authors[1,2] stress that the nurse must take into consideration not only the patient's beliefs and value system but also his or her own beliefs and values. The nurse must know about or develop resources to assist with understanding the different beliefs and religious practices of groups encountered in practice settings. Further understanding and assessment of a patient's beliefs can be ascertained by asking questions such as "How do you practice your religion?" or "Which beliefs and practices are important to you?"[3]

Studies have shown that the value of specific rituals such as prayer to the individuals who practice them is not affected by the fact that they can or cannot be proven scientifically.[4] As Potter and Perry[2] observe, the impact of values and beliefs is very great.

> When as much emphasis is placed on the symbolic and intuitive as on the analytical, consciousness develops more fully. The expansion of consciousness is what life and, therefore, health is all about and health can coexist with illness and even encompass it as a meaningful aspect. (page 404)

This can be seen in those individuals who consider suffering, illness, and even death as having "meaning in life" or as "God's will."

Many individuals believe that the only value of life, and the source of strength and power, is the will of the individual and that there is no need for assistance from the outside. This focus has been described as "a person's authority within himself."[4] This focus may actually revolve around work, physical activity, or self: "I can do anything I want to when I want to." According to Bayles,[5] there are three dominant indicators that must be considered when judging the value of continued life: mental capacity, physical capacity, and pain. This would indicate that life, in and of itself, is not intrinsically valuable to the possessor of it; instead, it is the quality of conscious life that is important.

In one phenomenological study,[6] the constituents of spirituality, as reported by the study subjects, included the following elements:

1. Realization of humanity of self or valued other
2. An event of nonhuman intervention
3. Receiving divine intervention
4. Visceral knowing
5. Willingness to sacrifice
6. Physical sensations
7. A personal experience
8. A reality experience not easily explained and different from or more than daily experience

Additional research is indicated to describe the experience of spirituality in different stages of the life-cycle.

Another study[7] provides insights regarding the interactive process of caring as it relates to spiritual needs. Trust, meaningful support systems, and a respect for personal beliefs were identified by participants as central to care.

Because of the conscious, subconscious, and unconscious components of the value-belief system, nurses must be continually alert for disruptions in the system. There is a need to be aware that every individual expresses disruptions in spirituality differently.[8] Some withdraw, some become more religious, and some become angry and defiant. Nurses need to be cognizant of the spiritual beliefs and needs they encounter in their patients. This awareness of and respect for the impact and influence values and beliefs have on the patient cannot be overemphasized in planning and providing quality care for the patient.

Developmental Considerations

The geographic, social, political, and home environment in which one lives has a major effect on how a person develops, how he or she will view health, and how spirituality, values, and beliefs are formulated. The values a person holds influence all facets of life. How one perceives the world about him or her, as well as his or her basic philosophy, guides all interactions with others and ultimately reflects a person's individuality.

INFANT

The infant is totally dependent on the parents and those about him or her and is busy building trust or mistrust.[9] Unable at this age to form values or distinguish spirituality, the infant is a mirror image of those about him or her. The parent's method of interaction, communication, and fulfillment of the emotional and physiologic needs of the infant forms the basis for value development.

TODDLER AND PRESCHOOLER

The toddler imitates those about him or her: parents, siblings, and other adults. The toddler develops by mimicking observed behavior and receiving either positive or negative reinforcement. Values begin to form as the toddler becomes aware of others and interacts with those around him or her. Values become known to individuals through the process of social cognition, which begins in early childhood. This arises not from objects or the subject but from the interaction between the subject and those objects.[10]

SCHOOL-AGE CHILD

The school-age child begins to be influenced by peers outside the family structure and begins to question and make choices. The school-age child actively participates in his or her own moral development. Individual reasoning develops through various stages, beginning in the elementary school years.[11] Play is the major mechanism of learning throughout this period.

ADOLESCENT

The adolescent searches for his or her own identity and begins to practice values that are separate and yet congruent with his or her family units. The adolescent is constantly questioning, trying, and searching for the "truth of life" and for his or her identity in the scheme of things. He or she sees values as being black-or-white, with no overlapping. The adolescent is still struggling with his or her own independence and formulating his or her own values, beliefs, and spirituality.

ADULT

Young adults are constantly examining, reformulating, and changing their values, beliefs, and spirituality. Often they completely change the values and beliefs they developed during adolescence, although it is important to note that they often keep the basic values and beliefs they learned during their younger years.

Adults usually strengthen the values and beliefs they have formed according to their life experiences. Adults are continually exploring and trying to see if their value system fits within their life-style. They are busy teaching children the values and beliefs that they want their children to adopt for their lives.

Older adults find great solace in their spirituality and the values and beliefs they have formed through a lifetime. In general, the older adult continues to use the values, beliefs, and spiritual patterns adopted in adulthood.

APPLICABLE NURSING DIAGNOSES
Spiritual Distress (Distress of the Human Spirit)
DEFINITION

Disruption in the life principle which pervades a person's entire being and which integrates and transcends one's biological and psychosocial nature.[12]

NANDA TAXONOMY: VALUING 4.1.1

DEFINING CHARACTERISTICS[12]

1. Major defining characteristics:
   a. Expresses concern with meaning of life and death and/or belief systems (*critical*)
   b. Anger toward God
   c. Questions meaning of suffering
   d. Verbalizes inner conflict about beliefs
   e. Verbalizes concern about relationship with deity
   f. Questions meaning of own existence
   g. Unable to participate in usual religious practices
   h. Seeks spiritual assistance
   i. Questions moral or ethical implications of therapeutic regimen
   j. Engages in gallows humor
   k. Displaces anger onto religious representatives
   l. Describes nightmares and sleep disturbances
   m. Exhibits alteration in behavior or mood: anger, crying, withdrawal, preoccupation, anxiety, hostility, apathy, and so on
2. Minor defining characteristics:
   None given

RELATED FACTORS[12]

1. Separation from religious or cultural ties
2. Challenged belief and value system because of moral or ethical implications of therapy, intense suffering, and so on

RELATED CLINICAL CONCERNS

1. Cancer
2. Severe head injury; brain death

3. Chronic illnesses: rheumatoid arthritis, multiple sclerosis, and so on
4. Mental retardation
5. Burns
6. Sudden infant death syndrome (SIDS)
7. Stillbirth, fetal demise
8. Infertility

HAVE YOU SELECTED THE CORRECT DIAGNOSIS?

Ineffective Individual Coping   Many individuals use religion or beliefs as a means of bargaining in unwanted life situations or denying their role in the situation by blaming it on a superior being. Others will find their source of strength and hope from their beliefs in a superior being or God and are able to live fully functional lives despite physical handicaps. If the patient mentions any of the defining characteristics of this diagnosis, then the primary diagnosis is Spiritual Distress, which must be attended to before trying to intervene for Ineffective Individual Coping. (See page 892.)

EXPECTED OUTCOMES

1. Will verbalize sense of spiritual peace by (date) and/or
2. Will describe at least (number) support systems to use when spiritual conflict arises by (date)

TARGET DATE

Because of the largely subconscious nature of spiritual beliefs and values, it is recommended the target date be at least 5 days from the date of diagnosis.

NURSING ACTIONS/INTERVENTIONS WITH RATIONALES

Adult Health

Actions/Interventions	Rationales
• Assist patient to identify and define his or her values, particularly in relation to health and illness, through the use of value clarification techniques such as sentence completion, rank ordering exercises, and completion of health-value scales.	Clarifies values and beliefs, and helps patient understand impact of values and beliefs on health and illness.
• Demonstrate respect for and acceptance of the patient's value and spiritual system by not judging, moralizaing, arguing, or advising changes in values or religious practices.	Spiritual values and beliefs are highly personal; a nurse's attitude can positively or negatively influence the therapeutic relationship.

- Adapt nursing therapeutics as necessary to incorporate values and religious beliefs: diet, administration of blood or blood products, rituals, and so on.

Maintains and respects patient's preferences during hospitalization.

- Schedule appropriate rituals as necessary: baptism, confession, communion, and so on.

Provides comfort for patient.

- Arrange visits from needed support persons: pastor, rabbi, priest, prayer group as needed.

Promotes comfort and reduces anxiety.

- Provide privacy for religious practices and rituals as necessary.

Allows for expression of religious practices.

- Encourage family to bring significant symbols to patient: Bible, rosary, prayer shawl, icons as needed.

Promotes comfort.

- Plan to spend at least 15 minutes twice a day at (times) with patient to allow verbalization, questioning, counseling, and support on a one-to-one basis.

Promotes mutual sharing and builds a trusting relationship.

- Assist patient to develop problem-solving behavior through practice of problem-solving techniques at least twice daily at (times) during hospitalization.

Involves patient in self-management activities; increases motivation.

Child Health

Actions/Interventions	Rationales
• Support the patient in attaining or maintaining spiritual integrity according to specific identified needs and developmental level. Remember to pay attention to the parental dyad's value-belief preferences: ○ Allow for appropriate privacy. ○ Allow time for self-reflection. ○ Allow time for prayer and practice of worship as permitted. ○ Support the child in expressing feelings about spiritual distress and related factors through use of open-ended questions and providing time for this at least twice a day at (times). ○ Act as advocate for the child and family when they are expressing differing beliefs from that of the staff, institution, or significant others.	Openness affords trust as the child grapples with the meaning of such stressors as illness and death.
• Answer value- and belief-related questions honestly according to patient's developmental level and after conferring with parents.	Sensitivity to needs within legal domains regarding appropriate standards of care honors the child's rights and attaches value to the family's cultural wishes.

Women's Health

Actions/Interventions	Rationales

• Allow mother and family to express feelings at the less-than-perfect pregnancy outcome:[13]
○ Stillborn or infant death:
  (1) Provide time for the mother and family to see, hold, and take pictures of infant if so desired.
  (2) Provide quiet, private place where mother and family can be with infant.
  (3) Arrange for religious practices requested: baptism, other rituals.
  (4) Contact religious or cultural leader as requested by the mother or family.
  (5) Refer to appropriate support groups within the community. (See Appendix B.)
	Allows family to receive religious and social support as a means of coping.

○ Spontaneous abortion:
  (1) Provide patient with factual information regarding etiology of spontaneous abortion.
  (2) Encourage verbal expressions of grief.
  (3) Allow expression of feelings such as anger.
  (4) Contact religious or cultural leader as requested by patient.
  (5) Provide referrals to appropriate support groups within the community. (See Appendix B.)
	Assists in reducing guilt, blame, etc.
	
	Provides information and support for family.

○ Less-than-perfect baby: sick baby, infant with anomaly:
  (1) Provide quiet, private place for mother and family to visit with infant.
  (2) Encourage verbalization of fears and asking of any question by providing time for one-to-one interactions at least twice a day at (times).
  (3) Encourage touching and holding of infant by mother and family.
  (4) Teach methods of caring for the infant, for example, special feeding techniques.
  (5) Teach methods for coping with the stress connected with caring for the infant, for example, planned alone time for relaxation techniques.	

(6) Assign one staff member to care for both mother and infant.

(7) Contact religious or cultural leader as requested by mother or family.

(8) Provide patient with information and referrals to appropriate support groups and community agencies. (See Appendix B.)

Provides support, gives information, and assists with coping.

- Provide support for the woman facing an unwanted pregnancy:
  - Encourage questions and verbalization of patient's life expectations by providing at least 15 minutes of one-to-one time at least twice a day at (times).
  - Provide information on options available to patient: adoption, abortion, keeping baby.
  - Assist patient in identifying life-style adjustments that each decision could entail: dealing with guilt, finances, and so on.
  - Involve significant others and include patient's religious or cultural leader, if so desired by patient, in discussion and problem-solving activities regarding life-style adjustments.

Provides information about choices and consequences of each choice which can assist with decision making. Gives long-term support by providing referrals.

- Assist patient facing gynecologic surgery to express her perceptions of life-style adjustments:
  - Provide explanation of surgical procedure and perioperative nursing care.
  - Provide factual information as to physiologic and psychologic reactions she may experience.
  - Allow patient to grieve loss of body image, inability to have a child, and so on.
  - Involve significant others in discussion and problem-solving activities regarding life-cycle changes that could affect self-concept and interpersonal relationships: hot flashes, sexual relationships, ability to have children.

Provides support and gives preoperative information that assists with postoperative recovery.

- Participate with patient in religious support activities, for example, praying, reading religious literature aloud.

Demonstrates visible support for the role these activities play in the patient's life.

Mental Health

Actions/Interventions	Rationales
• Remove items from the environment that increase problem behavior. (List specific items for each client: Bible, religious pictures, and so on.)	Environment will assist the client in demonstrating appropriate coping behaviors, which increases opportunities for succeeding with new coping behaviors. Success provides positive reinforcement, which encourages behavior and enhances self-esteem.
• Restrict visitors who increase problem behavior for the client. Discuss with family and other frequent visitors the necessity of not discussing the problem ideas with the client.	Promotes the client's sense of control.
• Request consultation from religious leader who has had education and experience in assisting clients to cope with this type of spiritual distress.	Meets the client's spiritual needs in a constructive manner.
• *Do not* discuss with client belief systems that are related to problem behavior. (State specifically what that content is here.)	These discussions only serve to reinforce client's misconceptions.
• *Do not* argue with client about religious belief system or behaviors that evolve from this system.	This would reinforce the dysfunctional belief system.
• *Do not* joke with client about belief system or behavior that evolves from this system.	Protects the client's self-esteem at a time when it is most vulnerable.
• Spend time with client when themes of conversation are not related to the problem behavior.	Presence of the nurse at this time provides positive reinforcement for this behavior, which encourages the behavior and enhances self-esteem.
• Limit topics of conversation to daily activities or situations that do not include religious beliefs.	Environmental structure helps client to focus away from problem areas, thus supporting their efforts to enlist more appropriate coping behaviors.

• Provide activities that decrease client time alone to reflect on the problem beliefs. Suggested activities include:
  ○ Physical exercise such as walks, bicycle riding, swimming, exercise classes
  ○ Group activities such as board games, meal preparation, sports, arts and crafts
	Provides the client with opportunities to practice alternative coping behaviors in a supportive environment.

Gerontic Health

Actions/Interventions	Rationales
• Encourage use of reminiscence to aid patient in examining life.[14]	Assists patient in finding meaning in life experiences and ego integrity.
• Discuss with patient possible sources of spiritual distress, and use problem-solving process as indicated.	Enables patient to identify problem areas and potential correctable measures to ameliorate distress.

Home Health

Actions/Interventions	Rationales
• Involve client and family in planning, implementing, and promoting spiritual well-being through: ○ Arranging family conferences to discuss spiritual values ○ Assisting with mutual goal setting for the client and family to enhance spiritual well-being: personal prayer; interactions with clergy, family, and nurses to find meaning during illness[15] ○ Assigning family members to specific tasks that assist in maintaining spiritual well-being: support person for client, companionship in meeting mutual goals, prayer, meditation, reading scripture, and so on[7] ○ Interviewing designed to provide opportunities for expression of spiritual needs[7]	Family and client involvement enhances the effectiveness of the interventions.
• Assist client to identify factors contributing to spiritual distress, for example, significant life experiences, treatment prescribed by health care team, inability to perform spiritual rituals.	Identification of contributing factors provides the opportunity for planning designed to decrease these factors.
• Assist client and family in life-style adjustments that may be required: diet, environmental changes, hygiene practices, and so on.	Life-style changes require change in behavior. Allows for self-evaluation and supports these changes.
• Refer to appropriate community resources as indicated. (See Appendix B.)	Challenges to one's value system may require long-term follow-up.

FLOW CHART EVALUATION
Flow Chart Expected Outcome 1

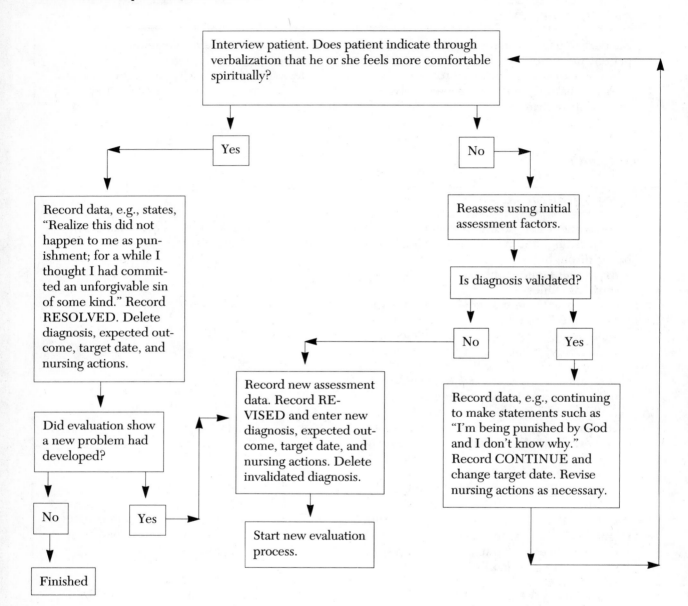

Flow Chart Expected Outcome 2

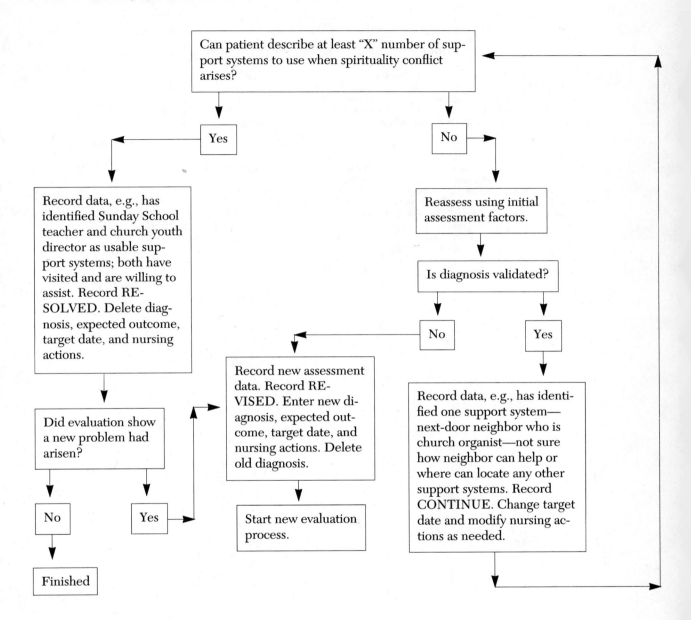

Can patient describe at least "X" number of support systems to use when spirituality conflict arises?

Yes

No

Record data, e.g., has identified Sunday School teacher and church youth director as usable support systems; both have visited and are willing to assist. Record RESOLVED. Delete diagnosis, expected outcome, target date, and nursing actions.

Reassess using initial assessment factors.

Is diagnosis validated?

No

Yes

Did evaluation show a new problem had arisen?

No

Yes

Record new assessment data. Record REVISED. Enter new diagnosis, expected outcome, target date, and nursing actions. Delete old diagnosis.

Record data, e.g., has identified one support system—next-door neighbor who is church organist—not sure how neighbor can help or where can locate any other support systems. Record CONTINUE. Change target date and modify nursing actions as needed.

Finished

Start new evaluation process.

References

1. Gordon, M: Nursing Diagnosis: Process and Application, ed 2. McGraw-Hill, New York, 1987.
2. Potter, PA and Perry, AG: Fundamentals of Nursing: Concepts, Process and Practice, ed 2. CV Mosby, St. Louis, 1989.
3. Corrine, BV, Valentin, M, Norontus, E, and Shirley, L: The unheard voices of women: Spiritual interventions in maternal-child health. MCN Am J Matern Child Nurs 17:141, 1992.
4. Stoll, RI: Guidelines for spiritual assessment. Am J Nurs 79:1574, 1979.
5. Bayles, MD: The value of life—by what standard? Am J Nurs 80:2226, 1980.
6. Burns, PB: Elements of spirituality and Watson's theory of transpersonal caring: Expansion of focus. In Chinn, P (ed): Anthology on Caring. National League for Nursing, New York, 1991.
7. Clark, CC, Cross, JR, Deane, DM, and Lowry, LW: Spirituality: Integral to quality care. Holist Nurs Pract 5:67, 1991.
8. Nagai-Jackson, MG and Buckhardt, MA: Spirituality: Cornerstone of holistic nursing practice. Holist Nurs Pract 3:18, 1989.
9. Erikson, EH: Childhood and Society. Triad/Paladin, St. Albans, England, 1978.
10. Chandler, JJ: Social cognition: A selective review of current research. In Overton, WF and Gallagher, JM (eds): Knowledge and Development, Vol 1, Research and Theory. Plenum, New York, 1977.
11. Kohlberg, L: The Philosophy of Moral Development. Harper & Row, San Francisco, 1981.
12. North American Nursing Diagnosis Association: Taxonomy I Revised 1990. Author, St. Louis, 1990.
13. Cox, BE: What if? Coping with unexpected outcomes. Childbirth Instructor 1:24, 1991.
14. Maas, M, Buckwalter, K, and Hardy, M: Nursing Diagnosis and Interventions for the Elderly. Addison-Wesley, Ft. Collins, CO, 1991.
15. Reed, PG: Preferences for spiritually related nursing interventions among terminally ill and nonterminally ill hospitalized adults and well adults. App Nurs Res 4:122, 1991.

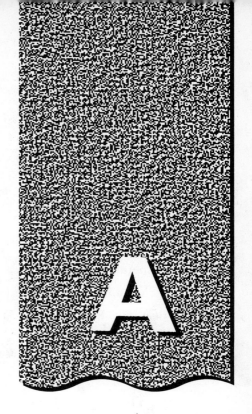

Admission Assessment and Example

Admission Assessment

DEMOGRAPHIC DATA   Date: _____   Time: _____

Name: _____

D.O.B.: _____   Age: _____   Sex: _____

Primary significant other: _____   Telephone: _____

Name of primary information source: _____

Admitting medical diagnosis: _____

VITAL SIGNS

Temperature: _____ F __ C __;   Oral __   Rectal __   Axillary __

    Tympanic __

Pulse rate: Radial _____   Apical _____;   Regular __   Irregular __

Respiratory rate: _____;   Abdominal __   Diaphragmatic __

Blood pressure: Left arm _____;   Right arm _____

                Sitting __   Standing __   Lying down __

Weight: _____ pounds; _____ kilograms

Height: _____ feet _____ inches; _____ meters

Do you have any allergies? No __   Yes __   What? _____

(Check reactions to medications, foods, cosmetics, insect bites, etc.)

Review admission CBC, urinalyses, and chest x-ray. Note any abnormalities here:

_____

HEALTH PERCEPTION-HEALTH MANAGEMENT PATTERN

Objective

1. Mental status (indicate assessment with an X)

   a. Oriented __   Disoriented __

     Time: Yes __   No __;   Place: Yes __   No __;   Person: Yes __   No __

   b. Sensorium

     Alert __   Drowsy __   Lethargic __   Stuporous __   Comatose __

     Cooperative __   Combative __   Delusional __

   c. Memory

     Recent: Yes __   No __;   Remote: Yes __   No __

2. Vision

   a. Visual acuity: Both eyes 20/ __;   Right 20/ __;   Left 20/ __;   Not

     assessed __

    b. Pupil size: Right: Normal ___ Abnormal ___; Left:

       Normal ___ Abnormal ___

       Description of abnormalities: _____

    c. Pupil reaction: Right: Normal ___ Abnormal ___; Left:

       Normal ___ Abnormal ___

       Description of abnormalities: _____

    d. Wears glasses: Yes ___ No ___; Contact lenses: Yes ___ No ___

3. Hearing

    a. Not assessed _____

    b. Right ear WNL ___ Impaired ___ Deaf ___; Left ear WNL ___ Impaired ___ Deaf ___

    c. Hearing aid: Yes ___ No ___

4. Taste

    a. Sweet: Normal ___ Abnormal ___ Describe: _____

    b. Sour: Normal ___ Abnormal ___ Describe: _____

    c. Tongue movement: Normal ___ Abnormal ___ Describe: _____

    d. Tongue appearance: Normal ___ Abnormal ___ Describe: _____

    _____

5. Touch

    a. Blunt: Normal ___ Abnormal ___ Describe: _____

    b. Sharp: Normal ___ Abnormal ___ Describe: _____

    c. Light touch sensation: Normal ___ Abnormal ___ Describe: _____

    _____

    d. Proprioception: Normal ___ Abnormal ___ Describe: _____

    e. Heat: Normal ___ Abnormal ___ Describe: _____

    f. Cold: Normal ___ Abnormal ___ Describe: _____

    g. Any numbness? No ___ Yes ___ Describe: _____

    h. Any tingling? No ___ Yes ___ Describe: _____

6. Smell

    a. Right nostril: Normal ___ Abnormal ___ Describe: _____

    b. Left nostril: Normal ___ Abnormal ___ Describe: _____

7. Cranial nerves: Normal ___ Abnormal ___ Describe deviations: _____

    _____

8. Cerebellar exam (Romberg, balance, gait, coordination, etc.)

   Normal ___ Abnormal ___ Describe: _____

   _____

9. Reflexes: Normal ___ Abnormal ___ Describe: _____

   _____

10. Any enlarged lymph nodes in the neck? No ___ Yes ___ Location and size:

    _____

    _____

11. General appearance

    a. Hair: _____

    b. Skin: _____

    c. Nails: _____

    d. Body odor: _____

Subjective

1. How would you describe your usual health status?

   Good ___ Fair ___ Poor ___

2. Are you satisfied with your usual health status?

   Yes ___ No ___ Source of dissatisfaction: _____

3. Tobacco use? No ___ Yes ___ Number of packs per day? _____

4. Alcohol use? No ___ Yes ___ How much and what kind? _____

5. Street drug use? No ___ Yes ___ What and how much? _____

6. Any history of chronic disease? No ___ Yes ___ Describe: _____

   _____

7. Immunization history: Tetanus _____ Pneumonia _____ Influenza _____ MMR _____ Polio _____ Hepatitus B _____

8. Have you sought any health care assistance in the past year? No ___ Yes ___ If yes, why? _____

9. Are you currently working? No ___ Yes ___ How would you rate your working conditions (e.g., safety, noise, space, heating, cooling, water, ventilation)? Excellent ___ Good ___ Fair ___ Poor ___ Describe any problem areas: _____

   _____

10. How would you rate living conditions at home? Excellent ___ Good ___ Fair ___ Poor ___ Describe any problem areas: _____

    _____

11. Do you have any difficulty securing any of the following services?

    Grocery store: Yes ___ No ___; Pharmacy: Yes ___ No ___; Health care facility: Yes ___ No ___; Transportation: Yes ___ No ___; Telephone (for police, fire, ambulance, etc.): Yes ___ No ___ If any difficulties, note referral here: _____

    _____

12. Medications (over-the-counter and prescription)

Name	Dosage	Times/Day	Reason for	Taking as Ordered
_____				Yes ___ No ___
_____				Yes ___ No ___
_____				Yes ___ No ___
_____				Yes ___ No ___
_____				Yes ___ No ___
_____				Yes ___ No ___
_____				Yes ___ No ___
_____				Yes ___ No ___

13. Have you followed the routine prescribed for you?

    Yes ___ No ___ Why not? _____

14. Did you think this prescribed routine was the best for you?

    Yes ___ No ___ What would be better? _____

15. Have you had any accidents/injuries/falls in the past year?

    No ___ Yes ___ Describe: _____

16. Have you had any problems with cuts healing? No ___ Yes ___ Describe:

    _____

17. Do you exercise on a regular basis? No ___ Yes ___ Type and frequency:

    _____

18. Have you experienced any ringing in the ears: Right ear: Yes ___ No ___

    Left ear: Yes ___ No ___

19. Have you experienced any vertigo: Yes ___ No ___ How often and when?

    _____

20. Do you regularly use seat belts? Yes ___ No ___

21. For infants and children: Are car seats used regularly? Yes ___ No ___

22. Do you have any suggestions or requests for improving your health? Yes ___ No ___ Describe: _____

_____

23. Do you do (breast/testicular) self-examination? No ___ Yes ___ How often? _____

Nutritional-Metabolic Pattern

Objective

1. Skin examination

   a. Warm ___ Cool ___ Moist ___ Dry ___

   b. Lesions: No ___ Yes ___ Describe: _____

   c. Rash: No ___ Yes ___ Describe: _____

   d. Turgor: Firm ___ Supple ___ Dehydrated ___ Fragile ___

   e. Color: Pale ___ Pink ___ Dusky ___ Cyanotic ___ Jaundiced ___

      Mottled ___ Other: _____

2. Mucous membranes

   a. Mouth

      (1) Moist ___ Dry ___

      (2) Lesions: No ___ Yes ___ Describe: _____

      (3) Color: Pale ___ Pink ___

      (4) Teeth: Normal ___ Abnormal ___ Describe: _____

      (5) Dentures: No ___ Yes ___ Upper ___ Lower ___ Partial ___

      (6) Gums: Normal ___ Abnormal ___ Describe: _____

      (7) Tongue: Norml ___ Abnormal ___ Describe: _____

   b. Eyes

      (1) Moist ___ Dry ___

      (2) Color of conjunctiva: Pale ___ Pink ___ Jaundiced ___

      (3) Lesions: No ___ Yes ___ Describe: _____

3. Edema

   a. General: No ___ Yes ___ Describe: _____

   _____

   Abdominal girth: _____ inches

   b. Periorbital: No __ Yes __ Describe: _____

   c. Dependent: No __ Yes __ Describe: _____

   Ankle girth: Right: ____ inches; Left: ____ inches

4. Thyroid: Normal __ Abnormal __ Describe: _____

5. Jugular vein distention: No __ Yes __

6. Gag reflex: Present __ Absent __

7. Can patient move self easily (turning, walking)? Yes __ No __

   Describe limitations: _____

8. Upon admission, was patient dressed appropriately for the weather?

   Yes __ No __ Describe: _____

For breast-feeding mothers only:

9. Breast exam: Normal __ Abnormal __ Describe: _____

_____

10. If mother is breast-feeding, have infant weighed. Is infant's weight within normal limits? Yes __ No __

Subjective

1. Any weight gain in last 6 months? No __ Yes __ Amount: _____

2. Any weight loss in last 6 months? No __ Yes __ Amount: _____

3. How would you describe your appetite? Good __ Fair __ Poor __

4. Do you have any food intolerance? No __ Yes __ Describe: _____

_____

5. Do you have any dietary restrictions? (Check for those that are a part of a prescribed regimen as well as those that patient restricts voluntarily, for example, to prevent flatus.) No __ Yes __ Describe: _____

6. Describe an average day's food intake for you (meals and snacks).

_____

_____

_____

_____

7. Describe an average day's fluid intake for you. _____

_____

8. Describe food likes and dislikes. _____

_____

9. Would you like to: Gain weight? __ Lose weight? __ Neither __

10. Any problems with:

    a. Nausea: No —— Yes —— Describe: _____

    b. Vomiting: No —— Yes —— Describe: _____

    c. Swallowing: No —— Yes —— Describe: _____

    d. Chewing: No —— Yes —— Describe: _____

    e. Indigestion: No —— Yes —— Describe: _____

11. Would you describe your usual lifestyle as: Active —— Sedate ——

For breast-feeding mothers only:

12. Do you have any concerns about breast-feeding? No —— Yes —— Describe:

_____

13. Are you having any problems with breast-feeding? No —— Yes —— Describe:

_____

ELIMINATION PATTERN

Objective

1. Auscultate abdomen:

    a. Bowel sounds: Normal —— Increased —— Decreased —— Absent ——

2. Palpate abdomen:

    a. Tender: No —— Yes —— Where? _____

    b. Soft: No —— Yes ——; Firm: No —— Yes ——

    c. Masses: No —— Yes —— Describe: _____

    d. Distention (include distended bladder): No —— Yes —— Describe: _____

_____

    e. Overflow urine when bladder palpated? Yes —— No ——

3. Rectal exam:

    a. Sphincter tone: Describe: _____

    b. Hemorrhoids: No —— Yes —— Describe: _____

    c. Stool in rectum: No —— Yes —— Describe: _____

    d. Impaction: No —— Yes —— Describe: _____

    e. Occult blood: No —— Yes ——

4. Ostomy present: No —— Yes —— Location: _____

Subjective

1. What is your usual frequency of bowel movements? _____

    a. Have to strain to have a bowel movement? No —— Yes ——

b. Same time each day? No _____ Yes __

2. Has the number of bowel movements changed in the past week? No __ Yes __ Increased? __ Decreased? __

3. Character of stool:

   a. Consistency: Hard __ Soft __ Liquid __

   b. Color: Brown __ Black __ Yellow __ Clay-colored __

   c. Bleeding with bowel movements: No __ Yes __

4. History of constipation: No __ Yes __ How often? _____

   Do you use bowel movement aids (laxatives, suppositories, diet)? No __ Yes __ Describe: _____

5. History of diarrhea: No __ Yes __ When? _____

6. History of incontinence: No __ Yes __ Related to increased abdominal pressure (coughing, laughing, sneezing)? No __ Yes __

7. History of recent travel: No __ Yes __ Where? _____

8. Usual voiding pattern:

   a. Frequency (times per day): _____ Decreased? __ Increased? __

   b. Change in awareness of need to void: No __ Yes __ Increased? __ Decreased? __

   c. Change in urge to void: No __ Yes __ Increased? __ Decreased? __

   d. Any change in amount: No __ Yes __ Increased? __ Decreased? __

   e. Color: Yellow __ Smokey __ Dark __

   f. Incontinence: No __ Yes __ When? _____

      Difficulty holding voiding when urge to void develops? No __ Yes __

      Have time to get to bathroom: Yes __ No __ How often does problem reaching bathroom occur? _____

   g. Retention: No __ Yes __ Describe: _____

   h. Pain/burning: No __ Yes __ Describe: _____

   i. Sensation of bladder spasms: No __ Yes __ When? _____

ACTIVITY-EXERCISE PATTERN

Objective

1. Cardiovascular

   a. Cyanosis: No __ Yes __ Where? _____

   b. Pulses: Easily palpable?

      Carotid: Yes __ No __; Jugular: Yes __ No __; Temporal: Yes __

No —; Radial: Yes — No —; Femoral: Yes — No —; Popliteal:

Yes — No —; Posttibial: Yes — No —; Dorsalis   pedis:

Yes — No —

c. Extremities:

(1) Temperature: Cold — Cool — Warm — Hot —

(2) Capillary refill: Normal — Delayed —

(3) Color: Pink — Pale — Cyanotic — Other —

Describe: _____

(4) Homan's sign: No — Yes —

(5) Nails: Normal — Abnormal — Describe: _____

(6) Hair distribution: Normal — Abnormal — Describe: _____

_____

(7) Claudication: No — Yes — Describe: _____

d. Heart: PMI location _____

(1) Abnormal rhythm: No — Yes — Describe: _____

_____

(2) Abnormal sounds: No — Yes — Describe: _____

_____

2. Respiratory

a. Rate: _____ Depth: Shallow — Deep — Abdominal —

Diaphragmatic —

b. Have patient cough. Any sputum? No — Yes — Describe: _____

_____

c. Fremitus: No — Yes —

d. Any chest excursion? No — Yes — Equal — Unequal —

e. Auscultate chest:

(1) Any abnormal sounds (rales, rhonchi)? No — Yes — Describe: _____

_____

f. Have patient walk in place for 3 minutes (if permissible):

(1) Any shortness of breath after activity? No — Yes —

(2) Any dyspnea? No — Yes —

(3) BP after activity: ____/____ in (right/left) arm

(4) Respiratory rate after activity: ____

(5) Pulse rate after activity: ____

3. Musculoskeletal

   a. Range of motion: Normal ___ Limited ___ Describe: _____

   b. Gait: Normal ___ Abnormal ___ Describe: _____

   c. Balance: Normal ___ Abnormal ___ Describe: _____

   d. Muscle mass/strength: Normal ___ Increased ___ Decreased ___ Describe:

   _____

   e. Hand grasp: Right: Normal ___ Decreased ___

      Left: Normal ___ Decreased ___

   f. Toe wiggle: Right: Normal ___ Decreased ___

      Left: Normal ___ Decreased ___

   g. Postural: Normal ___ Kyphosis ___ Lordosis ___

   h. Deformities: No ___ Yes ___ Describe: _____

   i. Missing limbs: No ___ Yes ___ Where? _____

   j. Uses mobility aids (walker, crutches, etc.)? No ___ Yes ___ Describe: ___

   _____

   k. Tremors: No ___ Yes ___ Describe: _____

   l. Traction or casts present: No ___ Yes ___ Describe: _____

4. Spinal cord injury: No ___ Yes ___ Level: _____

5. Paralysis present: No ___ Yes ___ Where? _____

6. Developmental assessment: Normal ___ Abnormal ___ Describe: _____

   _____

Subjective

1. Have patient rate each area of self-care on a scale of 0 to 4. (Scale has been adapted by NANDA from E. Jones, et al., Patient Classification for Long-Term Care: Users' Manual. HEW Publication No. HRA-74-3107, November 1974.)
   0 = Completely independenet
   1 = Requires use of equipment or device
   2 = Requires help from another person for assistance, supervision, or teaching
   3 = Requires help from another person and equipment device
   4 = Dependent, does not participate in activity

   Feeding ____; Bathing/hygiene ____; Dressing/grooming ____; Toilet-

   ing ____; Ambulation ____; Care of home ____; Shopping ____; Meal

   preparation ____; Laundry ____; Transportation ____

2. Oxygen use at home: No ___ Yes ___ Describe: _____

3. How many pillows do you use to sleep on? ___

4. Do you frequently experience fatigue? No ___ Yes ___ Describe: _____

   _____

5. How many stairs can you climb without experiencing any difficulty (can be individual number or number of flights)? _____

6. How far can you walk without experiencing any difficulty? _____

7. Has assistance at home for self-care and maintenance of home:

   No ___ Yes ___ Who? _____ If no, would like to have or believes needs

   to have assistance: No ___ Yes ___ With what activities? _____

8. Occupation (if retired, former occupation): _____

9. Describe your usual leisure-time activities/hobbies: _____

   _____

10. Any complaints of weakness or lack of energy? No ___ Yes ___ Describe:

    _____

11. Any difficulties in maintaining activities of daily living? No ___ Yes ___ Describe: _____

12. Any problems with concentration? No ___ Yes ___ Describe: _____

    _____

SLEEP-REST PATTERN

Objective

None.

Subjective

1. Usual sleep habits: Hours per night ___; Naps: No ___ Yes ___ a.m. ___ p.m. ___ Feel rested? Yes ___ No ___ Describe: _____

2. Any problems:

   a. Difficulty going to sleep? No ___ Yes ___

   b. Awakening during night? No ___ Yes ___

   c. Early awakening? No ___ Yes ___

   d. Insomnia? No ___ Yes ___ Describe: _____

3. Methods used to promote sleep: Medication: No ___ Yes ___ Name: _____;

   Warm fluids: No ___ Yes ___ What? _____; Relaxation techniques:

   No ___ Yes ___ Describe: _____

COGNITIVE-PERCEPTUAL PATTERN

Objective

1. Review sensory and mental status completed in Health Perception-Health Management Pattern.

2. Any overt signs of pain? No ___ Yes ___ Describe: _____

Subjective

1. Pain

   a. Location (have patient point to area): _____

   b. Intensity (have patient rank on scale of 0 to 10): ___

   c. Radiation: No ___ Yes ___ To where? _____

   d. Timing (how often; related to any specific events): _____

   _____

   e. Duration: _____

   f. What done to relieve at home? _____

   g. When did pain begin? _____

2. Decision making

   a. Decision making is: Easy ___ Moderately easy ___ Moderately difficult ___ Difficult ___

   b. Inclined to make decisions: Rapidly ___ Slowly ___ Delay ___

3. Knowledge level

   a. Can define what current problem is: Yes ___ No ___

   b. Can restate current therapeutic regimen: Yes ___ No ___

SELF-PERCEPTION AND SELF-CONCEPT PATTERN

Objective

1. During this assessment, does patient appear: Calm ___ Anxious ___ Irritable ___ Withdrawn ___ Restless ___

2. Did any physiologic parameters change? Face reddened: No ___ Yes ___; Voice volume changed: No ___ Yes ___ Louder ___ Softer ___; Voice quality changed: No ___ Yes ___ Quavering ___ Hesitation ___ Other: _____

   _____

3. Body language observed: _____

4. Is current admission going to result in a body structure or function change for the patient? No ___ Yes ___ Unsure at this time ___

Subjective

1. What is your major concern at the current time? _____

_____

2. Do you think this admission will cause any life-style changes for you? No ___ Yes ___ What? _____

3. Do you think this admission will result in any body changes for you? No ___ Yes ___ What? _____

4. My usual view of myself is: Positive ___ Neutral ___ Somewhat negative ___

5. Do you believe you will have any problems dealing with your current health situation? No ___ Yes ___ Describe: _____

6. On a scale of 0 to 5 rank your perception of your level of control in this situation:

_____

7. On a scale of 0 to 5 rank your usual assertiveness level: _____

ROLE-RELATIONSHIP PATTERN

Objective

1. Speech pattern

   a. Is English the patient's native language? Yes ___ No ___ Native language is: _____ Interpreter needed: No ___ Yes ___

   b. During interview have you noted any speech problems? No ___ Yes ___ Describe: _____

2. Family interaction

   a. During interview have you observed any dysfunctional family interactions? No ___ Yes ___ Describe: _____

   b. If patient is a child, is there any physical or emotional evidence of physical or psychosocial abuse? No ___ Yes ___ Describe: _____

Subjective

1. Does patient live alone? Yes ___ No ___ With whom? _____

2. Is patient married? Yes ___ No ___ Children? No ___ Yes ___ Ages of children: _____

3. How would you rate your parenting skills? Not applicable ___ No difficulty with ___ Average ___ Some difficulty with ___ Describe: _____

_____

4. Any losses (physical, psychologic, social) in past year? No ___ Yes ___ Describe: _____

5. How is patient handling this loss at this time?_____

_____

6. Do you believe this admission will result in any type of loss? No ___ Yes ___ Describe: _____

7. Ask both patient and family: Do you think this admission will cause any significant changes in (the patient's) usual family role? No ___ Yes ___ Describe:

_____

8. How would you rate your usual social activities? Very active ___ Active ___ Limited ___ None ___

9. How would you rate your comfort in social situations? Comfortable ___ Uncomfortable ___

10. What activities or jobs do you like to do? Describe:_____

_____

11. What activities or jobs do you dislike doing? Describe:_____

_____

SEXUALITY-REPRODUCTIVE PATTERN

Objective

Review admission physical exam for results of pelvic and rectal exams. If results not documented, nurse should perform exams. Check history to see if admission resulted from a rape.

Subjective

Female

1. Date of LMP: ___ Any pregnancies? Para ___ Gravida ___ Menopause? No ___ Yes ___ Year ___

2. Use of birth control measures? No ___ N/A ___ Yes ___ Type: _____

3. History of vaginal discharge, bleeding, lesions: No ___ Yes ___ Discharge:

_____

4. Pap smear annually: Yes ___ No ___ Date of last Pap smear _____

5. Date of last mammogram: _____

6. History of sexually transmitted disease: No __ Yes __ Describe: _____

_____

If admission is secondary to rape:

7. Is patient describing numerous physical symptoms? No __ Yes __

   Describe: _____

8. Is patient exhibiting numerous emotional reactions? No __ Yes __

   Describe: _____

9. What has been your primary coping mechanism in handling this rape episode?

   _____

10. Have you talked to persons from the rape crisis center? Yes __ No _____

    If no, want you to contact them for her? No __ Yes __

    If yes, was this contact of assistance? No __ Yes __

Male

1. History of prostate problems: No __ Yes __ Describe: _____

   _____

2. History of penile discharge, bleeding, lesions: No __ Yes __ Describe: __

   _____

3. Date of last prostate exam: _____

4. History of sexually transmitted disease: No __ Yes __ Describe: _____

   _____

Both

1. Are you experiencing any problems in sexual functioning? No __

   Yes __ Describe: _____

2. Are you satisfied with your sexual relationship? Yes __ No __ Describe:

   _____

3. Do you believe this admission will have any impact on sexual functioning?

   No __ Yes __ Describe: _____

COPING-STRESS TOLERANCE PATTERN

Objective

1. Observe behavior: Are there any overt signs of stress (crying, wringing of hands, clenched fists, etc.)? Describe:_____

   _____

Subjective

1. Have you experienced any stressful or traumatic events in the past year in addition to this admission? No ___ Yes ___ Describe: _____

_____

2. How would you rate your usual handling of stress? Good ___ Average ___ Poor ___

3. What is the primary way you deal with stress or problems? _____

_____

4. Have you or your family used any support or counseling groups in the past year? No ___ Yes ___ Group name: _____
Was support group helpful? Yes ___ No ___ Additional comments: _____

_____

5. What do you believe is the primary reason behind the need for this admission?

_____

6. How soon, after first noting symptoms, did you seek health care assistance? ___

_____

7. Are you satisfied with the care you have been receiving at home? Yes ___ No ___ Comments: _____

8. Ask primary caregiver: What is your understanding of the care that will be needed when the patient goes home? _____

_____

VALUE-BELIEF PATTERN

Objective

1. Observe behavior. Is the patient exhibiting any signs of alterations in mood (anger, crying, withdrawal, etc.)? Describe: _____

_____

Subjective

1. Satisfied with the way your life has been developing? Yes ___ No ___ Comments: _____

2. Will this admission interfere with your plans for the future? No ___ Yes ___ How? _____

3. Religion: Protestant ___ Catholic ___ Jewish ___ Muslim ___ Buddhist ___ None ___ Other _____

4. Will this admission interfere with your spiritual or religious practices? No ___ Yes ___ How? _____

5. Any religious restrictions to care (diet, blood transfusions)? No ___ Yes ___ Describe: _____

6. Would you like to have your (pastor/priest/rabbi/hospital chaplain) contacted to visit you? No ___ Yes ___ Who? _____

7. Have your religious beliefs helped you to deal with problems in the past? No ___ Yes ___ Comments: _____

GENERAL

1. Is there any information we need to have that I have not covered in this interview? No ___ Yes ___ Comments? _____

2. Do you have any questions you need to ask me concerning your health, plan of care, or this agency? No ___ Yes ___ Questions: _____
   _____

3. What is the first problem you would like to have help with? _____
   _____

Mr. Fred Carson

Mr. Fred Carson is a 63-year-old male who has been admitted with a medical diagnosis of hyperglycemia secondary to diabetes mellitus. He was first diagnosed as having adult-onset diabetes 2 years ago.

Upon admission Mr. Carson's vital signs are: temperature, 101.4°F orally; pulse, 98; respiration, 20; blood pressure, 98/70. Mr. Carson is 5 feet 9 inches tall and weighs 230 pounds. He states he has gained 20 pounds over the past 6 weeks. His fasting glucose is 200 mg/dl. His hemoglobin level is 20 g/dl, with a hematocrit of 56 vol/dl. Mr. Carson tells you he regulates his insulin according to what he eats and eats whatever he is hungry for. You find, in interviewing Mr. Carson, that he has been drinking 3 to 4 "ice-tea glasses" of water every hour, stating, "I'm always thirsty." He has been voiding at least once an hour. His urine specimen is dilute and a very pale yellow. Mr. Carson's urine glucose, as measure by a clinitest, is 4+. In the past 2 hours Mr. Carson voided 1500 ml in addition to the urine specimen and his intake has been 500 ml. Mr. Carson says he does not pay any attention to his urine tests—"They're just a waste of time"—but, he adds, "I've been peeing a lot more these past few days. Does this mean I'm not behaving?" Mr. Carson states he was taught about his diabetes but thinks, "They were just trying to scare me. I don't think I really have diabetes. Kids develop that—not old codgers like me. I only check in with the doctor when I feel like it. He wants me to come in every other month, but I think he's just trying to get more money." When asked to discuss what he was taught regarding his diabetes, Mr. Carson relates a high level of understanding of his prescribed regimen.

You find out this is Mr. Carson's fourth admission over the last 8 months. All of the admissions have been because of complications secondary to the diabetes. He exhibits anger upon each admission and refuses to have home health nurses visit him.

In examining Mr. Carson's skin you find that his toenails and fingernails are dry, thick, and brittle. Both his skin and mucous membranes are dry in spite of the amount of fluid Mr. Carson indicates he was drinking prior to admission. His extremities are shiny and cool to the touch, and his legs become cyanotic when they are kept in a dependent position. When elevated, his legs become pale and color is very slow to return when his legs are returned to a neutral position. His pedal pulses are difficult to locate and diminished in volume. He has a 10 cm+ size lesion on his left shin, and you can see that the lesion has begun to impact the muscle tissue. Mr. Carson tells you he hit his leg on a table 3 weeks ago. You note three round scars with atrophied skin on his right leg and one similar scar on his left leg. Mr. Carson describes a sensation of "pins and needles when walking, but if I stop, it goes away."

Admission Assessment

DEMOGRAPHIC DATA   Date: __10-25-92__   Time: __9:25 a.m.__

Name: __CARSON, FRED__

D.O.B.: __6-10-29__   Age: __63__   Sex: __MALE__

Primary significant other: __Wife — Ruth Carson__   Telephone __806-745-5689__

Name of primary information source: __Patient__

Admitting medical diagnosis: __Hyperglycemia Secondary to Insulin-Dependent Diabetes Mellitus__

VITAL SIGNS

Temperature: __101.4__ F __X__ C __—__; Oral __X__ Rectal __—__ Axillary __—__

Tympanic __—__

Pulse rate: Radial __98__ Apical __——__; Regular __X__ Irregular __—__

Respiratory rate: __20__; Abdominal __——__ Diaphragmatic __X__

Blood pressure: Left arm __98/60__; Right arm __100/64__

            Sitting __X__ Standing __—__ Lying down __—__

Weight: __230__ pounds; __—__ kilograms; Height: __5__ feet __9__ inches; __——__

meters

Do you have any allergies? No __X__ Yes __—__ What? _____

(Check reactions to medications, foods, cosmetics, insect bites, etc.)

Review admission CBC, urinalyses, and chest x-ray. Note any abnormalities here:

Fasting Glucose 200 mg/dl; HGB 20 g/dl; HCT 56 vol/dl

HEALTH PERCEPTION-HEALTH MANAGEMENT PATTERN

Objective

1. Mental status (indicate assessment with an X)

   a. Oriented __X__ Disoriented __

   Time: Yes __X__ No __; Place: Yes __X__ No __; Person: Yes __X__ No __

   b. Sensorium

   Alert __ Drowsy __X__ Lethargic __ Stuporous __ Comatose __

   Cooperative __X__ Combative __ Delusional __

   c. Memory: Recent: Yes __X__ No __; Remote: Yes __X__ No __

2. Vision

   a. Visual acuity: Both eyes 20/ __; Right 20/ __; Left 20/ __; Not assessed __X__

   b. Pupil size: Right: Normal __X__ Abnormal __

   Left: Normal __X__ Abnormal __

   Description of abnormalities: None _____

   c. Pupil reaction: Right: Normal __X__ Abnormal __

   Left: Normal __X__ Abnormal __

   Description of abnormalities: None _____

   d. Wears glasses: Yes __X__ No __; Contact lenses: Yes __ No __X__

3. Hearing

   a. Not assessed _____

   b. Right ear WNL __X__ Impaired __ Deaf __; Left ear WNL __X__ Impaired __ Deaf __

   c. Hearing aid: Yes __ No __X__

4. Taste

   a. Sweet: Normal __ Abnormal __ Describe: Not examined _____

   b. Sour: Normal __ Abnormal __ Describe: Not examined _____

   c. Tongue movement: Normal __X__ Abnormal __ Describe: Midline _____

   d. Tongue appearance: Normal __X__ Abnormal __ Describe: Pink; no lesions or exudate _____

5. Touch

   a. Blunt: Normal __X__ Abnormal __ Describe: Responds to touch on all extremities with flat tongue depressor _____

b. Sharp: Normal ___ Abnormal _X_

Describe: Diminished response on left foot

c. Light touch sensation: Normal ___ Abnormal _X_

Describe: Hyperesthesia left ankle and right leg

d. Proprioception: Normal _X_ Abnormal ___ Describe: _____

e. Heat: Normal ___ Abnormal _X_

Describe: Diminished response left foot

f. Cold: Normal ___ Abnormal _X_

Describe: Diminished response left foot

g. Any numbness? Yes _X_

Describe: Bilaterally in feet when walking   No ___

h. Any tingling? Yes _X_

Describe: "Pins and needles in feet" when walking   No ___

6. Smell

a. Right nostril: Normal _X_ Abnormal ___ Describe: _____

b. Left nostril: Normal _X_ Abnormal ___ Describe: _____

7. Cranial nerves: Normal _X_ Abnormal ___ Describe deviations: _____

_____

8. Cerebellar exam (Romberg, balance, gait, coordination, etc.)

Normal ___ Abnormal _X_

Describe: Romberg absent, balance good, does not bear full weight on light

foot

9. Reflexes: Normal _X_ Abnormal ___ Describe: _____

_____

10. Any enlarged lymph nodes in the neck? No _X_ Yes ___ Location and size:

_____

11. General appearance

a. Hair: Brown, thinning

b. Skin: Pale pink, dry, decreased turgor

c. Nails: Toenails and fingernails dry, thick, and brittle

d. Body odor: None

Subjective

1. How would you describe your usual health status?

Good ___ Fair _X_ Poor ___

2. Are you satisfied with your usual health status?

   Yes ___ No _X_ Source of dissatisfaction: "I'm always thirsty"

3. Tobacco use? No _X_ Yes ___ Number of packs per day? _____

4. Alcohol use? No _X_ Yes ___ How much and what kind? _____

5. Street drug use? No _X_ Yes ___ What and how much? _____

6. Any history of chronic diseases? No ___ Yes _X_ Describe: "The doctor says I have diabetes, but I don't believe it. Kids develop that, not old codgers like me."

7. Immunization history: Tetanus _1960_ Pneumonia _No_ Influenza _No_ MMR _Had diseases as child_ Polio _No_ Hepatitis B _No_

8. Have you sought any health care assistance in the past year? No ___ Yes _X_ If yes, why? "I'm thirsty all the time." "Sores on my legs." Four admissions in past 8 months for complications of diabetes.

9. Are you currently working? No _No, retired_ Yes ___ How would you rate your working conditions (e.g., safety, noise, space, heating, cooling, water, ventilation)? Excellent ___ Good ___ Fair ___ Poor ___ Describe any problem areas: _____

10. How would you rate living conditions at home? Excellent ___ Good _X_ Fair ___ Poor ___ Describe any problem areas: "Need another bathroom. We have only one, and I need to pee all the time."

11. Do you have any difficulty securing any of the following services? Grocery store: Yes ___ No _X_; Pharmacy: Yes ___ No _X_; Health care facility: Yes ___ No _X_; Transportation: Yes ___ No _X_; Telephone (for police, fire, ambulance, etc.): Yes ___ No _X_ If any difficulties, note referral here:

_____

12. Medications (over-the-counter and prescription)

Name	Dosage	Times/Day	Reason for	Taking as Ordered
Insulin	Regulates accord. to what he eats	1–3 times	Diabetes	Yes _X_ No ___
				Yes ___ No ___
				Yes ___ No ___
				Yes ___ No ___
				Yes ___ No ___
				Yes ___ No ___
				Yes ___ No ___

13. Have you followed the routine prescribed for you?

Yes __ No __X__ Why not? "I take the insulin, but I don't like the diet."

14. Did you think this prescribed routine was the best for you?

Yes __ No __X__ What would be better? "I eat what I want."

15. Have you had any accidents/injuries/falls in the past year?

No __ Yes __X__ Describe: "I hit my leg on the table a few weeks ago."

16. Have you had any problems with cuts healing? No __ Yes __X__ Describe: "This sore has been here since I hit it 3 weeks ago (points to left shin). These scars are from sores that took ages to heal." (points to right leg)

17. Do you exercise on a regular basis? No __X__ Yes __ Type and frequency: "I used to walk every afternoon, but since I have to pee so much, I can't leave the house."

18. Have you experienced any ringing in the ears: Right ear: Yes __ No __X__

Left ear: Yes __ No __X__

19. Have you experienced any vertigo: Yes __ No __X__ How often and when?

_____

20. Do you regularly use seat belts: Yes __ No __X__

21. For infants and children: Are car seats used regularly? Yes __ No __X__

22. Do you have any suggestions or requests for improving your health?

No __ Yes __X__ Describe: "I want to stop peeing so much."

23. Do you do (breast/testicular) self-examination? No __X__ Yes __

How often? _____

NUTRITIONAL-METABOLIC PATTERN

Objective

1. Skin examination

   a. Warm __ Cool __X__ Moist __ Dry __X__

   b. Lesions: No __ Yes __X__ Describe: 10 cm+ left shin several cm deep; red, three round scars with atrophied skin on right leg; 1 on left leg

   c. Rash: No __X__ Yes __ Describe: _____

   d. Turgor: Firm __ Supple __ Dehydrated __X__ Fragile __

   e. Color: Pale __ Pink __ Dusky __ Cyanotic __ Jaundiced __

   Mottled __ Other: Pink except for legs. Legs are cyanotic in dependent position, pale when elevated.

2. Mucous membranes

  a. Mouth

    (1) Moist __ Dry <u>X</u>

    (2) Lesions: No <u>X</u> Yes __ Describe: _____

    (3) Color: Pale <u>X</u> Pink __

    (4) Teeth: Normal <u>X</u> Abnormal __ Describe: <u>Bridge upper right; good repair.</u>

    (5) Dentures: No __ Yes __ Upper __ Lower __ Partial <u>X</u>

    (6) Gums: Normal <u>X</u> Abnormal __ Describe: _____

    (7) Tongue: Normal <u>X</u> Abnormal __ Describe: _____

  b. Eyes

    (1) Moist __ Dry <u>X</u>

    (2) Color of conjunctiva: Pale __ Pink <u>X</u> Jaundiced __

    (3) Lesions: No <u>X</u> Yes __ Describe: _____

3. Edema

  a. General: No <u>X</u> Yes __ Describe: _____

    Abdominal girth: _____ inches; Not measured <u>X</u>

  b. Periorbital: No <u>X</u> Yes __ Describe: _____

  c. Dependent: No __ Yes <u>X</u> Describe: <u>Bilateral ankles and feet when dependent; legs shiny; no pitting.</u>

    Ankle girth: Right: __ inches; Left: __ inches; Not measured: <u>X</u>

4. Thyroid: Normal <u>X</u> Abnormal __ Describe: _____

5. Jugular vein distention: No <u>X</u> Yes __

6. Gag reflex: Present <u>X</u> Absent __

7. Can patient move self easily (turning, walking)? Yes __ No <u>X</u>
Describe limitations: <u>Does not bear full weight on leg; turning OK.</u>

8. Upon admission was patient dressed appropriately for the weather?
Yes <u>X</u> No __ Describe: _____

For breast-feeding mothers only

9. Breast exam: Normal __ Abnormal __ Describe: _____

10. If mother is breast-feeding, have infant weighed. Is infant's weight within normal limits? Yes ___ No ___

Subjective

1. Any weight gain in last 6 months? No ___ Yes _X_ Amount: <u>20 lbs in last 6</u> weeks

2. Any weight loss in last 6 months? No _X_ Yes ___ Amount: _____

3. How would you describe your appetite? Good _X_ Fair ___ Poor ___

4. Do you have any food intolerances? No _X_ Yes ___ Describe: _____

5. Do you have any dietary restrictions? (Check for those that are a part of a prescribed regimen as well as those that patient restricts voluntarily, for example, to prevent flatus.) No ___ Yes _X_ Describe: <u>"Special diet my wife fixes</u> me for diabetes."

6. Describe an average day's food intake for you (meals and snacks).
   Breakfast: 3 pancakes with low-sugar syrup; juice; black coffee; sausage.
   Lunch: Sandwich; milk or sugar-free soft drink; potato chips; fruit; "sometimes a little cake or pie." *Dinner:* Casserole; iced tea; rolls with butter; vegetables; and dessert: "Sure do like my ice cream." *Snacks:* Cookies and juice.

7. Describe an average day's fluid intake for you. <u>"I drink all the time." At least</u> 4 large glasses per hour

8. Describe food likes and dislikes: <u>*Likes:* Meat, desserts, and potatoes. *Dislikes:*</u> Vegetables, low-sugar "stuff."

9. Would you like to: Gain weight? ___ Lose weight? _X_ Neither ___

10. Any problems with:
    a. Nausea: No _X_ Yes ___ Describe: _____
    b. Vomiting: No _X_ Yes ___ Describe: _____
    c. Swallowing: No _X_ Yes ___ Describe: _____
    d. Chewing: No _X_ Yes ___ Describe: _____
    e. Indigestion: No _X_ Yes ___ Describe: _____

11. Would you describe your usual life-style as: Active ___ Sedate _X_

For breast-feeding mothers only:

12. Do you have any concerns about breast-feeding? No ___ Yes ___
    Describe: _____

13. Are you having any problems with breast-feeding? No ___ Yes ___

Describe: _____

ELIMINATION PATTERN

Objective

1. Auscultate abdomen:

 a. Bowel sounds: Normal <u>X</u> Increased ___ Decreased ___ Absent ___

2. Palpate abdomen:

 a. Tender: No <u>X</u> Yes ___ Where? _____

 b. Soft: No ___ Yes <u>X</u>; Firm: No <u>X</u> Yes ___

 c. Masses: No <u>X</u> Yes ___ Describe: _____

 d. Distention (include distended bladder): No <u>X</u> Yes ___ Describe: _____

 _____

 e. Overflow urine when bladder palpated? Yes ___ No <u>X</u>

3. Rectal exam:

 a. Sphincter tone: Describe: <u>Within normal limits</u>

 b. Hemorrhoids: No <u>X</u> Yes ___ Describe: _____

 c. Stool in rectum: No ___ Yes <u>X</u> Describe: <u>Heme negative</u>

 d. Impaction: No <u>X</u> Yes ___ Describe: _____

 e. Occult blood: No <u>X</u> Yes ___

4. Ostomy present: No <u>X</u> Yes ___ Location: _____

Subjective

1. What is your usual frequency of bowel movements? <u>About 3 times per week</u>

 a. Have to strain to have a bowel movement? No <u>X</u> Yes ___

 b. Same time each day? No <u>X</u> Yes ___

2. Has the number of bowel movements changed in the past week? No <u>X</u> Yes ___

 Increased? ___ Decreased? ___

3. Character of stool:

 a. Consistency: Hard ___ Soft <u>X</u> Liquid ___

 b. Color: Brown <u>X</u> Black ___ Yellow ___ Clay-colored ___

 c. Bleeding with bowel movements: No <u>X</u> Yes ___

4. History of constipation: No <u>X</u> Yes ___ How often? ___

 Do you use bowel movement aids (laxatives, suppositories, diet)? No <u>X</u> Yes ___

 Describe: _____

5. History of diarrhea: No $\underline{X}$ Yes ___ When? _____

6. History of incontinence: No $\underline{X}$ Yes ___ Related to increased abdominal pressure (coughing, laughing, sneezing)? No ___ Yes ___

7. History of recent travel: No $\underline{X}$ Yes ___ Where? _____

8. Usual voiding pattern:

   a. Frequency (times per day): <u>For past 3 days, 3 to 4 times per hour</u>

      Decreased? ___ Increased? $\underline{X}$

   b. Change in awareness of need to void: No ___ Yes $\underline{X}$

      Increased? $\underline{X}$ Decreased? ___

   c. Change in urge to void: No ___ Yes $\underline{X}$ Increased? $\underline{X}$ Decreased? ___

   d. Any change in amount: No ___ Yes $\underline{X}$ Increased? $\underline{X}$ Decreased? ___

   e. Color: Yellow <u>Very pale</u> Smokey ___ Dark ___

   f. Incontinence: No ___ Yes $\underline{X}$ When? <u>"If too far from bathroom."</u>

      Difficulty holding voiding when urge to void develops: No ___ Yes $\underline{X}$

      Have time to get to bathroom: Yes ___ No $\underline{X}$ How often does problem

      reaching bathroom occur? <u>Every voiding</u>

   g. Retention: No $\underline{X}$ Yes ___ Describe: _____

   h. Pain/burning: No $\underline{X}$ Yes ___ Describe: _____

   i. Sensation of bladder spasms: No $\underline{X}$ Yes ___ When? _____

ACTIVITY-EXERCISE PATTERN

Objective

1. Cardiovascular

   a. Cyanosis: No ___ Yes $\underline{X}$ Where? <u>Legs when dependent</u>

   b. Pulses: Easily palpable?

      Carotid: Yes $\underline{X}$ No ___; Jugular: Yes $\underline{X}$ No ___; Temporal: Yes $\underline{X}$ No ___; Radial: Yes $\underline{X}$ No ___; Femoral: Yes $\underline{X}$ No ___; Popliteal: Yes $\underline{X}$ No ___; Posttibial: Yes ___ No $\underline{X}$; Dorsalis pedis: Yes ___ No $\underline{X}$

   c. Extremities:

      (1) Temperature: Cold ___ Cool $\underline{X}$ Warm ___ Hot ___

      (2) Capillary refill: Normal ___ Delayed $\underline{X}$

      (3) Color: Pink ___ Pale $\underline{X}$ Cyanotic $\underline{X}$ Other ___

         Describe: <u>Pale when raised; cyanotic when dependent</u>

      (4) Homan's sign: No $\underline{X}$ Yes ___

(5) Nails: Normal ___ Abnormal _X_ Describe: <u>Toenails and fingernails</u> <u>dry, thick, brittle</u>

(6) Hair distribution: Normal _X_ Abnormal ___ Describe: _____

(7) Claudication: No ___ Yes _X_ Describe: <u>Numbness and tingling in feet</u>

d. Heart: PMI location <u>4th ICS LCL</u>

   (1) Abnormal rhythm: No _X_ Yes ___ Describe: _____

   (2) Abnormal sounds: No _X_ Yes ___ Describe: _____

2. Respiratory

  a. Rate: <u>20/min</u> Depth: Shallow ___ Deep _X_ Abdominal ___ Diaphragmatic _X_

  b. Have patient cough. Any sputum? No _X_ Yes ___ Describe: _____

  c. Fremitus: No _X_ Yes ___

  d. Any chest excursion: No _X_ Yes ___ Equal ___ Unequal ___

  e. Auscultate chest:

   (1) Any abnormal sounds (rales, rhonchi)? No _X_ Yes ___

    Describe: _____

  f. Have patient walk in place for 3 minutes (if permissible):

   (1) Any shortness of breath after activity? No _X_ Yes ___

   (2) Any dyspnea? No _X_ Yes ___

   (3) BP after activity: <u>108</u> / <u>74</u> in (right/<u>left</u>) arm

   (4) Respiratory rate after activity: <u>25</u>

   (5) Pulse rate after activity: <u>110</u>

3. Musculoskeletal

  a. Range of motion: Normal ___ Limited _X_ Describe: <u>Limited in lower</u> <u>extremities</u>

  b. Gait: Normal ___ Abnormal _X_ Describe: <u>Does not bear full weight on</u> <u>left ankle</u>

  c. Balance: Normal _X_ Abnormal ___ Describe: _____

  d. Muscle mass/strength: Normal ___ Increased ___ Decreased _X_ Describe: <u>Atrophy in both legs, especially in area of wounds</u>

    e. Hand grasp: Right: Normal <u>X</u> Decreased __

                   Left: Normal <u>X</u> Decreased __

    f. Toe wiggle: Right: Normal <u>X</u> Decreased __

                   Left: Normal <u>X</u> Decreased __

    g. Posture: Normal <u>X</u> Kyphosis __ Lordosis __

    h. Deformities: No <u>X</u> Yes __ Describe: _____

    i. Missing limbs: No <u>X</u> Yes __ Where? _____

    j. Uses mobility aids (walker, crutches, etc.)? No <u>X</u> Yes __ Describe: ____

    _____

    k. Tremors: No <u>X</u> Yes __ Describe: _____

    l. Traction or casts present: No <u>X</u> Yes __ Describe: _____

4. Spinal cord injury: No <u>X</u> Yes __ Level: _____

5. Paralysis present: No <u>X</u> Yes __ Where? _____

6. Developmental assessment: Normal __ Abnormal __ Describe: <u>not done</u>

Subjective

1. Have patient rate each area of self-care on a scale of 0 to 4. (Scale has been adapted by NANDA from E. Jones, et al., Patient Classification for Long-Term Care: Users' Manual. HEW Publication No. HRA-74-3107, November 1974.)

    0 = Completely independent

    1 = Requires use of equipment or device

    2 = Requires help from another person for assistance, supervision, or teaching

    3 = Requires help from another person and equipment device

    4 = Dependent, does not participte in activity

    Feeding <u>0</u>; Bathing/hygiene <u>0</u>; Dressing/grooming <u>0</u>; Toileting <u>0</u>; Ambulation <u>0</u>; Care of home <u>Wife</u>; Shopping <u>Wife</u>; Meal preparation <u>Wife</u>; Laundry <u>Wife</u>; Transportation <u>0</u>.

2. Oxygen use at home: No <u>X</u> Yes __ Describe: _____

3. How many pillows do you use to sleep on? <u>1</u>.

4. Do you frequently experience fatigue? No __ Yes <u>X</u> Describe: <u>"I'm tired after going to the bathroom so much."</u>

5. How many stairs can you climb without experiencing any difficulty (can be individual number or number of flights)? <u>1 flight</u>

6. How far can you walk without experiencing any difficulty? <u>1 block. "My foot hurts if I try to walk too far."</u>

7. Has assistance at home for self-care and maintenance of home: No __ Yes <u>X</u> Who? <u>Wife</u>. If No, would like to

have or believes needs to have assistance: No ___ Yes ___ With what
activities? _____

8. Occupation (if retired, former occupation): <u>Mail carrier</u>

9. Describe your usual leisure time activities/hobbies: <u>Gardening, fishing,</u>
<u>reading</u>

10. Any complaints of weakness or lack of energy? No ___ Yes <u>X</u> Describe:
<u>Going to bathroom so much "wears me out"</u>

11. Any difficulties in maintaining activities of daily living? No ___ Yes <u>X</u> Describe: <u>"All I do is drink and pee."</u>

12. Any problems with concentration? No <u>X</u> Yes ___ Describe: _____
_____

SLEEP-REST PATTERN

Objective

None.

Subjective

1. Usual sleep habits: Hours per night <u>6</u>; Naps: No ___ Yes <u>X</u> a.m. ___
p.m. <u>X</u> Feel rested? Yes <u>X</u> No ___ Describe: _____

2. Any problems:
   a. Difficulty going to sleep? No <u>X</u> Yes ___
   b. Awakening during night? No ___ Yes <u>X (to go to bathroom)</u>
   c. Early awakening? No <u>X</u> Yes ___
   d. Insomnia? No <u>X</u> Yes ___ Describe: _____

3. Methods used to promote sleep: Medication No <u>X</u> Yes ___ Name: _____;
Warm fluids No <u>X</u> Yes ___ What? _____; Relaxation
techniques: No <u>X</u> Yes ___ Describe: _____

COGNITIVE-PERCEPTUAL PATTERN

Objective

1. Review sensory and mental status completed in Health Perception-Health Management Pattern.

2. Any overt signs of pain? No ___ Yes <u>X</u> Describe: <u>Winces when tries to bear</u>
<u>weight on left leg</u>

Subjective

1. Pain

   a. Location (have patient point to area): <u>Left shin</u>

   b. Intensity (have patient rank on scale of 0 to 10): <u>5</u>

   c. Radiation: No ___ Yes <u>X</u> To where? <u>Up leg</u>

   d. Timing (how often; related to any specific events) <u>"Aches all the time"; increased pain with walking or if touch wound</u>

   e. Duration: <u>As above</u>

   f. What done to relieve at home? <u>Elevate, take an Advil</u>

   g. When did pain begin? <u>"Two weeks ago"</u>

2. Decision making

   a. Decision making is: Easy <u>X</u> Moderately easy ___ Moderately difficult ___ Difficult ___

   b. Inclined to make decisions: Rapidly <u>X</u> Slowly ___ Delay ___

3. Knowledge level

   a. Can define what current problem is: Yes <u>X</u> No ___

   b. Can restate current therapeutic regimen: Yes <u>X</u> No ___

SELF-PERCEPTION AND SELF-CONCEPT PATTERN

Objective

1. During this assessment patient appears: Calm ___ Anxious ___ Irritable <u>X</u> Withdrawn ___ Restless ___

2. Did any physiologic parameters change? Face reddened: No <u>X</u> Yes ___; Voice volume changed: No <u>X</u> Yes ___ Louder ___ Softer ___; Voice quality changed: No <u>X</u> Yes ___ Quavering ___ Hesitation ___ Other: _____

3. Body language observed: <u>Guards left shin</u>

4. Is current admission going to result in a body structure or function change for the patient? No ___ Yes ___ Unsure at this time <u>X</u>

Subjective

1. What is your major concern at the current time? <u>"I'm tired of doing nothing but drinking and peeing."</u>

2. Do you think this admission will cause any life-style changes for you? No __ Yes _X_ What? "Help me get better" _____

3. Do you think this admission will result in any body changes for you? No __ Yes _X_ What? "Heal my leg" _____

4. My usual view of myself is: Positive _X_ Neutral __ Somewhat negative __

5. Do you believe you will have any problems dealing with your current health situation? No _X_ Yes __ Describe: _____

6. On a scale of 0 to 5 rank your perception of your level of control in this situation: _4_

7. On a scale of 0 to 5 rank your usual assertiveness level: _5_

ROLE-RELATIONSHIP PATTERN

Objective

1. Speech pattern
   a. Is English the patient's native language? Yes _X_ No __ Native language is: _____ Interpreter needed: No _X_ Yes __
   b. During interview have you noted any speech problems? No _X_ Yes __ Describe: _____

2. Family interaction
   a. During interview have you observed any dysfunctional family interactions? No _X_ Yes __ Describe: _____
   b. If patient is a child, is there any physical or emotional evidence of physical or psychosocial abuse? No __ Yes __ Describe: _____

Subjective

1. Does patient live alone? Yes __ No _X_ With whom? Wife _____

2. Is patient married: Yes _X_ No __ Children? No _X_ Yes __ Ages of children: _____

3. How would you rate your parenting skills? Not applicable _X_ No difficulty with __ Average __ Some difficulty with __ Describe: _____

4. Any losses (physical, psychologic, social) in past year? No __ Yes _X_ Describe: Early retirement _____

5. How is patient handling this loss at this time? <u>"Doing fine, just need to get feet in shape so I can do what I want to now that I have the time."</u>

6. Do you believe this admission will result in any type of loss? No <u>X</u> Yes __ Describe: _____

7. Ask both patient and family: Do you think this admission will cause any significant changes in (the patient's) usual family role? No <u>X</u> Yes __ Describe:

_____

8. How would you rate your usual social activities? Very active __ Active <u>X</u> Limited __ None __

9. How would you rate your comfort in social situations? Comfortable <u>X</u> Uncomfortable __

10. What activities or jobs do you like to do? Describe: <u>Gardening, fishing, playing cards and dominoes, reading</u>

11. What activities or jobs do you dislike doing? Describe: <u>Any housework or cooking and having to pee all the time</u>

SEXUALITY-REPRODUCTIVE PATTERN

Objective

Review admission physical exam for results of pelvic and rectal exams. If results not documented nurse should perform exams. Check history to see if admission resulted from a rape.

Subjective

Female

1. Date of LMP: ____ Any pregnancies? Para __ Gravida __ Menopause? No __ Yes __ Year ____

2. Use birth control measures? No __ N/A __ Yes __ Type: _____

3. History of vaginal discharge, bleeding, lesions: No __ Yes __ Discharge:

_____

4. Pap smear annually: Yes __ No __ Date of last Pap smear _____

5. Date of last mammogram: _____

6. History of sexually transmitted disease: No __ Yes __ Describe: _____

_____

If admission is secondary to rape:

7. Is patient describing numerous physical symptoms? No ___ Yes ___

   Describe: _____

8. Is patient exhibiting numerous emotional reactions? No ___ Yes ___

   Describe: _____

9. What has been your primary coping mechanism in handling this rape episode?

   _____

10. Have you talked to persons from the rape crisis center? Yes ___ No ___

    If no, want you to contact them for her? No ___ Yes ___

    If yes, was this contact of assistance? No ___ Yes ___

Male

1. History of prostate problems: No _X_ Yes ___ Describe: _____

   _____

2. History of penile discharge, bleeding, lesions: No _X_ Yes ___ Describe: ___

   _____

3. Date of last prostrate exam: Last admission _____

4. History of sexually transmitted disease: No _X_ Yes ___ Describe: _____

   _____

Both

1. Are you experiencing any problems in sexual functioning: No ___ Yes _X_

   Describe: Impotency for past several months _____

2. Are you satisfied with your sexual relationship? Yes ___ No _X_

   Describe: Impotent _____

3. Do you believe this admission will have any impact on sexual functioning?
   No ___ Yes _X_ Describe: "Get my diabetes under control and problem will be
   helped."

COPING-STRESS TOLERANCE PATTERN

Objective

1. Observe behavior. Are there any overt signs of stress (crying, wringing of hands,
   clenched fists, etc.)? Describe: Clenched fists _____

Subjective

1. Have you experienced any stressful or traumatic events in the past year in
   addition to this admission? No ___ Yes _X_ Describe: Numerous   admissions
   and I miss work some

2. How would you rate your usual handling of stress? Good ___ Average _X_ Poor ___

3. What is the primary way you deal with stress or problems? _Yell_ or _avoid situation. "I don't like to talk about it."_

4. Have you or your family used any support or counseling groups in the past year? No _X_ Yes ___ Group name: _____

   Was support group helpful? Yes ___ No ___ Additional comments: _____

   _____

5. What do you believe is the primary reason behind the need for this admission? _"To get my diabetes under control again; I guess I'm a slow learner."_

6. How soon, after first noting symptoms, did you seek health care assistance? _3 weeks_

7. Are you satisfied with the care you have been receiving at home? Yes _X_ No ___ Comments: _"My wife has always taken good care of me and I didn't want to have those people (VNA) coming to my house."_

8. Ask primary caregiver: What is your understanding of the care that will be needed when the patient goes home? _Wife not present at this time._

VALUE-BELIEF PATTERN

Objective

1. Observe behavior. Is the patient exhibiting any signs of alterations in mood (anger, crying, withdrawal, etc.)? Describe: _Clenched fists_

Subjective

1. Satisfied with the way your life has been developing? Yes ___ No _X_ Comments: _"Was OK until this diabetes developed."_

2. Will this admission interfere with your plans for the future? No _X_ Yes ___ How? _____

3. Religion: Protestant _X_ Catholic ___ Jewish ___ Muslim ___ Buddhist ___ None ___ Other _____

4. Will this admission interfere with your spiritual or religious practices? No _X_ Yes ___ How? _____

5. Any religious restrictions to care (diet, blood transfusions)? No _X_ Yes ___ Describe: _____

6. Would you like to have your (pastor, priest, rabbi, hospital chaplain) contacted to visit you? No _X_ Yes ___ Who? _____

7. Have your religious beliefs helped you to deal with problems in the past?
No ___ Yes _X_ Comments: _None_____

GENERAL

1. Is there any information we need to have that I have not covered in this interview? No _X_ Yes ___ Comments: _____

_____

2. Do you have any questions you need to ask me concerning your health, plan of care, or this agency? No _X_ Yes ___ Questions: _____

_____

3. What is the first problem you would like to have help with? _Stop me from having to go to the bathroom all the time_____

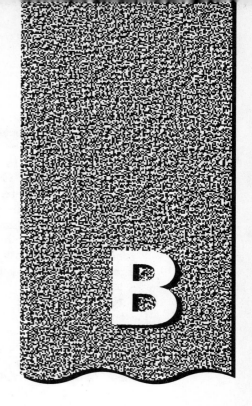

Community Resources

Community Resources

INDIVIDUAL

Acupuncturist: Locate through telephone directory.

Attorney (lawyer): Locate through telephone directory.

Audiologist: Locate through telephone directory or local speech and hearing clinic or check with local hospital. May also be listed under "Hearing Aids."

Childbirth educators: Contact local hospital offering obstetrical services about Lamaze classes, etc.

City and county commissioners: Look in telephone directory under Government, City or County

Community or public health nurse: Locate through local city, county, or state health department.

Computer expert: Locate in telephone directory under "Computers" or call local college.

Dentist, orthodontist: Locate in telephone directory.

Desensitization therapist: Locate through local college; try Department of Psychology first.

Drug and alcohol counselor: Locate through telephone directory, local hospital, or Department of Psychology at local college

Education counselor: Locate through local public school system or Department of Vocational Rehabilitation.

Electrician: Locate through telephone directory.

Enterstomal therapist: Locate through local hospital.

Family counselor or therapist: Locate through telephone directory, local college (Department of Family Studies or Psychology), local school system, nearest collegiate school of nursing, or local hospital.

Financial counselor: Locate through telephone directory; may also be listed under "Certified Public Accountants."

Health educator: Locate through local college, hospital, or school of nursing.

Heating and air conditioning contractor: Locate in telephone directory.

Hypnotherapist: Locate in telephone directory, through local college (Department of Psychology) or local hospital.

Job counselor: Locate in telephone directory, local state employment commission office, or local vocational rehabilitation department.

Lactation consultant: Locate in telephone directory or through local hospital.

Librarian: Check city, county, hospital, college, or health sciences center libraries.

Nurse midwife: Locate in telephone directory, through local hospital or nearest collegiate school of nursing.

Nurse practitioner or clinical nurse specialist: Locate through local hospital or nearest collegiate school of nursing. (Remember, there are multiple specializations for these nurses; pediatric, rehabilitation, psychiatric, adult, etc.)

Nutritionist or diet therapist: Locate through local hospital, college, health department, or home health agency.

Occupational therapist: Locate through local hospital, rehabilitation clinics, nearest health sciences center, college offering this major, or home health agency.

Ophthalmologist or optometrist: Locate through telephone directory.

Pharmacist: Locate through local hospital or at local pharmacies.

Physical therapist: Locate through local hospital, nearest health sciences center, telephone directory, nearest college offering this major, or local home health agency.

Physicians: Locate through telephone directory, local county medical society, local hospital, etc. (Remember all the various specialists and subspecialists: cardiologist, psychiatrist, neurologist, pediatrician, pediatric cardiologist.)

Play therapist: Locate through telephone directory (usually under "Psychologists"), local college (Department of Psychology), or local hospital.

Psychologist: Locate in telephone directory, local college (Department of Psychology), local hospital, or local home health agency.

Recreation therapist: Locate through telephone directory, local college (Department of Physical Education), or local hospital.

Relaxation trainer: Locate through telephone directory, local college (Department of Psychology), or local school of nursing.

Religious counselor: Locate through telephone directory or local churches.

Respiratory therapist: Locate through telephone directory, local hospital, or local home health agency.

Sex therapist: Locate through telephone directory, local hospital, or local college (Department of Psychology).

Speech therapist: Locate through telephone directory, local college (Department of Speech and Hearing), local hospital, or local home health agency.

Translators: Locate through local school system, local college, or local hospital.

ORGANIZATIONS

Agency for Health Care Policy and Research (National)
5600 Fishers Lane
Rockville, MD 20857
301-443-4100

Alcohol, Drug Abuse, and Mental Health Administration (National)
5600 Fishers Lane
Rockville, MD 20857
301-443-4797

Alcoholics Anonymous
PO Box 459
Grand Central Station
New York, NY 10163
212-686-1100

American Academy for Husband-Coached Childbirth (AAHCC)
Box 5224
Sherman Oaks, CA 91413
818-188-6662

American Academy of Orthotists and Prosthetists
717 Pendleton
Alexandria, VA 22314
703-836-7118

American Association for Protecting Children (Child Protective Services)
c/o American Humane Association
63 Inverness Drive E
Englewood, CO 80112
303-792-9900

American Association of Poison Control Centers
c/o Dr. Ted Tong
Arizona Poison and Drug Information Center
HSC Room 3204K
1501 N Campbell
Tucson, AZ 85725
602-626-1587
Also look in telephone directory, Yellow Pages or at front of directory
    under emergency numbers.

American Association of Retired Persons (AARP)
601 E Street NW
Washington, DC 20049
202-872-4700

American Cancer Society (I Can Cope Program, Reach to Recovery Program)
1599 Clifton Road NE
Atlanta, GA 30329
404-320-3333

American Cleft Palate–Craniofacial Association
1218 Grandview Avenue
Pittsburg, PA 15211
412-481-1376

American Diabetes Association
1660 Duke Street
PO Box 25757
Alexandria, VA 22314
703-549-1500

American Federation of Home Health Agencies
1320 Fenwick Lane
Suite 100
Silver Spring, MD 20910
301-588-1454

American Heart Association
7320 Greenville Avenue
Dallas, TX 75231
214-373-6300

American Liver Foundation
1425 Pompton Avenue
Cedar Grove, NJ 07009
201-256-2550

American Lung Association
1740 Broadway
New York, NY 10019
212-315-8700

American Pain Society
5700 Old Orchard Road
First Floor
Skokie, IL 60077-1024
708-966-5595

American Paraplegia Society
75-20 Astoria Boulevard
Jackson Heights, NY 11370
718-803-3782

American Parkinson's Disease Association
60 Bay Street
Suite 401
Staten Island, NY 10301
213-410-9732

American Red Cross (First Aid, CPR, Disaster Readiness)
17th and D Streets NW
Washington, DC 20006
202-737-8300

American Society for Psychoprophylaxis in Obstetrics (ASPO)
1411 K Street NW
Washington, DC 20005
703-524-7820

American Society of Childbirth Educators
PO Box 1630
Sedona, AZ 86336
602-284-9897

Candlelighters Childhood Cancer Foundation
1312 18th Street NW
No. 200
Washington, DC 20036
202-659-5136

Center for Attitudinal Healing
19 Main Street
Tilburon, CA 94920
415-435-5022

Centers for Disease Control
1600 Clifton Road NE
Atlanta, GA 30333
404-639-3311

Cesareans/Support Education and Concern (C/Sec)
22 Forest Road
Framingham, MA 01701
508-877-8266

Coalition on Smoking and Health
1615 New Hampshire Ave NW
2nd Floor
Washington, DC 20009
202-234-9375

Combined National Veterans Associations of America
5413C Backlick Road
Springfield, VA 22151
703-354-2140

Compassionate Friends
P.O. Box 3696
Oak Brook, IL 60522
708-990-0010

County Home Extension Service
Listed in telephone directory under "Government, County."

County Medical Society
Listed in telephone directory under (Name) "Medical Society"; name is
quite often the same as the county's name.

Crisis Intervention Hotlines
Listed in telephone directory under "Crisis."

Cystic Fibrosis Foundation
6931 Arlington Road
No. 20
Bethesda, MD 20814
301-951-4422

Department of Human Resources
Listed in telephone directory under "Government, State."

Easter Seal Research Foundation (formerly Crippled Children's Society)
70 E. Lake Street
Chicago, IL 60601
312-726-6200

Family Support Administration (National)
370 L'Enfant Promenade SW
Washington, DC 20447
202-252-4500

Fire Department
Usually listed on the first page of the telephone directory under "Emergency Numbers."

Food and Drug Administration (National)
   5600 Fishers Lane
   Rockville, MD 20857
   301-443-1544

Food Supplement Programs (Food Bank, WIC)
   Look in Yellow Pages under "Food Bank"; WIC is usually administered by
      city or county health department.

Government
   Look in telephone directory under "Government," then look for city,
      county, state, and federal listings.
   City Departments:
      Ambulance
      Animal Control
      County Extension Service
      Emergency Medical Services
      Health
         Board of Health
         Dental
         Environmental
         Family Planning
         Health Official
         HIV/AIDS
         Immunizations
         Laboratory Services
         Maternity
         Medicaid Information
         Medical Records
         Mosquito Spraying
         Nursing
         Public Health Administrator
         Rodent Control
         Sexually Transmitted Diseases
         Vital Statistics
         Water Tests
      Helpline
      Housing
         Assistance (Homeless)
         Rehabilitative Assistance
         Substandard Complaints
      Police
      Sanitation
      Senior Citizens Center
      Social Services
      Utilities
   State Departments:
      Genetic Screening
      Medical Examiners, State Board of
      Mental Health and Mental Retardation

State Commission for the Blind
State Department of Health
State Department of Human Services (or Resources)
    Aid to Families with Dependent Children
    Adult Protective Services
    Children's Protective Services
    Day Care Licensing
    EPSDT
    Family Services
    Food Stamps
    Institutional Licensing
    Medical Transportation
    Nursing, State Board of
    Nursing Home Care
    Nutritional Assistance
    Services for Aged and Disabled

National Departments: Branch offices of federal agencies may be located in your city. Look first under "United States Government" in your local telephone directory for these branches. The national numbers and addresses of agencies of interest to nurses are included in this appendix. When contacting the national office, also inquire as to the nearest regional office and contact person.

Group Homes
Look in Yellow Pages under "Social Service Organizations."

Habitat for Humanity
121 Habitat Street
Americus, GA 31709
912-924-6935

Health and Human Services
200 Independence Avenue SW
Washington, DC 20201
212-619-0257

Regional Offices
1. John F. Kennedy Federal Bldg.
   Boston, MA 02203
   617-565-1500
2. 26 Federal Plaza
   New York, NY 10278
   212-264-4600
3. 3535 Market Street
   Philadelphia, PA 19101
   215-596-6492
4. 101 Marietta Tower
   Atlanta, GA 30323
   404-331-2442
5. 105 W. Adams Street
   Chicago, IL 60603
   312-353-5160

6. 1200 Main Street
   Dallas, TX 75202
   214-757-3301
7. 601 E. 12th Street
   Kansas City, MO 64106
   816-426-2821
8. 1961 Stout Street
   Denver, CO 80294
   303-844-3372
9. Federal Office Bldg.
   50 United Nations Plaza
   San Francisco, CA 94102
   415-556-6746
10. Blanchard Plaza Bldg.
    2201 6th Avenue
    Seattle, WA 98121
    206-442-0420

Health Care Financing Administration (HCFA)
Department of Health and Human Services
200 Independence Avenue SW
Washington, DC 20201
202-245-6113

Health Resources and Services Administration
5600 Fishers Lane
Rockville, MD 20857
301-443-2086

Herpes Resources Center
PO Box 13827
Research Triangle Park, NC 27709
919-361-2120

Home Health Services (Homemaker, Home Health Aid)
Located in Yellow Pages under "Home Health."

Homeless Shelters
Located in Yellow Pages under "Social Services Organizations."

Hospice Association of America
519 C Street NE
Washington, DC 20002
202-546-4759

Hospitals: Infection Control Department
Contact local hospitals.

Indian Health Service (National)
5600 Fishers Lane
Rockville, MD 20857
301-443-1083

International Childbirth Education Association (ICEA)
PO Box 20048
Minneapolis, MN 55420
612-854-8660

La Leche League International (LLL)
9616 Minneapolis Avenue
Franklin Park, IL 60131
708-455-7730

Legal Aid.
Located in telephone directory under "Legal Aid."

Meals on Wheels
May be listed separately in the telephone directory, accessed through city or county government offices, or found under "Social Services Organizations."

Medical Equipment Suppliers
Located in Yellow Pages under "Medical Equipment."

Mothers Against Drunk Driving (MADD)
511 E John Carpenter Freeway
No. 70
Irving, TX 75062
214-744-6233

Mother's Day Out Programs
Located in telephone directory, usually under name of churches that provide the program.

Muscular Dystrophy Association
810 7th Avenue
New York, NY 10019
212-586-0808

Myasthenia Gravis Foundation
53 W. Jackson Boulevard
Suite 1352
Chicago, IL 60604
312-427-6252

NAACOG: The Organization for Obstetric, Gynecologic, and Neonatal Nurses
409 12th Street NW
Washington, DC 20024
202-638-0026

National AIDS Hot Line
800-342-AIDS

National Alzheimer's Association
919 N. Michigan Avenue
Suite 100
Chicago, IL 60611
1-800-272-3900

National Arthritis Foundation
1314 Spring Street NW
Atlanta, GA 30309
404-872-7100

National Association of Parents and Professionals for Safe Alternatives in Childbirth
Route 1, Box 646
Marble Hill, MO 63746
314-238-2010

National Association of People with AIDS
Washington, DC 20035
202-483-7970

National Association of Rehabilitation Facilities (Sheltered Workshops)
PO Box 17675
Washington, DC 20041
703-648-9300

National Association of Social Workers
7981 Eastern Avenue
Silver Spring, MD 20910
301-565-0333

National Coalition for the Homeless
1621 Connecticut Ave NW
No. 400
Washington, DC 20009
202-265-2371

National Head Injury Foundation
333 Turnpike Road
Southborough, MA 01772
508-485-9950

National Institute on Adult Daycare
c/o National Council on the Aging
600 Maryland Ave SW
West Wing 100
Washington, DC 20024
202-479-6680

National Institutes of Health
9000 Rockville Pike
Bethesda, MD 20892
301-496-4000

1. National Cancer Institute
   301-496-5737
2. National Center for Nursing Research
   301-496-0523
3. National Eye Institute
   301-496-7425

4. National Heart, Lung, and Blood Institute
301-496-2411
5. National Institute of Allergy and Infectious Disease
301-496-1521
6. National Institute of Arthritis and Musculoskeletal and Skin Diseases
301-496-4353
7. National Institute of Child Health and Human Development
301-496-3454
8. National Institute of Diabetes and Digestive and Kidney Diseases
301-496-5741
9. National Institute of General Medical Sciences
301-496-7714
10. National Institute of Neurological Disorders and Stroke
301-496-5751
11. National Institute on Aging
301-496-5345
12. National Institute on Deafness and Other Communication Disorders
301-496-7243
13. National Institute on Dental Research
301-496-6621
14. National Library of Medicine
301-496-6308

National Multiple Sclerosis Association
205 E. 42nd Street
New York, NY 10017
212-986-3240

National Organization of Mothers of Twins Clubs
12404 Princess Jeanne NE
Albuquerque, NM 87112
505-275-0955

National Rehabilitation Association
633 S. Washington Street
Alexandria, VA 22314
703-836-0850

National Spinal Cord Injury Association
600 W. Cummings Park
Suite 2000
Woburn, MA 01801
617-935-2722

National VD Hotline
800-227-8922
In California, 800-982-5883

National Wheelchair Athletes Association
3595 E. Fountain Boulevard
Suite L-10
Colorado Springs, CO 80910
719-574-1150

Occupational Safety and Health Administration (OSHA)
200 Constitution Avenue NW
Room N3603
Washington, DC 20210
202-523-7725

Outpatient Clinics (hospitals, city and state health departments)
Contact hospital or city or state health department. Hospitals will be listed in Yellow Pages. City and state health departments will be listed in Yellow Pages under "Government."

Overeaters Anonymous
PO Box 92870
Los Angeles, CA 90009
213-542-8363

Parents Anonymous
6733 S. Sepulveda
Suite 270
Los Angeles, CA 90045
213-410-9732

Planned Parenthood Federation of America
810 7th Avenue
New York, NY 10301
212-541-7800

Police
Usually listed on first page of telephone directory under "Emergency Numbers."

Prosthesis Manufacturers
Listed in Yellow Pages under "Prosthesis."

Public Health Service (National)
5600 Fishers Lane
Rockville, MD 20857
301-443-2404
or
200 Independence Avenue SW
Washington, DC 20201
202-619-1296

Public School Officials
Listed in Yellow Pages under "Schools."

Rape Crisis Center
Listed in telephone directory.

Social Security Administration (National)
6401 Security Boulevard
Baltimore, MD 21235
410-965-1234

Stop Smoking Clinics
   Contact local hospitals, YWCA, YMCA.

Support Groups (Parenting, Parents without Partners, Anorexia/Bulimia, Grief, Alcoholics Anonymous, AIDS, etc.)
   Look in Yellow Pages under "Social Services Organizations" or for individual title in white pages.

Take Off Pounds Sensibly (TOPS) Club
   4575 S. 5th Street
   PO Box 07360
   Milwaukee, WI 53207
   414-482-4620

Transportation Services (local churches, bus service, service organizations such as Elks, Lion's Club, etc.)
   Listed individually in the telephone directory.

United States Lighthouse for the Partially Sighted
   316 1/2 E. Mitchell Street
   Suite 4
   Petoskey, MI 49770
   616-347-1171

United Way of America
   701 N. Fairfax Street
   Alexandria, VA 22314
   703-836-7100

Vaginal Birth after Cesarean (VBAC) Information
   Nancy Cohen
   Great Plain Terrace
   Needham, MA 02192

Visiting Nurse Association of America
   3801 E Florida
   Suite 806
   Denver, CO 80210
   303-753-0218
   Also listed in the Yellow Pages of the telephone directory under "Home Health Services" or separately in white pages.

Vocational Rehabilitation Services
   Council of State Administrators of Vocational Rehabilitation
   P.O. Box 3776
   Washington, DC 20007
   202-638-4634

Weight Watchers International
   Jericho Atrium
   500 N. Broadway
   Jericho, NY 11753
   516-939-0400

Women's Shelter and Women's Protective Services
Listed in Yellow Pages.

YMCA (outdoor recreation and survival, water exercise)
National Council of YMCA of the U.S.A.
101 N. Wacker Drive
Chicago, IL 60606
312-977-0031

YWCA (outdoor recreation and survival, water exercise)
YWCA of the U.S.A.
726 Broadway
New York, NY 10003
212-614-2700
Listed in white pages of telephone directory.

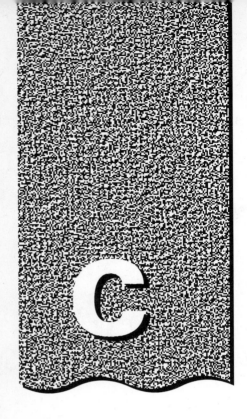

NANDA's Diagnostic Label Qualifiers

These qualifiers are listed in North American Nursing Diagnosis Association, Taxonomy I, Revised 1990. Author, St. Louis, 1990, p. 114.

Acute: Severe but of short duration.

Altered: A change from baseline.

Chronic: Lasting a long time; recurring; habitual; constant.

Decreased: Lessened, lesser in size, amount, or degree.

Deficient: Inadequate in amount, quality, or degree; defective; not sufficient; incomplete.

Depleted: Emptied wholly or partially; exhausted of.

Disturbed: Agitated; interrupted, interfered with.

Dysfunctional: Abnormal; incomplete functioning.

Excessive: Characterized by an amount or quantity that is greater than is necessary, desirable, or useful.

Increased: Greater in size, amount, or degree.

Ineffective: Not producing the desired effect.

Impaired: Made worse, weakened; damaged; reduced; deteriorated.

Intermittent: Stopping and starting again at intervals; periodic; cyclic.

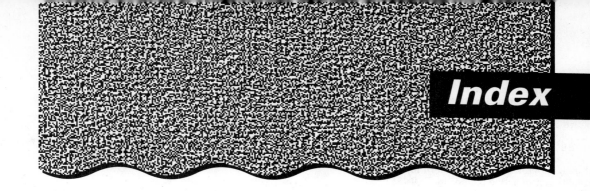

Index

Note: Page numbers followed by f indicate figures; those followed by t indicate tables.